Vascular Disease of the Central Nervous System

Vascular Disease of the Central Nervous System

Edited by

R. W. Ross Russell

MA MD DM FRCP

Consultant Physician to St Thomas' Hospital,
London; The National Hospital for Nervous
Diseases, Queen Square, London and Moorfields
Eye Hospital, City Road, London

SECOND EDITION

CHURCHILL LIVINGSTONE
EDINBURGH LONDON MELBOURNE AND NEW YORK 1983

CHURCHILL LIVINGSTONE
Medical Division of Longman Group Limited

Distributed in the United States of America by Churchill
Livingstone Inc., 1560 Broadway, New York, N.Y. 10036, and
by associated companies, branches and representatives
throughout the world.

First edition 1976
Second edition 1983

First edition published under
the title *Cerebral Arterial Disease.*

ISBN 0 443 02415 4

British Library Cataloguing in Publication Data
Vascular disease of the central nervous system.
 — 2nd ed.
 1. Cerebrovascular disease
 I. Ross Russell, R. W.   II. Cerebral arterial disease
 616.8′1   RC388.5

Library of Congress Cataloging in Publication Data
Main entry under title:
Vascular disease of the central nervous system.
 Includes index.
 1. Cerebrovascular disease. I. Ross, Russell,
 R. W. [DNLM: 1. Central nervous system
 diseases. 2. Cerebrovascular disorders.
 WL 355 V331]
 RC388.5.V37   1983   616.8′1   82-12866   (U.S.)

Typeset by CCC, printed and bound in Great Britain by
William Clowes (Beccles) Limited, Beccles and London

Preface

Since the first edition of this book was published in 1976 under the title of *Cerebral Arterial Disease* there have been a number of developments both of a practical and theoretical kind. At that time computerised scanning was just coming into general use and it has fully justified its initial promise to the extent that it is now essential in making the early critical decisions in the management of stroke — has the patient with an acute focal deficit had an infarct, a haemorrhage or some other non-vascular event? Not only does this enable therapy to be started earlier but the tightening of diagnostic criteria has enabled treatment and trials of new treatments to be put on a firmer basis.

The other major change in practical management is in the field of vascular surgery and here the position is still far from clear. The new technique of extracranial/intracranial anastomosis has developed rapidly and it is now apparent that an anastomosis can be established with safety and can effectively conduct blood from the scalp to the brain. Does the operation do any good? Probably it does if the patient has a region of brain with a precariously balanced blood supply which from time to time becomes insufficient; probably it does not in the patient with an established infarct; possibly it may in the patient who has made a good recovery following an internal carotid occlusion. The operation is in danger of being applied uncritically to patients in all these categories with no pause for proper assessment, and even the present controlled trial may be unable to answer some of the questions in the foreseeable future.

Medical therapy in acute stroke remains disappointing and the initial hopes which were entertained for the treatment of oedema with osmotic agents or corticosteroids have not been realised. Oedema can be a life threatening complication in massive hemisphere infarction but the effect of energetic treatment has too often been the survival of some severely disabled patients who would otherwise have died. In the posterior fossa however the situation is different; here the recognition and energetic treatment of oedema by both medical and surgical means continues to be well worthwhile.

Thanks largely to increasing awareness of the importance of hypertension and to more effective methods of antihypertensive treatment there are good reasons to expect a decline in stroke in middle-aged patients as well as a continuing reduction in cerebral haemorrhage. Faced with a slowly increasing proportion of elderly patients in the population there seems little likelihood that the overall incidence of stroke will decrease. The rehabilitation of established stroke patients is now claiming some overdue attention. Increasingly sophisticated aids and techniques are becoming available and there is literally no limit to the amount that can be spent on attempting to rehabilitate patients with cerebrovascular disease. In this situation it is essential to deploy limited resources to the best effect. This means looking critically at the results of different physical methods of rehabilitation in the various categories of stroke and comparing the cost-effectiveness in the light of the natural history. Expensive and complicated methods of rehabilitation may prove to be no more effective than simpler and cheaper ones.

In the theoretical field the most notable advance has been our increased understanding of the mechanisms of ischaemia and its effect on oxidative metabolism and regional blood flow made possible by positron emission tomography. This technique has revealed the complex disturbances which may be found around an ischaemic area and even in the opposite hemisphere — regions of depressed flow and metabolism, regions of absolute or relative hyperaemia, regions of relative vascular insufficiency with maintained metabolism, and even regions of hypermetabolism. The technology is so sophisticated and expensive as to be unsuitable for general use but it will provide an opportunity for assessment of claims made for vasoactive agents and metabolic stimulants to improve brain function at various stages after vascular occlusion. The development of similar isotopic techniques to label glucose, aminoacids, and drugs acting on the brain promises to open a new chapter in neuro-chemistry and neuro-pharmacology.

I am grateful to the team of distinguished contributors to this volume, both to those who have revised their chapters sometimes extensively and to those who have written new chapters. Their responses to my requests and amendments have been prompt, efficient and good-natured and have made editing a pleasure rather than a labour.

London 1983   R.W.R.R.

Acknowledgements

Acknowledgement is gratefully made to a number of authors, editors and publishers for permission to reproduce illustrations which have already appeared elsewhere. The source and author are indicated in the caption in each case.

A number of friends and colleagues have allowed me to use previously unpublished material — the source of each is again indicated.

My special thanks are due to Mrs Barbara Parker for an infinity of time and trouble in preparing the manuscript, and to my colleague Dr R. T. C. Pratt for much valuable help with proof-reading.

R.W.R.R.

Contributors

M. J. Aminoff
Associate Professor in Neurology, University of California, School of Medicine, San Francisco, California 94143, USA

H. J. M. Barnett
Professor of Clinical Neurological Sciences, University of Western Ontario, 399 Windermere Road, London, Canada N6A 5A5

W. Blackwood
Emeritus Professor of Neuropathology, University of London, 71 Seal Hollow Road, Sevenoaks, Kent, UK

D. P. de Bono
Consultant Physician, Department of Cardiology, The Royal Infirmary of Edinburgh, Edinburgh EH3 9YW, UK

N. Browse
Professor of Surgery, St Thomas' Hospital Medical School, London SE1 7EH, UK

J. J. Caronna
Professor of Clinical Neurology, Department of Neurology, Cornell University Medical College, 525 E68th Street, New York, New York 10021, USA

C. Fieschi
Professor of Neurology, I Institute of Neurology (IIIA Cattedra) Universita di Roma, Via dei 4 Cantoni, 6 Rome, Italy

W. M. Garraway
Department of Medical Statistics and Epidemiology, Mayo Clinic, Rochester, Minnesota 55901, USA

J. C. Gautier
Professor of Neurology, Hôpital de la Salpêtrière, 47 Bd de l'Hôpital, 75364 Paris, Cedex 13, France

M. J. G. Harrison
Consultant Neurologist and Director, Department of Neurology, Middlesex Hospital, Mortimer Street, London W1N 8AA, UK

K.-A. Hossman
Professor, Head, Forschungsstelle für Hirnkreislaufforschung, Max Planck Brain Research Institute, Ostmerheimer Strasse 200, 5000 Cologne 91, West Germany

E. C. Hutchinson
Professor, Department of Neurology, North Staffordshire Royal Infirmary, Princes Road, Hartshill, Stoke-on-Trent ST4 7LN, UK

W. B. Kannel
Professor of Medicine, Boston University Medical Center, School of Medicine, 80 East Concord Street, Boston, Massachusetts 02118, USA

R. Langton-Hewer
Consultant Neurologist, Neurological/Stroke Rehabilitation Unit, Frenchay Hospital, Bristol BS16 1LE, UK

G. L. Lenzi
Assistant Professor, I Institute of Neurology (IIIA Cattedra), Universita di Roma, Via dei 4 Cantoni, 6 Rome, Italy

J. Marquardsen
Professor of Neurology, Allborg Sygehus, Jutland, Denmark

J. C. Meadows
Consultant Neurologist, Atkinson Morley's Hospital, 31 Copse Hill, Wimbledon, London SW10 0NE, UK

M. D. O'Brien
Consultant Physician for Nervous Diseases, Department of Neurology, Guy's Hospital, St Thomas Street, London SE1 9RT, UK

M. R. Parsons
Consultant Neurologist, The General Infirmary at Leeds, Great George Street, Leeds LS1 3EX, UK

J. Pearce
Consultant Neurologist, Hull Royal Infirmary, Hull HU3 2JZ, UK

A. E. Richardson
Consultant Surgeon, Department of Neurosurgery, Atkinson Morley's Hospital, 31 Copse Hill, Wimbledon, London SW10 0NE, UK

R. W. Ross Russell
Consultant Physician, Department of Neurology, St Thomas' Hospital, London SE1 7EH; The National Hospital for Nervous Diseases, Queen Square, London WC1N 3BG, and Moorfields Eye Hospital, London EC1V 2PD, UK

L. Symon
Professor of Neurological Surgery, The National Hospital for Nervous Diseases, Queen Square, London WC1N 3BG, UK

D. J. Thomas
Consultant Neurologist, St Mary's Hospital, Praed Street, London W2 1NY, UK

P. A. Wolf
Professor of Neurology, Boston University Medical Center, School of Medicine, 80 East Concord Street, Boston, Massachusetts 02118, USA

Contents

1

Epidemiology of cerebrovascular disease

William B. Kannel and Philip A. Wolf

INTRODUCTION

Reduction of stroke incidence requires the identification and treatment of candidates for cerebrovascular disease. To await signs of a compromised cerebral circulation is to take an unacceptable risk since only ten percent of strokes are preceded by TIAs (Whisnant, 1974). There is little to suggest that the devastating consequences of stroke will be ameliorated by more expert medical or surgical management of the completed episode. A more fruitful approach is to deal with its precursors rather than to delay treatment until the stroke is imminent or has already occurred. Stroke is a consequence of a long-term process and not a chance or random event as the term 'cerebral vascular accident' implies. The association between brain infarction and atherosclerosis elsewhere indicates that it is part of a generalized vascular disease.

Epidemiologic investigation of the way cerebrovascular disease evolves in the general population has identified a number of host and environmental contributors. Major reductions in death and disability from stroke will come from prevention; such a program depends upon identification and treatment of the stroke-prone person.

Stroke does not as readily lend itself to epidemiologic study as does coronary heart disease because it generally occurs later in life and its incidence and mortality rates are substantially lower (Shurtleff, 1974) than those for coronary heart disease (CHD). In order to achieve equivalent results the cohorts studied must be larger and followed for longer periods. Alternatively, entry into the study at a later age may be considered, but this carries the liability of lower response rates and

loss of impact of risk factors presumably due to the overwhelming associative strength of age itself. Although neither as common nor as lethal as coronary heart disease, cerebrovascular disease is nevertheless the most devastating clinical manifestation of hypertension and atherosclerosis. The victim is often deprived of his dignity, ability to communicate, independence and physical capacity.

Diagnosis of an event, particularly as to specific type, is more difficult than for CHD because of less pathognomonic laboratory tests such as the ECG or enzyme abnormalities available for myocardial infarction. There are still no uniformly applied indications for the timing or performing of specific tests such as lumbar puncture, cerebral arteriography, CT-scan, brain scan, or noninvasive studies of carotid patency. Even at autopsy of fatal cases it may be difficult to differentiate accurately between intracerebral hemorrhage, hemorrhagic infarct and subarachnoid hemorrhage when there has been extensive destruction of brain and vascular structures. Ischemic brain infarction may be due to thrombosis or embolism and it is often difficult to distinguish between the two alternatives.

Despite these problems epidemiology studies have been carried out yielding useful information about the way strokes evolve, their precursors and prognosis.

Information has been obtained from prospective epidemiologic studies such as that at Framingham on the incidence of strokes in the general population, the way they evolve, hallmarks of vulnerability, a profile of potential candidates, clues to its pathogenesis and the disability and mortality which ensues. The importance of stroke as a cause of morbidity and mortality in the increasingly elderly population warrants an exploration of each of these features of the epidermiology of stroke, using data from the Framingham Study and elsewhere.

EPIDEMIOLOGIC ASSESSMENT OF THE STROKE ENTITY

Prevalence

Estimates of the prevalence from general population samples are sparse and the figures obtained are rather diverse (Table 1.1). There were some 1.8

is necessary because there is little hope of reversing established brain damage. The potential for salvage is particularly important in the case of stroke, which has a high incidence of permanent disability among survivors. The fatality rate in the acute stage is only 15 percent, but of the survivors, 50 percent suffer permanent disability. Of the estimated two million cases of post-stroke disability in the United States, one-third are age 35–65 wage earners who have become unemployable because of their stroke disability. The estimated annual cost

Table 1.1 Cerebrovascular disease: age-specific prevalence rates both sexes

*Rochester, Minnesota 1970 (a)**		*English General Practices 1955–6 (b)7*		*U.S. Health interviews 1978†*	
Age	*Prevalence/ 100 000 populations*	*Age*	*Prevalence/ 100 000 population*	*Age*	*Prevalence/ 1000 population*
<35	10	15–44	30	<45	1.1
35–44	200				
45–54	440				
		45–64	400	45–64	12.3
55–64	810				
65–74	3560	65+	2930		
75+	5970			65+	44.9
Total	612	Total	486	All ages	8.0
Age-adjusted (to U.S. 1960)	556	Age-adjusted (to U.S. 1960)	363		
(Cases)	(303)	(Cases)	(1862)	(Interviews)	(134 000)

(a) Matsumoto et al 1973.
(b) Logan and Cushion 1958.
* Modified from Kurtzke 1976a.
† Modified from National Center for Health Statistics 1978.

million strokes estimated by the American Heart Association in 1977; a prevalence roughly equal to that of rheumatic heart disease and almost half that of coronary heart disease (Fig. 1.1). The prevalence increases with age and is substantially higher for blacks, particularly at younger ages (Kurtzke, 1976a).

Cerebrovascular disease is also a major contributor to disability accounting for half the patients hospitalized for neurologic disease. In the Framingham Study, 31 percent of stroke survivors needed assistance in self-care, 20 percent required assistance in ambulation and 71 percent had an impaired vocational capacity when examined an average of 7 years after stroke (Gresham et al, 1975; Gresham et al, 1979). Some 16 percent remain institutionalized.

A preventive approach to cerebrovascular disease

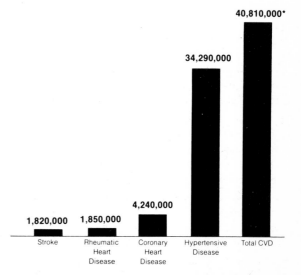

Fig. 1.1 Estimated prevalence of the major cardiovascular diseases (United States, 1977).

of care for stroke disability is three billion dollars. There are further costs of care during the acute stage of hospitalization. Thus, the potential rewards, in both health care and resources, of detection of stroke candidates and preventive treatment are obvious.

Incidence

About 500 000 new strokes occur annually within the United States. The incidence reaches major proportions only after age 55, but no age group is completely spared. The reported incidence rates vary depending on whether the sample was derived from the general population or hospitalization, its age composition and whether recurrent strokes were included.

The incidence of strokes generally, and atherothrombotic brain infarctions (ABI) specifically, in the Framingham Study increased with age in both sexes but more precipitously in women than in men (Table 1.2). Only under age 55 is the male

Table 1.2 Incidence of stroke and myocardial infarction by age and sex, 20 year follow-up. Framingham study. Men and women, age 45–74

Age	Average annual incidence per 10 000					
	Strokes — all types		Atherothrombotic brain infarctions		Myocardial infarctions	
	Men	Women	Men	Women	Men	Women
45–54	20	9	10	6	48	9
55–64	32	29	20	18	91	19
65–74	84	86	52	55	111	51
45–74	34	29	20	18	72	19

preponderance characteristic of atherosclerotic disease apparent. Comparing brain and myocardial infarction, there is a marked male predominance at all ages for myocardial infarction and almost four myocardial infarctions occur in men for each brain infarction. For women, the incidence of each is virtually identical. For reasons which are not clear, ABI is the only major clinical atherosclerotic manifestation which fails to exhibit a preference for males. This may stem from the fact that cerebral atherosclerosis, which begins later in life than in other vascular territories, does not reach major proportions until women have already lost their premenopausal immunity to atherosclerotic vascular disease.

Kurtzke estimated an incidence rate of 2 per 1000 per year for all ages combined (Kurtzke, 1976b). The Joint Committee for Stroke Facilities estimated that stroke death rates in 1972 increased from 1 per 1000 at ages 45–54, to 3.5 per 1000 at 55–64 and to 9 per 1000 at ages 65–74 (Table 1.3).

Table 1.3 Estimated annual incidence rates for stroke per 1000 population (both sexes, all races)★

Age group	Probable minimum	Midpoint	Probable maximum
35–44	—	0.25	—
45–54	0.6	1.00	1.8
55–64	2.5	3.50	5.0
65–74	6.0	9.00	12.0
75–84	15.0	20.00	25.0
85 and older	—	40.00	—

Notes on use of estimated incidence rates:
1. Rates for males tend to approach the maximum and those for females the minimum estimates.
2. Rates for blacks are probably generally higher than for whites.
3. These rates for the most part are based on studies of first events only, so that to derive a figure for total case load, an adjustment should be made for recurrent strokes. Our best estimate is that the rates would be 25 percent higher if recurrent cases are included.
★ (Report of the Joint Committee for Stroke Facilities, 1972).

These estimates are similar to those prospectively obtained in the Framingham Study (Table 1.2). Framingham data suggest that the chances of suffering a stroke before age 70 are one in twenty. Although strokes occur most often late in life, 20 percent occur in persons under age 65.

Frequency of strokes by type

The prevalence of the major varieties of cerebral vascular disease is uncertain and varies depending on the source of the data. Because of its lethal nature, parenchymal brain hemorrhage is over-represented in autopsy data. Data from hospitals and neurology clinics are subject to selective bias and are likely to over-emphasize strokes that are severe and require hospitalization. General population survey data are more representative but often suffer from small numbers of the less common types of stroke, making precise estimates of frequency difficult (Kurtzke, 1976a).

The Harvard Cooperative Stroke Registry suggests that about half of strokes (53 percent) are 'thrombotic'; and of these about two-thirds involve large arteries producing infarctions while the remaining third affects small penetrating arteries causing the small deep brain infarcts known as lacunes (Mohr et al, 1978). Of the thrombotic strokes, 18 percent of all events are a result of atherothrombotic disease of the carotid artery, 16 percent from disease of vertebral and basilar arteries and 19 percent lacunar infarcts. Embolism appears to account for 31 percent of all strokes and intracranial hemorrhage from hypertension or ruptured aneurysm accounts for 10 percent and 6 percent respectively.

Data from the Framingham Study, based on a general population survey routinely assessed for strokes at biennial intervals, are in close agreement with the Stroke Registry as to the frequency of atherothrombotic brain infarcts and intracranial hemorrhages (Wolf et al, 1978a). See Fig. 1.2.

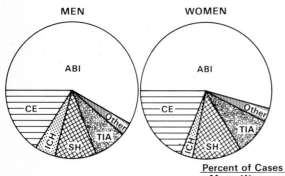

| | | Percent of Cases | |
		Men	Women
ABI	Atherothrombotic Brain Infarction	58%	54%
CE	Cerebral Embolus	16%	19%
ICH	Intracerebral Hemorrhage	5%	3%
SH	Subarachnoid Hemorrhage	10%	12%
TIA	Transient Ischemic Attacks Only	8%	9%
Other		3%	3%

Fig. 1.2 Frequency of stroke by type. Men and women age 65–74: the Framingham study, 26 year follow-up.

Because uncomplicated TIAs are also included, the percentages may be somewhat understated. It is interesting that the frequency of the various types is quite similar in the two sexes. It is also noteworthy that, even in the same advanced age group (65–74), there is a predominance of myo-cardial infarction in males over females (Fig. 1.3) while in the same cohort brain infarction frequen-cies are quite similar. It is difficult to determine the precise proportion of strokes that are due to extracranial vascular disease. Carotid artery disease appears to account for some 18 percent of strokes. It is likely that the frequency of small intracerebral

hemorrhages is greater than indicated in these data and will be found to be larger when CT scan data become more readily available.

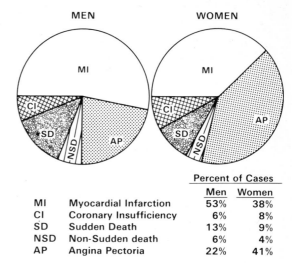

| | | Percent of Cases | |
		Men	Women
MI	Myocardial Infarction	53%	38%
CI	Coronary Insufficiency	6%	8%
SD	Sudden Death	13%	9%
NSD	Non-Sudden death	6%	4%
AP	Angina Pectoria	22%	41%

Fig. 1.3 Frequency of coronary heart disease by type. Men and women age 65–74, the Framingham study, 26 year follow-up.

Autopsy studies of the relative frequencies of stroke types give very different results but they may be unreliable (Kuller, 1978). It is likely that hospital-based data are also fallible. The best data must be presumed to be the community-based incidence studies. From these Kurtzke has esti-mated that 8 percent of stroke incidence is due to subarachnoid hemorrhage, 12 percent intracere-bral hemorrhage and 69 percent thromboembolism of which 3–8 percent are due to embolism. The remaining 11 percent are ill-defined strokes (Kurtzke, 1976a).

Mortality

In 1977, cerebrovascular disease accounted for nearly 182 000 deaths in the USA comprising nearly a tenth of the total mortality (Vital Statistics of the United States, 1977) See Fig 1.4. This may be an underestimate because death certificates by underlying cause often fails to note the contribution of a past stroke. Stroke fatalities rank third among all causes of death in most affluent countries, exceeded only by heart disease and cancer.

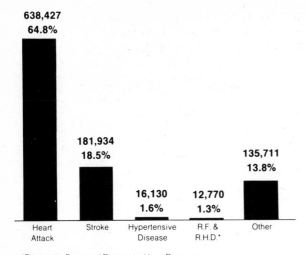

638,427
64.8%

181,934
18.5%

135,711
13.8%

16,130
1.6%

12,770
1.3%

Heart Attack | Stroke | Hypertensive Disease | R.F. & R.H.D.* | Other

*Rheumatic Fever and Rheumatic Heart Disease
Source: National Center for Health Statistics, USPHS, DHEW

Fig. 1.4 Deaths due to cardiovascular diseases by major type of disorder (United States, 1977).

RISK FACTORS

Major reductions in disability and death from stroke will come from prevention rather than from more effective medical or surgical treatment. It is a universal finding among all epidemiologic studies that the most important risk factor for stroke, whether infarction or hemorrhage, is hypertension.

There is also general agreement that both elevated pressure and cardiac abnormalities are powerful contributors to stroke incidence. Factors which have been inconsistently incriminated are glucose intolerance, blood lipids, elevated hematocrit and cigarette smoking. Further confirmation is needed concerning the suggestion that *lower* serum cholesterol and LDL-cholesterol may be associated with increased risk of brain infarction in women and intracerebral hemorrhage in men. The association of alcohol with an increased risk of stroke is highly suggestive. Few environmental factors have been conclusively linked to stroke incidence.

Because ABI, the most common variety of stroke shares a common pathology with CHD, it might be expected that they would also share common risk factors. However, there are a number of differences which are both noteworthy and unex-

plained. Although subjects with CHD are at a five-fold increased risk of stroke and CHD risk profiles will identify stroke candidates with equal or greater efficiency (Kannel, 1978), the impact of some CHD risk factors are surprisingly weak. Thus, hypertension predisposes to both. Serum total cholesterol, obesity and cigarettes are rather weak stroke risk factors. This may derive from the advanced age at which strokes occur, when even for CHD these risk factors lose their impact (McGee, 1973).

At the present time the main risk factors for ABI are: hypertension, CHD, CHF, ECG abnormalities, diabetes, certain systemic diseases affecting cerebral blood flow, blood viscosity and coagulation, complications of operations on the heart and great vessels and certain medications such as oral contraceptives.

Cerebral embolism is chiefly a consequence of valvular disease, myocardial infarction and irregularities in cardiac rhythm (chiefly atrial fibrillation) or complications of cardiac operations.

Intracranial hemorrhage is a consequence of congenital anomalies, AV malformations, hypertension and interference with blood clotting.

Atherogenic personal attributes

Hypertension

Of the various risk attributes known to contribute to the occurrence of strokes, hypertension has been shown to play a dominant role (Whisnant, 1974; Kannel, 1971; Kannel, 1976; Kannel and Wolf, 1975; Kannel et al, 1978; Kannel et al, 1971). The relationship seems to be just as strong for non-embolic cerebral infarction as it is for intracranial hemorrhage. Not only is hypertension the most powerful contributor to stroke incidence, but it is also a highly prevalent one so that the attributable risk is greatest for hypertension as well. The risk of stroke is related to the height of the blood pressure, not only among hypertensives but throughout the range of blood pressure, with no discernible critical value of systolic or diastolic pressure which delineates the stroke candidate from the general population (Whisnant, 1974; Kannel, 1971; Kannel, 1976; Kannel & Wolf, 1975; Kannel et al,

1978). There is no evidence that the influence of blood pressure diminishes with advancing age.

Systolic hypertension

Both stroke and hypertension reach major proportions in the elderly. Since there is a disproportionate rise in systolic pressure with advancing age, systolic hypertension is common in the elderly. For some time this was regarded as a harmless consequence of progressive rigidity of the arteries in advanced age. It has now been shown that this isolated systolic hypertension is far from innocuous and it is accompanied by a 2–4 fold increased risk of stroke (Colandrea et al, 1970). Some remain sceptical, however, suggesting that the systolic hypertension is only a sign of a rigid diseased vessel which is the true culprit. This distinction is important if we are to make proper decisions about prophylactic treatment of isolated systolic hypertension (O'Malley & O'Brien, 1980).

This issue has been examined in the Framingham Study. It was found that the prevalence of isolated systolic hypertension (>160/ <95 mmHg) increased from 2 percent in those 60–69 to 11 percent among those 70–79. An excess occurrence of strokes was noted among those with isolated systolic hypertension in all age-sex subgroups which was generally of the same order of magnitude as observed in those with elevations of both systolic and diastolic pressure. The data indicated that not only is the use of diastolic pressure in the elderly stroke candidate less efficient but may actually be misleading in persons with elevated systolic pressure. This may be because diastolic pressure is less accurately determined by the indirect method in the elderly than is the systolic pressure (Master & Lasser, 1961).

Analysis, using the depth of the dicrotic notch as an indication of elastic recoil of the arterial circulation, carried out in the Framingham cohort, strongly suggests that the elevated systolic pressure is more than an innocent sign of rigid arteries and makes an independent contribution to risk (Kannel et al, in press JAMA). Multivariate analysis including the systolic pressure, age and arterial rigidity judged from the pulse wave configuration shows a strong effect of pressure taking rigidity and age into account.

Comparison of stroke risk gradients based on systolic versus diastolic pressure gives no indication of a closer relationship to the diastolic component even in the elderly (Kannel et al, 1976).

Thus systolic hypertension appears to be a neglected contributor to stroke (Table 1.4). Elevation of systolic pressure can no longer be regarded as a normal concomitant of aging simply because it increases more with age than the diastolic component. The fact that hypertension in the elderly is predominantly systolic in character cannot be taken to mean that it is innocuous, and there is no *a priori* reason why hypertensive damage should derive more from the diastolic than systolic pressure.

Table 1.4 Two-year incidence of stroke according to level of systolic and diastolic blood pressure men and women, age 50 to 79: the Framingham study, 24-year follow-up

Diastolic blood pressure	Systolic blood pressure					
	<140		140–159		160+	
	At risk	Rate/1000 age adj.	At risk	Rate/1000 age adj.	At risk	Rate/1000 age adj.
Men						
<90	6735	5.3	1816	7.4	544	21.0
90–94	478	6.5	911	12.1	499	10.8
95+	137	13.1	761	12.3	1372	24.8
Women						
<90	7827	3.8	2894	6.6	1295	9.6
90–94	344	0.0	1195	8.3	1009	11.9
95+	91	0.0	684	18.6	2192	16.8

While it is clear that isolated systolic hypertension constitutes a substantial risk factor for stroke, it is still uncertain whether this situation can be corrected by antihypertensive treatment and at what cost in side effects. Treatment is less often successful for systolic than diastolic hypertension in the elderly and it is sometimes necessary to reduce diastolic pressures to very low values in order to achieve the desired lowering of systolic pressure (Koch-Weser, 1976; Seligman et al, 1977).

Since the evidence available now indicates that the increased risk of strokes associated with systolic hypertension is probably a direct result of the pressure, it seems likely that lowering the systolic pressure would be efficacious. However, only a controlled trial can determine the indications, best drugs, dosage, side effects, benefits and hazards of such an endeavor. Because of the high risk of stroke in persons with isolated systolic hypertension such a trial seems long overdue.

Lipids

The relationship of serum lipids to development of coronary disease is well established; the association for stroke has been inconsistent. This has been attributed to the advanced age at which strokes generally occur since even in coronary disease the relationship of serum total cholesterol to risk becomes markedly attenuated beyond age 55. For coronary disease the relationship re-emerges when the cholesterol is fractionated into lipoprotein components.

At the time of the eleventh biennial examination of the Framingham cohort, a complete lipid profile was obtained on all subjects, still free of cerebrovascular disease. In the course of the subsequent six years of follow-up 55 strokes occurred among the men and 44 among the women, with 30 of these being brain infarctions in the men and 21 in the women. In this 49–82 year old age group there was a striking *positive* relationship of the LDL-cholesterol to risk of coronary disease even when other risk factors are taken into account, and in both sexes. For stroke (Table 1.5), there was a *negative* relationship to LDL-cholesterol which was substantial and highly significant in women (Kannel et al, in press, Stroke). This strong negative relationship was demonstrable both for

brain infarction and for all other types of stroke combined. For HDL-cholesterol, as in coronary disease, there was a modest *negative* relationship for both sexes; the coefficients, however, were not statistically significant. For VLDL-cholesterol, no substantial or significant relationship to stroke incidence was noted in either sex.

Clearly more data are needed on cholesterol lipoprotein fractions in stroke, both from Framingham and elsewhere. However, thus far it must be concluded that the relation of lipoprotein cholesterol fractions to stroke may well differ from that for CHD. There is evidently a strong *negative* relationship for the atherogenic LDL-cholesterol component to both strokes in general and brain infarctions in particular, which requires explanation. This is curious in view of the *positive* correlation for CHD demonstrable as expected in the same cohort within the same advanced age range. For stroke as for CHD, HDL-cholesterol appears to exert a modest protective effect as anticipated.

The inverse relationship of LDL-cholesterol and stroke incidence in these data on older subjects is consistent with findings reported from a study of Japanese in Hawaii, where an inverse relation between total cholesterol and stroke incidence was found (Kagan et al, 1980). In these studies, however, the inverse relationship applied only to hemorrhagic strokes.

Diabetes

The discovery of insulin in 1921 provided the means of preventing the ketoacidosis and coma of diabetes, but has not greatly influenced the atherosclerotic sequelae of diabetes. The cardiovascular hazards of diabetes are widely acknowledged but there has been some uncertainty as to whether it is truly an independent risk factor. Only recently have prospective epidemiologic data begun to clarify the role of diabetes in cardiovascular morbidity (Blacket et al, 1973; Tibblin et al, 1975; Garcia et al, 1973).

Prospective population studies such as the Framingham Study indicate that the greatest impact of diabetes is on occlusive peripheral arterial disease (Table 1.6). The reason for this is obscure considering that the arterial lesions produced in

Table 1.5 Incidence of stroke and ABI by serum total cholesterol level 20 year follow-up. Framingham study. Men and Women 65–74

Serum total cholesterol level (mg/dl)	Person-years at risk	Stroke incidence			
		No. of cases		Rate/1000 year	
		Stroke	ABI	Stroke	ABI
Men					
<190	690	12	8	174	116
190–234	1920	12	7	62	36
235–294	1700	7	5	41	29
295+	304	5	4	164	132
Women					
<190	254	9	6	354	236
190–234	1122	12	5	107	45
235–294	3490	22	14	63	40
295+	1410	12	10	85	71

ABI = Atherothrombotic Brain Infarction.
Stroke = Stroke (all types).

Table 1.6 Incidence of cardiovascular events according to diabetic status, men and women, age 45–74: the Framingham study

| | Age-adjusted average annual incidence per 1000 | | | | | |
| | Men | | | Women | | |
	Diabetic	Non-diabetic	Risk ratio	Diabetic	Non-diabetic	Risk ratio
Cardiac failure	7.6	3.5	2.2	11.4	2.2	5.2
Intermittent claudication	12.6	3.3	3.8	8.4	1.3	6.3
Brain infarction	4.7	1.9	2.5	6.2	1.7	3.7
Coronary disease	24.8	14.9	1.7	17.8	6.9	2.6

the head, heart and limbs are similar. The relative impact of diabetes for atherothrombotic brain infarction is, however, substantial, greater in women than in men, and exceeds that of coronary heart disease, the most common sequel of diabetes on an absolute scale. In terms of attributable risk, which takes into account the prevalence of diabetes as well as its potency as a risk factor, diabetes also accounts for a greater proportion of brain infarctions than myocardial infarctions (Table 1.7).

Table 1.7 Population attributable risk of diabetes for cardiovascular events, men and women, age 45–74: the Framingham study

| | Attributable fraction | |
	Men	Women
Brain infarction	10.1	14.3
Coronary disease	3.8	7.7
Intermittent claudication	13.6	2.7
Cardiac failure	7.7	18.6

Attributable fraction $= (R_2-R_1) \times P/R$
R_2 = Age-adjusted cardiovascular disease rate in those with diabetes
R_1 = Rate in those without diabetes
R = Rate in total population
P = Prevalence of diabetes

Table 1.8 Probability (per 1000) of brain infarction in 8 years among diabetics according to level of other risk factors, men and women, 55 years of age the Framingham study, 18-year follow-up

| | Men | | | | | | | | |
| Chol | Systolic blood pressure | | | | Chol | Systolic blood pressure | | | |
	105	135	165	195		105	135	165	195
185	5	11	25	57	185	6	13	30	67
235	6	14	32	71	235	7	16	37	83
285	7	17	39	87	285	9	20	46	102
335	9	22	49	107	335	11	25	58	125
	ECG-LVH negative					ECG-LVH positive			
	Women								
Chol	Systolic blood pressure				Chol	Systolic blood pressure			
	105	135	165	195		105	135	165	195
185	2	4	7	13	185	5	9	16	27
235	3	6	11	19	235	7	13	23	40
285	5	9	15	27	285	11	19	33	57
335	7	13	22	39	335	15	27	47	81
	ECG-LVH negative					ECG-LVH positive			

Average risk of brain infarction for 55 year old men, 11/1000; women 10/1000.

Diabetes exerts an impact on the incidence of brain infarction, which is independent of other risk factors. After adjustment for differences in other associated cardiovascular risk factors (systolic blood pressure, serum total cholesterol, cigarette smoking and LVH by ECG) the relative impact of diabetes on brain infarction incidence is the same 2.2-fold increase in each sex.

There is considerable variability in the incidence of brain infarction among diabetics depending on the level of other risk factors (Table 1.8). Although the higher level of cardiovascular risk factors in diabetics could conceivably account for the increased risk of brain infarction, the increased propensity to stroke is not entirely a function of the associated risk factors. Multivariate analysis indicates a significant two-fold net effect of diabetes taking correlated risk factors into account.

Environmental factors

Despite reported sizeable geographic variation and secular trends in stroke mortality, only a few environmental contributors to the occurrence of stroke have been identified.

Personality, type of work and lifestyle have all been suggested as possible factors. Diets too rich in calories, saturated fat and cholesterol and deficient in fiber and complex carbohydrates have been incriminated in hyperlipidemia. High salt intake in susceptible persons may promote hypertension. Cigarette smoking, while not a strong stroke risk factor, nonetheless contributes to the problem by promoting coronary heart disease which in turn predisposes to stroke. Alcohol appears to contribute by raising blood pressure.

Cigarette smoking

Cigarette smoking, which so clearly is related to the rate of development of CHD and occlusive peripheral arterial disease, is unaccountably only weakly associated with stroke. The correlation is confined to men under age 65, with maximum impact below age 55 (Table 1.9). This is reminiscent of CHD where the risk also decreases with advancing age and cannot be demonstrated beyond age 65. Since most strokes occur beyond age 65, cigarette smoking does not rank high among the risk factors for stroke. It is curious that this does not apply for atherosclerotic disease involving the legs where even women beyond age 65 who smoke are at substantially increased risk.

Table 1.9 Risk of occlusive arterial disease and atherothrombotic brain infarction according to cigarette habit. The Framingham study. 20 year follow-up, men, age 45–74

| Cigarettes smoked/day | Average annual incidence per 10 000 | | | | | |
| | Intermittent claudication | | | Atherothrombotic brain infarction | | |
	Age 45–54	55–64	65–74	Age 45–54	55–64	65–74
None	10	30	58	5	17	52
Under 20	15	45	65	8	20	52
20	21	67	74	12	24	52
Over 20	30	100	83	18	28	53

Although the impact is modest, marginally significant, and confined to men below age 65, the effect where it exists is an independent one, not accounted for by the associated risk factors.

Diet

Comparison of national differences in diet, feeding experiments in animals and human metabolic studies have all suggested that an excess of calories, saturated fat and cholesterol may be responsible for the hypercholesterolemia regularly found in populations where CHD is highly prevalent (National Diet-Heart Study Final Report, 1968). Although dietary factors may influence atherogenesis, perhaps by elevating LDL-cholesterol values, evidence that alterations in diet reduce stroke risk is lacking.

Coffee

An association between coffee drinking and coronary disease has been alleged, based on retrospective studies. This has not stood up to prospective study scrutiny and appears to derive from difficulties with controls and failure adequately to take into account the associated cigarette habit. The relationship to stroke is even more tenuous (Dawber et al, 1974).

Obesity

The Framingham Study findings on the relation of stroke incidence to body weight throws some light on pathogenesis. In general, stroke incidence in Framingham tends to increase with weight, more prominently in women, in whom the relationship is statistically significant. Multivariate analysis suggests that the association derives from higher pressures (and possibly blood sugars) in the obese. Hence, a high stroke incidence in the obese is not unexpected. However, in the elderly (65–74), there is a *negative* trend in stroke incidence in relation to relative weight which may be related to the inverse association of LDL-cholesterol with stroke incidence.

Water

An association between soft water and atherosclerotic cardiovascular mortality including stroke has been noted and a cause and effect relationship suggested (Schroeder, 1960). A recent review has failed to demonstrate an independent effect on vascular disease mortality (Hammer & Heyden, 1980.)

Alcohol

Although a *negative* association between alcohol intake and coronary heart disease incidence has been found, some have also noted an increased risk of CHD among excessive drinkers. A possible explanation for this beneficial effect is a strong positive association of moderate alcohol intake with HDL-cholesterol and a negative association with atherogenic LDL-cholesterol. Curiously, there are indications that, if anything, alcohol promotes strokes. This observation may be related to the association between alcohol and hypertension.

The Hisayama Study in Japan, studies in Honolulu Japanese and in Caucasians in Alabama have shown an increase risk of hemorrhagic strokes (Marshall, 1971; Peacock et al, 1972; Omae et al, 1976; Kagan et al, 1980). The Framingham Study data also have suggested an association between alcohol intake and stroke, including brain infarction (Table 1.10).

Table 1.10 Risk of stroke according to alcohol intake: the Framingham study men, age 35–64

Oz. alcohol per month	Age-adjusted incidence per 1000	
	Strokes (all types)	Brain infarction
None	58	22
1–10	61	26
11–30	68	30
31–400	79	51

Physical activity

An association between physical inactivity and the risk of CHD was first demonstrated by Logan (1952) and by Morris and co-workers in 1953. While it can be argued with some conviction that there is a beneficial effect of physical activity to CHD incidence and mortality, the relationship to stroke is tenuous (Paffenbarger et al, 1978). Sedentary work activity has not been associated with an increased incidence of stroke in spite of the associated enhanced risk of MI (Marquardsen, 1969). Framingham data show an inverse relationship but this is neither substantial nor statistically significant.

Climate

Climate appears to influence both stroke and coronary heart disease mortality; death from either is apparently lowest in areas where environmental temperatures range between 60–79°F (Rogot & Padgett, 1976). Death rates from both diseases rise with declining temperature and abundant snow fall. Apparently either extreme of temperature promotes strokes and heart attacks, because the rates also increase when ambient temperatures exceed 79°F. These temperatures correlations are particularly evident for elderly persons.

The reasons for seasonal variation in stroke incidence are unclear. The lower incidence in summer in northern climates may provide a clue to ways of reducing the risk of stroke (Schuman et al, 1964).

Migration

From carefully controlled collaborative studies it seems clear that Japanese immigrants to the USA and their offspring have a substantially lower prevalence and mortality from stroke than do ethnically similar residents in Japan (Worth et al, 1975; Kagan et al, 1976). Since there is little difference in the prevalence of hypertension, but a substantial difference in fat and protein intake between migrant and indigenous Japanese, protein and fat malnutrition has been cited as predisposing to stroke (Kagan et al, 1974; Kimura, 1976). There is some experimental evidence derived from feeding spontaneously hypertensive rats which supports this contention (Yamori et al, 1976).

It is interesting that the lower prevalence of stroke in migrants from Japan is associated with a higher occurrence of CHD, another atherosclerotic vascular disease (Marmot et al, 1975; Robertson et al, 1977).

Other host factors

Impaired cardiac function

Hypertensives are especially prone to develop cardiac impairments such as ECG abnormalities, cardiac enlargement on X-ray and arrhythmias such as atrial fibrillation. They are also more likely to develop coronary heart disease and congestive heart failure (Shurtleff, 1974; Kannel & Sorlie, 1975). On this account alone, cardiac impairments should be associated with an increased risk of stroke, and they are (Fig. 1.5).

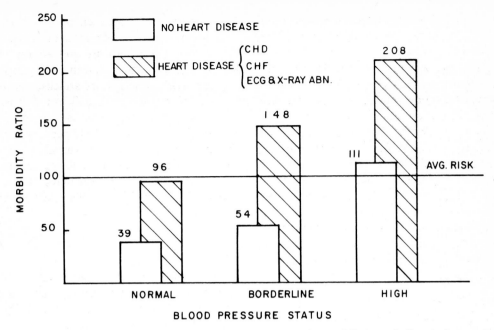

Fig. 1.5 Risk of stroke according to blood pressure and cardiac impairment, 24 year follow-up, the Framingham study.

Coronary heart disease frequently occurs in persons who appear well. This is not the case in brain infarction where 70 percent have established hypertension (20 percent associated with left ventricular hypertrophy), 30 percent co-existing coronary heart disease, 15 percent congestive heart failure, 30 percent occlusive peripheral arterial disease and 15 percent diabetes.

Infarctions in the heart and brain often co-exist and their co-existence increases with age. Kagan reported that 40 percent of those dying from stroke had a myocardial scar (Kagan, 1976). Cardiac impairments which have been found to contribute independently to stroke include: left ventricular hypertrophy on ECG, cardiac enlargement on X-ray, coronary heart disease, congestive heart failure and atrial fibrillation. Myocardial infarction not only predisposes to stroke but also is the most frequent cause of death in patients who experience a stroke, TIAs or carotid bruits (Toole et al, 1975).

In addition to reflecting sustained hypertension and its damaging effects on the vascular system, it seems likely that poor cardiac function directly precipitates strokes in persons with a compromised cerebral circulation. Persons with coronary heart disease were found to have almost a threefold increased risk of stroke and those whose cardiac disease progressed to the point of overt congestive failure had almost a fivefold increased risk. In neither case was this solely a consequence of the often associated hypertension, since the excess risk could be demonstrated even after the blood pressure elevation was taken into account.

Not only does overt cardiac disease contribute independently to stroke incidence, but even more subtle asymptomatic cardiac impairments do as well. ECG-LVH, in particular, was found to be associated with almost a fivefold increased risk, a hazard as great as actual heart failure. This, to some extent, reflects the severity and duration of associated hypertension. It also very likely reflects myocardial ischemia and impaired cardiac function because at any level of blood pressure those with ECG-LVH have a higher risk than those without it (Colandra et al, 1970). Cardiac enlargement without symptoms also further increases risk in hypertensive but more likely if ECG-LVH is also present. Three of every four stroke victims have one or more of these cardiac impairments.

Other cardiac disorders such as chronic rheumatic valvular disease, infective and marantic endocarditis, prolapsed mitral valve (Barnett et al, 1976), and cardiac myxoma are also associated with an increased risk of embolic stroke. Stroke, predominantly embolic, occurs as a complication of cardiac catherization, following installation of prosthetic heart valves and during cardiac surgery employing circulatory bypass methods.

Atrial fibrillation

Embolism from the left atrium occurs frequently in atrial fibrillation with mitral stenosis (Daley et al, 1951; Askey & Bernstein, 1960). While this is widely recognized, there was disagreement as to the risk of cerebral embolism in persons with chronic atrial fibrillation in the absence of rheumatic valvular disease (Beer & Ghitman, 1961; Hurst et al, 1964). Data from the Framingham Study leave little doubt that chronic atrial fibrillation, with or without RHD is an important stroke precursor (Wolf et al, 1978b). This is supported by other epidemiologic prospective evidence (Friedman et al, 1968). It is also supported by clinical and autopsy evidence (Hinto Hinton et al, 1977; Fairfax et al, 1976).

Chronic atrial fibrillation was assessed as a possible precursor of stroke over 24 years of follow-up in the Framingham Study. Persons with chronic atrial fibrillation with or without co-existing RHD were found to be at greatly increased risk of strokes, probably due to embolism. In the absence of RHD, chronic atrial fibrillation was found to be associated with almost a sixfold increase in stroke incidence (Table 1.11). This arrhythmia when accompanying RHD was associated with a 17-fold excess risk.

stroke, it was not appreciated until the Framingham Study that this also applied within the normal range of hematocrits (Fig. 1.6). Much of this relationship was attributable to concomitant blood pressure elevation, also related to hematocrit (Kannel et al, 1972; Wolf et al, 1978a). Evidence supporting this relationship was also found in a Japanese hospital study of fatal strokes (Tohgi et al, 1978).

The mechanism is uncertain but it is known that viscosity increases progressively with increments of hematocrit within the normal range (Thomas et al 1977; Pearson & Thomas, 1979). Rheological factors become critical in the small calibre penetrating vessels and also in larger vessels severely stenosed by atherosclerosis.

There is evidence that a raised hematocrit, not necessarily accompanied by an increased red cell mass may also predispose to vascular disease (Lawrence & Berlin, 1952; Kaung & Peterson, 1962; Burge et al 1975). It is thus possible that the increased incidence of brain infarction in patients with high hematocrits results from retardation of cerebral blood flow which tends to lead to arterial thrombosis (Begg & Hearns, 1966).

Cerebral blood flow has been found to be significantly lower in patients with hematocrit values in the range of 45–53 percent than in those with hematocrits between 36–46 percent (Thomas et al 1977). Also, after reduction of hematocrit by venesection, flow was found to increase by 50 percent (Thomas et al, 1977). This improvement

Table 1.11 Stroke risk by atrial fibrillation (AF) and rheumatic heart disease (RHD) status. The Framingham study. 20 year follow-up; men and women, age 30–62

| AF and RHD status | Age-sex-blood pressure adjusted rate† | | | |
	Number of strokes	Observed rate	Expected rate	Observed/ Expected
Neither	311	2.9	3.1	0.9
AF Alone	20	41.5	7.4	5.6*
AF plus RHD	7	45.5	2.6	17.5*

* $p < 0.01$
† Per 1000 person-years

Hematocrit

Although pathologically elevated hematocrits were long recognized as a predisposing condition for

in flow may be partly attributable to a reduction in viscosity, as well as to the homeostatic mechanism maintaining oxygen delivery at a level appropriate to cerebral metabolism.

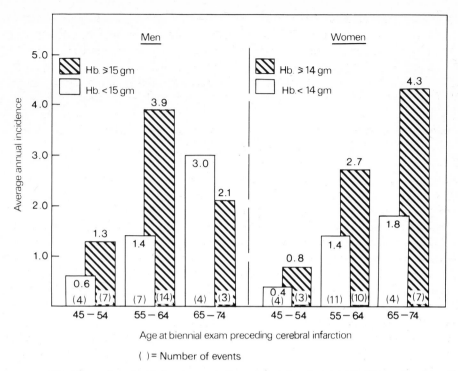

Fig. 1.6 Average annual incidence of cerebral infarction according to antecedent hemoglobin. Men and women, 45–74, the Framingham study 16 year follow-up.

It thus appears that hematocrits at the upper limit of the normal range may be a contributor to occlusive cerebral vascular disease.

Race

Mortality data have long suggested that blacks are more prone to stroke than whites of the same age and sex living in the same geographic area of the U.S.A. (Heyman et al, 1971). Incidence data also strongly suggest a greater incidence of strokes in blacks. Although the findings are fairly consistent, the estimates are based on rather modest numbers of cases and the case ascertainment methods are often crude. Nevertheless, it seems very likely that there is an excess of strokes in blacks consistent with the higher prevalence of hypertension.

A high mortality from cerebrovascular disease is characteristic of Japanese statistics. A high mortality from intracerebral hemorrhage in particular has been reported. The Hisayama Study which was prospective with a high autopsy rate demonstrated that stroke is indeed more common than heart disease and showed that cerebral hemorrhage accounted for about 30 percent of the strokes. In this study, there was a clear excess of strokes in men compared to women at all ages (Omae et al, 1976). Recent Japanese vital statistics attribute about one-fourth of total deaths to stroke. While cerebral hemorrhage has been declining over the years, the rate of cerebral infarction has been increasing. It is not clear how much of this is a change in fashions in diagnosis of stroke death and how much is actually a change in the pattern of stroke.

The Ni-Hon-San Study, using the same case ascertainment methods in these areas, found higher rates in Japanese in Japan, than in Hawaii or California (Kagan et al, 1976; Kagan et al, 1980). This strongly suggests differences in diet, lifestyle and environment are responsible rather than race.

Oral contraceptives

In the 1960s neurologists became aware of vascular brain syndromes in young women using birth control pills (Bickerstaff, 1975). Subsequent planned prospective studies have substantiated an increased risk of transient cerebral and retinal ischemic attacks, and embolic, thrombotic and hemorrhagic infarcts of the brain. These infarcts result from *in situ* thrombi, emboli and hemorrhage from aneurysm as well as from venous occlusive disease (Vessey & Doll, 1969). Atherosclerosis is rarely present. It is estimated that there is a tenfold increase in stroke risk compared to women of the same age not taking the oral contraceptive pill (Collaborative Group for the Study of Stroke in Young Women, 1973). While the relative risk is great, the absolute risk is small (1 in 10 000). The risk is further enhanced by co-existing hypertension, a history of migraine (particularly ophthalmic or hemiplegic varieties), age exceeding 35 years and prolonged use of the pill, the presence of diabetes or hyperlipidemia, and, in particular, by cigarette smoking. The risk seems greatest in high estrogen dose oral contraceptive pills (Handin, 1974). Some reviews suggest that the evidence of pill-associated stroke is inconclusive. The stroke incidence in the age group 15 to 45 is equal in men and women, and no substantial increase in fatal stroke in these ages has been noted in death data since the pill became available (Kuller, 1978).

Most large neurology centers encounter a small number of unexplained nonpuerperal strokes each year in otherwise healthy persons ages 15 to 45. Tally of these cases fails to disclose any substantial increase in number or of an increase in the ratio of women to men, which is approximately 1.0 (Illis et al, 1965; Jennett & Cross, 1967; Heyman et al, 1969; Schoenberg et al, 1970; Comer et al, 1975). There may be a tendency for physicians to overdiagnose a neurologic illness as stroke when confronted with a patient currently taking oral contraceptives, just as thrombophlebitis was overdiagnosed in women on the pill in another study (Barnes et al, 1978).

Environmental factors

Despite reported sizeable geographic variation and secular trends in stroke mortality, only a few environmental contributors to the occurrence of stroke have been identified.

Personality, type of work and life style have all been suggested as possible factors. Diets too rich in calories, saturated fat and cholesterol and deficient in fiber and complex carbohydrate have been incriminated in hyperlipidemia. High salt intake in susceptible persons may promote hypertension. Cigarette smoking, while not a strong stroke risk factor, nonetheless contributes to the problem by promoting coronary heart disease which in turn predisposes to stroke. Alcohol appears to contribute by raising blood pressure.

Heredity

Reports on familial occurrence of strokes have often consisted of descriptions of families with an unusual number of strokes. Precisely because such families are unusual these anecdotal reports are of limited value for analysis of genetic influences. The occurrence of strokes in the general population is sufficiently common so that chance familial aggregation is likely (Marshall, 1971). 'Cerebral apoplexy' has been shown to be significantly more common in the relatives of hypertensives as compared to the general population (Alter & Kluznik, 1972). However, case ascertainment in the two groups may not have been equivalent.

The excess of strokes in the family of patients compared to the spouse's family seems confined to siblings and no other family members emerge as being at extremely high risk. Thus close relatives of a stroke patient are at only slightly greater risk than genetically nonrelated persons (Alter & Kluznik, 1972; Heyden, et al 1969; Davidenkova et al, 1966; Slack & Evans, 1966; Gifford, 1966; Issaeva & Mikheeva, 1967; Gertler et al, 1968). No single Mendelian genetic pattern has been discerned, but there is a suggestion that hereditary factors are operative in stroke.

However, it is not clear what it is that is inherited. Hypertension and diabetes which predispose to strokes are subject to inherent susceptibility (Alter & Kluznik, 1972; Slack & Evans, 1966; Platt, 1963; Miall & Olham, 1963; Winkelstein et al, 1966). These predisposing conditions might account for much of the excess of strokes in relatives of stroke patients. Prospective studies to obtain a true assessment of whether strokes tend to occur in families are too sparse to allow a conclusion. Although direct prospective evidence that a family history of stroke is of itself a predisposing factor is unsatisfactory, it would still seem reasonable to regard a family history of premature stroke as a sign of increased vulnerability.

THE STROKE RISK PROFILE

Risk factor information can be efficiently synthesized into composite risk estimate using multiple logistic equations. These describe the conditional probability of a cerebrovascular event for any given set of risk variables from their known coefficients of regression on incidence and constants for the intercept (Gordon et al, 1971). This allows a more logical selection of patients for preventive treatment and avoids underestimating the risk of persons with multiple marginal 'abnormalities' according to categorical assessments of 'risk factors'. It also avoids over-reacting to those with only a single 'abnormality'.

Using such formulations risk estimates can be obtained over a wide range depending on the combined strength of the ingredients. Using an efficient set of ingredients (systolic blood pressure, serum cholesterol, glucose tolerance, cigarette habit and ECG-LVH) one-tenth of the asymptomatic population can be identified from which

about half the ABIs will emerge. This segment of the population has a 40 to 47 percent chance of an ABI in eight years (Table 1.12).

Such an approach is feasible for computerized health agencies screening the normal population. Since such multiple logistic formulations can seldom be applied in medical office practice, handbooks have been computed which display the risk for a wide range of combinations of relevant risk factors (McGee, 1973). This makes it feasible to estimate the risk of an ABI for any combination of factors at any given age in either sex. For example, a 60 year old man who does not smoke cigarettes, has no glucose intolerance or ECG-LVH, but has a systolic blood pressure of 165 mmHg and a serum cholesterol of 185 mg percent will have a 20/1000 probability of developing an ABI in eight years (Fig. 1.7). A man of the same age with a similar blood pressure, but with a cholesterol of 335 mg percent who smokes, has glucose intolerance and ECG-LVH has a risk of 113/1000, about five times as great. These compare with an average risk of 16/1000 for men this age.

The variables selected are an efficient set of independent contributors to risk. They also have

Table 1.12 Risk of specified cardiovascular events according to decile of risk score. Men and women, 35 to 74. (from Kannel, 1976)

| Decile of risk | Average probability (in thousands) | | | | |
	Coronary disease	Brain infarction	Intermittent claudication	Hypertensive heart failure	Total C-V disease
Men					
1	16.4	0.2	1.4	0.4	18.9
2	31.1	0.6	3.2	1.0	36.5
3	44.6	1.3	5.3	1.6	53.9
4	59.0	2.3	7.6	2.4	72.8
5	73.6	3.6	10.2	3.3	92.7
6	88.9	5.5	13.2	4.7	115.1
7	105.3	7.9	17.7	6.5	140.1
8	124.0	11.2	24.3	8.8	170.7
9	150.3	17.1	34.9	13.6	215.0
10	225.6	47.4	68.5	44.4	343.6
Women					
1	3.2	0.2	0.9	0.4	6.5
2	6.7	0.5	1.6	0.7	12.2
3	10.7	1.1	2.4	1.2	18.3
4	16.1	1.9	3.2	1.8	26.2
5	23.9	3.4	4.3	2.6	37.4
6	34.5	5.4	6.0	3.7	52.1
7	46.6	8.0	7.9	5.5	70.2
8	62.8	11.5	10.6	8.0	95.0
9	82.2	16.8	14.8	12.9	127.5
10	140.9	39.8	37.0	37.9	224.4

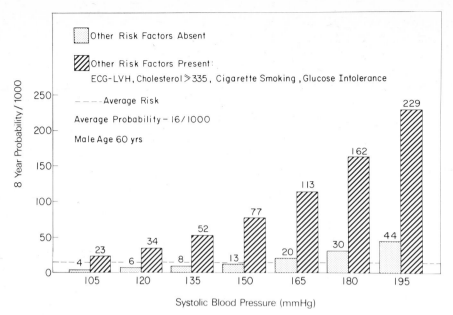

Fig. 1.7 Estimation of risk of an ABI in a male age 60 years.

the virtue of being objective, obtainable from an unprepared, non-fasting patient, without trauma or undue expense, and, most important, they apply to other cardiovascular outcomes as well (McGee, 1973).

The table is based on a population free of all major cardiovascular diseases such as coronary and rheumatic heart disease, intermittent claudication, congestive heart failure and previous strokes. Persons with such diseases have a markedly enhanced risk of strokes by virtue of these alone. The variables chosen are not the only set for the reasons given above. Other information which should be taken into account in evaluating risk includes: other ECG abnormalities, cardiac dysrhythmias, cardiac enlargement on X-ray, congestive heart failure, overweight and elevated hemoglobin values.

SIGNS OF COMPROMISED CEREBRAL CIRCULATION

Once a completed stroke has occurred the victim is left with a permanent neurologic deficit which cannot be corrected. Now that medical and surgical procedures are available to restore flow through or around a blocked extracranial blood supply to the brain, there is a growing interest in the early detection of a compromised cerebral circulation. There is also an interest in correctable precipitating factors for stroke.

There are two clinical findings which indicate that a compromised cerebral circulation may be present — asymptomatic carotid bruits and transient cerebral ischemic attacks. Modern medical technology is also becoming available to non-invasively detect obstructions and measure flow in the extracranial cerebral circulation.

Asymptomatic carotid bruits

There is uncertainty about the prognostic importance and management of persons with asymptomatic carotid bruits. It is not clear what proportion of strokes are heralded by carotid bruits or whether, when present, the stroke was actually caused by the obstructive disease in the vessel involved. Carotid bruits may be associated with a greater incidence of strokes either because they are directly involved in the pathogenesis of the ictus or only because they are non-specific indicators of generalized atherosclerosis which often includes the intracerebral vessels. It is also not clear how often asymptomatic carotid bruits lead to transient ischemic cerebral attacks and whether those that do are more specifically related to the subsequent occurrence of strokes. In the Framingham Study, beginning with the ninth biennial examination in 1966 and on all subsequent examinations, carotid bruits were routinely sought out by auscultation. Over eight years, carotid bruits appeared in 171 subjects, 66 in men and 105 in women, all of whom were asymptomatic and free of bruit on Exam 9. The prevalence of bruits increased with age and was equal in men and women, rising from 3.5 percent at ages 45–54, to 7.0 percent at ages 67–79 (Wolf et al, JAMA, in press). The prevalence was greater in subjects with hypertension and with the presence of coronary heart disease and diabetes. TIA appeared in 8 (2 alone) and strokes in 21 of the 171, a stroke rate twice expected for age and sex. More often than not, however, the cerebral infarction occurred in a vascular territory different from that of the carotid bruit, often in the posterior circulation, and ruptured aneurysm, embolism from the heart and lacunar infarction was the mechanism of stroke in nearly half the cases. Interestingly, the incidence of myocardial infarction was also increased twofold in those with asymptomatic carotid bruit (Fig. 1.8). General mortality was also increased; 1.7-fold in men, and 1.9-fold in women, with 79 percent of the deaths due to cardiovascular disease, including stroke.

Carotid bruit is clearly an indicator of increased stroke risk; however, in asymptomatic populations, the bruit is chiefly a nonspecific sign of advanced atherosclerotic disease and not necessarily an indicator of a local arterial lesion which will lead to cerebral infarction in the territory of the vessel (Heyman et al, 1980).

TRANSIENT ISCHEMIC ATTACKS (TIA)

Transient ischemic attacks are reversible focal neurologic deficits, lasting minutes to 24 hours. Based on retrospective clinical data from patients who have sustained a stroke, TIAs are believed frequently to precede development of brain infarction. However, best estimates indicate that only 10 percent of strokes are preceded by TIAs (Whisnant, 1974; Mohr, 1978; Hass, 1977).

It is estimated that surgically accessible carotid artery atherothrombotic disease of the extracranial circulation to the brain accounts for less than 15 percent of strokes, and that atherothrombotic disease of the large extracranial arteries, including

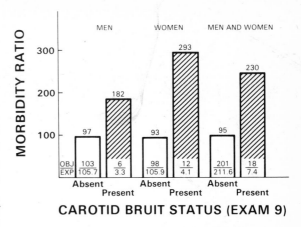

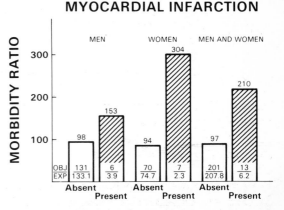

Fig. 1.8 Age adjusted 2 year incidence of stroke and myocardial infarction by carotid bruit status in men and women 50–79 years, the Framingham study.

the carotid, altogether produces about 34 percent of strokes (Mohr, 1978).

The incidence of TIAs is uncertain because of non-uniform definitions and case ascertainment. The best estimate is that the incidence approaches one per 1000 per year in the elderly. Over 65 percent of patients who experienced TIAs before stroke had carotid artery disease, but it is estimated that only 30 percent of patients with carotid territory TIAs have clinical signs of extracranial carotid disease on careful examination.

The risk of stroke is believed to be increased tenfold in those who experience TIAs. Fully 35 percent can expect a stroke within four years (Mohr, 1978). It is estimated that the risk of a stroke in persons with a well defined TIA is approximately 7 percent per year (Haas, 1977). Risk of a stroke appears to be greater in carotid than vertebrobasilar territories. If a stroke is to occur it is likely to do so within a few months of onset of TIAs. Although risk of a stroke is substantially increased, survival is little altered compared to persons the same age in the general population (Whisnant, 1974).

The prognosis for those with carotid territory TIAs without demonstrable vascular abnormality is almost as ominous as in those with stenotic occlusion. This suggests that embolic events, hypercoagulable states and other causes may be responsible.

The risk of TIAs and the risk of their evolving into brain infarctions is best discerned from prospective study of a general population sample. In the Framingham Study, 5184 adult men and women free of stroke or TIAs have been followed biennially for the development of TIAs and strokes. After 26 years, 393 strokes occurred, 197 in men and 196 in women. Brain infarction, the commonest type of stroke (56 percent), was preceded by TIAs in 12 percent of the cases.

The average annual incidence of TIAs was similar in men and women. Also like brain infarction, the incidence rose with age from four per 100 000 for those under age 40 at entry, to eight per 100 000 at age 40 to 49 to 14 per 100 000 at age 50 to 62. Only 20 percent of persons with symptoms suggesting TIAs fulfilled minimal criteria.

Of the 67 persons with TIA, stroke developed in 27 (40 percent). Half of the brain infarctions which followed TIAs occurred within three months of the onset of the TIAs and two-thirds within six months. In most cases, there were less than four TIAs preceding the stroke. It thus appears that 40 percent of subjects with TIAs will develop brain infarctions, and that if they are to occur it will happen soon after the episodes begin. This suggests that the onset of TIAs constitutes an urgent situation requiring prompt medical or surgical intervention.

SECULAR TRENDS AND THE DECLINING INCIDENCE OF STROKE

Mortality trends in Western nations including the United States indicates a recent decline in stroke mortality (Acheson, 1960; Wylie, 1962; Borhani, 1965; Prineas, 1971; Metropolitan Life Insurance Co., 1975; Haberman et al, 1978; Levy, 1979). This decline seems real despite recognized limitations imposed by fashions in death certification and inaccuracies in death diagnoses (Florey et al, 1967; Israel & Klebba, 1969). Morbidity statistics on the actual incidence of strokes are sparse and the comparability of case ascertainment over time is questionable (Eisenberg et al, 1964; Aho & Fogelholm, 1974; Abu-Zeid et al, 1975; Christie, 1976; Hansen & Marquardsen, 1977). Study of secular trends in stroke incidence in Framingham where uniform criteria and case ascertainment has been maintained over three decades confirms a decline in stroke incidence but only in women (Wolf et al, 1978c).

Stroke is part of a larger problem of cardiovascular disease (CVD) and time trends must be examined from the perspective of overall mortality. Age adjusted cardiovascular mortality rates in the U.S.A. have declined almost 32 percent over the past 30 years. This decrease has accelerated over the past decade, accounting for two-thirds of the 30 year decline. Despite an ageing population of increasing size, the total number of deaths attributed to CVD recently fell below one million for the first time in almost a decade. The decline in cardiovascular mortality has occurred in both sexes, in non-whites as well as whites and at all adult ages.

Over nine years following 1968, mortality rates from coronary heart disease, the leading cause of death in the United States declined 23 percent and for stroke the decline was 32 percent. A downward trend in stroke mortality has been apparent for more than 50 years but has accelerated in recent years (Soltero et al, 1978). Death rates for stroke have fallen more rapidly than other components of cardiovascular disease. In the 1940s and 1950s stroke mortality in the U.S.A. declined at a rate of 1 percent per year. Since 1972, the rate of decline has been 5 percent per annum (Levy, 1979).

The sizeable geographic differences in reported stroke death rates in the U.S.A. have narrowed and stroke death rates from all regions have fallen over the past 15 years (Soltero et al, 1978; Moriyama et al, 1971). The decline has been especially notable in non-whites and the 48.5 percent fall in stroke mortality for non-white females (1960–1975) represents a dramatic change in the racial patterns of stroke mortality.

It is not possible to determine at present whether the mortality is declining because of a fall in the incidence rate or because better treatment has lowered case fatality rates. It is not even clear whether the rates are declining for hospitalized or out of hospital deaths. It is likely, however, that the decline is real and not simply a result of changes in death certification practices. It is also likely that both primary prevention and better medical care have contributed to the decline.

Hypertension, a demonstrated contributor to stroke incidence and mortality, is being more effectively controlled; hence, the decline in stroke mortality is not unexpected (Levy, 1979). The Veterans Administration Cooperative Study (1967, 1970) leaves little doubt that treatment of hypertension can prevent strokes. However, this cannot be accepted unequivocally since stroke mortality was declining for years before effective antihypertensive therapy became available. It is interesting that in the Framingham Study a decline in stroke incidence could be shown only for women; and women have had more effective blood pressure treatment and control than men (Wolf et al, 1978). It is difficult to escape the conclusion that hypertension control efforts have contributed to stroke death rate declines. In the United States, from 1972–1977, age-adjusted death rates for hypertension-related cardiovascular disease declined 20 percent whereas unrelated cardiovascular disease declined only 9 percent.

Incidence of stroke, nonfatal as well as fatal, is difficult to determine accurately. Few defined populations are available where stroke has been studied over a sufficiently long time to draw conclusions about temporal trends. To discern changes in incidence of specific stroke types, i.e., thrombosis, embolism, intracerebral or subarachnoid hemorrhage, a degree of diagnostic sophistication is required. Studies in Rochester, Minnesota suggest a decline in stroke occurrence during the period 1945 to 1974. Average annual incidence rates for all types of stroke combined and adjusted for age and sex have fallen from 190 per 100 000 in the 1945–1949 period to 104 per 100 000 in 1970–1974 (Garraway et al, 1979). This decline seems to

have occurred in two phases over the 30 year period. From 1945–49 to 1955–59 the rate fell 3.1 per 100 000 per year; there was a plateau in rates from 1955–59 to 1960–64 following which the decline resumed and accelerated to fall annually by 5.3 per 100 000 from 1965–69 to 1970–74.

Clinicians have noted that hypertensive encephalopathy, a fairly commonly encountered condition prior to 1950 is now a rarity (Wolff & Lindeman, 1966; Carter, 1970). Massive hypertensive intracerebral hemorrhage has also become less frequently seen in hospital emergency rooms and autopsy tables. In 1964, clinicians in Goteberg Sweden noted this decline in the number of patients seen with hypertensive intracerebral hemorrhage, particularly below the age of 55 (Aurell & Hood, 1964). Those with intracerebral hemorrhage turned out to be untreated hypertensives with markedly elevated blood pressures. In a comparison of autopsy records representing 97 percent of all hospital deaths, cerebral hemorrhage rates were lower below age 65 than in prior years. Median age at hemorrhage was five years older in 1961 than it had been in 1948.

This decline in intracerebral hemorrhage was also noted in studies in Rochester, Minnesota where incidence rates fell by 34 percent when the 15 year period from 1961 to 1976 is compared with the period from 1945 to 1960. Median age at onset of stroke also increased; from 67 years in 1945–52 to 71 years in 1969–76.

This decrement in intracerebral hemorrhage rates predates the advent of the Computerized Tomographic (CT) Scan of the head. The CT scan has demonstrated that many more restricted hemorrhages occur than had been suspected. These strokes were previously thought to be infarcts since the event was nonlethal, the deficit restricted and the spinal fluid free of blood. Whether the rate of smaller hypertensive hemorrhages is changing may be determined in future years.

CONTROL OF HYPERTENSION AND STROKE PREVENTION

On the basis of clinical observations among groups of patients with treated and untreated severe hypertension, clinicians have noted improvement in outcome among the treated (Wolff & Lindeman, 1966; Carter, 1970). The Veterans Administration Cooperative Study, in a controlled clinical trial demonstrated a highly significant benefit in stroke prevention and in survival among treated *severe* hypertensives whose pretreatment diastolic blood pressure levels were above 115 mmHg (Veterans Administration Cooperative Study, Group on Antihypertensive Agents, 1967). Similar benefits in stroke prevention were found in the treated group of men with *moderate* hypertension whose average pretreatment diastolic blood pressure levels were 105–114 mmHg (Veterans Administration Cooperative Study, Group on Antihypertensive Agents, 1970). The degree of benefit correlated with levels of prerandomization blood pressure and with degree of blood pressure control (Taguchi & Freis, 1974). In the moderate hypertensives with pretreatment diastolic blood pressure between 104 and 115 mmHg, there was one fourth the number of strokes among the treated as in the placebo (control) group during the average 3.8 year follow-up period.

That control of moderate and severe hypertension prevents or reduces stroke occurrence has been confirmed repeatedly and with few exceptions (Beevers et al, 1978). In a recent community-based randomized controlled trial involving nearly 11 000 persons with high blood pressure including *mild* hypertension, five year mortality was significantly lower in the systemically treated and controlled antihypertensive treatment group than in those given standard care (Hypertension Detection and Follow-up Progress Cooperative Group, 1979). In the group with mild hypertension, (entry diastolic blood pressure 90 to 104), mortality was significantly reduced by 20 percent in the systematic treatment group. This benefit was due to a reduction in death from cardiovascular disease including a 45 percent reduction in stroke and a 46 percent decrease in acute MI. In the systematic treatment group, control of blood pressure was consistently better at all ages, in blacks and whites and in both sexes. This hypertension control was matched by a corresponding reduction in mortality in the older age groups, in white men and in black men and women. These findings have enormous potential significance for disease prevention since about 70 percent of hypertensives in the United States fall in the mild hypertension category with diastolic blood pressures averaging between 90 and 104 mmHg. Sixty percent of the excess mortality attributable to hypertension occurs among persons in this blood pressure range.

PREVENTIVE IMPLICATIONS

The appearance of stroke or TIA should be regarded as a failure of prevention. Measures to diagnose and treat the stroke patient at this point are, for the most part, too little too late. In the case of cerebral infarction and cerebral hemorrhage, physicians must shift their attention from high technology instrumentation to the more mundane business of modifying risk factors for disease prevention in the presymptomatic stage. This requires attending to what are often considered medical trivia — modest elevations of blood pressure, early signs of cardiac impairment and the application of general hygenic measures to obesity, cigarette smoking and physical inactivity to try to prevent cardiovascular disease.

For stroke, prospects for prevention would be greatly improved by the demonstration of correctable environmental incidence factors. Unfortunately, there are few powerful environmental contributors to stroke mortality.

Acceleration in the decline in the incidence and mortality from cerebrovascular disease in recent years is a clear indication that stroke is not an inevitable consequence of ageing or genetic constitution. Diminution of stroke mortality has occurred at all ages including the eighth and ninth decades of life, providing evidence that control of hypertension and changes in environmental factors can effect changes in stroke occurrence.

Each physician can identify 'prime' candidates for stroke among his asymptomatic patients. Control of severe and moderately severe hypertension will definitely prevent stroke. Patients with these levels of blood pressure require vigorous and sustained therapy to maintain normotension. However, the greatest impact of elevated blood pressure on the public health is attributable to *mild* elevations of pressure because this abnormality is so common. Medical treatment of the 40 percent of the adult population of the U.S.A. known to have mild hypertension, (with diastolic pressure between 90 and 104 mmHg), is an extraordinary therapeutic and financial endeavour. The drugs have significant adverse effects limiting their acceptance. Needed are hygenic measures that can be practised by the individual to reduce the risk of cardiovascular disease including stroke. Weight loss, reduction of salt in the diet, giving up cigarette smoking are measures that can be advocated for most people. In addition, the practising physician, on the basis of a few historical, clinical and laboratory tests, can identify 10 percent of the population in whom the majority of strokes will occur. Utilizing a history of cigarette smoking, an ECG, a blood sugar, systolic blood pressure and serum cholesterol, a cardiovascular risk profile can be determined for each person and risk of subsequent stroke, CHD or peripheral arterial disease determined. It is to those persons comprising 10 percent of the population, whose cardiovascular or stroke risk profiles fall in the uppermost decile, that vigorous antihypertensive therapy should be applied.

The appearance of impaired cardiac function (LVH by ECG, CHF, enlarged heart on X-ray, intraventricular block, AF or CHD), heralds a definite increment in risk of stroke and marks the person as definitely stroke-prone. Initiation of antihypertensive therapy including a diuretic prior to the appearance of frank cardiac failure might help prevent stroke. Overt signs of a compromised cerebral circulation (the appearance of a carotid bruit or TIA), should alert the physician to the extreme hazard his patient faces. Forty percent of patients with TIAs develop stroke, half within three months of TIA onset. Ten percent of persons developing carotid bruit have a stroke within eight years of its appearance. These persons need all the risk reduction measures at the physician's disposal, particularly control of elevated blood pressure. Physicians have been loth to lower blood pressure of patients following stroke of TIA for fear of precipitating a stroke. Reduction in blood pressure among hypertensives with prior stroke or TIA has been shown in fact to increase cerebral blood flow (Meyer et al, 1968).

It can be clearly stated that the benefits outweigh the hazards. *Control of blood pressure elevation is the single most effective means of stroke prevention.* Prevention of stroke recurrence also rests on antihypertensive therapy (Rabkin, et al., 1978).

Acknowledgment

This work was supported in part by contracts numbers NIH–NO1–HV–92922 and NIH–NO1–HV–52971 (William B. Kannel, M.D., National Heart, Lung and Blood Institute); and grant NIH 1PO INS–16367 with Contract NO1–NS–8–2398 (Philip A. Wolf, M.D., National Institute of Neurological Communicative Diseases and Stroke).

REFERENCES

Abu-Zeid H A H, Choi N W, Nelson N A 1975 Epidemiologic features of cerebrovascular disease in Manitoba: Incidence by age, sex and residence, with etiologic implications. Canadian Medical Association Journal 113:379

Acheson R M 1960 Mortality from cerebrovascular accident and hypertension in the Republic of Ireland. British Journal of Preventive and Social Medicine 14:139

Aho K, Fogelholm R 1974 Incidence and early prognosis of stroke in Espoo-Kauniainen area, Finland, in 1972. Stroke 5:258

Alter M, Kluznik J 1972 Genetics of cerebrovascular accidents. Stroke 3:41

Askey J M, Bernstein S 1960–1961 The management of rheumatic heart disease in relation to systemic arterial embolism. Progress in Cardiovascular Disease 3:220

Aurell M, Hood B 1964 Cerebral hemorrhage in a population after a decade of active anti-hypertensive treatment. Acta Medica Scandinavica 176:377

Barnes R W, Krapf T, Hoak J C 1978 Erroneous clinical diagnosis of leg vein thrombosis in women on oral contraceptives. Obstetrics and Gynecology 51:556

Barnett H J M, Jones M W, Boughner D R, Kostuk W J 1976 Cerebral ischemic events associated with prolapsing mitral valve. Archives of Neurology 33:777

Beer D T, Ghitman B 1961 Embolization from the atria in arteriosclerotic heart disease. Journal of the American Medical Association 177:287

Beevers D G, Johnston J, Devine B L et al 1978 Relation between prognosis and the blood pressures before and during treatment of hypertensive patients. Clinical Science and Molecular Medicine 55 (Suppl):333s

Begg T B, Hearns J B 1966 Components in blood viscosity. The relative contribution of haematocrit, plasma fibrinogen and other proteins. Clinical Science 31:87

Bickerstaff E R 1975 Neurological complications of oral contraceptives, Clarendon Press, Oxford, England

Blacket R B, Leelarthaepin B, Palmer A J, Woodhill J M 1973

Coronary heart disease in young men: a study of 70 patients with a critical review of etiological factors. Australian and New Zealand Journal of Medicine 3:39

Borhani N O 1965 Changes and geographic distribution of mortality from cerebrovascular disease. American Journal of Public Health 55:673

Burge P S, Johnson W S, Prankerd T A J 1975 Morbidity and mortality in pseudo-polycythaemia. Lancet 1:1266

Carter A B 1970 Hypotensive therapy in stroke survivors. Lancet 1:485

Christie D 1976 Stroke in Melbourne: a study of the relationship between a teaching hospital and the community. Medical Journal of Australia 1:565

Colandrea M A, Friedman G D, Nichaman M Z, Lynd C N 1970 Systolic hypertension in the elderly. An epidemiology assessment. Circulation 41:239

Collaborative Group for the Study of Stroke in Young Women 1973 Oral contraception and increased risk of cerebral ischemia or thrombosis. New England Journal of Medicine 288:871

Comer T P, Tuerck D G, Bilas R A, Clow S F, Falero F, Raskind R R 1975 Comparison of strokes in women of childbearing age in Rochester, Minnesota and Bakersfield, California. Angiology 26:351

Daley R, Mattingly T W, Hold C L et al 1951 Systemic arterial embolism in rheumatic heart disease. American Heart Journal 42:566

Davidenkova E F, Babkova A V, Godinova A M et al 1966 A clinico-genetic study of patients with thrombosis of cerebral vessels. Klinicheskaia Meditsina (Moskva) 44:27

Dawber T R, Kannel W B, Gordon T 1974 Coffee and cardiovascular disease observation from the Framingham Study. New England Journal of Medicine 291:871

Eisenberg H, Morrison J T, Sullivan A et al 1964 Cerebrovascular accidents: Incidence and survival rates in a defined population, Middlesex County, Connecticut. Journal of the American Medical Association 189:883

Fairfax A J, Lambert C D, Leatham A 1976 Systemic embolism in chronic sinoatrial disorder. New England Journal of Medicine 295:190

Florey C D V, Senter M G, Acheson R M 1967 A study of the validity of the diagnosis of stroke in mortality data. I. Certificate analysis. Yale Journal of Biology and Medicine 40:148

Friedman G D, Loveland D B, Ehrlich S P 1968 Relationship of stroke to other cardiovascular disease. Circulation 38:533

Garcia M, McNamara P, Gordon T, Kannel W B 1973 Cardiovascular implications in diabetics. Advances in Metabolic Disorders, Suppl 2:493

Garraway W, Whisnant J P, Furlan A J et al 1979 The declining incidence of stroke. New England Journal of Medicine 300:449

Gertler M M, Rusk H A, Whiter H H et al 1968 Ischemic cerebrovascular disease: the assessment of risk factors. Geriatrics 23:135

Gifford A J 1966 An epidemiological study of cerebrovascular disease. American Journal of Public Health 58:452

Gordon T, Sorlie P, Kannel W B 1971 An epidemiological investigation of cardiovascular disease. Coronary heart disease, atherothrombotic brain infarction, intermittent claudication. A multivariate analysis of some factors related to their incidence. In: The Framingham Study, 16 Year Follow-up. Washington DC, United States Government Printing Office

Gresham G E, Fitzpatrick T E, Wolf P A, McNamara P M,

Kannel W B, Dawber T R 1975 Residual disability in survivors of stroke — the Framingham Study. New England Journal of Medicine 293:954

Gresham G E, Phillips T F, Wolf P A, McNamara P M, Kannel W B, Dawber T R 1979 Epidemiologic profile of long-term stroke disability: the Framingham Study. Archives of Physical Medicine and Rehabilitation 60:487

Haberman S, Capildeo R, Rose F C 1978 The changing mortality of cerebrovascular disease. Quarterly Journal of Medicine 47:71

Handin R 1974 Thromboembolic complications of pregnancy and oral contraceptives. Progress in Cardiovascular Diseases 16:395

Hansen B S, Marquardsen J 1977 Incidence of stroke in Frederiksberg, Denmark. Stroke 8:663

Hammer D I, Heyden S 1980 Water hardness and cardiovascular mortality. An idea that has served its purpose. Journal of the American Medical Association 243:2399

Hass W K 1977 Aspirin for the limping brain. Editorial. Stroke 8:299

Heyden S, Heyman A, Camplong L 1969 Mortality patterns among parents of patients with atherosclerotic cerebrovascular disease. Journal of Chronic Diseases 22:105

Heyman A, Arons M, Quinn M, Camplong L 1969 The role of oral contraceptive agents in cerebral arterial occlusion. Neurology 19:519

Heyman A, Karp H R, Heyden S et al 1971 Cerebrovascular disease in the biracial population of Evans County, Georgia. Stroke 2:509

Heyman A, Wilkenson W E, Heyden S et al 1980 Risk of stroke in asymptomatic persons with cervical arterial bruits. New England Journal of Medicine 302:838

Hinton R C, Kistler J P, Fallon J T et al 1977 Influence of etiology of atrial fibrillation on incidence of systemic embolism. American Journal of Cardiology 40:509

Hurst J W, Paulk E A, Proctor H D et al 1964 Management of patients with atrial fibrillation. American Journal of Medicine 37:728

Hypertension Detection and Follow-up Program Cooperative Group 1979 Five-year findings of the Hypertension Detection and Follow-up Programs. I. Reduction in mortality of persons with blood pressure, including mild hypertension. Journal of the American Medical Association 242:2562

Illis L, Kocen R S, McDonald W I, Mondkar V P 1965 Oral contraceptives and cerebral arterial occlusion. British Medical Journal 2:1164

Israel R A, Klobba A J 1969 A preliminary report on the effect of eighth revision ICDA on cause of death statistics. American Journal of Public Health 59:1651

Issaeva I I, Mikheeva V F 1967 The role of hereditary factors in the evolution of apoplexy. Zhurnal Nevropathologii i Psikhiatrii imeni S. S. Korsakova 67:22

Jennett W B, Cross J N 1967 Influence of pregnancy and oral contraception on the incidence of strokes in women of childbearing age. Lancet 1:1019

Kagan A, Harris B R, Winkelstein W et al 1974 Epidemiologic studies of coronary heart disease and stroke in Japanese men living in Japan, Hawaii and California: Demographic, physical, dietary and biochemical characteristics. Journal of Chronic Diseases 27:345

Kagan A R 1976 Atherosclerotic and myocardial lesions in subjects dying from fresh cerebrovascular disease. Bulletin of the World Health Organization 53:597

Kagan W, Popper J, Rhoads G G et al 1976 Epidemiologic studies of coronary heart disease and stroke in Japanese men living in Japan, Hawaii and California: Prevalence of stroke. In: Scheinberg P (ed) Cerebrovascular Diseases. Raven Press, New York, p 267

Kagan A, Popper J S, Rhoads G C 1980 Factors related to stroke incidence in Hawaii Japanese men. The Honolulu Heart Study. Stroke 11:14

Kannel W B 1971 Current status of the epidemiology of brain infarction associated with occlusive arterial disease. Stroke 2:295

Kannel W B, Blaisdel F W, Gofford R, Hass W, McDowell F, Meyer J S, Millikan C H, Rentz L E, Seltzer R 1971 Risk factors in stroke due to cerebral infarction. Stroke 2:423

Kannel W B, Gordon T, Wolf P A, McNamara P M 1972 Hemoglobin and the risk of cerebral infarction: the Framingham Study. Stroke 3:409

Kannel W B, Sorlie P 1975 Hypertension in Framingham. In Paul O (ed) Epidemiology and control of hypertension. Symposia Specialists, Miami, p 553

Kannel W B, Wolf P A 1975 Risk factors in atherothrombotic cerebrovascular disease. In: Meyer J S (ed) Modern concepts of cerebrovascular disease. Spectrum Publications, Inc., New York, p 113

Kannel W B 1976 Epidemiology of cerebrovascular disease. In: Ross Russell R W (ed) Cerebral Arterial Disease. 1st edn. Churchill Livingstone, London

Kannel W B, Dawber T R, Sorlie P, Wolf P A 1976 Components of blood pressure and risk of atherothrombotic brain infarction: the Framingham Study. Stroke 7:327

Kannel W B 1978 Status of coronary heart disease risk factors. Journal of Nutrition Education 10:10

Kannel W B, Wolf P A, Dawber T R 1978 Hypertension and cardiac impairments increase stroke risk. Geriatrics 33:71

Kannel W B, Wolf P A, Gordon T, Castelli W P In press. Cholesterol-lipoprotein fractions and risk of stroke: the Framingham Study. Stroke

Kannel W B, Wolf P A, McGee D L, Dawber T R, McNamara P M, Castelli W P In press. Systolic blood pressure, arterial rigidity and risk of stroke; the Framingham Study. Journal of the American Medical Association

Kaung D T, Peterson R E 1962 'Relative polycythemia' — or 'pseudopolycythemia' Archives of Internal Medicine 110:456

Kimura N 1976 Epidemiology of hypertension and stroke in Asia. In: Hatano S, Shigematsu I, Strasser T (eds) Hypertension and stroke control in the community. WHO, Geneva, p 55

Koch-Weser J 1976 Modern approaches to the treatment of hypertension. In: Gouveia W A, Tognono G, Kleign E V D (eds) Elsevier/North Holland Biomedical Press, Amsterdam, p 93

Kuller L H 1978 Epidemiology of stroke. In: Schoenberg B S (ed) Advances in Neurology, Volume 19: Neurological epidemiology: principles and clinical applications. Raven Press, New York, p 281

Kurtzke J F 1976a Epidemiology of cerebrovascular disease. In: Cerebrovascular survey report for joint council subcommittee on cerebrovascular disease, National Institute of Neurological and Communicative Disorders and Stroke and National Heart and Lung Institute. Whiting Press Inc., Rochester, Minnesota, p 213

Kurtzke J F 1976b An introduction to the epidemiology of cerebrovascular disease. In: Scheinberg P (ed)

Cerebrovascular diseases. Raven Press, New York, p 239

Lawrence J G, Berlin N I 1952 Relative polycythemia — the polycythemia of stress. Yale Journal of Biology and Medicine 24:498

Levy R I 1979 Stroke decline; Implications and prospects. New England Journal of Medicine 300:490

Logan W P D 1952 Mortality from coronary and myocardial disease in different social classes. Lancet 1:758

Logan W P D, Cushion A A 1958 Studies on medical and population subjects no. 14. Morbidity statistics from general practice. Volume I (General). H M Stationery Office, London

Marmot M G, Syme S L, Kagan A et al 1975 Epidemiologic studies of coronary heart disease and stroke in Japanese men living in Japan, Hawaii and California: prevalence of coronary and hypertensive heart disease and associated risk factors. American Journal of Epidemiology 102:514

Marquardsen J 1969 The natural history of acute cerebrovascular disease. A retrospective study of 769 patients. Acta Neurologica Scandinavica 45 (Suppl 38):11

Marshall J 1971 Familial incidence of cerebrovascular disease. Journal of Medical Genetics 8:84

Master A M, Lasser R P 1961 Blood pressure elevation in the elderly. In: Brest A N, Moyer J H (eds) Hypertension. Recent Advances. Lea & Febiger, Philadelphia, p 24

Matsumoto N, Whisnant J P, Kurland L T, Okazaki H 1973 Natural history of stroke in Rochester, Minnesota, 1955 through 1969: an extension of a previous study, 1945 through 1954. Stroke 4:20

McGee D 1973 The probability of developing cardiovascular disease in eight years at specified values of some characteristics. In: Kannel W B, Gordon T (eds) The Framingham study, An epidemiological investigation of cardiovascular diseases. Section 28. US Government Printing Office, Washington DC

Metropolitan Life Insurance Company 1975 Recent trends in mortality from cerebrovascular disease. Statistical Bulletin 56:2 November

Meyer J S, Sawada T, Kitamura A, Toyoda M 1968 Cerebral blood flow after control of hypertension in stroke. Neurology 18:772

Miall W E, Oldham P D 1963 The hereditary factor in arterial blood pressure. British Medical Journal 1:75

Mohr J P 1978 Transient ischemic attacks and the prevention of strokes. Editorial. New England Journal of Medicine 299:93

Mohr J P, Caplan L R, Melski J W, Goldstein R J, Duncan G W, Kistler J P, Pessin M S, Bleich H L 1978 The Harvard Cooperative Stroke Registry; A prospective registry. Neurology 28:754

Moriyama I M, Drueger D E, Stamer F 1971 Cerebrovascular diseases in the United States. Harvard University Press, Cambridge, Massachusetts

Morris J N, Heady J A, Raffle P A B, Roberts C G, Parks J W 1953 Coronary heart disease and physical activity of work. Lancet 2:1053,1111

National Diet-Heart Study Final Report 1968 American Heart Association Monograph 18. Circulation 37 (Suppl 1):1

Omae T, Takeshita M, Hirota Y 1976 The Hisayama Study and Joint Study on cerebrovascular diseases in Japan. In: Scheinberg P (ed) Cerebrovascular Diseases. Raven Press, New York, p 255

O'Malley K, O'Brien E 1980 Drug therapy; management of hypertension in the elderly. New England Journal of

Medicine 302:397

Paffenbarger R S, Wing A L, Hyde R T 1978 Physical activity as an index of heart attack risk in college alumni. American Journal of Epidemiology 103:161

Peacock P B, Riley C P, Lampton T D, Raffel S S, Walker J S 1972 In: Stewart C T (ed) Charles C. Thomas, Springfield, Illinois, p 231

Pearson T C, Thomas D J 1979 Physiological and pharmacological factors influencing blood viscosity and cerebral blood flow. In: Tognomi G, Geratini S (eds) Drug treatment and prevention in cerebrovascular disorders. Elsevier/North-Holland, Amsterdam, p 33

Platt R 1963 Heredity in hypertension. Lancet 1:899

Prineas R J 1971 Cerebrovascular disease occurrence in Australia. Medical Journal of Australia 2:509

Rabkin S W, Mathewson F A L, Tate R B 1978 The relation of blood pressure to stroke prognosis. Annals of Internal Medicine 89:15

Report of the Joint Committee for Stroke Facilities 1972 I. Epidemiology for stroke facilities planning. Stroke 3:359

Robertson T L, Kato H, Rhoads G G et al 1977 Epidemiologic studies of coronary heart disease and stroke in Japanese men living in Japan, Hawaii and California. Incidence of myocardial infarction and death from coronary heart disease. American Journal of Cardiology 39:239

Rogot E, Padgett S J 1976 Association of coronary and stroke mortality with temperatures and snowfall in selected areas of the United States, 1962–1966. American Journal of Epidemiology 103:565

Schoenberg B S, Whisnant J P, Taylor W F, Kempers R D 1970 Strokes in women of childbearing age. A population study. Neurology 20:181

Schroeder H A 1960 Relation between mortality from cardiovascular disease and treated water supplies. Journal of the American Medical Association 172:1902

Schuman S H, Anderson C P, Oliver J T 1964 Epidemiology of successive heat waves in Michigan in 1962 and 1963. Journal of the American Medical Association 189:773

Seligman A W, Alderman M H, Engelland A L, Davis T K 1977 Treatment of systolic hypertension. Clinical Research 25:254a (Abstract)

Shurtleff D 1974 Some characteristics related to the incidence of cardiovascular disease and death: Framingham Study, 18-year follow-up. In: Kannel W B, Gordon T (eds) The Framingham Study, An Epidemiological Investigation of Cardiovascular Disease. Section 30. US Government Printing Office, Washington DC, DHEW Publication No. (NIH) 74–599

Slack J, Evans K A 1966 The increased risk of death from ischaemic heart disease in first degree relatives of 121 men and 96 women with ischaemic heart disease. Journal of Medical Genetics 3:239

Soltero I, Kiu K, Cooper R et al 1978 Trends in mortality from cerebrovascular diseases in the United States, 1960 to 1975. Stroke 9:549

Taguchi J, Freis E D 1974 Partial reduction of blood pressure and prevention of complications in hypertension. New England Journal of Medicine 291:329

Thomas D J, Marshall J, Ross Russel R W, Wetherley-Mein G, DuBoulay G H, Pearson T C, Symon L, Zilkha E 1977 Effect of haematocrit on cerebral blood-flow in man.

Lancet 2:941

Tibblin G. Wilhelmsen L, Werko L 1975 Risk factors for myocardial infarction and death due to ischemic heart disease and other causes. American Journal of Cardiology 35:514

Tohgi H, Yamanouchi H, Mrakami M, Kameyama M 1978 Importance of the hematocrit as a risk factor in cerebral infarction. Stroke 9:369

Toole J F, Janeway R, Choi K, Cordell R, Davis C, Johnston F, Miller H S 1975 Transient ischemic attacks due to atherosclerosis. A prospective study of 160 patients. Archives of Neurology 32:5

Vessey M P, Doll R 1969 Investigation of relation between use of oral contraceptives and thromboembolic disease. A further report. British Medical Journal 2:651

Veterans Administration Cooperative Study Group on Antihypertensive Agents. 1967 Effects of treatment on morbidity in hypertension. I. Results in patients with diastolic blood pressures averaging 115 through 129 mmHg. Journal of the American Medical Association 202:1028

Veterans Administration Cooperative Study Group on Antihypertensive Agents. 1970 Effects of treatment of morbidity in hypertension. II. Results in patients with diastolic blood pressure averaging 90 through 114 mmHg. Journal of the American Medical Association 213:1143

Whisnant J P 1974 Epidemiology of stroke: emphasis on transient cerebral ischemia attacks and hypertension. Stroke 5:68

Winkelstein W, Kantor S, Ibrahim M et al 1966 Familial aggregation of blood pressure. Preliminary report. Journal of the American Medical Association 195:848

Wolf P A, Kannel W B, Dawber T R 1978a Prospective investigations; the Framingham Study and the epidemiology of stroke. In: Schoenberg B S (ed) Advances in neurology, volume 19: Neurological epidemiology: principles and clinical applications. Raven Press, New York, p 107

Wolf P A, Dawber T R, Thomas H E, Kannel W B 1978b Epidemiological assessment of chronic atrial fibrillation and risk of stroke: the Framingham Study. Neurology 28:973

Wolf P A, Dawber T R, Thomas H E, Colton T, Nickerson R, Pool J 1978c The declining incidence of stroke: the Framingham Study. Stroke 9:97 (Abstract)

Wolf P A, Kannel W B, Sorlie P, McNamara P In press Asymptomatic carotid bruit and risk of stroke: the Framingham Study. Journal of the American Medical Association

Wolff F W, Lindeman R D 1966 Effects of treatment in hypertension results of a controlled study. Journal of Chronic Diseases 19:227

Worth R M, Kato H, Rhoads G G et al 1975 Epidemiologic studies of coronary heart disease and stroke in Japanese men living in Japan, Hawaii and California: Mortality. American Journal of Epidemiology 102:481

Wylie C M 1962 Cerebrovascular accident deaths in the United States and in England and Wales. Journal of Chronic Diseases 15:85

Yamori Y, Horie R, Sato M et al 1976 Stroke-prone SHR. A study of pathogenesis and prevention of stroke using animal model. Nippon Rinsho 34:25 (In Japanese)

istory and prognosis of cerebrovascular

...rovascular disease, being a frequent ... of death and disability, is now a major public ...th problem in most parts of the world. An accurate knowledge of the natural history of cerebrovascular disorders is therefore necessary not only for the reliable prediction of the outcome in individual cases, but also for the evaluation of new methods of prevention and treatment and for the planning of comprehensive health services aimed at the control of vascular diseases in the community. Many reports on the subject have been published over the past 15 years; the present chapter, dealing exclusively with acute cerebrovascular disorders, is based on these reports and on the author's personal experience.

The term 'acute cerebrovascular disease', synonymous with 'cerebrovascular accident' or 'stroke', is used here according to the definition adopted by the World Health Organization (WHO), i.e., 'rapidly developed clinical sign of a focal disturbance of cerebral function of presumed vascular origin and of more than 24 hours' duration'. This purely clinical definition includes most cases of intracerebral haemorrhage, subarachnoid haemorrhage, and cerebral infarction (with or without demonstrable arterial occlusion), but not cases of transient cerebral ischaemia or diffuse cerebrovascular disease of insidious onset. The prognosis of subarachnoid haemorrhage, being dealt with in another chapter of the book, will be commented on very briefly here.

IMMEDIATE PROGNOSIS FOR LIFE

In spite of modern advances in the management of cerebrovascular disease a stroke is still an immediate threat to life. Of patients admitted to general hospitals in the acute phase of stroke about 30 to 60 per cent have been reported to die within three or four weeks of the ictus (Boyle & Reid, 1965; Marquardsen, 1969; Acheson & Fairbairn, 1970; Shafer et al, 1973). The widely varying rates reflect the fact that few, if any, hospital series are representative of the general run of cerebrovascular accidents. In the hitherto published community studies of cerebrovascular disease — based on experience both in hospital and in general practice — about one-fourth to one-third of the strokes were fatal (Eisenberg et al, 1964; Acheson et al, 1968; Whisnant et al, 1971; Aho, 1975; Terént, 1980). Fatality rates of similar magnitude were recently observed in an international WHO stroke project, based on the prospective registration of cerebrovascular accidents in selected communities in different parts of the world (Aho et al, 1980).

In individual cases the immediate outlook for life depends on several factors, such as the age of the patient and the type, size, and anatomical site of the cerebrovascular lesion. Very high fatality rates, ranging from 60 to 90 per cent, have been observed in series of patients with a clinical diagnosis of intracerebral haemorrhage (Eisenberg, 1964; Acheson & Fairbairn, 1970; Aho, 1975; Frithz & Werner, 1976). More recently, however, it has been demonstrated that many small, non-fatal haemorrhages, presenting a clinical picture similar to that of cerebral infarction, can be safely diagnosed only by means of CT-scanning. In the pre-scan era such cases were probably misdiagnosed as infarcts. It is therefore not surprising that a more favourable prognosis for life has been found in series of patients with a diagnosis of cerebral haemorrhage based on CT-scanning. In one such series of ganglionic-thalamic haemorrhages no more than 25 per cent of the patients died (Weisberg, 1979a). A further contribution of CT-scanning has been to demonstrate that, contrary to common belief, many patients recover from intraventricular haemorrhages (Wiggins et al, 1978), and some patients actually survive primary brain stem haemorrhages (Müller et al, 1975; Dhopesh et al, 1980). Acute cerebellar haematomas are fatal in most instances, unless surgical evacuation of the clot can be undertaken immediately (McKissock et al, 1960).

Ischaemic lesions carry a better prognosis than do haemorrhagic ones. About one-fifth to one-third of patients with a clinical diagnosis of atheromatous cerebral infarction die from the stroke (Carter, 1964; Matsumoto et al, 1973; Aho, 1975; Oxbury et al, 1975; Frithz & Werner, 1976). Most of the fatal ischaemic lesions are either extensive hemispheric infarcts with brain oedema or large brain stem lesions. By contrast, the immediate prognosis is very favourable in cases of so-called 'lacunar strokes'; this term refers to various vascular syndromes — such as 'pure motor hemiplegia' — caused by small lesions in the basal ganglia or the pons (Fisher, 1967), usually a softening, but occasionally a small haemorrhage, as demonstrated by CT-scanning (Weisberg, 1979 b).

Attempts have been made to relate the immediate mortality of ischaemic strokes to the presence of arterial occlusion as demonstrated by angiography. Strokes due to occlusion of the middle cerebral artery appear to become fatal more often than those associated with occlusion of the internal carotid artery, or those without angiographically demonstrable occlusion (Thygesen et al, 1964; Rompel & Wiedermann, 1970).

A special type of ischaemic stroke is that caused by embolism as a manifestation of certain heart diseases, e.g., rheumatic endocarditis. About one-fourth of such patients have been reported to die from the cerebral episode (Carter, 1965). What characterises these patients as a separate prognostic group is that they are comparatively young people who, because of previously intact cerebral vessels, are more likely to establish a collateral blood supply than are patients with atheromatous cerebral infarction. In the vast majority of cerebral infarcts it is difficult to distinguish between thrombotic and embolic occlusions. According to clinico-pathological evidence, however, most occlusions of intracranial arteries are caused by embolism, the source of which may be mural thrombi from the heart or the large arteries in the neck (Blackwood et al, 1969).

The type of cerebral lesion influences not only the ultimate outcome but also the length of the survival time. More than half of the patients who succumb to cerebral haemorrhage die within two days of the onset of symptoms, and about 80 per cent die within one week. In contrast, less than one-third of deaths due to cerebral infarction occur within a week of the stroke (Brown & Glassenberg, 1973). The difference clearly reflects the fact that in most cases of cerebral haemorrhage the cerebral lesion itself is the immediate cause of death, whereas many patients with cerebral infarction, after having actually survived the cerebral catastrophe *per se*, are left in a precarious condition that makes them easy victims of incidental causes of death, such as pneumonia or heart failure. In a personal series of 340 fatal cases of stroke (haemorrhages as well as infarcts) the causes of death were analysed. In little over half of these cases the cerebral lesion was thought to be the immediate or direct cause of death; nearly all such fatalities occurred within a few days of the stroke. The remaining cases were either severely paralysed patients who eventually succumbed to extracerebral complications or patients who were apparently recovering from the immediate effects of the stroke but died from acute cardiopulmonary disease, e.g., unexpected pulmonary embolism. It is of practical interest to note that the last-mentioned category of potentially preventable deaths accounted for one-fifth of all the fatal cases.

A short comment on the relation between cerebrovascular disease and 'sudden death' seems appropriate. Although large intracranial haemorrhages can be very rapidly fatal, death only rarely occurs earlier than one or two hours after onset. In cases of instantaneous, unexpected death the cause 'cerebral apoplexy' is sometimes given by the certifying physician, but in fact such instances are nearly always caused by sudden cardiopulmonary events.

In every case of fatal cerebral lesion, irrespective of its type and primary site, the direct cause of death is irreversible failure of vital functions of the brain stem. Primary subtentorial haemorrhages or infarcts are therefore often rapidly fatal, as they affect the brain stem directly, producing either disruption, necrosis, or compression. In supratentorial lesions, on the other hand, any brain stem damage is a secondary phenomenon, resulting either from caudal expansion of the pathological process itself, or from transtentorial herniation of the brain. The latter term implies a downward displacement of the brain through the tentorial notch, accompanied by vasoparalysis and oedema proceeding caudally to diencephalic, midbrain, pontine, and finally medullary structures, thereby producing serial functional transections (Plum & Posner, 1972).

In most supratentorial lesions the question of death or survival depends mainly on whether or not a transtentorial herniation will follow; when herniation has actually started, the speed of the process is the main factor deciding the length of survival. The propagation usually takes some time, except in cases of massive intraventricular haemorrhage, where the sudden extravasation of blood probably creates a pressure wave that immediately propagates downwards to the fourth ventricle, causing compression of the surrounding brain stem tissue. This explains why many patients die shortly after rupture of a haemorrhage into the ventricular system. In some instances, on the other hand, the partial evacuation of a haematoma into the ventricles may actually relieve the local pressure on the brain tissue and thus have a favourable effect on the clinical condition. In contrast to haemorrhagic lesions, a hemisphere infarct, however large, becomes fatal only if a secondary oedematous swelling of the brain causes transtentorial herniation. Such swelling, reaching a maximum in three to five days, seems to occur only when an infarct involves the entire territory of the internal carotid artery (Ng & Nimmannitya, 1970).

Clinical signs of prognostic value

A clinician who wants to assess his patient's chances of surviving a recent stroke must focus his attention on such neurological signs that are known to be suggestive of impending brain stem damage. Most important, and easily recognisable, is impairment of consciousness. Figure 2.1 clearly illustrates the prognostic significance of the level of consciousness, as observed in a large series of hospitalised stroke patients. Nearly all the patients who were deeply comatose at the time of admission died, most of them within 24 hours of the stroke. Those who were semicomatose — i.e., inaccessible to questioning but responsive to painful stimuli — also fared badly, whereas the vast majority of the initially alert patients survived the acute phase.

Although the immediate outlook for life can be estimated with fair reliability on the basis of the conscious level alone, more detailed information

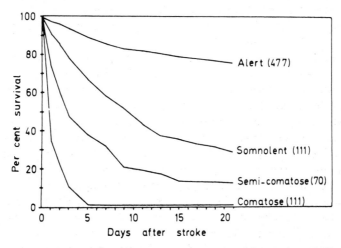

Fig. 2.1 Immediate survival after stroke by level of consciousness on admission (Marquardsen, 1969). (The figures in parentheses indicate the number of patients.)

can be gained by observing certain ocular, respiratory, and motor signs. Thus the caudal propagation of a supratentorial lesion is accompanied by pupillary constriction, which may be replaced by unilateral or bilateral mydriasis, with loss of reaction to light. Patients in whom this sequence of pupillary changes is observed are unlikely to survive for more than a few hours. An enlarged pupil on the side of the cerebral lesion indicates herniation of the homolateral temporal lobe through the tentorial notch, often caused by a rapidly expanding hemispheric haemorrhage. In the personal series referred to above, this sign was observed in 23 patients, 19 of whom died within 24 hours of the stroke.

The pupillary changes may be accompanied by abnormal respiratory patterns such as Cheyne-Stokes respiration, central hyperventilation, ataxic breathing, etc., all of which are of ominous prognostic significance. This has been demonstrated also by means of analyses of respiratory gases and acid-base balance in the blood; out of 11 stroke patients with a Pco_2 of less than 35 mmHg and a pH of more than 7.46 in the arterial blood, only one survived (Rout et al, 1971).

In the motor system, as a result of the downward progression of the lesion, the originally unilateral defect becomes bilateral; decorticate and later decerebrate rigidity may develop, indicating irreversible brain stem damage.

The signs enumerated above are only some of several clinical manifestations that occur in various combinations, each of which reflects a particular stage in the process of transtentorial herniation. For a full account of these clinical syndromes the reader is referred to the monograph of Plum & Posner (1972).

In patients who are fully alert and who are therefore unlikely to die from the cerebral lesion itself, the prognosis for life depends on the presence or absence of complicating extracerebral disease, in particular cardiac, pulmonary and renal disorders. A number of clinical findings, such as tachycardia, fever, anaemia, and ECG changes have thus been found to correlate with a high immediate mortality (Aho, 1975; Terént, 1980).

Finally, some authors have tried to express the chances of survival numerically by combining a number of neurological signs in a prognostic score (Frithz & Werner, 1976; Britton et al, 1980). It appears that a fairly reliable prediction of the outcome can be obtained in this way, but the ultimate role of such scoring systems in clinical practice is still uncertain.

PROGNOSIS FOR FUNCTIONAL RECOVERY

When a patient has survived the acute phase of stroke, the next step in the prognostic evaluation is to assess the chances of recovery of function. Such an assessment meets with certain difficulties, mainly concerned with the definition and measurement of 'recovery'. In theory, the natural history of cerebrovascular accidents could be recorded in terms of the more or less complete restoration of normal anatomical and physiological conditions in the brain. In practice, however, the current state of cerebral dysfunction, being inaccessible to direct observation, can only be measured indirectly, usually by means of the resulting neurological deficit. This type of prognostic evaluation, based on repeated neurological examinations, is very useful in the individual case, but has serious drawbacks as a basis for the statistical analysis of large series of patients. In particular, the method requires for each patient a detailed, quantitative registration of numerous neurological modalities, subsequently to be fitted into a scoring system. Many elaborate systems for stroke patients have in fact been devised but none of them has gained universal acceptance.

The simplest yardstick by which to measure recovery after stroke is the overall functional capacity of the patient, as illustrated by his ability to perform the ordinary activities of daily living. This method of evaluation, which has been used in most reports on the functional prognosis, only requires a rating scale for the grouping of the patients. A simple and practical scale is that of Rankin (1957) using five grades of disability:

Grade I. No disability: able to carry out all usual activities.

Grade II. Slight disability: unable to carry out some previous activities, but able to look after own affairs without assistance.

Grade III. Moderate disability: able to walk unaided, but needing some help with dressing.

Grade IV. Moderately severe disability: requiring help with both walking and self-care.

Grade V. Severe disability: bedfast or chairfast, usually incontinent; requiring constant nursing care and attention.

In the author's series of 404 immediate survivors from stroke the final functional levels achieved by the patients are shown in Table 2.1. About 15 per

Table 2.1 Maximum functional capacity achieved by 404 immediate survivors[a] by age and sex

Age (years)	*Males* Disability grade I	II	III	IV	V	Died within 2 months	Total
–59	10	25	7	4	2	—	48
60–69	12	22	8	5	2	2	51
70–79	5	12	13	9	3	—	42
80–	1	1	2	—	2	1	7
Total	28	60	30	18	9	3	148
%	18.9	40.5	20.3	12.2	6.1	2.0	100.0

Age (years)	*Females* Disability grade I	II	III	IV	V	Died within 2 months	Total
–59	9	24	3	10	4	—	50
60–69	13	34	10	8	9	3	77
70–79	10	28	17	19	16	10	100
80–	1	3	3	7	9	6	29
Total	33	89	33	44	38	19	256
%	12.9	34.8	12.9	17.2	14.8	7.4	100.0

[a] In three cases the disability grade was unascertainable.

cent of the patients made apparently complete recoveries (Grade I); 37 per cent remained slightly disabled (Grade II); 16 per cent were moderately disabled (Grade III) whereas the remaining 32 per cent either became more severely disabled or died within a couple of months. These results are in accordance with those of other follow-up examinations of hospitalised stroke patients (Rankin, 1957; Adams & Merret, 1961; Katz et al, 1966; Shafer et al, 1973; Britton et al, 1980). Briefly summarised, these studies show that 50 to 75 per cent of stroke survivors become able to walk unaided; 20 to 30 per cent become permanently and severely handicapped. In community-based studies complete recovery from stroke has been found to be more frequent than in hospital series,

presumably because of a larger representation of mild cases (Aho, 1975; Gresham et al, 1975).

An important question is to what extent the functional recovery from stroke can be influenced by therapeutic procedures. It is not surprising that excellent results have been obtained in rehabilitation centres, since most of the patients admitted are relatively young persons who have been specially selected as suitable candidates for rehabilitation. Indeed, the study of Feldman et al (1962), has shown that the majority of hemiparetic stroke victims can be adequately rehabilitated in ordinary medical or neurological wards without formal rehabilitation services, if proper attention is given to ambulation and self-care. Quite recently, Garraway et al (1980a) reported the preliminary results of a randomised, controlled trial, comparing the management of elderly stroke patients in a special stroke unit and in medical units. The proportion of patients who obtained independence was found to be significantly higher in the former group than in the latter, but one year after discharge the difference was found to have disappeared (Garraway, 1980b).

Factors influencing the functional recovery

Type of stroke. Since haemorrhagic strokes are less frequent but much more lethal than ischaemic ones, all representative series of survivors from stroke consist mainly of cases of cerebral infarction. Little is actually known about the functional prognosis after intracerebral haemorrhage, but there is no reason to believe that recovery should be less complete after cerebral haemorrhage than after cerebral infarction. In the category of primary subarachnoid haemorrhage the prospect for physical recovery is generally excellent, obviously because most of the survivors are younger people with mild, if any, motor deficits. Patients with cerebral infarction caused by occlusion of major intracranial arteries have been reported to fare worse than those without angiographically demonstrable occlusion (Thygesen et al, 1964). It has often been demonstrated, however, that even complete occlusion of the middle cerebral artery does not preclude excellent recovery (Kaste & Waltimo, 1976), obviously because the extent of cerebral damage after arterial occlusion depends on the availability of collateral blood supply more than on the type or the site of the occlusion.

Extent and site of the lesion. The single most important factor governing the recovery from stroke is the extent of permanent cerebral damage. The larger a lesion is, the higher is the risk not only of interruption of motor pathways but, still more important, of widespread cortical or subcortical damage with loss of a variety of higher cerebral functions, all of which are involved in the process of recovery.

In addition to the size, the *site* of the lesion is prognostically relevant. Patients with ischaemic lesions in the brain stem, if they survive at all, are more likely to overcome a severe hemiparesis than are those with supratentorial lesions, the reason being that the cortical functions are intact in the former category but often damaged in the latter. A typical example of small, strategically placed lesions are the 'lacunar strokes' which, whether situated in the pons or in the basal ganglia, usually carry a favourable prognosis for recovery (Fisher, 1967).

The question of the prognostic significance of the *laterality* of supratentorial lesions has been a subject of some controversy. It was originally assumed that lesions of the dominant hemisphere, because of the accompanying disorders of language, might be more disabling than those affecting the other half of the brain. However, more recent reports suggest that the defects in visuomotor, temporal and spatial concepts that often accompany lesions of the non-dominant hemisphere are more ominous prognostic signs than loss of speech. Thus, 21 per cent of the author's female patients with left-sided paresis became severely disabled, as compared with only 9 per cent of those with right-sided deficit.

Clinical predictors of functional outcome

Already at the initial neurological examination of the stroke patient the chances of recovery can be roughly estimated on the basis of the neurological deficit, which reflects the size of the cerebral lesion. At this very early stage, however, it is difficult to distinguish between permanent damage caused by neuronal loss and temporary dysfunction caused by reversible cerebral oedema. The clinical prognostication is therefore more reliable when based on a neurological examination performed one or two weeks after the stroke, or even later. Referring particularly to old and more handicapped survivors, Adams (1974) stated that confident predictions about their prospects can seldom be given in less than 12 or 16 weeks, nor can the ultimate grade of recovery be assessed in under 24 to 30 weeks.

In the following paragraphs a short account is given of some clinical signs which, separately or in combination, have significant prognostic implications.

Motor deficit. It is almost self-evident that the risk of becoming permanently disabled by a hemiplegia is directly proportional to the grade of paresis. However, there is some indication that the time elapsed before recovery begins is still more significant as a prognostic indicator than the initial severity of the motor deficit. This was first mentioned by Gowers (1888), who stated that patients in whom improvement begins within three days of onset will almost certainly become able to walk unaided, whereas a paralysis that is still complete after three months is likely to remain severe. Later reports suggest that even one month without improvement indicates an unfavourable prognosis. In the present author's series, for example, the ability to walk alone was regained by only 15 per cent of the patients who had not improved at the end of four weeks. In the upper limb, progress is likely to be poor if there is no voluntary movement within three weeks.

A special type of motor deficit is paralysis of conjugate ocular movements. This sign, being observed mostly in the initial phase of the stroke, often in combination with severe hemiplegia and impairment of consciousness, indicates that the patient's chances of regaining independence are less than 50 per cent.

Sensory deficit. The importance of sensory regulation of movement patterns has often been stressed, and it is generally assumed that recovery from hemiplegia is severely impeded by loss of sensation in the paralysed limbs. Although this is probably true, a significant correlation between sensory loss and persistent motor handicap has not yet been satisfactorily established in stroke patients. In the author's series, independence in self-care was regained by 46 per cent of the patients with initial sensory deficit, and by 54 per cent of those with normal sensation; the difference is not significant. Similarly, in the series of severely disabled stroke patients reported by Isaacs & Marks (1973), the presence of hemianaesthesia or proprioceptive loss did not apparently influence the ultimate outcome. On the other hand, Moskowitz et al (1972) found that stroke patients with hemisensory loss, despite significant motor recovery in many cases, did not attain the same ambulatory levels as those without such sensory disorders. It seems, therefore, that definite conclusions regarding the prognostic value of sensory deficit must await the results of further studies.

Visual disturbances. When these are present in surviving stroke patients, they obviously add to the difficulties of rehabilitation. It is particularly noteworthy that the presence of homonymous hemianopia, in spite of preserved central vision, is associated with poor recovery from hemiplegia (Haerer, 1973). The explanation may be that the hemianopia simply implies a larger lesion and therefore a poorer rehabilitative potential, or that the visual field defect is often accompanied by other more subtle perceptual defects, which are more serious handicaps than the hemianopia itself.

Disorders of higher nervous function. It is a common experience that some stroke patients fail to regain independence, although motor function improves and adverse prognostic factors are apparently absent. Many of these therapeutic failures — traditionally often ascribed to dementia or 'lack of motivation' — are the results of disorders of highly specialised mental functions, caused by focal lesions of cortical or subcortical structures. Adams & Hurwitz (1963) were able to demonstrate such 'mental barriers to the recovery from stroke' in one-half of a series of chronic hemiplegic invalids; among the disorders were: defect in comprehension, neglect of the hemiparetic limbs, denial of disease, disturbance of body-image, apraxia, motor perseveration, memory loss of recent events.

Of the above disorders, those characterised by unrealistic attitudes towards illness have attracted particular attention. In severe cases such defects cause striking and bizarre clinical pictures, dominated by the patient's complete denial of ownership of the paralysed limbs or by his unawareness of the motor deficit. Such patients, whose vascular lesions affect the parietal lobe of the non-dominant hemisphere, are usually inaccessible to rehabilitative treatment. In contrast to these dramatic manifestations the milder forms of parietal lobe dysfunction, causing only partial neglect of the hemiplegia, may easily escape notice; suspicion should arise whenever an acute neurological deficit fails to evoke an adequate emotional response in the patient. Other signs of parietal lobe dysfunction of prognostic importance are the defects in the patient's concept of space, speed and time; again, such signs may remain unnoticed, if not particularly looked for at the neurological examination.

Dysphasia. This is present in about one-third of immediate survivors from stroke, and is another disorder that may impede recovery. This is true particularly when the dysphasia is of the receptive type, thus preventing the patient from understanding instruction; in addition, the loss of communication often results in severe frustration, which further adds to the patient's difficulties. Nevertheless, the presence of dysphasia does not preclude a satisfactory functional recovery, as observed in the author's series of survivors with right hemiplegia: independence in walking was attained by 61 per cent of those who were dysphasic, as compared with 71 per cent of those without this defect. Generally speaking, the perceptual defects caused by lesions of the non-dominant hemisphere are more ominous as prognostic indicators than are disorders of language.

Dementia. This indicates diffuse cerebral damage and is undoubtedly the most severe 'mental barrier' to recovery. Stroke patients with marked mental deterioration, particularly those presenting urinary incontinence and/or episodes of confusion, will almost certainly remain disabled and helpless.

Combinations of prognostic factors. It follows from the preceding paragraphs that, even in the acute phase of stroke, the chances of functional recovery can be assessed by paying due attention to the following adverse prognostic factors: old age, severe motor deficit, impairment of consciousness, disorders of higher nervous function, and conjugate ocular deviation. These signs, which are indicators of the extent of cerebral dysfunction, may occur in many combinations, each of which has a more or less distinct prognostic significance. As an example, for a patient under the age of 70 who has a complete or severe hemiplegia but without other signs of extensive lesion, the chances are two to one that he will regain independence in both walking and self-care. On the other hand, if more signs of extensive lesion are present, and particularly if any type of subsequent complication occurs, the patient is likely to remain incapacitated.

Social readaptation after stroke

An important part of the prognostic evaluation is the estimation of the patient's chances of ultimately returning home and of resuming his usual activities. Because of the high average age of patients with cerebrovascular disease, *vocational* rehabilitation after stroke is the exception rather than the rule. Of the patients who were in employment at the time of the stroke no more than one-third can be expected to go back to work (Marquardsen, 1969; Fugl-Meyer et al, 1975). In most cases, therefore, the realistic goal of rehabilitation is not re-employment but self-care and return home. According to reports from European and American hospitals, 60 to 80 per cent of survivors from stroke can finally be discharged home, whereas the remaining patients have to be transferred to nursing institutions.

In the individual case the chances of returning home, although primarily depending on the degree of functional recovery, are strongly influenced by such factors as the sex of the patient, the domestic structure and the socio-economic status. This is illustrated by Table 2.2, which shows the discharge placement of the survivors in the author's series. Female patients living with a spouse were much more likely to return home than were those who were living with other relatives or alone. For males,

on the other hand, the chances of being discharged home were apparently independent of the domestic structure.

When seen in the global perspective, the most decisive factor influencing social readaptation after stroke is the general structure of the community of which the patients are members. Of particular importance are the patterns of family life and the prevailing attitudes towards handicapped people. It should thus be emphasised that the discharge rates given above are probably representative of the conditions in the highly industrialised and urbanised countries in Western Europe and in the U.S.A., but not of those in many other parts of the world. In the Far East, where large families live together as closely knit units, virtually all surviving stroke patients, no matter how disabled, are discharged home and subsequently cared for by their children or other relatives (Aho et al, 1980). It is a sobering thought that in such countries, now referred to as 'developing', social re-integration of handicapped patients may become more difficult with increasing industrialisation and prosperity.

LATE SURVIVAL

Over the past 20 years numerous follow-up studies of stroke victims have been reported (Marshall & Shaw, 1959; Adams & Merrett, 1961; Carter, 1964; Droller, 1965; Marquardsen, 1969; Robinson et al, 1969; Matsumoto et al, 1973; Hutchinson & Acheson, 1975; Abu-Zeid et al, 1978). These studies have shown that the late mortality of survivors from stroke is much higher than that observed in the general population. In Figure 2.2 the survival data have been plotted on a semilogarithmic scale, which means that for any annual interval after the stroke the slope of the graph is a direct measure of the probability of dying within the interval. The excess mortality of the stroke patients is immediately apparent: for male patients, for example, the observed three-year survival rate is only 54 per cent, as compared with an expected rate of 88 per cent; after 5 years the actual number of survivors is one-half of that expected, after 10 years a mere one-fourth. The median survival time, i.e., the length of time required for 50 per cent of the patients to have died, is less than 4 years

Table 2.2 Discharge rates by domestic structure

Household composition	No. of patients	Mean age (years)	Discharged home Number	%
Males				
Living with spouse	102	62.4	89	87.3
Living with relatives	14	70.7	12	85.7
Living alone	24	67.9	19	79.2
Females				
Living with spouse	85	63.6	74	87.0
Living with relatives	62	69.9	35	56.5
Living alone	93	70.8	64	68.8

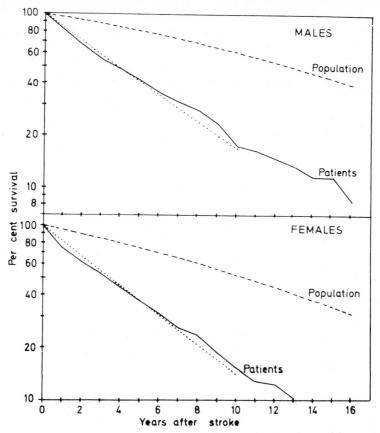

Fig. 2.2 Long-term survival after stroke, 150 males and 257 females (Marquardsen, 1969). (The dotted lines represent the average annual probabilities of dying.)

for patients of either sex, whereas in the general population it exceeds 10 years. It is further noted that the accelerated rate of death is found not only in the first year after the stroke, but throughout the period of observation. In fact, the annual death rate of the patients — represented by the slope of the survival curve — remains almost constant, irrespective of the time that has elapsed since the stroke. It is therefore convenient, for purposes of comparison, to describe the long-term mortality in any particular group of stroke patients by simply giving the average annual death rate observed over a specified period of time. Thus in the series on which Figure 2.2 is based the number of survivors decreased at an average annual rate of 16 per cent in males, 18 per cent in females.

In most of the previous reports the survival data were plotted on an ordinary arithmetic scale. The tailing off of such survival curves has led some writers to believe that a 'cessation of activity' of cerebrovascular disease might occur after a period of 5 or more years. In actual fact, however, all reports based on large series of stroke patients followed for more than 10 years have shown that the annual probability of dying remains strikingly constant over the years. It is therefore fair to conclude that the excess mortality of patients who have recovered from stroke is not due to the effect of the cerebral lesion, but reflects the steady progression of an underlying vascular disease. This is borne out by an analysis of the causes of death: in the follow-up studies referred to above the most frequent causes of death were recurrent stroke (accounting for 20 to 50 per cent of the deaths), myocardial infarction and congestive heart failure. At least three-quarters of all the deaths were caused by such vascular diseases.

The validity of the general mortality trends

described here is uninfluenced by the fact that there is a minority of patients whose cerebral lesion is caused by a non-progressive, or even transient, pathological process and whose life-expectancy may thus be equal to that of the normal population.

Factors influencing the long-term mortality

As expected, the age of the patient is an important prognostic factor. Thus for each successive year after the stroke the annual death rate is twice as high for patients aged 70 to 79 years as for those 20 years younger. The *excess* mortality, on the other hand, is highest in the younger groups. Thus, stroke patients aged 50 to 60 years die at an annual rate equal to that which, according to official life-tables, is expected for persons 25 years older, whereas the survival of patients aged 70 to 79 years is similar to that of persons only 15 years older. The explanation of this trend must be that in the general population, with which the stroke patients are compared, the incidence of vascular disease rises steeply with advancing age. With respect to vascular mortality, therefore, old patients with cerebrovascular disease differ less from their 'normal' contemporaries than do young ones.

Cardiovascular disease. Evidence of pre-existing *heart disease* — whether obtained by history taking, by observation of relevant clinical signs, or by electrocardiography — is an adverse factor in the long-term prognosis after stroke. A comparison of the survival curves for patients with and without abnormal ECGs thus shows that the presence of any type of ECG abnormality reduces the patient's chances of surviving for 3 years by nearly 50 per cent; after that time, however, the survival curves become nearly parallel. The reason for this may be that most of the patients with severe heart disease die within a few years of the stroke, leaving a group of survivors with a more benign type of cardiac disorder. The prognostic implications of all types of heart disease, but particularly of coronary artery disease, is more marked in males than in females.

Arterial hypertension. The role of hypertension in the prognosis after cerebrovascular accidents has been the subject of many discussions and the cause of some controversy. As is well known from the vast literature on hypertension, no definite answer

can be given to such basic questions as where to draw the dividing line between normal and elevated blood pressure; whether to base the assessment on the systolic or the diastolic pressure; and whether to prefer resting or 'casual' pressures. For patients with cerebrovascular accidents the issue is further confused by the fact that a stroke may produce considerable changes in the blood pressure level; in the period of convalescence after stroke it is therefore particularly difficult to classify patients as either hypertensives or normotensives. Nevertheless, most workers who have published follow-up studies of patients with stroke, although using different definitions of hypertension, seem to agree that patients with blood pressures exceeding a given level fare much worse than those with lower pressures, the trend being observed particularly in males (Marshall & Kaeser, 1961; Carter, 1964; Marquardsen, 1969; Hutchinson & Acheson, 1975). Other studies, some of which were based on geriatric patients, failed to demonstrate such an adverse prognostic effect of hypertension (Adams, 1965; Droller, 1965; Robinson et al, 1969; Abu-Zeid et al, 1978). The discrepancies are probably explained by differences in the definition of hypertension and in the age and sex structure of the various series. It appears from Figure 2.3 that at ages under 70 years patients with blood pressures over 180/100 mmHg survive for a shorter time than those with lower pressures; at ages over 70 the difference between the two categories, although less marked, is still present in males, but almost absent in females. The remarkable immunity of old women to the effects of hypertension has been observed in numerous studies of the prognosis in essential hypertension.

The height of the blood pressure influences not only the actual length of survival but also the eventual cause of death. In particular, a close relationship exists between the presence of hypertension at the time of the original stroke and the risk of dying from recurrent cerebrovascular accident. In the author's series the proportion of late deaths due to recurrent stroke rose from 18 per cent in patients with diastolic blood pressures below 100 mmHg to 41 per cent in those whose pressures were 120 mmHg or over. Moreover, in the group with low pressures the recurrent accidents were more often infarcts than haemorrhages,

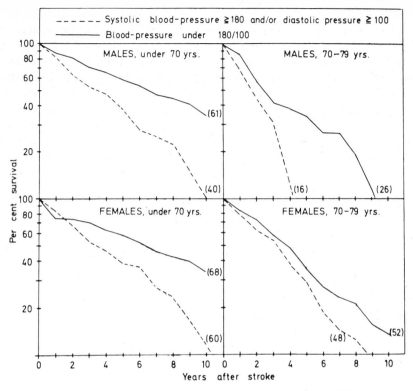

Fig. 2.3 Survival by height of blood pressure (Marquardsen, 1969).

whereas in the hypertensive group the reverse was the case. It should be noted that certain causes of death were found to be inversely related to the blood pressure level; for example, fatal pulmonary embolism occurred almost exclusively in patients whose diastolic pressures were under 100 mmHg.

Valuable prognostic information is gained by taking both blood pressure and ECG findings into consideration. Figure 2.4 shows that the ECG findings were particularly important in the estimation of the patients' chances of surviving for one or two years, whereas the long-term outlook seemed to depend more on the blood pressure level. Patients in whom both blood pressure and ECG were normal had a remarkably favourable prognosis, the three-year survival rate being almost equal to that of the general population. In contrast, patients with abnormal ECGs and high blood pressures fared badly: about 60 per cent of these patients died within three years of the stroke.

Characteristics of the cerebral lesion. Once the acute phase of the stroke is over, the pathological type of the cerebral lesion is no longer a prognostic

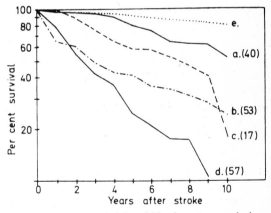

Fig. 2.4 Survival by height of blood pressure and electrocardiographic findings (Marquardsen, 1969). (Patients under 70 years; both sexes.) a. BP < 180/100; ECG normal (mean age 59.2 years). b. BP < 180/100; ECG abnormal (mean 59.3 years). c. BP ≥ 180/100; ECG normal (mean age 57.7 years). d. BP ≥ 180/100; ECG abnormal (mean age 60.5 years). e. Sample of general Danish population, age 59 years.

factor of major importance. Survivors from intracerebral haemorrhage thus appear to survive longer than those with cerebral infarction, probably because of a lower prevalence of generalised cardiovascular disease (Eisenberg, 1964; Matsumoto et al, 1973; Abu-Zeid et al, 1978). Certain categories of patients present specific problems. In survivors from subarachnoid haemorrhage, for example, the prognosis depends mainly on whether or not recurrent bleeding from an aneurysm will occur; when no aneurysm can be demonstrated by angiography, the prognosis is good (Pakarinen, 1967). In cases of cerebral infarction the angiographical findings seem to have some bearing on the prognosis. Patients with normal angiograms survive longer than those who present arteriosclerotic stenosis or occlusion (Shenkin et al, 1965; Acheson et al, 1969). This seems to be in keeping with the view that the extent of arterial disease is the dominating prognostic factor.

The natural history of occlusion of the internal carotid artery or other extracranial arteries has attracted particular attention because of the possibility that vascular surgery might improve the long-term prognosis in cases of this type. A difficulty arises from the fact that most published series of patients with carotid occlusion comprise highly selected groups of relatively young patients admitted to neurological or neurosurgical departments. Such series are of course not directly comparable with the ordinary types of patients with strokes. Nevertheless, it should be noted that in a joint study of extracranial arterial occlusion (Bauer et al, 1969) the three-year survival rate observed in the 'non-surgical group' was exactly the same as that experienced by the patients of similar age in the author's series of unspecified stroke cases. It seems therefore, that the late mortality of patients with extracranial arterial occlusion conforms to the general pattern seen in cerebral infarction.

The strong influence of selective factors is illustrated by the survival observed in two series of patients with an angiographical diagnosis of middle cerebral artery occlusion. The five-year survival rate was 78 per cent in a group of youngish patients referred to a university department of neurology (Kaste & Waltimo, 1976), but only 42 per cent in a series of patients admitted to a general hospital in the acute phase of stroke (personal observation).

The *extent* of the cerebral lesion is a reliable indicator not only of the immediate prognosis for life, as already mentioned, but also of the late survival. A convenient, although indirect, measure of the extent of permanent cerebral damage is the resulting physical disability of the patient. Figure 2.5 illustrates the relevance of this factor. Patients who regained the ability to walk unaided fared much better than those who could walk only with assistance. Patients who became permanently bedfast or chairbound experienced a strikingly high mortality, the median survival time being less than one year.

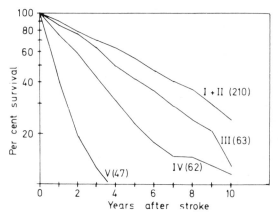

Fig. 2.5 Survival by ultimate disability grade (Marquardsen, 1969). (Patients under 80; both sexes.) I & II. Independent in self-care (mean age 63.4 years). III. Requires some help, but walks without assistance (mean age 68.5 years). IV. Dependent on others; can walk only with assistance (mean age 67.8 years). V. Bedfast or chairfast (mean age 76.5 years).

Combinations of prognostic factors. An analysis of the author's series gave the result that for patients who have recovered from the immediate effects of a stroke the probability of surviving for 5 years can be estimated with fair reliability on the basis of only three factors; age at onset, a history of cardiac symptoms and blood pressure level. Thus, irrespective of the severity of the stroke, the following proportions of patients under 70 years of age were alive after 5 years: three-fourths of those who had neither cardiac symptoms nor blood pressure over 180/100 mmHg; half of those in whom only one of these factors was present; one-fourth of those with both cardiac symptoms and hypertension. Such prognostic criteria are useful in the ordinary type of arteriosclerotic or hypertensive stroke but are not applicable to specific categories of stroke such as cerebral embolism from rheumatic endocarditis or subarachnoid haemorrhage from intracranial aneurysm or angioma.

RECURRENCE RATE

Many clinicians concerned with the management of cerebrovascular disease have been puzzled by the observation that some survivors from stroke suffer very early recurrences, whereas others remain free from further attacks for many years. It is of obvious clinical importance to obtain statistical information about the risk of recurrences in different types of stroke and to study the factors that influence the recurrence rate. In series of patients with cerebral infarction, or with unspecified stroke, recurrent episodes have been reported in 15 to 38 per cent of the individuals, about half of the recurrences being fatal (Marshall & Kaeser, 1961; Baker et al, 1962; Carter, 1964; Droller, 1965; Marquardsen, 1969). The differences in these overall rates clearly reflect the widely varying lengths of observation. The influence of this factor can be eliminated by calculating, for each series, the number of recurrences observed in 100 patient-years. When this is done, the results of different studies are remarkably similar, with recurrence rates ranging from 8 to 11 per 100 patient-years. In one prospective study (Hutchinson & Acheson, 1975) no fewer than 91 per cent of the patients experienced at least one further episode within 5 years; many of them had several recurrences. One of the reasons for this extraordinarily high recurrence rate seems to be that the authors accepted any episode of more than one hour as representing a stroke.

It seems to be a widespread belief that recurrent attacks are particularly frequent in the first year after the original stroke and that the risk decreases in later years. However, in the author's series the annual rate of recurrence remained at the initial level for at least 10 years after the stroke, the average annual rate being 8.9 per cent for males, 10.6 for females. An annual recurrence rate of this magnitude means that, in the absence of deaths from causes other than cerebrovascular accident, 75 per cent of the patients can be expected to have a recurrent episode within 15 years of the original stroke. It is suggested, therefore, that any stroke patient who survives long enough is likely to have a further cerebral accident. It is evident, however, that with a relatively low annual risk of recurrence and a high mortality from other causes, the majority of the patients will die from intercurrent disease before having had another attack. This explains why the overall recurrence rate observed in follow-up studies rarely exceeds 30 per cent, and why few patients actually suffer more than two recurrences.

There is some evidence that recurrent attacks are more often fatal than are initial strokes, but the difference may be a statistical artefact, since non-fatal recurrences are more likely to escape notice than fatal ones. An analysis of the author's series showed that recurrent lesions of the previously affected hemisphere carried a lower fatality rate than contralateral lesions. The difference results from the fact that cerebral haemorrhages, which constituted about half of the recurrent lesions, tended to occur in the hitherto unaffected side of the brain. A possible explanation of this trend is that occlusions or arteriosclerotic stenoses in the proximal part of the carotid arterial system may to some extent protect the ipsilateral hemisphere against the effects of systemic hypertension. Such an explanation is supported by the observation, made by several vascular surgeons, that cerebral haemorrhage sometimes occurs as a post-operative complication of carotid endarterectomy. The fact that localised intracerebral haematomas, sometimes mimicking cerebral infarcts, may be responsible for recurrent episodes after stroke has been stressed by Hutchinson & Acheson (1975).

Factors influencing the recurrence rate

Type of initial cerebral lesion. Particularly high recurrence rates have been observed in patients with cerebral embolism from rheumatic heart disease. According to Carter (1964), such patients have at least a 50 per cent chance of recurrence, especially if atrial fibrillation is present. Recurrent emboli are more often in the same hemisphere as the original episode than in the contralateral one. The same author felt that emboli tend to come in showers, the rate being highest in the first few months after the first attacks; this was ascribed to some change of consistency in an atrial or auricular mural thrombus or to some alteration in cardiac rhythm.

Arteriosclerotic occlusion or stenosis of the internal carotid artery as demonstrated by angiography seems to be associated with a higher recurrence rate than occlusion of the middle cerebral artery. The cause of this difference may be that the former type of lesion remains a potential source of emboli that may enter the intracranial circulation, whereas an occlusion of the middle cerebral artery effectively blocks the path of any future emboli to that territory.

Survivors from cerebral haemorrhage are too few to justify any statements concerning the risk of recurrence in this type of stroke. It is interesting, however, that in most of the above-mentioned cases of secondary haemorrhagic strokes the original accident had been diagnosed as cerebral infarction. This gives some support to the view that recurrent cerebrovascular accidents, whether infarcts or haemorrhages, may have a common aetiology, the underlying diseases being arteriosclerosis and hypertension.

Clinical factors. The risk of sustaining further strokes is inversely related to the severity of the neurological deficit caused by the primary lesion. Recurrences are thus rarely seen in patients who are completely and permanently disabled after their first stroke. This is hardly surprising, since in this category of patients a new vascular episode, at least when affecting the same hemisphere, can add little to the damage already done, and may therefore be clinically 'silent'.

In the author's series a history of heart failure or the presence of ECG abnormalities at the time of the first stroke were associated with an annual recurrence rate of about 15 per cent, which is twice the rate found in survivors without indication of heart disease. Patients with atrial fibrillation had only slightly higher recurrence rates than those with other types of ECG abnormality. An analysis of the fatal recurrences verified by necropsy showed that recurrent strokes suffered by patients with antecedent heart failure were most likely to be cerebral infarctions; cerebral haemorrhages occurred almost exclusively in patients without clinical signs of heart disease.

As expected, the risk of recurrences increases with the height of the blood pressure, particularly

in males (Hutchinson & Acheson, 1975). In the author's personal series the patients whose diastolic pressures at the time of the initial stroke were over 120 mmHg presented recurrence rates exceeding 20 per cent per year; all the fatal recurrences in this group were haemorrhages.

Combination of factors. Particularly high recurrence rates are observed in patients who present a combination of two or more of the above prognostic factors. For example, in patients with both hypertension and atrial fibrillation the risk of having a further stroke within one year is about 50 per cent. It should be realised, however, that such associations, although statistically significant, are of limited value in the assessment of the prognosis in individual cases. No investigator has hitherto succeeded in making a sharp distinction between patients who are likely to have recurrences and those who are not.

CONCLUSIONS

Even with modern standards of medical care, cerebrovascular accidents often result in death or permanent disability, and even those patients who have apparently recovered from the stroke experience a high excess mortality and excess morbidity, which remain remarkably constant over the subsequent years. The obvious explanation is that a stroke, apart from being in itself a serious brain disorder, is a more or less incidental manifestation of a steadily progressing generalised vascular disease, most often of the arteriosclerotic or hypertensive type. This statement refers particularly to the natural history of cerebral infarction, but may be true also of cerebral haemorrhage, with the exception of bleeding aneurysms or other strictly local defects.

It has been demonstrated in this survey that in most cases of stroke a reliable assessment of the prognosis can be made on the basis of two categories of clinical signs, reflecting the extent and site of the cerebral lesion and the severity of generalised cardiovascular disease, respectively. Reservation must be made for the minority of patients whose strokes are complications of diseases other than arteriosclerosis or hypertension, e.g., rheumatic heart disease, blood dyscrasias, various types of arteritis, etc.

In view of the serious consequences of cerebrovascular accidents, both for the individual and for the community, it is important to decide whether it is possible, by eliminating some of the adverse prognostic factors, to improve the outlook. On theoretical grounds, stroke patients should be expected to benefit from several types of treatment, an obvious example being antihypertensive therapy. It is a regrettable fact, however, that little is known about the actual prognostic consequences of admission to hospital, of many drugs, of surgical operations and of special rehabilitation techniques, etc. Controlled trials are badly needed in order to fill the gaps in our knowledge and thus contribute to a better control of cerebrovascular disease in the community.

REFERENCES

Abu-Zeid H A H, Choi N W, Hsu P H, Maini K K 1978 Prognostic factors in the survival of 1484 stroke cases observed for 30 to 48 months. Archives of Neurology 35:121, 213

Acheson J, Acheson H W K, Tellwright J M 1968 The incidence and pattern of cerebrovascular disease in general practice. Journal of the Royal College of General Practitioners 16:428

Acheson J, Boyd W N, Hugh A E, Hutchinson E C 1969 Cerebral angiography in ischaemic cerebrovascular disease. Archives of Neurology 20:527

Acheson R M, Fairbairn A S 1970 Burden of cerebrovascular disease in the Oxford Area in 1963 and 1964. British Medical Journal i:621

Adams G F 1965 Prospects for patients with strokes. British Medical Journal ii:253

Adams G F 1974 Cerebrovascular Disability and the Ageing Brain. Churchill Livingstone, London

Adams G F, Hurwitz L J 1963 Mental barriers to recovery from strokes. Lancet ii:533

Adams G F, Merrett J D 1961 Prognosis and survival after strokes. British Medical Journal i:309

Aho K 1975 Incidence, profile and early prognosis of stroke. Academic Dissertation, Helsinki

Aho K, Harmsen P, Hatano S, Marquardsen J, Smirnov V E, Strasser T 1980 Cerebrovascular disease in the community: results of a WHO collaborative study. Bulletin of the World Health Organization 58:113

Baker R N, Broward J A, Fang H C, Fisher C M, Groch S N, Heyman A, Karp H R, McDevitt E, Scheinberg P, Schwartz W, Toole J F 1962 Anticoagulant therapy in cerebral infarction. Neurology 12:823

Bauer R B, Meyer J S, Fields W S, Remington R, Macdonald M C, Callen P 1969 Joint study of extracranial arterial occlusion. Journal of the American Medical Association 208:509

Blackwood W, Hallpike J F, Kocen R S, Mair W G P 1969 Atheromatous disease of the carotid arterial system and embolism from the heart in cerebral infarction: a morbid anatomical study. Brain 92:897

Boyle R W, Reid M 1965 What happens to the stroke victim? Geriatrics 20:949

Britton M, de Faire U, Helmers C, Miah K 1980 Prognostication in acute cerebrovascular disease. Acta Medica Scandinavica 207:37

Brown M, Glassenberg M 1973 Mortality factors in patients with acute stroke. Journal of the American Medical Association 224:1493

Carter A B 1964 Cerebral infarction. Pergamon Press, London

Carter A B 1965 Prognosis of cerebral embolism. Lancet ii:514

Dhopesh U P, Greenberg J O, Cohen M M 1980 Computed tomography in brainstem haemorrhage. Journal of Computer Assisted Tomography 4:603

Droller H 1965 The outlook in hemiplegia. Geriatrics 20:630

Eisenberg H, Morrison J T, Sullivan P, Foote F M 1964 Cerebrovascular accidents. Journal of the American Medical Association 189:883

Feldman D J, Lee P R, Untereker J, Lloyd K, Rusk H A, Toole A 1962 A comparison of functionally oriented medical care and formal rehabilitation in the management of patients with hemiplegia due to cerebrovascular disease. Journal of Chronic Diseases 15:297

Fisher C M 1967 A lacunar stroke. Neurology 17:614

Frithz G, Werner I 1976 Studies on cerebrovascular strokes. Clinical findings and short-term prognosis. Acta Medica Scandinavica 199:133

Fugl-Meyer A, Jaasko L, Norlin V 1975 The post-stroke hemiplegic patient. Scandinavian Journal of Rehabilitation Medicine 7:73

Garraway W M, Akhtar A J, Prescott R J, Hockey L 1980a Management of acute stroke in the elderly: preliminary results of a controlled trial. British Medical Journal i:1040

Garraway W M, Akhtar A J, Hockey L, Prescott R J 1980b Management of acute stroke in the elderly: follow-up of a controlled trial. British Medical Journal ii:827

Gowers W R 1888 A manual of diseases of the nervous system. Churchill, London

Gresham G E, Fitzpatrick T E, Wolf P A, McNamara P M, Kannel W B, Dawber T R 1975 Residual disability in survivors of stroke. The Framingham Study. New England Journal of Medicine 293:954

Haerer A F 1973 Visual field defects and the prognosis of stroke patients. Stroke 4:163

Hutchinson E C, Acheson A J 1975 Strokes. Natural history, pathology and surgical treatment. W B Saunders, London

Isaacs B, Marks R 1973 Determinants of outcome of stroke rehabilitation. Age and Ageing 2:139

Kaste M, Waltimo O 1976 Prognosis of patients with middle cerebral artery occlusion. Stroke 7:482

Katz S, Ford A B, Chinn A B, Newill W A 1966 Prognosis after strokes. Medicine (Baltimore) 45:236

Marquardsen J 1969 The natural history of acute cerebrovascular disease: a retrospective study of 769 patients. Munksgaard, Copenhagen

Marshall J, Kaeser A C 1961 Survival after non-haemorrhagic cerebrovascular accidents. British Medical Journal ii:73

Marshall J, Shaw D A 1959 The natural history of

cerebrovascular disease. British Medical Journal i:1614

Matsumoto N, Whisnant J P, Kurland T, Akazaki H 1973 Natural history of stroke in Rochester, Minnesota, 1955 through 1969. Stroke 4:20

McKissock W, Richardson A, Walsh L 1960 Spontaneous cerebellar haemorrhage: a study of 34 consecutive cases treated surgically. Brain 83:1

McKissock W, Richardson A, Taylor J 1961 Primary intracerebral haemorrhage. Lancet ii:221

Moskowitz E, Lightbody F E H, Freitag N S 1972 Long-term follow-up of the poststroke patient. Archives of Physical Medicine and rehabilitation 53:167

Müller H R, Wüthrich R, Wiggli U, Hünig R, Elke M 1975 The contribution of computerized axial tomography to the diagnosis of cerebellar and pontine hematomas. Stroke 6:467

Ng L K Y, Nimmannitya J 1970 Massive cerebral infarction with severe brain swelling. Stroke 1:158

Oxbury J M, Greenhall R C D, Grainger K M R 1975 Predicting the outcome of stroke: acute stage after cerebral infarction. British Medical Journal ii:125

Pakarinen S 1967 Incidence, aetiology and prognosis of primary subarachnoid haemorrhage. Munksgaard, Copenhagen

Plum F, Posner J B 1972 The diagnosis of stupor and coma. 2nd edn. F A Davis, Philadelphia

Rankin J 1957 Cerebral vascular accidents in patients over age of 60. Part II, Prognosis. Scottish Medical Journal 2:200

Robinson R W, Demirel M, LeBeau R J 1969 Natural history of cerebral thrombosis. Nine to Nineteen year follow-up. Journal of Chronic Disease 21:221

Rompel K, Wiedenmann 1970 Restitution und Letalitat bei Verschlussen zerebraler Gefasse. Medizinische Klinik 65:1334

Rout M W, Lane D J, Wolner L 1971 Prognosis in acute cerebrovascular accidents in relation to respiratory pattern and blood gas tensions. British Medical Journal iii:7

Shafer S Q, Bruun B, Richter R W 1973 The outcome of stroke at hospital discharge in New York City blacks. Stroke 4:782

Shenkin H A, Haft H, Somach F M 1965 Prognostic significance of arteriography in nonhaemorrhagic strokes. Journal of the American Medical Association 194:612

Terént A 1980 Acute cerebrovascular diseases. Abstract of Uppsala dissertations from the faculty of medicine, 376. Uppsala

Thygesen P, Christensen E, Dyrbye M, Eiken M, Frantzen E, Gormsen J, Lademann A, Lennox-Buchthal M, Rønnov-Jessen V, Therkelsen J 1964 Cerebral apoplexy. Danish Medical Bulletin 11:233

Weisberg L A 1979a Computerized tomography in intracranial hemorrhage. Archives of Neurology 36:422

Weisberg L A 1979b Computed tomography and pure motor hemiparesis. Neurology 29:490

Whisnant J P, Fitzgibbons J P, Kurland L T, Sayre G P 1971 Natural history of stroke in Rochester, Minnesota, 1945 through 1954. Stroke 2:11

Wiggins W S, Moody D M, Toole J F, Laster D W, Ball M R 1978 Clinical and computerized tomographic study of hypertensive intracerebral hemorrhage. Archives of Neurology 35:832

3

Pathological aspects of cerebral and spinal vascular disease

William Blackwood

HYPOXIA AND ISCHAEMIA

The nutrition of nerve cells depends essentially upon oxygen and glucose and so indirectly on an adequate cerebral blood flow conveyed by arteries (Figs 3.1 & 3.2) arterioles and capillaries and carried away by venules, veins and dural sinuses. Oxygen is more rapidly exhausted than glucose and it is customary to speak of circulatory disorders, in which nerve cells are prevented from receiving or utilizing adequate supplies of oxygen, as producing *hypoxia*, or in extreme, *anoxia*. When the disorder of heart and/or blood vessels causes an impairment of blood flow, but the arterial blood is

normal in oxygen tension and oxygen content, this is called *stagnant* (oligaemic or ischaemic) hypoxia. When the primary disorder is diminished oxygen tension in otherwise normal blood, as in suffocation, then this is called *hypoxic* or *anoxic* hypoxia. Other varieties are *anaemic* hypoxia, where the amount of haemoglobin is too small, or its oxygen carrying ability is reduced, as in carbon monoxide

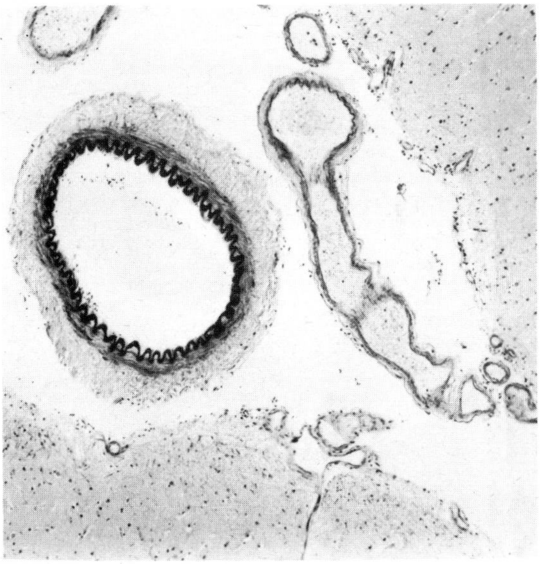

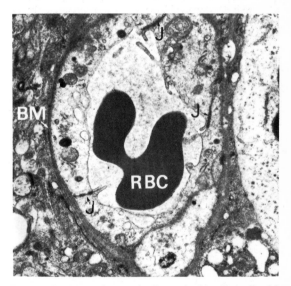

Fig. 3.2 Electron micrograph of a cerebral capillary, lined by flattened polygonal endothelial cells, enclosed by a well defined basement membrane (BM) and covered by the expanded footplates of astrocytes. Except in certain regions, the endothelial cells are joined together by tight junctions (J) and normally lack pinocytic vesicles in their cytoplasm, characteristics which underlie the main blood brain barrier phenomenon. The role of the astrocytic processes is uncertain (Bradbury, 1979). In places pericytes lie within the basement membrane. It is at capillary level that oxygen, glucose and other metabolites are transferred from the blood to the nervous tissue. The prolongations of the subarachnoid space, the Virchow-Robin spaces, extend as far as, but do not surround, the capillaries. (Greenfield's Neuropathology, 3rd edn. Arnold, London.)

Fig. 3.1 Normal leptomeningeal arteries and arterioles. Note the wavy internal elastic lamina, the dark staining muscularis, no external elastic lamina, small amount of adventitia. Celloidin; Weigert's elastic van Gieson × 64. (Greenfield's Neuropathology, 3rd edn. Arnold, London.)

poisoning and *histotoxic* hypoxia as in poisoning by barbiturates, hypnotics or anaesthetic agents where tissue uptake of oxygen is abnormal. In *hypoglycaemia* the brain is unable to utilize oxygen because of a deficiency of glucose. In the human these categories are not mutually exclusive e.g. if the causative process, such as carbon monoxide inhalation, damages the myocardium there will be an element of stagnant (oligaemic) as well as anaemic hypoxia which further damages the brain. Furthermore, after or before complete cardiac arrest there may be a damaging period of severely reduced tissue perfusion (Adams, 1976; Brierley, 1976).

Impairment of blood flow to the nervous system may be *generalised*, as in systemic hypotension or cardiac arrest, or *focal*, as beyond a stenosed or occluded artery. In the other categories of hypoxia the deficiency will be generalised.

The ill effects of stagnant (oligaemic) hypoxia on the brain are, to a certain extent, mitigated by the autoregulatory capacity of the cerebral arterioles. As the systemic arterial blood pressure falls, the arterioles dilate, so that the cerebral blood flow does not diminish. At a mean arterial blood pressure of about 60 mmHg, in a normotensive man, the arterioles are fully dilated (Larsen & Lassen, 1979) so that below this pressure autoregulation is ineffective and blood flow fails (vasoparalysis). Even when this happens, hypoxic damage to cerebral tissues is further postponed by the extraction of larger amounts of oxygen from blood, thus increasing the arteriovenous oxygen difference. Only when the cerebral blood flow is reduced to approximately 25 per cent of normal do signs of cellular metabolic failure appear.

The structural changes which result from a hypoxic injury depend in part on the degree and duration of hypoxia and in part on the length of time which has elapsed. Even with severe hypoxia a short period of survival is necessary before any structural changes at all are visible and if mild, the degree and duration of hypoxia may only be sufficient to cause transient functional impairment without structural change. Anoxia may cause irreversible damage only to nerve cells (selective neuronal necrosis); and because some nerve cells are more vulnerable to anoxia than others, only certain groups may be affected. Broadly speaking,

the order of vulnerability is cerebral cortex, basal ganglia, brainstem and cord.

In generalised hypoxia the cerebral neocortex is most vulnerable, damage being worse in the parietal and occipital lobes than in the temporal and frontal lobes. Within any region changes are usually more pronounced in the depths of the sulci. Of cortical layers the third, fifth and sixth are most vulnerable. In the allocortex, the cornu ammonis, the Sommer sector and the endfolium are the most vulnerable (Figs 3.3 & 3.4).

In the basal ganglia the amygdaloid nucleus, the outer halves of the caudate nucleus and putamen are vulnerable (and the globus pallidus noticeably in CO poisoning). In the thalamus the anterior, dorso-medial and ventrolateral nuclei are most at risk. In the cerebellum the Purkinje cells are the most susceptible while in the brainstem the substantia nigra, inferior colliculus and inferior olive are relatively so. In the infant and young child there may be damage to the 3rd nerve nuclei, the spinal nuclei of the 5th nerves, the cochlear and vestibular nuclei, nucleus ambiguus, nucleus gracilis and cuneatus. All lesions are bilateral.

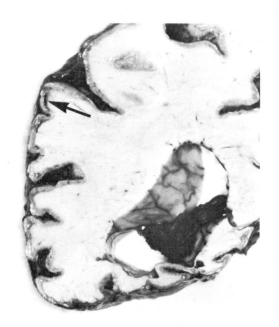

Fig. 3.3 Coronal section of cerebral hemisphere, posterior parietal region, male aged 58 dying 5 months after cardiac arrest. There is shrinkage of both cortex and white matter which are often separated by a cleft (arrow) at their junction. (Greenfield's Neuropathology, 3rd edn. Arnold, London.)

With increasing hypoxia the vulnerability of components of the nervous system other than nerve cells becomes apparent, in the order of oligodendrocytes, astrocytes and capillaries. The severest grades of hypoxia will cause necrosis of all elements, a process which is called *ischaemic necrosis or infarction.*

General patterns of involvement

Generalised hypoxia, especially generalised stagnant hypoxia, produces certain patterns of involvement, which are summarized below. Since the various categories of hypoxia are not mutually exclusive, differences in individual cases may not be as clear cut as the table suggests.

Effects of hypoxia on neurons, glia and mesodermal tissues

Neurons

An hour after hypoxia, in the human, the mitochondria are the principal sites of structural alteration. They swell and their cristae are disorganized. The tubules and cisternae of the endoplasmic reticulum also enlarge, with *microvacuolation* of the cytoplasm. (Brierley, 1976). Due presumably to failure of the ion exchange pumps,

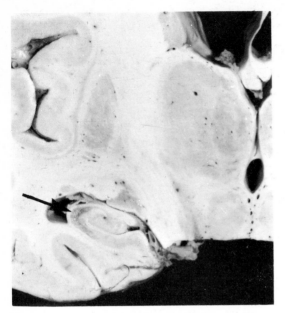

Fig. 3.4 Same case as Figure 3.3. The Sommer sector (arrow) of the hippocampus is a crescent of spongy tissue. (Greenfield's Neuropathology, 3rd edn. Arnold, London.)

Table 3.1 Patterns of damage in survivors from generalised hypoxia

Category of hypoxia	Special clinical feautures	Cortex	Basal ganglia	Cornu Ammonis	Cerebellar cortex
Stagnant A. Oligaemic	Generalised hypotension				
	(1) Episode of major abrupt hypotension. Rapid return to normal B.P.	Boundary zone lesions. Parieto-occipital especially. Figs 3.3 & 3.4	Upper ⅔ head caudate and upper ⅓ putamen moderate. Thalamus slight	Slight	Boundary zone
	(2) Hypotension of relatively slow onset but long · duration (uncommon)	Diffuse lesions	Thalamus	Slight	Diffuse
	(3) Abrupt initial hypotension followed by prolonged period less severe hypotension	Diffuse lesions accentuated at boundary zones	Severe	Slight	Severe diffuse
B. Ischaemic	Cardiac arrest	Diffuse lesions Fig. 3.5	Considerable	Marked Fig. 3.6	Diffuse
Hypoxic	Suffocation	Diffuse lesions	Severe	Slight	Diffuse
Anaemic	Carbon monoxide	Diffuse lesions. Sometimes more in white matter	Globus pallidus involved	Moderate	Diffuse
Histotoxic	Barbiturate hypnotic anaesthetic poisoning	No particular pattern			
Hypoglycaemia	Diabetic patients after treatment with insulin Idiopathic hypoglycaemia	Similar to Stagnant (ischaemic) but with sparing of Purkinje cells			

K⁺ ions leak into the perineuronal extracellular
fluid and there is oedematous swelling of the
processes of adjacent astrocytes (Tower, 1979).

Up to six hours after a hypoxic episode the
affected neurons will show *ischaemic cell change*. In
a pyramidal cell there will be shrinkage of the cell
body and the proximal portions of the axon and the
dendrites, which stain darkly with aniline dyes.
The Nissl substance is dispersed and granular, the
cytoplasm is usually noticeably eosinophilic: the
nucleus is triangular, basophilic and without a
noticeable nucleolus. After this the cytoplasm
continues to shrink; both nucleus and cytoplasm
stain darkly. The cytoplasm is invaginated by the
swollen astrocytic processes and the projecting
portions of dark cytoplasm between these processes
appear, under the light microscope, as incrustations on the surface of the ischaemic neuron. (Figs
3.5 & 3.6). At the next stage the nueron has a
uniformly eosinophilic cytoplasm and a shrunken
or disintegrating nucleus. This change, known as

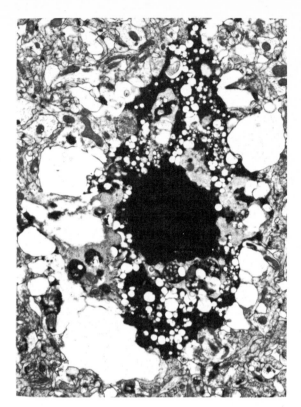

Fig. 3.6 Electron micrograph of ischaemic pyramidal nerve
cell of a rat which survived for 2 hours after 40 minutes
intermittent exposure to nitrogen. Around the nucleus the
vacuolated electron-dense cytoplasm contrasts with the less
dense membrane-limited areas. Some of the electron-dense
portions of the perikaryon and dendrites correspond to the
incrustations of the light microscope. The neuron is surrounded
by swollen astrocytic processes. × 5800. (Greenfield's Neuropathology, 3rd edn. Arnold, London.)

homogenizing cell change is characteristically seen in
Purkinje cells.

Glia. Swelling of perineuronal and perivascular
astrocytic processes is an early change. Two to
twelve hours after a period of hypoxia there is
swelling of astrocytic nuclei, which proliferate,
maximally at four to six days. In regions where
damage is confined to nerve cells, the microglia
change their shape into rod-cells, then multiply
and become lipid-phagocytes. Those lying close to
dying nerve cells, multiply and form 'glial stars'.
Oligodendroglia and capillaries usually show little
change.

Border zone lesions

This expression refers to the ischaemic lesions
which are sometimes found in the cerebrum and

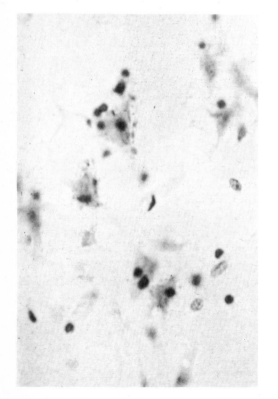

Fig. 3.5 Ischaemic pyramidal cortical nerve cells showing
incrustations at the periphery of the nerve cells. Nissl
preparation.

the cerebellum. In the cerebrum they are localised to the periphery of the cortical fields of supply of the anterior, middle and posterior cerebral arteries (Figs 3.7 & 3.8), regions where there are anastomotic vessels between the fields (Vander Eecken, 1959). Most vulnerable is the parieto-occipital region, which is furthest from the origins of the anterior, middle and posterior cerebral arteries. The lesions may extend anteriorly to involve the region of the middle frontal gyrus. The border zones in the cortex of the convexity of the temporal

lobe and in the supraorbital frontal region are least often involved. In the cerebellum the site is on the postero-inferior aspect, between the fields of supply of the superior and posterior inferior cerebellar arteries. Such lesions are characteristically found bilaterally after generalised hypotension (oligaemic stagnant hypoxia, type (1)) but they may also be found in patients where the flow to the anterior and middle cerebral arterial territories is critically diminished due to carotid stenosis or occlusion. The reason for this localization, at

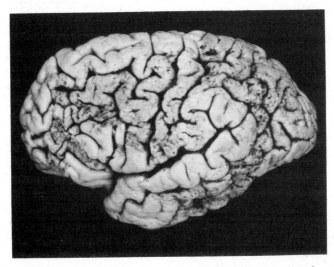

Fig. 3.7 Lateral aspect of cerebral hemisphere with leptomeninges removed to show scarring of cortex due to old microinfarcts in boundary zones between the anterior, middle and posterior cerebral arterial distributions.

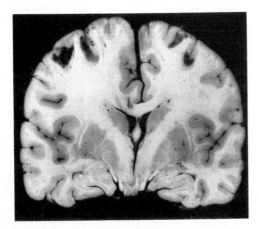

Fig. 3.8 Coronal section of cerebral hemispheres to show recent haemorrhagic infarction in the boundary zone regions between the anterior and middle cerebral arterial territories. (Gradwohl's Legal Medicine, 3rd edn. Wright, Bristol.)

the periphery of the fields, is that here the blood pressure will be lowest and the flow becomes sluggish or static.

In the newborn, ischaemic lesions may be found in the white matter bordering the lateral aspects of the anterior horns, bodies and occipital horns of the lateral ventricles. Larroche (1977) considers that they occur in the border zone between the fields of irrigation of the deep branches of the superficial cerebral arteries and those of the periventricular branches of the choroidal arteries.

Cerebral arteries in the border zones. In patients with systemic hypotension or stenosis of the large arteries in the neck and with small infarcts in the border zone region of the brain, one occasionally finds a solid chalky-white or translucent greyish appearance of some of the leptomeningeal arteries, often over a considerable length (Fig. 3.9). The walls of these arteries appear healthy, but the lumen is narrowed or occluded (Fig. 3.10). Romanul & Abramowicz (1964) found that the chalky-white appearance was due to recent change, when platelet aggregations were adherent to the arterial wall, were sometimes covered by endothelium, or were organizing. Usually a lumen was still present. The translucent greyish arteries represented older lesions, when the lumen was filled with a loose web of collagen or appeared to be recanalized. The internal elastic lamina was noticeably folded. It is generally agreed that the changes seen here are not due to a primary disease of small arteries. Romanul and Abramowicz were satisfied that the early platelet masses were locally deposited and were not embolic. They were in favour of the lesions being produced by a decrease in the blood flow through major cerebral vessels with 'prolonged stasis in their most distal branches and anastomoses which did not serve as sources of collateral blood supply'. Whilst agreeing with most

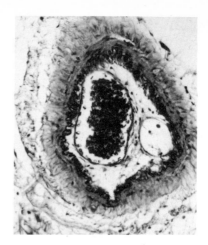

Fig. 3.10 Solid looking artery from same case as Figure 3.9. The internal elastic lamina is noticeably folded, the lumen contains a loose collagenous web in which blood channels are present. Elastic van Gieson × 100.

of their conclusions one could question the word 'stasis', for platelet masses require flowing blood from which to be deposited. In support of this view, a lumen was often visible.

Detail of infarction in the central nervous system

When a large artery of the brain is obstructed, especially if the obstruction is rapid, as by an embolus, the region affected will be all except the periphery of the arterial territory. Both grey and white matter will be involved. Initially all regions are pale in colour. Within a short time, if the embolus fragments and moves on, or if the blood pressure in the collateral circulation is high enough, blood flow returns to the periphery of the infarct and blood leaks out through the devitalized vessels in the grey matter, producing a *haemorrhagic infarct* (Figs 3.11 & 3.12). The white matter always remains pale. Whether pale or haemorrhagic, the infarct begins to swell. This swelling is maximal at 4 days and then gradually decreases, until by three weeks it is no longer present. (Figs 3.13, 3.14 & 3.15). If the infarct is large and in the territory of the middle cerebral artery, it can produce as much as 11 mm of contralateral shift and this, together with caudal displacement of midline structures, results in secondary vascular changes (ischaemic or haemorrhagic) in the rostral brainstem, changes

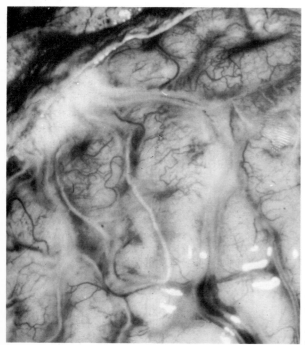

Fig. 3.9 Solid looking arteries on the superior parietal convexity of the cerebrum of a man who had periods of arterial hypotension during the last two months of his life. With severe polyneuritis, he was in an intensive care unit. Autopsy revealed myocardial fibrosis and solitary plasma cell myeloma.

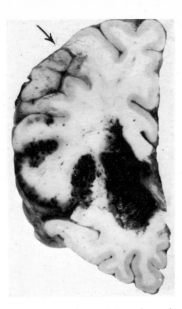

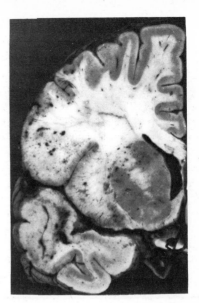

Fig. 3.11 Coronal section, frontal lobe, atherosclerotic carotid artery. In the lower part of the picture is recent, embolic, haemorrhagic infarction of the cortex. The underlying white matter is also necrotic, although this is not clearly visible. This part of the brain is swollen and the line of demarcation between cortex and white matter is ill-defined. In the upper part of the picture (arrow) is an older lesion, of about 6 weeks' duration. (Greenfield's Neuropathology, 3rd edn. Arnold, London.)

Fig. 3.13 Embolic occlusion of middle cerebral artery, of 3 weeks' duration, from thrombus overlying atherosclerotic myocardial infarct of left ventricle. The necrotic grey matter, which is friable, is not clearly defined from the white matter. In the centrum semi-ovale the edge of the necrotic white matter is visible. The inferomedial half of the corpus striatum (supplied by the recurrent artery of Heubner) is not necrotic. (Greenfield's Neuropathology, 3rd edn. Arnold, London.)

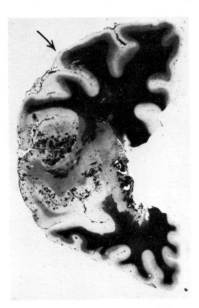

which kill the patient. If the infarct is not lethal, the dead tissue in it begins to disintegrate and to be replaced and removed by swollen phagocytes. This change commences at the edge of the infarct. After about six weeks a narrow channel, filled with fluid, is clearly visible to the naked eye outlining the infarct. Gradually the rest of the infarct is removed

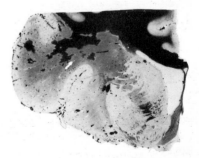

Fig. 3.12 Myelin preparation of Figure 3.11. Note the sharp edge to the necrotic white matter, which does not stain. In some places only the subcortical U-fibres are necrotic; in other places the deep white matter is damaged. Note the older lesions (arrow). (Greenfield's Neuropathology, 3rd edn. Arnold, London.)

Fig. 3.14 Myelin preparation of middle part of Figure 3.13. Note the sharp edge to the necrotic white matter. (Greenfield's Neuropathology, 3rd edn. Arnold, London.)

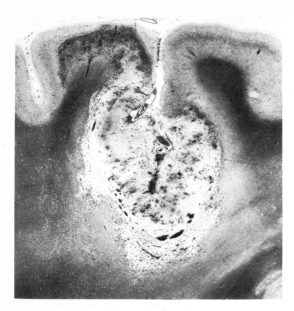

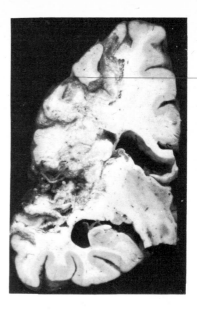

Fig. 3.15 Isolated embolic cerebral infarct, 3 weeks' duration, same case as Figures 3.13 and 3.14. The central portion of the infarct shows coagulative necrosis. At the periphery there is cellular reaction, which is more marked in the grey matter. Organizing thrombus is visible in the cortical arteriole within the sulcus. Celloidin, haematoxylin van Gieson. (Greenfield's Neuropathology, 3rd edn. Arnold, London.)

Fig. 3.16 Old infarct (clinically 5 months) due to atherosclerotic carotid artery occlusion. The products of tissue destruction have been largely removed, leaving cystic spaces. Note that the edge of the infarct, which goes down to the ventricular wall, is clearly defined. The hemisphere is shrunken, the ventricle dilated. Middle cerebral artery distribution. (Greenfield's Neuropathology, 3rd edn. Arnold, London.)

and its place is taken by cerebro-spinal fluid. (Figs 3.16 & 3.17). At the periphery of this cystic lesion the astrocytes multiply and lay down fibrils. Blood vessels, least vulnerable to hypoxia, often project into the cystic space.

Distribution of significant atherosclerosis between the arch of the aorta and the branches of the circle of Willis

Atherosclerosis is often found in these arteries, but large lesions have certain sites of predeliction (*v. infra*). They become significant when they seriously impair or arrest the blood flow by stenosis, or occlusion, or act as sources of emboli. Occlusion is usually the result of thrombosis of the lumen at the site of a tight stenosis. Embolism frequently occurs in the carotid system but less often in the vertebral system. Serious stenosis or occlusion was found by Yates & Hutchinson (1961) to be present in both internal carotid and vertebral systems in 33 of their 100 cases, in the internal carotid arteries alone in 18 cases and in the vertebral arteries alone in 7 cases.

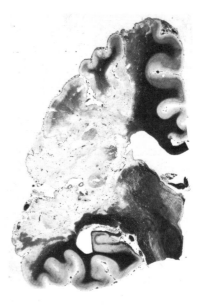

Fig. 3.17 Myelin preparation of Figure 3.16 showing well-defined margin of the infarct. (Greenfield's Neuropathology, 3rd edn. Arnold, London.)

Significant atherosclerosis occurs in:

Arch of the aorta, where it is unlikely to cause symptoms unless there is ulceration and thrombosis, from which emboli pass predominantly into the carotid system.

Innominate artery, which can be stenosed or occluded proximal to the vertebral artery, in which case the *subclavian* artery may receive blood which has flowed in a reverse direction down the ipsilateral vertebral artery.

Common carotid arteries at their origins.

Internal carotid arteries. The most frequent site of origin of emboli or of stenosis or occlusion in the carotico-vertebral system is in the region of the carotid sinus (Fig. 3.18). Much less frequently it is in the osseous, cavernous or the intradural portions of these arteries.

Vertebral arteries, where it is more diffusely spread than in the carotid arteries. Yates & Hutchinson found significant atherosclerosis in the 1st part in 36 cases, in the 2nd (intraspinous) part in 17 cases, in the 3rd part in 8 cases and in the 4th (intradural) part in 4 cases. One has the impression that embolization from such plaques is infrequent.

Basilar artery which is often diffusely affected. Correlation of regions of infarction in the brainstem with the sites of occlusion of branches of the basilar artery is technically easier if the brainstem is sectioned in the coronal plane (Fisher, 1977).

Collateral circulation

Development of collateral circulation is favoured by a gradual obstruction of the artery, or arteries, in question and by the presence, calibre and patency of pre-existent collateral channels. Obstruction of the lumen of the *aorta* distal to the left subclavian artery, with potential ischaemia of the caudal spinal cord, as in the adult type of coarctation of the aorta, may be compensated for by an increased flow of blood down the anterior spinal artery. Obstruction of a *subclavian artery* proximal to the origin of a *vertebral artery* results, especially during exercise of the upper limb, in a reverse flow down the ipsilateral vertebral artery, blood being diverted from the contralateral vertebral and possibly basilar artery — subclavian steal. Local muscle collaterals from the interna mammary and thyrocervical trunk also enlarge to by-pass blocked segments.

Obstruction of a *common carotid artery* may also result in retrograde flow, usually down the ipsilat-

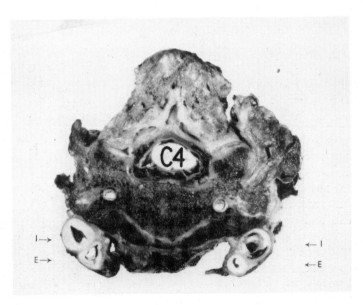

Fig. 3.18 Horizontal slice of the cervical vertebrae just above the level of the bifurcation of the common carotid arteries. In the lower part of the figure the stenosed, atherosclerotic, smaller external (E) and larger internal (I) carotid arteries are visible. On the right of the picture recent haemorrhage is present into the plaque in the I.C.A. About midway between the carotid arteries and the spinal cord are the patent vertebral arteries. (From Atlas of Neuropathology published by E. & S. Livingstone Ltd.)

eral internal carotid artery and into the external carotid bed. The capacity of the contralateral artery is such that clinical symptoms seldom result. The retrograde flow may be down the ipsilateral external carotid artery which attracts blood from the ipsilateral subclavian flow through the anastomoses which are present between the superior thyroid branches of the external carotid and the inferior thyroid branches of the thyro-cervical trunk, a branch of the subclavian. It attracts some of the ipsilateral vertebral flow through the anastomoses between the muscular branches of the vertebral and those of the occipital branch of the external carotid artery. Anastomoses also open up, across the midline, between branches of the ipsilateral and the contralateral external carotid artery.

Obstruction of an *internal carotid artery* first of all calls into operation the anastomotic ring of the circle of Willis and draws blood from the contralateral internal carotid artery via the anterior communicating artery and/or from a posterior cerebral artery via the posterior communicating artery. If this is inadequate it calls upon anastomoses between the internal and external carotid systems. If the obstruction is in the inferior part of the internal carotid, the collateral circulation is from the external carotid artery via its internal maxillary branch. This gives off the sphenopalatine artery which anastomoses with branches of the posterior ethmoidal artery (a branch of the ophthalmic artery) and by reverse flow delivers blood to the supraclinoid portion of the internal carotid artery. Less frequently the supraclinoid portion of the carotid artery may draw blood from the external carotid artery by utilizing the branches of the facial and superficial temporal arteries which anastomose with the dorsal nasal, frontal and supraorbital branches of the ophthalmic artery, in which the flow will again be reversed. Still less frequently it may draw blood from the external carotid artery along its internal maxillary division, along the middle meningeal artery and its anterior division which anastomoses with the lacrimal branch of the ophthalmic artery. An anastomosis can open up between the middle meningeal artery and the artery of the inferior cavernous sinus. This last is a branch of the meningohypophyseal trunk, one of the three small branches of the cavernous

portion of the internal carotid artery (Parkinson, 1965). There is another branch of the meningohypophyseal trunk, called the dorsal meningeal branch, which may utilize its anastomosis with either the middle meningeal artery or with anterior meningeal branches of the vertebral artery.

In obstruction of a *vertebral artery*, and this is most frequently in its proximal part, use is made of the anastomoses of its distal part with (1) deep and superficial branches of the thyrocervical trunk (a branch of the subclavian artery) (2) muscular branches of the occipital artery (a branch of the external carotid artery) in the suboccipital region. (3) The contralateral vertebral artery.

Dural collaterals. In relation to some arteriovenous angiomata, which may have a greatly increased blood flow, and in moya-moya, where there is occlusion of the distal carotid arteries and circle of Willis, the arterial supply to the brain makes use of collateral channels which can develop by dilatation of the many small interconnected arteries which normally supply the dura. These arteries come from both the external and internal carotid arteries and from the vertebral artery. From the *external carotid artery*, (1) the middle meningeal branch of the internal maxillary supplies the dura of the convexity (2) the meningeal branches of the ascending pharyngeal artery supply some of the dura of the posterior and middle fossae (3) meningeal branches of the occipital artery supply the dura of the lateral aspect of the posterior fossa. From the *internal carotid artery* (1) the tentorial and dorsal meningeal branches of the meningohypophyseal trunk, a branch of the cavernous carotid, supply the medial dura of the middle and posterior fossa (2) the ethmoidal branches of the ophthalmic artery supply the floor of the anterior fossa and the anterior part of the falx cerebri (3) the recurrent meningeal branch of the lachrimal branch of the ophthalmic artery may supply the dura of the middle fossa. From the *vertebral arteries* (1) meningeal branches, arising near the foramen magnum supply the dura of the posterior fossa (2) infratentorial meningeal arteries from the posterior cerebral arteries supply the midline of the tentorium cerebelli. In certain pathological conditions, such as the above, collateral vessels can usually be demonstrated angiographically, uniting dural arteries and leptomeningeal arteries across the subdural space (Mishkin & Schreiber, 1974; Newton & Troost, 1974; Taveras & Wood, 1976).

Pial collateral circulation

The extent of infarction in the brain, following occlusion of an extracranial or intracranial artery, is often less than the anatomical distribution of the artery, especially in respect of the cortex and subadjacent white matter. If stenosis or occlusion develops slowly, the collateral vessels dilate, blood flow remains adequate and significant hypoxia does not occur. When the occlusion is sudden, restoration of blood flow depends on the blood pressure and the adequacy of collateral channels. Van der Eecken (1959) has shown that, in respect of the basal ganglia and brainstem, there are communications between the arteries of supply, but only at capillary and arteriolar level and rarely above 150 micron calibre. Such anastomoses do not appear to be adequate. In respect of the cortical distribution of the anterior, middle and posterior cerebral arteries and of the three cerebellar arteries, he found direct end-to-end and side-by-side anastomoses, between branches of the individual arteries in the cerebral group, lying in the depths of the sulci, along the border zones of their respective distributions, measuring 312 microns calibre on average (range 200–760 microns) and explicable on an embryological basis. Anastomoses between the cerebellar arteries were even more frequent and averaged 278 microns (calibre range 180–543 microns). The blood flow through the collaterals is often sufficient to enable the cortex, at the periphery of the field of distribution, to survive.

Occlusive vascular disease — atherosclerosis

Atherosclerosis is typically found in the large elastic arteries and the muscular distributing arteries. The normal arterial wall consists of intima, media and adventitia. The *intima* consists of an inner single layer of endothelial cells and a peripheral fenestrated sheet of elastic fibres. The endothelial cells are linked together by highly interdigitated margins and form a barrier to the passage of blood constituents into the arterial wall. Between the two layers are various components of extracellular connective tissue and occasional smooth-muscle cells which increase in amount and number with age. The *media* consists of diagonally orientated smooth-muscle cells surrounded by variable amounts of collagen, small elastic fibres and proteoglycans. The proportions of elastic tissue is greater in elastic arteries such as the aorta and carotid arteries. Fibroblasts are not present and the morphology of the media does not alter with age.

The adventitia consists of fibroblasts, smooth muscle cells, bundles of collagen and proteoglycans. The arteries of the nervous system have a very thin adventitia and lack a definite external elastic lamina which elsewhere usually separates media and adventitia.

Atherosclerosis primarily affects the intima, the media may be secondarily affected. Classically three different categories are recognized (1) the fatty streak (2) the fibro-musculo-elastic plaque (3) the complicated lesion.

The fatty streak commonly seen in the aorta of young persons consists of focal accumulations of relatively small numbers of intimal smooth-muscle cells, containing and surrounded by deposits of lipid (cholesterol and cholesterol esters).

The fibro-musculo-elastic plaque consists principally of a subendothelial accumulation of proliferated, intimal, smooth-muscle cells laden with lipid (cholesterol and cholesterol esters). These cells are surrounded by lipid, by collagen, elastic fibres and proteoglycans. The cells and the extracellular matrix components form a fibrous cap which later covers a deeper deposit of free extracellular lipid intermixed with cell debris.

The complicated lesion is a fibro-musculo-elastic plaque containing intramural haemorrhage and/or collections of atheromatous debris, with surface ulceration or luminal thrombus (Fig. 3.19).

Atherosclerotic lesions have in common:

(1) Proliferation of intimal smooth muscle cells
(2) Deposition of intracellular and extracellular lipid
(3) Accumulation of extracellular matrix components including collagen, elastic fibres and proteoglycans

There is evidence that in at least a proportion of atherosclerotic lesions the plaques have enlarged by the incorporation in them of mural thrombus

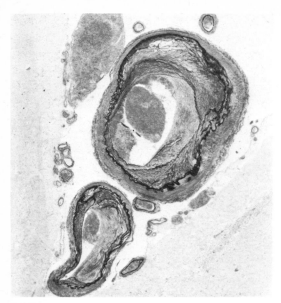

Fig. 3.19 Leptomeningeal arteries from a normotensive patient with marked atherosclerosis. The arteries are eccentrically narrowed by plaques composed of fibrous and elastic tissue. In places the media is thin. Celloidin; Weigerts elastic van Gieson. × 24. (Reproduced by courtesy of Dr W. G. P. Mair.)

(Woolf, 1978a). The exact nature of the process which initiates atherosclerosis in the human is not yet certain (Woolf, 1978b) though the climate of opinion has veered towards considering that damage to endothelial cells is the key factor. Experimentally it has been shown that injury to endothelial cells, as by direct trauma or haemodynamic factors, results in adherence and aggregation of platelets which release a factor (Ross & Gomsett, 1976) which causes proliferation of smooth muscle cells. These cells are capable of synthesizing the extracellular connective tissue matrix, of collagen, elastic fibres and proteoglycans, which is an important constituent of the fibromusculo-elastic plaque of atherosclerosis (Wolf, 1978b; Mustard, 1977). If the stress is withdrawn the lesion will heal, but if it is continuous or repeated there will be further proliferation of smooth muscle cells and accumulation of connective tissue and lipid.

For a review of the role of lipoproteins in atherosclerosis see Steinberg (1981).

Cholesterol emboli or athero-emboli

Advanced atheromatous plaques contain lipid material consisting of cholesterol, partly in crys-talline form, 30 per cent, cholesterol esters 50 per cent, phospholipids 15 per cent, triglycerides 5 per cent. When released into the circulation, by rupture of the plaque, fragments of this material may be large enough and structurally stable enough to form emboli which occlude smaller arteries in the vertebral or carotid circulation. Rail et al (1981) have shown experimentally that these substances are individually harmless when injected into the carotid arteries of rats or rabbits, but when mixed together in the above proportions they cause embolic cerebral infarction. The important factor appears to be the aggregation of the crystals of cholesterol by oily cholesterol esters. When mixed together 'in vitro' these two form a range of very glutinous aggregates. In the human plaque phospholipids and triglycerides are additionally present and modify the cholesterol/ester aggregates. Triglycerides favour aggregation, though in high concentration they reduce the mutual adhesiveness of the aggregates in the presence of mechanical forces, such as turbulence. Phospholipids, acting like an emulsifying agent, promote dispersion of the aggregates. With so many factors involved it is not surprising that, when an atherosclerotic plaque is present and ruptures, there can be great variation in the size and number of aggregates. In some cases there are no clinical effects, in some transient occlusion of small retinal vessels causes amaurosis fugax, in some there is permanent occlusion of small leptomeningeal arteries (McDonald, 1967) (Fig. 3.20).

Sites of impaction of atheromatous emboli

Soloway & Aronson in 1964 studied the sites and sizes of the arteries in which atheromatous emboli were found at autopsy. In 71 cases emboli were all found in the terminal leptomeningeal arteries of the cerebrum and cerebellum except for one small artery in the basal ganglia and in two cases in the spinal cord. The majority of the emboli were in arteries with a calibre less than 100 μm (range 17–585 μm, Alexander & Putnam's (1938) orders of magnitude 4 and 5).

Atherosclerotic stenosis **and** *occlusion* **at the** *bifurcation of the common carotid artery*

Examination of autopsy (Yates & Hutchinson,

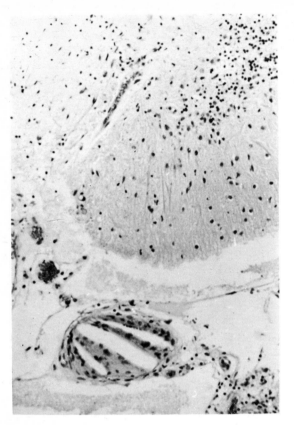

Fig. 3.20 Occlusion of small cerebellar artery by organized atheroembolus containing three cholesterol crystals. Small old infarct of adjacent cortex. (Greenfield's Neuropathology, 3rd edn. Arnold, London.)

1961) and operative (Imparato et al, 1979) material reveals all the stages from a healthy common carotid bifurcation through fibro-musculo-elastic mural thickening to a complicated atheromatous lesion involving the distal common and proximal internal and external carotid arteries over a length of 1–3 cm each (Fig. 3.18). Until the lumen is reduced to about 80 per cent of its original calibre there will probably not be any significant impairment of blood flow to the brain. At this stage the plaques are sometimes of simple fibro-musculo-elastic type upon which intimal thrombus may or may not be present. The irregularity of outline and the stenosis of the lumen result in turbulence which is conducive to thrombus formation. Many fibrous plaques have atheromatous debris in their depths. This debris is often associated with evidence of old haemorrhage. Imparato et al, in their

operative specimens, found that impaired blood flow was associated, most often on the side appropriate to focal symptoms, with significant intraplaque haemorrhage (at least 50 per cent of thickness of the plaque). Yates and Hutchinson support this finding. The surface of such a plaque was ulcerated in a third of such cases and intimal thrombus was adherent to about half the ulcerated and about 1/7th of the non-ulcerated haemorrhagic plaques. Large collections of atheromatous debris, with or without ulceration and intimal thrombus were less often present. Impairment of blood flow was least often associated with mural thrombus covering a fibrous plaque.

The intimal thrombus, which forms in flowing blood, is sometimes recent and is composed of platelet aggregations (white thrombus) at other times it is older and contains alternating bands of platelets and fibrin with entrapped red blood corpuscles (mixed thrombus). Later still it becomes organised and endothelium may grow again over the surface. The initial deposition of platelets is probably due to damage to the endothelial cells and exposure of collagen. Production of anti-aggregatory prostacylin is impaired, the platelets adhere to the sub-endothelial tissues release pro-aggregatory thromboxane A2 and thereby induce further platelets to aggregate. At this stage the thrombus is relatively unstable. Portions of it may fragment and form emboli. The aggregations are usually so small that they impact only temporarily in the small arteries of the brain or retina. The next stage is the formation of fibrin which binds the thrombus more firmly together, so that if fragments break off and form emboli these are more stable, impact in larger vessels and disintegrate less easily.

The thrombus which forms upon the atheromatous lesion is called the primary thrombus. With a stenosed carotid sinus, blood will continue to flow through the internal carotid artery until the lumen is occluded. Once this has occurred secondary thrombus develops, in an anterograde and a (usually shorter) retrograde fashion, in the now stagnant columns of blood. Secondary thrombus, developing in stagnant blood, is dark red in colour and composed of a mass of red and white blood cells surrounded by an outer layer of platelets. It fills the internal carotid artery, usually as far as the first collateral branch — the ophthalmic artery.

Here the thrombus encounters flowing blood and is capped by a white thrombus. Quite often the anterograde thrombus spreads as far as the circle of Willis or even into the stems of the middle and anterior cerebral arteries. Gautier (1979) considers that, in some cases, the thrombus may spread from the origin of the internal carotid artery to the circle of Willis in 4–6 hours.

Embolism from the heart

Embolism from the heart is the cause of cerebral infarction in one-third to one-half of cases of stroke. The emboli arise from bacterial endocarditis of the mitral or aortic valves, non-bacterial thrombotic endocarditis, myocardial infarction (recent or healed), atrial fibrillation, following cardiac surgery, or cardiac myxoma. Gautier (1979) considered that the cause in 136 cases was idiopathic atrial fibrillation 89, valvulopathy and atrial fibrillation 29, thyrotoxicosis and atrial fibrillation 3, myocardial infarction 9, other causes 6. At autopsy about 60 per cent of such cases can be expected to have infarcts in spleen and/or kidneys.

About 10 per cent of the emboli will impact in the vertebro-basilar circulation, about 90 per cent in the carotid circulation. The emboli vary in size and fragility. In 17 autopsied cases of embolism from the heart, in which the cervical arteries had been examined, Blackwood et al (1969) found impaction at the bifurcation of the common carotid artery in 2 cases, with extensive anterograde thrombus in the internal carotid artery: impaction at the bifurcation of the internal carotid artery in 1 case: at the first major branching of the middle cerebral artery in 6 cases: in a small peripheral artery in 3 cases and in 5 cases infarction was extensive but no embolus was found. These last confirm the angiographic evidence that emboli tend to impact and then fragment and disappear

(Dalal et al, 1965). Histologically, emboli may be difficult to distinguish from local thrombosis, especially when the embolus has been impacted for some time.

Frequency of thrombotic and embolic occlusion of cerebral arteries

Table 3.2, from Escourolle & Poirier (1978), supports the view that the internal carotid, vertebral and basilar arteries are most often occluded by local athero-thrombosis. The anterior, middle and posterior cerebral arteries are most often occluded by embolism, or by the growth of anterograde thrombus from primary athero-thrombosis of the internal carotid: local athero-thrombosis is less frequent.

Giant cell (temporal) arteritis

This is a subacute inflammatory disease affecting arteries of all sizes from the aorta downwards, usually in people over the age of 55 years. When it affects the superficial temporal arteries they become swollen, tender, tortuous and nodular. Pulsation is usually diminished or lost. The involvement is segmental so that a biopsy may be falsely negative. (Allsop & Gallagher, 1980). The coronary arteries, the cervical portion of the internal carotid, the vertebral, ophthalmic (Wilkinson & Russell, 1972), the central artery of the retina and the ciliary arteries (Crompton, 1959) may be involved. Infarction in the brain is usually the result of thrombosis of, or thrombo-embolism from, the internal carotid or vertebral artery. Intracranial arteries are seldom involved.

Microscopically, in the acute or subacute phase, all coats are involved. Deep to the internal elastic lamina, cellular proliferation narrows the lumen. Often this sub-intimal layer consists of an inner,

Table 3.2

Artery and number of cases	Internal carotid (61)%	Middle cerebral (41)%	Anterior cerebral (31)%	Vertebral (25)%	Basilar (18)%	Posterior cerebral (30)%
Primary thrombotic occlusion	62	5	13	68	83	1
Occluded by anterograde thrombus of proximal source	0	23	26	12	11	26
Embolic occlusion	21	64	52	16	0.5	53

thicker zone of loosely packed cellular fibrous tissue and mucoid intercellular substance, and of an outer, thinner zone composed of vascular granulomatous tissue infiltrated by small and large mononuclear cells, plasma cells and a few neutrophil polymorphonuclear leucocytes. The internal elastic lamina is always damaged, focally. The media is infiltrated by large and small mononuclear cells and close to the damaged, often fragmented, elastica are multinucleated giant cells. In the adventitia is a lesser degree of inflammatory cell infiltration (Fig. 3.21).

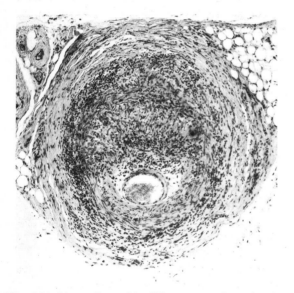

Fig. 3.21 Giant cell arteritis. Ciliary artery of eye showing intimal proliferation and cellular infiltration, including multinucleated giant cells close to the irregularly damaged internal elastic lamina. There is mononuclear infiltration of the media and, to a lesser extent, of the adventitia. Celloidin; haematoxylin van Gieson. × 64. (Greenfield's Neuropathology, 3rd edn. Arnold, London.)

Aortic arch syndrome

Takayasu's arteritis

In this condition there is a gradual obstruction of the aortic arch, the innominate, the common carotid and subclavian arteries. In children the descending thoracic or abdominal aorta and its branches are affected. Radiological studies have shown that nearly all the arteries of the body may be involved, apart from those of the lower limbs, of the heart and of the brain, which may however show evidence of embolism. It was originally described in young Japanese women. Nasu (1963) found that all layers of the arterial wall were irregularly thickened and hardened, especially the intima which might be up to five times the thickness of the media. Inflammatory changes were most marked in the media. Here there might be granulomata with giant cells, with or without coagulation necrosis, or diffuse inflammatory infiltration by lymphocytes and plasma cells. Elastic tissue was damaged, fragmented or lost. The adventitia showed less inflammatory change. In the intima there was a great increase of basophilic ground substance. Young connective tissue and probably smooth muscle cells were increased in number and at the periphery, fine elastic fibres were present. In later cases fibrous tissue replaced the damaged coats.

Dalal (1973) found a less florid type quite common in India. There was irregular or diffuse thickening of the intima, by firm, pearly white material. These thickenings often protruded into the ostia of the arteries of the arch of the aorta. Microscopically the intima was greatly thickened by connective tissue: on its surface organising thrombi were present. The internal elastic membrane was fragmented and occasional giant cells were present nearby. The media was somewhat thin and elastic tissue was fragmented. The adventitia was focally thickened by fibrous tissue.

Transient emboligenic aortoarteritis, a disease process confined to the aortic arch and its branches and in the authors' opinion, a different entity from Takayasu's arteritis, was first described by Wickremasinge et al in 1978. In their ten patients, aged 16–36 yrs, there were active or healed inflammatory lesions situated in the arch of the aorta and its main branches, with overlying thrombus from which thrombo-emboli had occluded cerebral arteries, causing such symptoms as hemiparesis and hemiplegia of sudden onset. The acute inflammatory lesions affected the middle and outer thirds of the media, with foci of fragmentation and depletion of elastica, dilatation of vasa vasorum which were surrounded by polymorphonuclear leucocytes, macrophages which sometimes had large lobulated nuclei, lymphocytes and occasional plasma cells. The overlying intima was oedematous, with connective tissue hyperplasia and with organizing thrombus adherent to its luminal surface. Healing occurred in a few weeks, when there was fibrous replacement of the inflammatory lesions and the intimal thrombus was organizing or fibrosed. The arteries elsewhere were not diseased but pulmonary or cervical glandular tuberculosis was present more often than in unselected autopsies.

Dissecting aneurysm of aorta

Dissecting aneurysm of the aorta, usually in hypertensive patients, is the result of extensive haemorrhage into the media, usually previously weakened by idiopathic cystic medionecrosis. The haemorrhage usually commences at a tear in the ascending aorta and extends into the abdominal aorta. In Marfan's syndrome, only the ascending aorta is involved. In another quite frequent type, the aneurysm commences beyond the left subclavian artery and may or may not be confined to the thoracic aorta. In the first type the dissection may continue out in the media of the innominate, carotid or femoral arteries, narrowing the lumen and impairing the blood flow. The haemorrhage may surround, stretch or even tear apart the intercostal and lumbar arteries, with thrombosis or obliteration of the lumen. An intimal tear may communicate with the lumen of the artery at the distal end of the dissection. The neurological complications have been divided into those:

(1) With ischaemic lesions of the brain. This is the least frequent complication. It is usually associated with extension of the dissection into the innominate or carotid arteries.

(2) With ischaemic lesions of the spinal cord. The mid and lower thoracic region of the cord, supplied by the intercostal arteries, is most frequently and severely involved. The rostral cord is seldom involved. When the dissection has been more extensive the lumbosacral cord may be damaged. The ischaemic necrosis always involves the grey matter and the adjacent white matter. Often the white matter at the periphery of the cord is spared, but in some cases, at some levels, the whole cross-section of the cord may be necrotic.

(3) With ischaemic lesions of peripheral nerves. This is the most frequent neurological complication and is associated with extension of the

dissection out into the subclavian or iliac arteries (Stehbens, 1972; Cochrane & LeBlanc, 1980).

Dissecting aneurysms of the carotid arteries in the neck

Dissecting aneurysm of the cervical portion of the internal carotid artery and its major intracranial branches, may develop spontaneously, or may extend from a proximal spontaneous dissection, or it may be traumatic following external violence to the head and neck, or follow carotid puncture for angiography.

In spontaneous cases, the dissecting haematoma starts at an intimal tear, at a variable distance from the origin of the artery and is either in the outer layers of the media or between the media and adventitia. Cystic medial necrosis is frequently but not invariably present, occasional cases showing fibromuscular dysplasia, or a disorganized appearance of the medial elastica and muscle (Ojemann et al, 1972). Stehbens (1972) points out that a sufficient quantity of control material should be examined before interpreting the changes which may be seen in the elastic tissue and muscle in such cases as abnormal. Local thrombosis may occlude the remaining lumen of the artery, with antero-grade spread into intracranial arteries and cerebral infarction.

Dissecting aneurysms of the vertebral arteries in the neck are exceedingly rare.

Dissecting aneurysms of the intracranial arteries

These are usually found in the 2nd, 3rd and 4th decades, though they do occur earlier or later. They have been ascribed to closed head injury without fracture, as a complication of intracranial surgery, to atherosclerosis in older persons, to migraine, infection, homocystinuria, congenital medial defects, panarteritis, fibromuscular dysplasia and strenuous physical exercise. In many cases no cause was found.

The dissecting haematoma usually lies just external to the internal elastic lamina. The involved vessel is enlarged, the lumen is narrowed and may be thrombosed. Infarction in the field of supply or subarachnoid haemorrhage are often the presenting lesions. The subarachnoid haemorrhage may organize and result in communicating hydrocephalus. Most intracranial arteries have been affected. In 58 cases which have been published, the terminal internal carotid and its branches have been involved in 13 cases, the middle cerebral artery alone in 17 and the basilar artery alone in 12 cases (I.C. alone 4, I.C.+M.C. 4, one bilateral, I.C.+M.C.+A.C. 4, I.C.+M.C.+A.C.+P.C. 1: M.C. alone 17, A.C. alone 4, A.C.+M.C. 1: V. alone 4, V.+B. 4, B. alone 12, B.+P.C. 2, B.+2P.C. 1) (Stehbens, 1972; Alexander et al, 1979).

Polyarteritis nodosa

This is an acute and subacute disease of medium and small sized arteries usually affecting the kidneys, the heart and the gastrointestinal system, sometimes the peripheral nerves (20–50%) muscle (40–80%), and the central nervous system (10–20% of cases). The primary lesion appears to be subendothelial oedema followed by fibrinoid or hyaline necrosis of the media, destruction of the internal elastic lamina and infiltration of all coats by inflammatory cells. These changes often involve only part of the circumference of the artery, as seen on cross-section. The cellular infiltration is most abundant in the adventitia. It is composed of neutrophil polymorphonuclear leucocytes, large and small mononuclear cells and eosinophil leucocytes which may be very numerous (Fig. 3.22). Secondary thrombus may occlude the vessel; nodular dilatation or, seldom, aneurysm formation or rupture may occur. In the central nervous system the walls of the arteries are so thin that rupture with haemorrhage frequently occurs. In the healing or healed stage the damaged structures are replaced by fibrous tissue and there is intimal narrowing. Polyarteritis nodosa may follow streptococcal infection, drug sensitivity and rheumatoid arthritis and is of the nature of a hypersensitivity reaction (Goetz, 1980).

Systemic lupus erythematosus (S.L.E.)

A neurological complication in S.L.E. is a frequent occurrence. Disorders of mental function, epilepsy, cranial nerve lesions, hemiparesis, disorders of movement, myelopathy or peripheral neuropathies

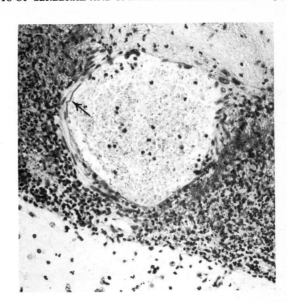

Fig. 3.22 Polyarteritis nodosa. Dilated small leptomeningeal artery. Only a portion of the internal elastic lamina is visible (arrow) and most of the muscularis is destroyed. Polymorphonuclear leucocytes infiltrate the outer coats of the artery and the adjacent leptomeninges. Celloidin; haematoxylin van Gieson. ×75. (Greenfield's Neuropathology, 3rd edn. Arnold, London.)

indicate widespread lesions. Such patients may have renal disease or be hypertensive. Radiological occlusions of major cervical and intracranial arteries have occasionally been seen (Trevor et al, 1972). These patients may have Libman–Sachs endocarditis, from which some authors (Fox et al, 1980) consider that emboli can arise; emboli which having impacted and caused infarction could then either remain or disintegrate and vanish. In patients in whom, at autopsy, cerebral lesions are expected, there is often nothing macroscopically visible, or there may be large or multiple small intracerebral haemorrhages or large often haemorrhagic, infarcts. A carotid artery in the neck may be thrombosed (Bennett et al, 1972), or old or recent fibro-cellular intimal narrowing or occlusion of major cerebral, or small leptomeningeal arteries (Morsier, 1962) may be present (Figs 3.23 & 3.24), or various combinations of necrosis with fibrinoid degeneration and proliferative thickening of small arteries (less than 100 μm diam.) may be visible microscopically (Richardson, 1980). Usually however the lesions are less marked. In 20 out of their series of 24 autopsied cases (Johnson &

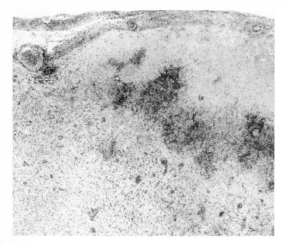

Fig. 3.23 Systemic lupus erythematosus. Cortical lesion of a coagulative necrotic nature infiltrated peripherally by mononuclear cells and nuclear debris. Small vessels have thickened walls with cellular infiltration. Celloidin; haematoxylin and eosin.

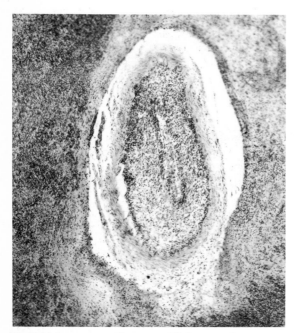

Fig. 3.24 Same case as Figure 3.23. Died 6 years after presence of numerous L.E. cells confirmed diagnosis. Despite treatment disease remained active. At autopsy there was a haemorrhagic occipital infarct within distribution of this leptomeningeal artery in which there is cellular endarteritic stenosis. The adjacent cortex is infarcted. Celloidin; haematoxylin and eosin. × 24.

Richardson, 1968), there were multiple micro-infarcts or increased pericapillary microglia. The almost universal change was prominence of the endothelial cells of the capillaries. Sometimes the arterioles showed fibrinoid degeneration or hyalinization. The changes in the arterioles and capillaries were considered by them to be morphologically similar to those seen in hypertensive encephalopathy and thrombocytopenic purpura. The damaged vascular walls were not infiltrated by inflammatory cells and did not resemble the changes seen in polyarteritis nodosa. It is not possible to point to any single distinctive or definitely diagnostic neuropathological feature in S.L.E., though the features in combination seem to have a pattern which is not quite like any other condition. Deposits of immune complexes or immunoglobulins in the walls of the diseased vessels have not so far been found, but, in patients with neuropsychiatric manifestations, immune complex deposits, closely resembling those found in the glomeruli in lupus nephritis, have been shown in the choroid plexus (Richardson, 1980).

Granulomatous angiitis. This rare condition, of unknown aetiology, is usually restricted to the central nervous system, but it may be a generalised disease. It affects individuals of either sex from the 2nd decade onwards. It may run an acute course or may persist for nine months to five years. In the brain and cord it involves all sizes of arteries and sometimes veins, especially small leptomeningeal vessels. The extracranial carotid and vertebral arteries are occasionally involved. The vessel walls are surrounded (Fig. 3.25) or infiltrated by small and large mononuclear cells and multinucleated giant cells. Sometimes the vessel walls are necrotic with fibrinoid infiltration. In older lesions, collagen replaces the damaged wall and narrows the lumen. Infarcts of various ages and sizes are found in the nervous parenchyma. It differs from giant celled (temporal) arteritis in involving small arteries and veins and from sarcoidosis in that vessel walls are sometimes necrotic. The cerebrospinal fluid is under raised pressure and it usually contains an excess of cells and of protein (Jellinger, 1977).

Arteritis and aneurysms caused by fungal infections

Fungal arteritis and aneurysms of the brain may be blood borne from a primary focus usually in the lungs, or they may be secondary to local infection

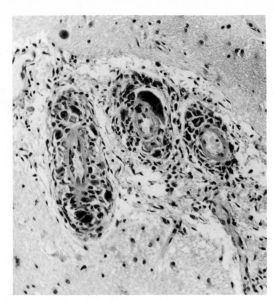

Fig. 3.25 Granulomatous angiitis. Small leptomeningeal arteries cuffed by multinucleate giant cells and large and small mononuclear cells. PAS and haematoxylin. × 125.

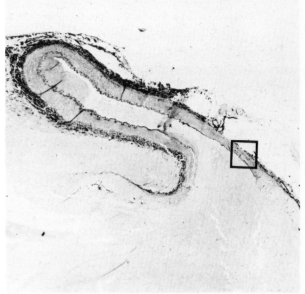

Fig. 3.26 Intracranial vertebral artery involved in meningovascular infection, by aspergillus flavus. Top left of picture the mycotic aneurysm has ruptured. Grocott's methenamine silver technique for fungi, which also impregnates collagen and elastica. × 24.

in the paranasal air sinuses. Under suitable warm condition fungal spores are numerous in the environment. Usually man is resistant but, in drug addicts, or in those exposed to abundant infected dust or when suffering from debilitating disease or under treatment with immunosuppresive drugs, the lungs or air sinuses may be infected. Certain fungi appear to have a predeliction for spreading in the walls of blood vessels and these may cause aneurysms and haemorrhage or thrombosis with infarction.

Aspergillus, fumigatus or *flavus,* often spreads from a granuloma of the orbit or paranasal air sinuses and may involve the wall of arteries such as the internal carotid, middle cerebral or vertebral (Figs 3.26 & 3.27). (Partridge & Chin, 1981.) The organisms, with septate hyphae of fairly uniform size, 3–6 µm diam., produce a granulomatous reaction, with caseation, mononuclear cells, plasma cells, eosinophil leucocytes and multinucleated giant cells. When the fungus comes from a focus in the lung it is more likely to affect small arteries, producing haemorrhagic infarction in cortex and white matter. Such cases may resemble acute haemorrhagic leucoencephalitis macroscopically (Burston & Blackwood, 1963).

Mucormycosis (phycomycosis). Here the infection

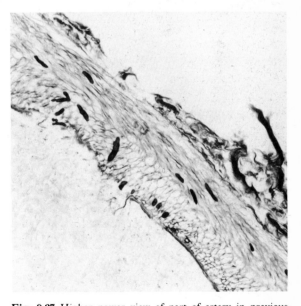

Fig. 3.27 Higher power view of part of artery in previous picture (square) showing fungi in vessel wall. The granulomatous cellular response is not visible in these preparations impregnated by Grocott's methenamine silver technique. × 196.

usually starts in the paranasal air sinuses and
spreads, by the arterial walls, to orbit, meninges
and brain. The arterial wall is invaded by the fungi
and becomes necrotic. The lumen is often occluded
by infected thrombus. There is an acute inflammatory cell infiltration of the vessel wall; mono-
nuclears and giant cells may be present. The fungi
have large, branching, non-septate hyphae 3–
12 μm diameter.

Candida albicans reaches the brain by the blood
stream. It may come from the lungs or gastrointestinal tract and it may cause leptomeningitis,
abscesses with a predominantly lymphocytic, plas-
mocytic reaction, or granulomata, with invasion of
the walls of the cortical blood vessels and secondary
thrombosis, infarction or multiple petechiae. It
may also reach the brain in the form of infected
vegetations from mycotic endocarditis, a complication of cardiac surgery. In such a case death may
be due to a ruptured mycotic aneurysm.

Nocardia asteroides usually comes from a pulmonary focus and causes abscesses. These are not
well encapsulated and in their walls is a feltwork of
numerous delicate tangled hyphae, about 1 μm
diam., which are occasionally branched. The
cellular response is usually neutrophil polymorph
leucocytic (Stehbens, 1972; Fetter et al, 1967).

Thrombotic microangiopathy

This is a rare generalised condition affecting
adolescents and young adults more often than older
persons, with the clinical features of fever, purpura,
haemolytic anaemia and thrombo-cytopenia. The
central nervous system is frequently involved. Here
Adams et al (1948) found that the lesions were
predominantly in the grey matter, consisting of
hyperplasia of endothelial and probably of adventitial cells, of terminal arterioles and capillaries
(Figs 3.28 & 3.29). The diameter of the vessels was
increased, sometimes the walls of the vessels were
necrotic. The vessels were occluded by acidophilic
thrombi. There were foci of damage to nerve cells,
occasional proliferation of glia, but proportionately
less than the vascular involvement. Petechial
haemorrhages were sometimes present. The
thrombi are mainly composed of platelet aggregates, with a variable quantity of fibrin. Neame et
al (1976), considered that the condition was one in

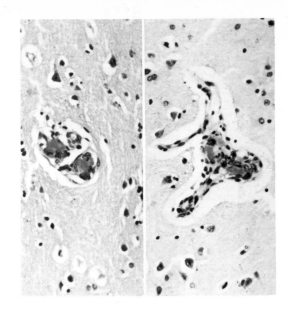

Figs 3.28 & 3.29 Thrombotic micro-angiopathy. Hyaline
eosinophilic thrombus obstructs the dilated lumen at the
arteriolocapillary junction zone where there is endothelial
hyperplasia. The adjacent grey matter does not show any
significant abnormality. Paraffin; haematoxylin and eosin.
× 200. (Reproduced by courtesy of Professor W. Symmers.)

which intravascular consumption of platelets results in disseminated platelet thrombosis. Lian et
al (1979) suggest that there is a deficiency of an
unspecified 'platelet aggregating factor inhibitor',
resulting in a widespread formation of platelet
thrombi in the microcirculation. Some of the
pathological features have been seen in systemic
lupus erythematosus and the two conditions have
been found together.

Disseminated intravascular coagulation
(consumption coagulopathy, intravascular
coagulation fibrinolysis syndrome, acquired
hypofibrinogenaemia)

This condition may follow tissue damage due to
trauma, including trauma to the brain, surgical
operations, heat stroke, burns, dissecting aneurysms, infection by bacteria, viruses, protozoa or
rickettsia, immunological disturbances such as
immune-complex disorders, allograft rejection,
incompatible blood transfusions, obstetric disorders such as abruptio placentae, amniotic fluid
embolism, retained foetal products, eclampsia,

diabetic keto-acidosis, mucin secreting adenocarcinomata, leukaemia, cyanotic congenital heart disease, cavernous haemangioma, shock, snake bite or fat embolism. In many of these conditions there is damage to body tissue, including the endothelial cells of blood vessels, which releases thromboplastic substances into the blood. Injury to red blood corpuscles releases phospholipids which are known to accelerate clotting. Fibrin, either soluble or insoluble, is formed, especially in brain, kidneys, gastro-intestinal tract and lungs, and intravascular coagulation occurs, with ischaemic lesions. Clotting factors and platelets are locally consumed, so that they are decreased in the circulating blood. Often there is a secondary fibrinolytic response, with an increase, in the circulating blood, of fibrin degradation products which have anticoagulant properties of their own. These features often swing the balance so that haemorrhagic rather than coagulative, ischaemic, lesions are found. Distorted or fragmented red blood corpuscles are often observed in the blood during life, features which suggest that they have been damaged in passing through the deposited strands of fibrin in the vessels. Should the patient with cerebral symptoms, come to autopsy there may be no visible change, there may be scattered dusky ischaemic regions deep in the cortical sulci, there may be small infarcts, petechial haemorrhages or even massive intracerebral haemorrhage.

Microscopically the vessels may appear healthy, possibly due to postmortem fibrinolysis or because the coagulative process had got no further than the formation of soluble fibrin. Diagnostically, however, fibrin-rich thrombi are seen in short lengths of arterioles, capillaries and venules; it seems likely that these originally formed in the systemic circulation, as fibrin aggregates, which then became impacted in the smaller vessels. Globules of fibrin are sometimes seen, lying free in larger and smaller vessels. The surrounding tissue may show various degrees of damage, from focal neuronal and glial vacuolation, or perivascular demyelination or necrosis, to regions of complete necrosis with or without haemorrhage. In young people, where the fibrinolytic response is usually vigorous the changes may be mostly haemorrhagic, with little or no evidence of fibrin in vessels (Hamilton et al, 1978; Davies-Jones et al, 1980).

Moya-moya disease

('A hazy scene, of smoke floating or trailing' Jap.) This unusual variety of cerebro-vascular disease (Figs 3.30, 3.31 & 3.32) is named after the angiographic appearance of an extensive fine anastomotic network in the region of the basal perforating and pial arteries. There is subtotal or non-filling of the circle of Willis and narrowing or occlusion of the terminal portions of both internal carotid arteries (Figs 3.30, 3.31 & 3.32). Kudo (1968) described twelve such cases, eight juvenile (age of onset 4–13 yrs), four adult (age of onset 40–56 yrs). Since then some 600 cases from Japan and some 70 cases from outside Japan, sometimes familial, have been reported (Kitahara et al, 1979; Coakham et al, 1979).

In the juvenile cases the symptoms are of milder onset but recurrent and are associated with infarcts, whilst in adults there is often subarachnoid or intracerebral haemorrhage. Adequate postmortem studies have been few. The surface arteries have been described as being generally hypoplastic, or with hypoplasia of one or other constituent of the arterial wall. The internal elastic lamina has either been excessively infolded and thickened or was intermittent or absent. The circle of Willis, or the anterior half of the circle of Willis, and the internal carotid arteries have been described as hypoplastic or narrowed by fibro-cellular intimal thickening.

In Coakham et al's case (aged 51), the pial anastomotic network was very noticeable. Engorged vessels, of up to 1 mm diameter, were visible in the basal ganglia and deep white matter, which microscopically were of capillary or venular type. Intermittent lengths of one anterior cerebral, both middle cerebral and one posterior communicating artery were thin and white with a markedly folded internal elastic lamina and a lumen which was occluded by a fine connective tissue web, (appearances reminiscent of those seen, in border zone arteries following hypotension, by Romanul & Abramowicz, 1964). The main arteries were accompanied by leashes of numerous thin walled vessels with which they communicated. The posterior cerebral and basilar arteries were unaffected; one vertebral artery was occluded by recent thrombus. The intracranial portions of the internal

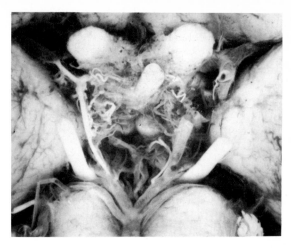

Figs 3.30, 3.31 & 3.32 Case of moya-moya disease, marked on right side, where there was fibro-cellular occlusion of the intracranial internal carotid and the posterior communicating arteries. The left posterior communicating artery (Fig. 3.32) has been accidently cut. The intracranial vertebral arteries were stenosed. From the terminal basilar artery and the proximal posterior cerebral arteries there was hypertrophy of the paramedian perforating arteries (Fig. 3.32). Figure 3.31 shows the atrophy of the right cerebral hemisphere due to old infarction and the dilated lenticulostriate arteries. Patient had normal birth, fits at 3 weeks, later left hemiplegia recognised, mentally retarded. Right carotid angiogram at age 13 years revealed a moya-moya picture (Dr. J. A. E. Ambrose). The patient died at 17 yrs.

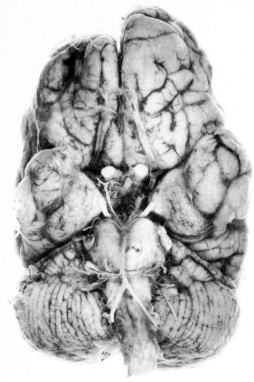

Fig. 3.30

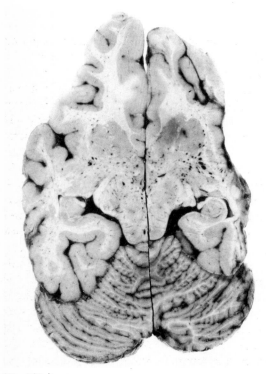

Fig. 3.31

carotid arteries were not stenosed, an uncharacteristic finding in Moya-moya.

The above findings belong to the much more numerous idiopathic group, of which there are not, as yet, enough adequate clinicopathological studies (Nishimoto & Takeuchi, 1972) to allow us to decide whether the striking anastomotic arterial network at the base of the brain develops from a congenital abnormality, or from obstruction of the circle of Willis, or from both, or from some other cause. There is a much smaller group in which a rich collateral circulation has been seen, secondary to an optic nerve glioma in neurofibromatosis, to stenotic neoplasms, to basal meningitis (tuberculous or pyogenic) or to atherosclerosis.

Endarteritis obliterans

When the leptomeninges, especially at the base of the brain, are involved by a chronic or low grade bacterial leptomeningitis, the arteries may show a considerable narrowing of the lumen as a result of subendothelial cellular infiltration.

Tuberculous arteritis (Figs 3.33 & 3.34). The meshes of the pia-arachnoid are infiltrated by lymphocytes, plasma cells, large mononuclear cells

and abundant fibrin. Close to the vessels the exudate is caseous. Vascular changes are prominent. The arteries, and often the veins, show infiltration of the adventitia and to a lesser extent, the media by lymphocytes, plasma cells and

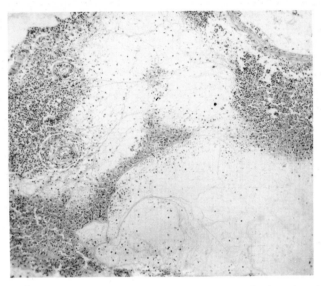

Fig. 3.33 Tuberculous arteritis. Exudate in the subarachnoid space in a case of tuberculous leptomeningitis showing the abundance of fibrin, the copious cellular exudate and the arterial involvement.

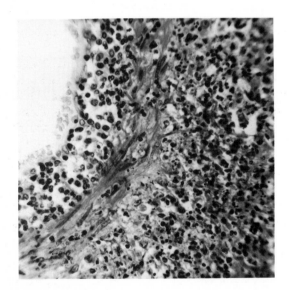

Fig. 3.34 Higher power of an artery in tuberculous leptomeningitis showing infiltration of the subendothelial layer, the media and the adventitia by lymphocytes and histocytes. Necrosis of the arterial wall and thrombosis in the lumen are common sequelae, with ischaemic damage in the adjacent brain. Haematoxylin and eosin. × 350.

mononuclear cells. The endothelium is separated from the usually intact internal elastic lamina by inflammatory cells, so that the lumen is narrowed. Fibrinoid necrosis of the vessel wall and thrombosis occur. Regions of ischaemic necrosis may be found in the distribution of the perforating arteries. If treatment is instituted late or is inadequate, collagenous tissue replaces the inflamed regions, in particular around the narrowed lumen.

Syphilitic arteritis (Fig. 3.35). The classical type (Heubner's arteritis), which is found in meningovascular syphilis, affects large and medium sized meningeal vessels. The adventitia is thickened and infiltrated by lymphocytes and plasma cells. The media is fibrosed or thinned and may be infiltrated with inflammatory cells. The internal elastic lamina is usually intact. The intima is concentrically or eccentrically thickened by fibroblastic or collagenous tissue, so that the lumen is reduced in size. Thrombosis may occur and there are ischaemic lesions in its zone of supply. Gummatous necrosis, which is necrosis of collagenous tissue,

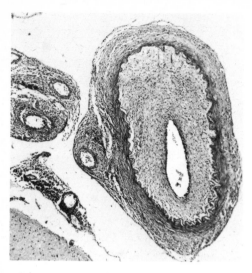

Fig. 3.35 Syphilitic arteritis. Cerebral artery in meningo-vascular syphilis showing marked concentric intimal fibrosis. The internal elastic lamina appears intact. The media is damaged but less noticeably. All regions are infiltrated by lymphocytes and plasma cells. Haematoxylin and eosin. × 40.

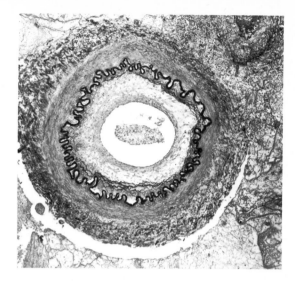

Fig. 3.36 Artery at the base of the brain, pneumococcal leptomeningitis, treated sulpha drugs, one month duration. Fibrinous exudate is present around the artery which shows a thickened adventitia, a normal looking media and internal elastic lamina and concentric fibro-cellular intimal thickening. An adjacent artery, top right of picture, shows necrosis and cellular infiltration of its wall. Weigert's elastic van Gieson. × 57. (Greenfield's Neuropathology, 3rd edn. Arnold, London.)

may occur in the adventitia and media (Harriman, 1976).

Pyogenic arteritis. In subacute or chronic pyogenic meningitis, due to avirulent organisms or to unsuccessful antibiotic or chemical treatment, the arteries in the basal cisterns and over the surface of the cord are surrounded by inflammatory exudate for a long period and proliferative fibrous endoarteritis occurs (Fig. 3.36). Cairns & Russell (1946) found such changes in pneumococcal meningitis treated with sulphapyridine, sulphadiazine and/or penicillin. In addition smaller arteries showed fibrinoid necrosis of their walls.

ANEURYSMS — SACCULAR

Almost all saccular aneurysms of the circle of Willis arise at, or very close to, the regions of division of arteries. About 30 per cent are found on the 1st or 2nd point of branching of the middle cerebral artery in the Sylvian fissure, about 25 per cent are at the junction of the anterior cerebral and anterior communicating arteries, about 20 per cent are at the junction of the internal carotid and posterior communicating arteries and about 12–15 per cent are at the junction of the basilar artery and

its branches. In 20–30 per cent of patients they are multiple. It is unlikely that they are present at birth, few occur under the age of 20 years, the majority present between the ages of 40 and 70 years, with peak incidence between 50–60.

Saccular aneurysms are found in the region where there is a developmental gap in the muscularis. The endothelium, internal elastic membrane and the thin adventitia bulge outwards. Proximal to the neck of an aneurysm, inelastic intimal thickenings or pads are found. These contain an increased number of smooth muscle cells, fine elastic fibrils and fibrous tissue, an appearance similar to atheroma. These pads are present not only near to aneurysms, but similar smaller pads are found proximal to, at and distal to the point of bifurcation of arteries of the circle of Willis in younger persons and in bifurcations without aneurysms (Sheffield & Weller, 1980).

Further into the aneurysm the elastica is no longer present and the wall is composed only of collagen, which is continuous with the thin adventitia of the parent artery. Initially endothelial cells line the sac but later this lining is incomplete. Angiography usually reveals that there is some blood flow through the aneurysm, but it is slowed and is unlikely to be laminar. Thrombus is deposited on the wall of the sac, giving rise to atheromatous change. In large aneurysms calcification may outline the sac, whilst the lumen may be largely occupied by laminated thrombus. Focal weakness of the wall leads to multiloculation.

Saccular aneurysms usually rupture near the fundus, whence the blood may pass:

(1) into the subarachnoid space
(2) into the overlying brain, forming a haematoma or rupturing into a ventricle
(3) infrequently, into the subdural space, having torn apart the adhesions, the sequel to previous leaks, which bind the aneurysmal sac to the arachnoid.

Rupture of an aneurysm is often associated with pale ischaemic lesions, in cortex and white matter, not only in the field of supply of the parent artery but often in other territories. If the patient survives a generalised subarachnoid haemorrhage, this may organize and produce communicating hydrocephalus.

Many factors have to be considered in the development of a saccular aneurysm of the circle of Willis. It develops in a region where there is usually and normally a gap in the media, a gap which increases in size with age. Though these gaps are found in other arteries of the body, the cerebral arteries lack the support of an external elastic lamina and the adventitial coat is thin and is supported only by the cerebro-spinal fluid and the leptomeninges. In cerebral arteries inelastic intimal pads develop which increase in size with age, and they may well produce alterations in normal blood flow and stresses at the bifurcations. Evidence is now accumulating that hypertension is no more likely to be present in aneurysm cases than in an age matched general population, except for females aged 18–54 years, in whom the mean diastolic is raised 10–15 mmHg and in persons with multiple aneurysms (Andrews & Spiegel, 1979). It is surprising that aneurysms are more often single than multiple (Stehbens, 1972; Yates, 1976; Crompton, 1976; Sheffield & Weller, 1980).

The carotid artery in the cavernous sinus has four small branches and is surrounded by venous blood. A communication may develop between the arterial and venous streams, secondary to fracture of the base of the skull, to rupture of a small intracavernous saccular carotid aneurysm, or in association with atherosclerotic degeneration of the carotid artery. Arterial blood enters the venous sinus and its tributaries, there is proptosis of the eye, a bruit and paralysis of the 3rd, 4th and 6th cranial nerves. Spontaneous cure sometimes occurs, probably the result of thrombosis closing the fistula (Stern, 1976).

Aneurysms associated with micro-organisms may be bacterial, fungal (mycotic) or amoebic. Bacterial aneurysms may be embolic or metastatic in origin, or they may be secondary to local infection. In *embolic* aneurysms the source of the embolus may be bacterial endocarditis, a septic lesion in the lung, a complication of septicaemia, or pyaemia, or cardiac surgery, or the intravenous fluid line. The aneurysm is usually small and found on the branches of the middle cerebral artery, either in the lateral fissure, or on peripheral small pial branches and then is often multiple. The embolus becomes adherent to the vessel wall which shows a focal, acute, often eccentric, inflammatory reaction. The organisms, such as *strep.viridans, staph aureus, albus, pneumococci, strep.faecalis* or *haemophilus influenzae,* multiply, the arterial wall weakens, bulges and may rupture (Figs 3.37 & 3.38).

Bacterial aneurysms may, very infrequently, be *secondary* to local infection, such as influenzal or pneumococcal meningitis, meningitis secondary to fracture of the skull, or septic cavernous sinus thrombosis, as a sequel to sphenoidal sinusitis, or to subcutaneous infection of its drainage region of the face (Stehbens, 1972).

INTRACRANIAL VASCULAR MALFORMATIONS

Capillary telangiectases are composed of a 'berried bush' like collection of capillary type vessels, with saccular and fusiform dilatations (Fig. 3.39), separated from one another by normal nervous tissue. They are usually small and solitary and are situated in the brainstem, usually pons, in the subcortical cerebral white matter, or in the basal

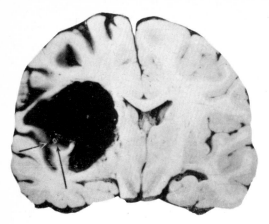

Fig. 3.37 Coronal slice of brain at the level of the substantia nigra, showing massive intracerebral haemorrhage. The arrows point to the middle cerebral artery whose wall has ruptured at this point due to secondary infection from an infected embolus from the heart.

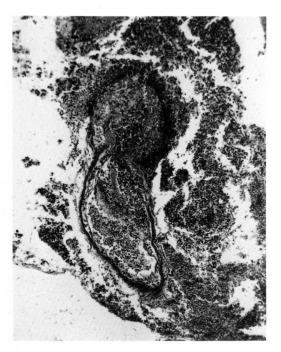

Fig. 3.38 Cerebral artery showing an embolic pyogenic aneurysm. The organisms in the infected embolus are present in the dark stained region at the periphery of the embolus. The arterial wall is weakened and bulging (upwards and to the right) and there has been leakage of blood. Haematoxylin and eosin. × 80.

ganglia. They are usually clinically silent and are found incidentally at autopsy, where they are seen as a focal prominence of small veins and an ill defined, reddish, peppered appearance of the

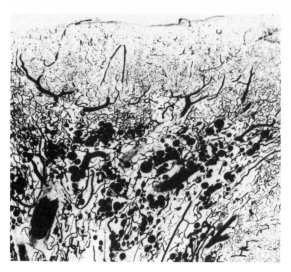

Fig. 3.39 Capillary telangiectasis. Frozen section 200 mμ thick stained by Pickworth's benzidine method to show red blood corpuscles filling the dilated capillaries of a telangiectasis in the occipital cortex and white matter. × 8.

nervous tissue. Feeding vessels are not noticeable. Rarely, if large and suitably situated, they may be associated with clinical signs. Even less often are they recorded as having bled or being associated with fatal haemorrhage (Stehbens, 1972).

Cavernous angiomata are composed of a honeycomb like arrangement of macroscopically small blood filled spaces separated by thin collagenous walls, which are lined by endothelium. Only at the periphery are the walls separated from each other by astrocytic tissue, which is often pigmented by old haemorrhage. They vary in size from minute to massive. Prominent feeding or draining vessels are not present. They occur most often in the cerebrum, subcortically, in the region of the central sulcus, in the basal ganglia, or in the walls of the 3rd ventricle: less often in the pons. They may show signs of thrombosis, organization, calcification or ossification. They are found over a wide age range; in about 25 per cent of cases they are multiple (Russell & Rubinstein, 1977). They may show clinical signs, there is often evidence of old small haemorrhages, some are associated with fatal haemorrhage.

Arteriovenous malformations

The old name of 'serpentine' angioma well describes the tangled mass of dilated vascular channels which is most often found, in the distribution of the middle cerebral artery, extending from the leptomeningeal surface in a pyramidal shape into the depths of the cerebrum. The malformation may be fed, not only by a considerably dilated middle cerebral artery, but also by dilated anterior and posterior cerebral arteries. Saccular aneurysms, sometimes multiple, may be present either on the feeding artery or on apparently uninvolved arteries of the circle of Willis. Haemorrhage can occur from such an aneurysm or from the main mass. The malformations can also be frontal, or occipital, or brainstem in situation. Dissection will often reveal narrow anastomotic vessels, with both elastic and muscle in their walls, connecting arteries and veins. Some of the vessels in the main mass of the angioma have the characteristics of arteries, some of veins, whilst some, which resemble veins, have such an increase of elastic tissue that they merit the name of arterialized veins. The walls of some of the dilated vessels show pathological change, such as fibrosis, adherent intimal thrombus, atheromatous change or calcification. Atrophy of the ipsilateral cerebral hemisphere may be present. The draining dural sinus or sinuses may be enlarged. Secondary cardiac hypertrophy is infrequent, except in young infants (Lagos, 1977; Takashima & Becker, 1980).

Arteriovenous malformation of the vein of Galen

This malformation, which may also become evident over a wide range of ages, is usually supplied by one or both posterior cerebral arteries, which, by means of a relatively small collection of small anastomosing vessels, or an arteriovenous angioma, drain into the vein of Galen, which becomes distended, sometimes to an enormous size. In early infant life there is usually cardiac hypertrophy and failure, after 5 months of age compression of the aqueduct of Sylvius produces obstructive hydrocephalus, at a later age headache or subarachnoid haemorrhage are the principal features (Lagos, 1977; Takashima & Becker, 1980).

Cryptic angiomatous malformations

Occasionally, intracerebral haemorrhage occurs in young normotensive persons and, even if it is fatal

and an autopsy is carried out, one may have great difficulty or fail to find the cause of the haemorrhage. In 20 such cases, all under 40, 15 under 20, Crawford & Russell (1956) were able to demonstrate arteriovenous, or much less often venous, angiomata in the cerebral convexity, or central cerebral region, or the cerebellum.

Neurological complications of the adult type of coarctation of the aorta

In this condition, of unknown aetiology, there is a localized narrowing of the aorta, distal to the origin of the left subclavian artery, at or just below the aortic insertion of the ductus arteriosus, which is almost always obliterated. The blood pressure in the arterial system proximal to the stenosis is raised and the heart is hypertrophied. In the lower part of the body there is arterial hypotension.

In the brain, atheroma of cerebral arteries is well marked and fusiform aneurysms may be present (Stehbens, 1972). Saccular aneurysms, often multiple, which rupture, and spontaneous intracerebral haemorrhage are frequent complications, usually during the third decade (Cochrane & LeBlanc, 1980).

The stenosis of the aorta impedes the arterial blood from reaching the lower part of the body by the usual route. An anastomotic circulation develops, which includes blood passing via the subclavian arteries to the vertebral arteries to the cranial end of the anterior spinal artery, also via the ascending cervical branches of the inferior thyroid arteries and the branches of the thyro-cervical trunks into the upper radicular tributaries of the anterior spinal artery. The blood then flows down the anterior spinal artery to reach the spinal branches of the aortic intercostal arteries below the obstruction. The anterior spinal artery becomes enlarged and tortuous (Edwards et al, 1948). The cord beneath the dilated artery may be softened or spontaneous haemorrhage may occur (Hughes, 1976).

CEREBRAL THROMBOPHLEBITIS AND VENOUS SINUS THROMBOSIS

One of the above may occur alone or they may be combined. The condition may be *primary*, probably due to an abnormality in the circulating blood and not infected. *Secondary*, to pyogenic infection either local or distant may or may not be infected.

Primary thrombosis may complicate malnutrition, dehydration, fever, disease of the heart usually with right heart failure (Barnett & Hyland, 1953), the post-operative state (excluding intracranial operations), head injury, cerebral arterial occlusion, intracerebral haemorrhage, leukaemia, polycythaemia rubra vera, in puerperal women following abortion, and in women taking contraceptive pills. In some of these conditions the blood is more viscous and the blood flow may be slow. In the puerperium there is an increase in plasma fibrinogen (Plass & Matthews, 1926) and both then and following surgical operations the platelets are both increased in number and adhesiveness (Wright, 1942) commencing on the fourth and maximal on the tenth day. During pregnancy the condition is most frequent during the first three months, when the hormonal state has started to change, a feature which probably underlies the association between hormonal contraceptive pill treatment and thrombosis (Atkinson et al, 1970).

The superior longitudinal sinus, where the blood enters against the blood flow, is the most frequently involved sinus and the clot may extend into the lateral sinus. The veins, which drain into the venous sinuses, anastomose freely, so that thrombosis of a short segment of a sinus does not necessarily cause much impairment of the venous drainage of the brain. Extensive thrombosis of a sinus, which is usually associated with thrombosis of the veins which drain into it, causes infarction of the cortex. This infarction is more haemorrhagic than that seen after arterial occlusion (Figs 3.40 & 3.41) and is not sharply limited to the cortex, regions of haemorrhage being present in the underlying white matter.

Secondary thrombosis occurs as a sequel to subdural abscess or to pyogenic infection of the frontal air sinuses (superior sagittal sinus), the mastoid air spaces or middle ear (lateral sinus), pyogenic infection of the eye, cheek, nose, upper jaw, ethmoidal or sphenoidal air sinus (cavernous sinus). Involvement of the sinus may follow involvement of its wall by an adjacent pyogenic process, or may be by retrograde venous thrombosis. If the thrombus in the sinus is infected,

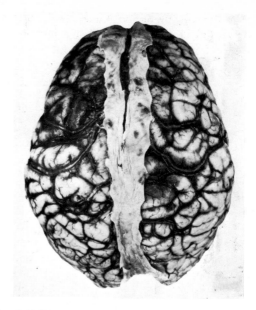

Fig. 3.40 Thrombosis of the superior sagittal sinus, and thrombophlebitis of the cortical veins which are distended by partly pale, partly dark thrombus. Note the marked perivenular subarachnoid haemorrhage. Clinically three days' duration. Puerperal woman with breast abscess. (Greenfield's Neuropathology, 3rd edn. Arnold, London.)

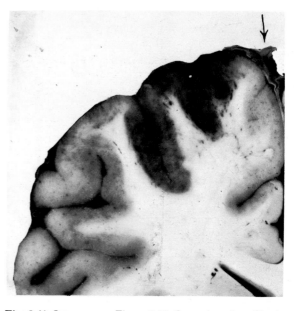

Fig. 3.41 Same case as Figure 3.40. Coronal section of brain showing thrombus in the superior sagittal sinus (arrow), with swelling and gross haemorrhagic streaking of the cortex and the underlying white matter. (Greenfield's Neuropathology, 3rd edn. Arnold, London.)

portions of it may be carried in the bloodstream to the heart and lungs, giving rise to pyaemia and abscesses (Yates, 1976).

SPINAL CORD

Blood supply. Branches of the anterior spinal artery supply all the spinal cord except the posterior white columns and the posterior grey horns which are supplied by the two posterior spinal arteries. The anterior spinal artery is formed initially by the fusion of the anterior spinal branches of the vertebral arteries. In its course down the spinal cord it receives a variable number of contributions from the radicular arteries. Above the 2nd thoracic segment these come from branches of the subclavian artery, below they come from branches of the aorta. In the region of the cauda equina the anterior spinal artery anastomoses with the two posterior spinal arteries in which the blood flow is rostral as high as the upper thoracic level. Cranially the two posterior spinal arteries arise from the vertebral or posterior inferior cerebellar arteries and the flow is caudal. Numerous radicular tributaries join the posterior spinal arteries. The venous drainage of the cord is through abundant and anastomosing vessels (Stehbens, 1972; Hughes, 1978).

Even allowing for its lesser volume, the spinal cord has less often been recorded as suffering from hypoxic or ischaemic lesions than the brain, except in the case of caisson disease, which particularly affects the white matter of the rostral thoracic cord (Haymaker, 1957). In particular, hypertensive changes are less marked; hypertensive haemorrhages have not been recorded. The complications of atherosclerosis, even in respect of its main and often atheromatous sources of supply, the vertebral and subclavian arteries and the aorta, are infrequent. The circulatory disorders which affect the spinal cord may be considered on an anatomical basis. As with those which affect the brain one should first think of the heart, even though spinal lesions due to generalized hypotension or cardiac emboli have seldom been published.

Lesions of aortic origin. Atheromatous (cholesterol) embolism to the spinal cord, but without softening, presumably from an aortic atheromatous ulcer, was seen by Soloway & Aronson (1964).

Wolman & Bradshaw (1967), in a similar case, considered that the atheromatous emboli were arrested at the origins or bifurcations of radicular arteries. In the affected cord (D2–10) the main lesion consisted of a crescentic region of infarction lying in the border zone of distribution between the central branches of the anterior spinal artery and the penetrating branches of the peripheral circumferential pial arteries.

Occlusions of the aorta during surgical procedures. Adams & van Geertruyden (1956) concluded that if the occlusion is above the origin of the renal arteries then ischaemia of the spinal cord may occur, if below the origin of the renal arteries then the cord escapes.

Vertebral arterial occlusion. The vertebral arteries are at risk as they run through the foramina in the transverse processes (C1–6). In Hughes' (1964) two cases, undue movement of the mobile lower cervical spine had torn the C5–6 intervertebral disc, both vertebral arteries were compressed and the lower cervical cord was infarcted.

Radicular arterial occlusion can be caused by atheromatous embolism, neoplasms invading intervertebral foramina, or tuberculous infection.

Anterior spinal artery occlusion. In the earlier reports syphilitic arteritis was the usual cause; nowadays it is more likely to be due to trauma or cervical spondylosis. Atheroma is a very rare cause (Hughes, 1978). Embolism of fibrocartilage, into both the anterior spinal artery and into veins from the nucleus pulposus, has been reported (Hubert et al, 1974). When the anterior spinal artery is occluded, the infarction is in the distribution of the artery, always involving the anterior grey horns and the grey commissure, usually the anterior white columns, and a variable amount of the lateral white columns.

Posterior spinal arterial occlusion was initially reported to be caused by syphilitic arteritis, more recently by indirect trauma, atheromatous embolization, or the injection of intrathecal phenol (Hughes, 1978).

Arteriosclerosis

Jellinger & Neumeyer (1962) and Hughes & Brownell (1966) have described patients of 65 and over, with 8 months to 10 years of progressive impairment of both upper and lower motor neuronal function, with severe aortic atheroma, who had ischaemic lesions in the spinal cord, especially in the anterior horns. Jellinger (1967) pointed out that the lesions were most marked between C5 and T2, the region of overlap between the vertebral, subclavian and the aortic supplies. He noted the fibrous thickening and stenosis of the small intraspinal arteries, which must diminish the vascular reserve in the presence of hypotension.

Acute venous infarction. This rare condition, secondary to generalized sepsis, spinal cord neoplasia or a thrombotic state, manifests itself in spinal, or extra spinal, venous thrombosis and necrosis of the cord, which is very haemorrhagic even to the extent of haematoma formation. The infarction is more extensive than that following arterial obstruction, the necrosis is less complete and the margin is less distinct (Hughes, 1971).

Chronic spinal thrombophlebitis. Subacute necrotic myelitis or Foix-Alajouanine disease, is now considered by most authors to be a misnomer for a spinal arteriovenous malformation (Pia & Djindjian, 1978).

Acknowledgements

We are indebted to Professor W. Symmers, Drs J. V. Diengdoh, R. O. Barnard, C. Hunter-Craig, W. G. P. Mair and R. Sarvesvaren for histological material; to the editors and publishers of Brain for Figure 3.25, to the editor of the Post-graduate Medical Journal for Figures 3.33–3.35, 3.37 and 3.38; to Professor J. H. Adams and to John Wright and Sons, publishers of Gradwohl's Legal Medicine 3rd edition 1976 for Figure 3.8; to Professor P. O. Yates (Fig. 3.2), to Dr J. B. Brierley (Figs 3.3, 3.4 and 3.6) and to Edward Arnold, publishers of Greenfield's Neuropathology 3rd edition 1976 for Figures 3.1, 3.2, 3.3, 3.4, 3.6, 3.11–3.17, 3.20–3.22, 3.36, 3.40 and 3.41; to Beryl Bailey, Marion Jackson, Elizabeth Lorentzen and Betty Travers, librarians, Marion Hudson, James Mills, Mary Pugh and Robert Wade, photographers, Keith Laker and Roy Stanbury, medical laboratory scientific officers and Sheila Reynolds, secretary, for all their help.

REFERENCES

Adams J H 1976 The neuropathy of cerebral hypoxia. In: Camps F E (ed) Gradwohl's legal medicine, 3rd edn. Wright, Bristol, ch 18

Adams H D, van Geertruydin H H 1956 Neurologic complications of aortic surgery. Annals of Surgery 144:574–610

Adams R D, Cammermeyer J, Fitzgerald P J 1948 Neuropathological aspects of thrombocytic acroangiothrombosis clinico-anatomical study of generalised platelet thrombosis. Journal of Neurology Neurosurgery and Psychiatry 11:27–43

Alexander C B, Burger P C, Goree J A 1979 Dissecting aneurysms of the basilar artery in 2 patients. Stroke 10:294–299

Alexander L, Putnam T J 1938 Pathological alterations in cerebral vascular patterns. Proceedings Association for Research in Nervous and Mental Disease 18:471–543 Williams & Wilkins, Baltimore

Allsop C J, Gallagher P J 1981 Temporal artery biopsy in giant cell arteritis — a reappraisal. American Journal of Surgical Pathology 5:317–323

Andrew R J, Spiegel P K 1979 Intracranial aneurysms: age, sex, blood pressure and multiplicity in an unselected series of patients. Journal of Neurosurgery 51:27–32

Atkinson E A, Fairburn B, Heathfield K W 1970 Intracranial venous thrombosis as complication of oral contraception. Lancet i:914–918

Barnett H J M, Hyland H H 1953 Non-infective intracranial venous thrombosis. Brain 76:36–49

Bennett R, Hughes G R V, Bywaters E G L, Holt P J L 1972 Neuropsychiatric problems in systemic lupus erythematosus. British Medical Journal 4:342–345

Blackwood W, Hallpike J F, Kocen R S, Mair W G P 1969 Atheromatous disease of the carotid arterial system and embolism from the heart in cerebral infarction: a morbid anatomical study. Brain 92:897–910

Bradbury M 1979 The concept of a blood-brain barrier. Wiley, Chichester

Brierley J B 1976 Cerebral hypoxia. In: Blackwood W, Corsellis J A N (eds) Greenfield's neuropathology, 3rd edn. Arnold, London

Burston J, Blackwood W 1963 A case of aspergillus infection of the brain. Journal of Pathology and Bacteriology 86:225–229

Cairns H, Russell D S 1946 Cerebral arteritis and phlebitis in pneumococcal meningitis. Journal of Pathology and Bacteriology 58:649–665

Coakham H B, Duchen L W, Scaravilli F 1979 Moya-moya disease clinical and pathological report of a case with associated myopathy. Journal of Neurology Neurosurgery and Psychiatry 42:289–297

Cochrane D D, LeBlanc F E 1980 Lesions of the aorta and their neurological complications. In: Vinken P J, Bruyn G W (eds) Handbook of clinical neurology. North Holland Publishing Co, Amsterdam, vol 39

Crawford J V, Russell D S 1956 Cryptic arteriovenous and venous hamartomas of brain. Journal of Neurology Neurosurgery and Psychiatry 19:1–11

Crompton M R 1959 The visual changes in (temporal) giant cell arteritis. Brain 82:377–390

Crompton M R 1976 Pathology of degenerative cerebral arterial disease. In: Russell R W R (ed) Cerebral arterial disease. Churchill Livingstone, Edinburgh

Dalal P M 1973 The aortic arch syndrome. In: Spillane J D (ed) Tropical neurology. Oxford University Press, Oxford

Dalal P M, Shah P M, Aiyar R R 1965 Arteriographic study of cerebral embolism. Lancet 2:358–361

Davies-Jones G A B, Preston F E, Timperley W R 1980 Neurological complications in clinical haematology. Blackwell, Oxford

Edwards J E, Clagett O T, Drake R L, Christensen N A 1948 Collateral circulation in co-arctation of the aorta. Proceedings of the Mayo Clinic 23:333–334

Escourelle R, Poirier J 1978 Manual of basic neuropathology, 2nd edn. Saunders, Philadelphia

Fetter B F, Klintworth G K, Hendry W S 1967 Mycoses of the central nervous system. William & Wilkins, Baltimore

Fisher C M 1977 Bilateral occlusion of basilar artery branches. Journal of Neurology Neurosurgery and Psychiatry 40:1182–1189

Fox I S, Spence A M, Wheelis R F, Healey L A 1980 Cerebral embolism in Libman-Sacks endocarditis. Neurology 30:487–491

Gautier J C 1979 Arterial pathology in cerebral ischaemia and infarction. In: Greenhalgh R M, Rose F C (eds) Progress in stroke research. Pitman Medical Publishing, Tunbridge Wells, ch 3

Goetz C G 1980 Polyarteritis nodosa. In: Vinken P J and Bruyn G W (eds) Handbook of clinical neurology. North Holland Publishing Co, Amsterdam, vol 39

Hamilton P J, Stalker A L, Douglas A S 1978 Disseminated intravascular coagulation: a review. Journal of Clinical Pathology 31:609–619

Harriman D G F 1976 Bacterial infections of the nervous system. In: Blackwood W, Corsellis J A N (eds) Greenfields neuropathology, 3rd edn. Arnold, London

Haymaker W 1957 Decompression sickness. In: W. Scholz (ed) Handbuch der Speziellen Pathologischen Anatomie und Histologie. Springer, Berlin, vol XIII/IB, p 1600–1672

Hubert J-P, Ectors M, Ketelbant-Balasse P, Flamant-Durand J 1974 Fibrocartilaginous venous and arterial emboli from the nucleus pulposus in the anterior spinal system. European Neurology 11:164–171

Hughes J T 1964 Vertebral artery insufficiency in acute cervical spinal trauma. International Journal of Paraplegia 1:1–14

Hughes J T 1971 Venous infarction of the cord. Neurology (Minneapolis) 21:794–800

Hughes J T 1976 Disease of the spine and spinal cord. In: Blackwood W, Corsellis J A N (ed) Greenfield's neuropathology, 3rd edn. Arnold, London

Hughes J T 1978 Pathology of the spinal cord, 2nd edn. Lloyd-Luke, London

Hughes J T, Brownell B 1966 Spinal cord ischaemia due to arteriosclerosis. Archives of Neurology (Chicago) 15:189–202

Imparato A M, Riles T S, Gorstein F 1979 The carotid bifurcation plaque: pathologic findings associated with cerebral ischaemia. Stroke 10:238–245

Jellinger K 1967 Spinal cord arteriosclerosis and progressive vascular myelopathy. Journal of Neurology Neurosurgery and Psychiatry 30:195–206

Jellinger K 1977 Giant cell granulomatous angiitis of the central nervous system. Journal of Neurology 215:175–190

Jellinger K, Neumayer E 1962 Myelopathie progressive d'origine vasculaire, Contribution anatomoclinique aux syndromes d'une hypovascularization chronique de la moelle. Acta Neurologica Belgica 62:944–956

Johnson R T, Richardson E P 1968 The neurological manifestations of systemic lupus erythematosus. Medicine 47:337–369

Kitahara T, Ariga N, Yamaura A, Makino H, Maki Y 1979 Familial occurrence of moya-moya disease: report of three Japanese families, Journal of Neurology Neurosurgery and Psychiatry 42:208–214

Kudo T 1968 Spontaneous occlusion of the circle of Willis a disease apparently confined to the Japanese. Neurology 18:485–496

Lagos J C 1977 Congenital aneurysms and arterovenous malformations. In: Vinken P J, Bruyn G W (ed) Handbook of clinical neurology. North Holland Publishing Company, Amsterdam, vol 31

Larroche J-C 1977 Developmental pathology of the neonate. Elsevier/North Holland Biomedical Press, Amsterdam, p 403

Larsen B, Lassen N A 1979 Regulation of cerebral blood flow in health and disease. In: Goldstein M, et al (eds) Advances in neurology, vol 25. Raven Press, New York

Lian E C-Y, Harkness D R, Byrnes J J, Wallach H, Nunez R 1979 Presence of a platelet aggregating factor in the plasma of patients with thrombotic thrombocytopoenic purpura (TTP) and its inhibition by normal plasma. Blood 53:333–338

McDonald W I 1967 Recurrent cholesterol embolism as a cause of fluctuating cerebral symptoms. Journal of Neurology Neurosurgery and Psychiatry 30:489–496

Mishkin M M, Schreiber M N 1974 Collateral circulation. In: Newton T H, Potts D G (eds) Radiology of the brain and skull, vol 2, book 4

de Morsier G 1962 Lupus erythemateux disseminé avec lesions encephalo-medullaires et troubles mentaux. World Neurology 3:629–658

Mustard J F 1977 Atherosclerosis thrombosis and clinical complications in thromboembolism. A new approach to therapy. Mitchell J R A, Domenet J G (ed) Academic Press, New York

Nasu T 1963 Pathology of pulseless disease. Angiology 14:225–242

Neame P B, Hirsh J, Browman G, Denburg J, D'Souza T J, Gallus A, Brain M C 1976 Thrombotic thrombocytopoenic purpura; a syndrome of intravascular platelet consumption. Canadian Medical Association Journal 114:1108–1112

Newton T H, Troost B T 1974 Arteriovenous malformations and fistulae. In: Newton T H, Potts D G (eds) Radiology of the skull and brain, vol 2, book 4

Nishimoto A, Takeuchi 1972 Moya-moya disease: abnormal cerebrovascular network in the cerebral basal region. In: Vinken P J, Bruyn G W (eds) Handbook of clinical neurology. North Holland Publishing Co, Amsterdam, vol 12

Ojemann R G, Fisher C M, Roch J C 1972 Spontaneous dissecting aneurysm of the internal carotid artery. Stroke 3:434–440

Parkinson D 1965 A surgical approach to the cavernous portion of the carotid artery. Anatomical studies and a case report. Journal of Neurosurgery 23:474–483

Partridge B M, Chin A T L 1981 Cerebral aspergilloma. Postgraduate Medical Journal 57:439–442

Pia H W, Djindjian R 1978 Spinal angiomas. Advances in diagnosis and therapy. Springer Verlag, Berlin

Plass E D, Mathew C W 1926 Plasma protein factors in normal pregnancy, labor and puerperium. American Journal of Obstetrics and Gynecology 12:346–358

Rail D L H, Steiner T J, Rose F C 1981 The differential contributions of the major lipid components of atheroma to the outcome of cerebral atheroembolism. A study in an animal model. Stroke (in press)

Richardson E P Jnr 1980 Systemic lupus erythematosus. In: Vinken P J, Bruyn G W (eds) Handbook of clinical neurology. North Holland Publishing Co, Amsterdam, vol 39

Romanul F C, Abramowicz A 1964 Changes in brain and pial vessels in arterial border zones; a study of 13 cases. Archives of Neurology (Chicago) 11:40–65

Ross R, Gomsett J A 1976 The pathogenesis of atherosclerosis. New England Journal of Medicine 295:369–377 and 420–425

Russell D S, Rubinstein 1977 Pathology of tumours of the nervous system, 4th edn. Arnold, London

Sheffield E A, Weller R O 1980 Age changes at cerebral artery bifurcations and the pathogenesis of berry aneurysms. Journal of the Neurological Sciences 46:341–352

Solway H B, Aronson S M 1964 Atheromatous emboli to central nervous system. Report of 16 cases. Archives of Neurology (Chicago) 11:657–667

Stehbens W E 1972 Pathology of the cerebral blood vessels. Mosby Co, St Louis

Steinberg D 1981 Journal of Pathology 133:75–87

Stern W E 1976 Carotid cavernous fistula. In: Vinken P J, Bruyn G W (eds) Handbook of clinical neurology. North Holland Publishing Co, Amsterdam, vol 24

Takashima S, Becker L E 1980 Neuropathology of cerebral arteriovenous malformations in children. Journal of Neurology Neurosurgery and Psychiatry 43:380–385

Taveras J M, Wood E H 1976 Diagnostic radiology, 2nd edn. Williams & Wilkins, Baltimore, vol 2

Tower D B 1979 Effects of ischaemia or tissue hypoxia on the neuron. In: M Goldstein et al (eds) Advances in Neurology, vol 25. Raven Press, New York

Trevor R P, Sondheimer F K, Fessel W J, Wolpert S M 1972 Angiographic demonstration of major cerebral vessel occlusion in systemic lupus erythematosus. Neuroradiology 4:202–207

Vander Eecken H M 1959 The anastomoses between the leptomeningeal arteries of the brain. Thomas, Springfield

Wickremasinghe H R, Peiris J B, Thenabadu P N, Sheriffdeen A H 1978 Transient emboligenic aortoarteritis. Archives of Neurology (Chicago) 35:416–422

Wilkinson I M S, Russell R W R 1972 Arteries of the head and neck in giant cell arteritis. Archives of Neurology 27:378–391

Wolman L, Bradshaw P 1967 Spinal cord embolism. Journal of Neurology Neurosurgery and Psychiatry 30:446–454

Woolf N 1978 Thrombosis and atherosclerosis. British Medical Bulletin 34:137–142

Woolf N 1978 The origins of atherosclerosis. Postgraduate Medical Journal 54:156–161

Wright H P 1942 Changes in adhesiveness of blood platelets following parturition and surgical operations. Journal of Pathology and Bacteriology 54:461–468

Yates P O 1976 Vascular disease of the central nervous system. In: Blackwood W, Corsellis J A N (eds) Greenfield's neuropathology, 3rd edn. Arnold, London, p 136–138

Yates P O, Hutchinson E C 1961 Cerebral infarction. The role of stenosis of the extracranial cerebral arteries. MRC special report series No. 300 HMSO, London

4

Experimental aspects of stroke

K-A. Hossmann

INTRODUCTION

Since the early animal experiments performed by Petersen & Evans (1937), the pathophysiology, biochemistry and morphology of stroke have been extensively studied by many investigators. Numbers of experimental models in different animal species have been developed and used to investigate various aspects of regional ischemic brain damage (Table 4.1). Methods of vascular occlusion have included ligation, clipping or embolization with plastic material, steel balls and iron filings; the animal species were rats, gerbils, cats, monkeys, goats and others, and the experiments were performed either under anesthesia with a variety of anesthetic drugs, or in unanesthetized animals with or without curarization. It is evident that the results obtained under these different experimental conditions are not readily comparable. Anesthesia plays a major role. Depending on the agent used there may be either an ameliorating or a detrimental effect on ischemic brain damage. The size of vessel occluded is a further factor influencing the type of brain edema developing after the onset of ischemia. In models with occlusion of large cerebral vessels such as the middle cerebral artery, edema is primarily of the cytotoxic type (Hossmann & Schuier, 1979a, b), followed by the vasogenic type after several hours (O'Brien et al, 1974). In contrast, multiple small vessel occlusion by microembolism causes primary brain vasogenic edema and secondary edema of the cytotoxic type (Vise et al, 1977, Schuier et al, 1978).

In order to avoid confusion between the pathophysiology of these different forms of ischemia, the following description will be based on the results obtained in one standardized ischemic

Table 4.1 Experimental stroke models

Species	Methods	Authors
Rat	carotid artery ligation and asphyxia	Levine 1960
Rat	microembolism	Kogure et al, 1974
Rat	arachidonate injection	Furlow & Bass, 1976
Rat	macroembolism	Turner, 1975
Rat	middle cerebral artery ligation	Tamura et al, 1980
Hypertensive rats	carotid artery ligation	Choki et al, 1977
Stroke-prone hypertensive rats	spontaneous infarcts	Okamoto et al, 1974
Gerbil	carotid artery ligation	Levine & Payan, 1966
Gerbil	common carotid and (contralateral) external carotid ligation	Bosma et al, 1981
Dog	macroembolism of middle cerebral artery	Molinari, 1970
Dog	macroembolism of basilary artery	Oki et al, 1979
Dog	retro-orbital middle cerebral artery ligation	Anthony et al, 1963
Dog	transorbital middle cerebral artery ligation	Fisk et al, 1969
Goat	internal maxillary artery occlusion	Miletich et al, 1975
Rabbit	pial artery occlusion	Ross Russell, 1971
Cat	microembolism	Vise et al, 1977
Cat	retro-orbital middle cerebral artery ligation	Sundt & Waltz, 1966
Cat	transorbital middle cerebral artery ligation	O'Brien & Waltz, 1973b
Monkey	macroembolism of middle cerebral artery	Molinari et al, 1974
Monkey	intracranial middle cerebral artery ligation	Meyer & Denny-Brown, 1957
Monkey	transorbital middle cerebral artery ligation	Hudgins & Garcia, 1970
Monkey	occlusion common carotid artery following ligation of anterior and posterior cerebral arteries	West & Matsen, 1972

model, acute occlusion of the middle cerebral artery. This model has been extensively used since the original description by Peterson & Evans (1937). It is a valid counterpart of human acute non-hemorrhagic ischemic stroke and data are available about the most pertinent problems relating to ischemic brain damage. However, not all of the conclusions drawn from this experimental model can be applied to other forms of cerebrovascular disease. For this reason the major differences in the pathophysiology and pathobiochemistry between this and the other models summarized in Table 4.1 will also be discussed briefly and reference will be given to more detailed descriptions of these experiments.

MIDDLE CEREBRAL ARTERY OCCLUSION

Anatomical considerations

The angioarchitecture of the monkey, cat and dog brain has been described by Watanabe et al (1977a), Kamijyo & Garcia (1975) and Habermehl (1973), respectively. In all three species the middle cerebral artery originates from the circle of Willis near the junction with the internal carotid artery. A few millimetres distally, it gives off several ascending branches to the basal ganglia (lenticulo-striate arteries), then turns laterally and ramifies over the surface of the cerebral hemisphere. There it gives off numerous branches which penetrate the cortex.

The branches to the basal ganglia are end-arteries, i.e., they do not make significant collateral connexions with other arterial territories. The cortical branches, in contrast, are interconnected among each other and with the cortical branches of the anterior and posterior cerebral arteries via the pial arterial network on the cortical surface (Heubner's leptomeningeal anastomoses).

In the cat and the dog, the territory of the middle cerebral artery covers approximately 60 to 70 per cent of the hemisphere, and the bordering zone between the middle cerebral artery and the anterior cerebral artery is close to the midline (gyrus parasagittalis). In the monkey, the middle cerebral artery supplies about 50 per cent of the hemisphere and the borderzone shifts laterally to the suprasylvian gyrus. This territory is still large in comparison

to man, in whom the territory of the middle cerebral artery is about 40 per cent of the hemisphere volume. Occlusion of the middle cerebral artery, in consequence, results in larger infarcts in lower animal species than in higher ones, a fact which should be considered when experimental and clinical strokes are compared (Waltz, 1979).

Another factor which is of importance for the configuration of the infarct is the position of the clip on the middle cerebral artery. Since the branches to the basal ganglia are end-arteries, collateral blood supply is small, particularly when the occlusion is proximal to or directly at the point of branching. The peripheral cortical region, by contrast, can be supplied from the adjacent anterior and posterior cerebral artery territories via the leptomeningeal anastomoses. For this reason, infarcts are large and include the basal ganglia when the occlusion is close to the origin of the middle cerebral artery but are smaller when the clip is positioned more laterally (Meyer & Denny-Brown, 1957, Tamura et al, 1979). The size of the cortical lesion also depends on the individual collateral blood supply and therefore varies considerably from animal to animal.

Surgical procedure

Three techniques are available for the exposure of the middle cerebral artery: the intracranial approach along the sphenoidal wing, the extradural retro-orbital and the transorbital access. The intracranial exposure of the middle cerebral artery was used in the early experimental studies by Petersen & Evans (1937), Rasmussen & Harvey (1951) and Denny-Brown & Meyer (1957). It was later modified by Sundt & Waltz (1966) for an extradural approach, using an operating microscope. The surgical procedure is relatively simple; a small craniotomy is performed between the lateral wall of the orbit and the internal auditory meatus, the temporal lobe is lifted with a spatula and the middle cerebral artery is exposed close to its origin from the internal carotid artery through a small incision of the dura. The main argument against the operation is the fact that lifting the temporal lobe may cause compression trauma of this part of the brain, resulting in vasogenic edema and also, when pressure is applied for a sufficient period, local ischemia. The effects of vascular occlusion, therefore, may be complicated by local brain trauma.

In order to avoid this problem, transorbital access for exposing the middle cerebral artery was developed by Hudgins & Garcia (1970). The operation is carried out in the following way: first, the globe is either removed or deflated by aspiration of the vitreous, giving access to the optic foramen. The optic nerve is transected and the optic foramen enlarged with a dental drill. Using an operating microscope, the dura is split with fine scissors and the middle cerebral artery exposed at its origin from the internal carotid artery. This operation can be carried out in monkeys (Hudgins & Garcia, 1970), cats (O'Brien & Waltz, 1973b) or dogs (Fisk et al, 1969), and vascular occlusion is performed either by ligation or by applying a small vessel clip. For chronic experiments in unanesthetized animals, simple devices have been designed which can be implanted into the orbit and which permit the occlusion of the artery at a later time by external manipulation (Hayakawa & Waltz, 1975b, Little, 1977). Care has to be taken that always the same vascular segment is occluded because a lateral placement of the vessel clip results in smaller infarcts than a more medial one.

The main advantage of the transorbital approach is the avoidance of local trauma to brain tissue. However, bulbectomy *per se* is a highly traumatizing surgical procedure and transection of the optic nerve may produce acute uncontrollable disturbances of functional activity of the brain which may be associated with undesired metabolic and hemodynamic changes. Some authors, therefore, perform this experiment only in chronic preparations (Hayakawa & Waltz, 1975b, Little, 1977).

Another problem inherent to both the transorbital and the retro-orbital approach is the incision of the dura which is necessary to expose the main trunk of the middle cerebral artery. This causes a leakage of cerebrospinal fluid with subsequent penetration of air into the basal cisterns. In order to avoid this complication, a watertight closure of the opening should be performed. It is evident that this is of benefit only in the chronic experimental situation because sufficient time has to elapse after the surgical intervention for resorption of pene-

trated air. However, most of the experimental investigations are performed under acute conditions and whenever discrepancies between the experimental and clinical situations are encountered, this fact should be considered as a possible explanation.

A problem which has been rarely considered is the lesion produced by the clamp itself. After four hours nerve bundles of the middle cerebral artery are damaged to such an extent that temporary or permanent impairment of neurogenic innervation may result distal to the clip (Dodson et al, 1976b).

The control of the physiological state of the animals after middle cerebral artery occlusion generally does not present any difficulties. In the anesthetized, immobilized and artificially ventilated animal, cardiovascular or pulmonary symptoms are absent (Hossmann & Schuier, 1979b). In the awake animal neurological symptoms will appear shortly after vascular occlusion (see below), but there is no major interference with respiration or the cardiovascular state.

Hemodynamic observations

Pial microcirculation. Acute occlusion of the middle cerebral artery in the normotensive anesthetized monkey or cat has surprisingly little immediate effect on the cerebral microcirculation, as judged from the microscopic observation of the cortical surface (Waltz & Sundt, 1967, Sundt & Waltz, 1967). In pial arteries pulsations cease but blood flow stops only in a few venous or arterial vessels. In some of these, flow after a period of stasis is resumed in the same or opposite direction. The earliest consistent finding is the darkening of the colour of venous blood, followed by a decrease in blood flow velocity and aggregation of formed blood elements (sludging). Pallor of the cortex (as a consequence of anemic ischemia) does not develop earlier than a few minutes after middle cerebral artery occlusion, and may be delayed for 1 to 3 hours. Arteries generally constrict, possibly as a consequence of increased extracellular potassium (Wade et al, 1975). Reversal of vasoconstriction is possible by topical application of papaverin (Waltz & Sundt, 1967) or calcium antagonists such as nifedipine (Brandt et al, 1980).

At varying intervals after occlusion, ranging

from minutes to hours, white platelet thrombi accumulate in some superficial veins, whereas in others bright red venous blood appears, indicating grossly inhomogeneous perfusion with cessation of flow in some and luxury perfusion in other vessels. Inhomogeneity of blood flow is also caused by the opening of arterio-venous shunts which allow the passage of microspheres as large as 76 microns (Prosenz, 1971).

Infarct size. The extent of ischemia is difficult to assess during the experiment, but can be easily delineated at the time of sacrifice, using antipyrine autoradiography (Blair & Waltz, 1970), microangiography (Garcia & Kamijyo, 1974) or systemic injection of dyes (single dye passage according to Weber et al, 1974, Fig. 4.1). When the animal

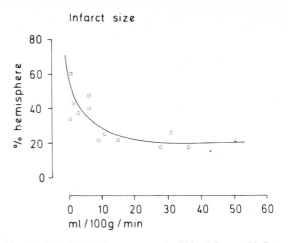

Infarct size

Fig. 4.2 Relationship between cerebral blood flow and infarct size 1–4 hours following middle cerebral artery occlusion in cats. Blood flow was measured in the cortex of the middle cerebral artery territory. Infarct size was determined planimetrically on coronal brain sections (from Hossmann & Schuier, 1980).

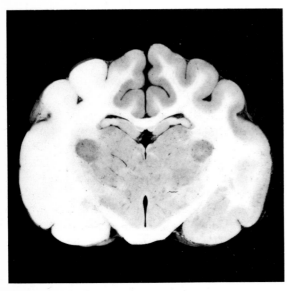

Fig. 4.1 Experimental stroke following transorbital occlusion of the middle cerebral artery of cat. The ischemic territory is identified by its failure to stain with intra-arterially injected carbon black (from Hossmann & Schuier, 1980).

survives for more than 12–24 hours, the ischemic territory can be identified unequivocally using standard histological staining procedures (Garcia & Kamijyo, 1974).

The size of the ischemic territory may vary considerably from animal to animal, depending on the location of the vascular clip and the individual efficiency of collateral circulation (Fig. 4.2). Critical factors are the anatomical situation, blood

pressure, vascular tone, blood viscosity and the development of ischemic brain edema. The volume of the infarcted region may thus vary between 10 and 100 per cent of the territory of the middle cerebral artery (Hossmann & Schuier, 1980). The most frequently affected part is the center of the basal ganglia, and the least sensitive region the peripheral parts of the cortical territory, i.e., the borderzones between the middle, posterior and anterior cerebral arteries (Dodson et al, 1975a).

Blood flow. The variability of the infarct size is associated with considerable quantitative differences in the flow rate within the ischemic territory. Both the pre-ischemic and post-ischemic blood flows vary, depending on species, anesthesia and the methods of flow measurement used; this almost precludes any correlation between different experimental series (Table 4.2). However, despite this variability a relatively close correlation exists between the absolute flow values and the functional and biochemical consequences (see below). This suggests that regardless of the experimental situation, the absolute and not the relative decrease of flow rate is a limiting factor for ischemic damage. Estimation of percentage flow decrease alone, therefore, is of little relevance.

For the quantitative measurement of cerebral blood flow after middle cerebral artery occlusion,

Table 4.2 Cerebral blood flow after middle cerebral artery occlusion

Methods	Species	Anesthesia	Before occlusion	Time	After occlusion	Authors
[133]xenon	baboon	pentobarbital	—	4 hours	26 ± 2[a]	Abraham et al, 1975
[133]xenon	baboon	phencyclidin	35	—	25[a]	Reivich et al, 1978
[133]xenon	squirrel	pentobarbital	40 ± 4	1 hour	29 ± 4[a]	Donley et al, 1975
[133]xenon	squirrel	pentobarbital	84 ± 9	—	61 ± 8[a]	Hanson et al, 1975
[85]krypton	rhesus	phencyclidin	83 ± 3	—	49 ± 4[b]	Simeone et al, 1979
[85]krypton	squirrel	pentobarbital	140 ± 27	—	49 ± 10[b]	Hanson et al, 1975
[85]krypton	cat	halothane	114 ± 23	—	92 ± 19[b]	Waltz, 1970
[85]krypton	cat	halothane	—	—	81 ± 17[b]	Regli et al, 1971c
[14]C-antipyrine	squirrel	pentobarbital	118 ± 25	—	80 ± 16	Blair & Waltz, 1970
[14]C-antipyrine	cat	pentobarbital	101 ± 37	0–180 days	51 ± 27[b]	Yamaguchi et al, 1971b
[14]C-antipyrine	cat	pentobarbital	82 ± 20	2–15 min	12 ± 4[b]	Ginsberg et al, 1976
Hydrogen	monkeys	pentobarbital	26 ± 9	—	23 ± 9	Meyer et al, 1972
Hydrogen	baboon	chloralose	45 ± 10	—	6 ± 8[b]	Crockard et al, 1976
Hydrogen	baboon	chloralose	42 ± 12	—	7 ± 5[b]	Symon et al, 1979
Hydrogen	dog	pentobarbital	53 ± 8	1 hour	39 ± 11[b]	Shima et al, 1979
Hydrogen	cat	pentobarbital/nitrous oxide	84 ± 27	—	16 ± 13[b]	Traupe & Heiss, 1980
Microspheres	cat	pentobarbital	41 ± 4	4 hours	15 ± 4[b]	Hossmann & Schuier, 1980
Microspheres	cat	halothane/nitrous oxide	62 ± 5	2 hours	13 ± 4[b]	Matsuoka et al, in preparation

a = mean flow,
b = cortical flow. Flow values are expressed as ml/100 g/min.

different techniques have been used. Although the variety of these methods may appear confusing, each one has particular advantages and disadvantages which restrict its use to a limited number of specific problems.

The *intra-arterial* [85]*krypton injection technique* (Ingvar & Lassen, 1962) allows repetitive measurements of flow in the cortical grey matter with external detectors. [85]Krypton is a beta-emitting isotope, and the cortex, therefore, must be exposed to avoid absorption of radioactivity by the bony calvarium. The *intra-arterial* [133]*xenon injection technique* (Hoedt-Rasmussen et al, 1966) can be used in the intact skull preparation because [133]xenon is a gamma-emitting isotope. However, it should be applied only in primates and not in dogs, cats or smaller mammals because in these species the brain is supplied both by the internal and external carotid arteries, making it impossible to avoid extracranial contamination. In addition, the so-called 'look-through' artefact (Donley et al, 1975, Hanson et al, 1975) represents a major problem. It is due to the low concentration of the isotope in the ischemic territory, which leads to an activation of external detectors mainly by perifocal non-ischemic tissue, and thus to an overestimation of the actual flow rate.

Hydrogen electrodes (Pasztor et al, 1973), in contrast, give highly regional results and flow measurements can be repeated many times, but the number of electrodes is limited and a traumatic effect cannot be fully excluded. Probably the best available technique for three-dimensional evaluation of flow is quantitative autoradiography using [14]*C-iodo-antipyrine* (Sakurada et al, 1978). In large animals, however, the costs of such a measurement are exceedingly high and flow measurements can only be performed once. This precludes the possibility of assessing kinetic changes. In our laboratory, blood flow has been measured for several years using the *intracardiac microsphere injection* technique (Rudolph & Heymann, 1967), as a compromise between regional and temporal resolution. Microspheres can be labeled with different nuclides, and three up to six flow measurements can be performed in the same animal. The tissue sample may be as small as 100 to 150 mg, which is sufficient to differentiate between white and grey matter of ischemic and non-ischemic brain regions. The major advantage of the technique is the fact that the same tissue sample which is used for flow measurement can also be assessed for tissue constituents, such as water and electrolyte content or biochemical substrates (Hossmann & Schuier, 1979a, b).

Some of the results obtained with these different methods are summarized in Table 4.2. Immediately after middle cerebral artery occlusion, a wide range of flow values were measured: highest values were close to normal and lowest below a few ml/100g/min. However, complete cessation of flow was only occasionally seen and, when present, was restricted to the center of the ischemic territory. There is good evidence that the density of ischemia progresses during the early period after vascular occlusion. Factors responsible are development of edema (O'Brien et al, 1974, Schuier & Hossmann, 1980), release of serotonin or thromboxane A_2 from aggregated platelets (Welch et al, 1973, Hallenbeck & Furlow, 1979), and the increase of extracellular potassium (Wade et al, 1975). It has been reported that not only the density but also the size of the infarct gradually increases because of progressing ischemia in the borderzone of the infarct (Welch et al, 1973). If this is true, one would expect a gradual deterioration of blood flow in this zone. In our series of experiments blood flow, in fact, slightly decreased during the first hour in the borderzone, but it subsequently stabilized, indicating that growth of infarcts is restricted to the early period of ischemia (Fig. 4.3).

When middle cerebral artery occlusion persists for a prolonged period, different flow patterns ensue, the pathophysiology of which remains unclear. Empirically, a certain relationship exists between these flow patterns and the resulting neurological deficits (Heiss et al, 1976b). Functional damage was least in those animals in which a persistent, moderate ischemia was observed or in which delayed hyperemia developed. In contrast, the most severe deficits occurred in animals with persistent severe ischemia and in animals in which hyperemia developed spontaneously shortly after vascular occlusion.

After *reversible* middle cerebral artery occlusion, regional flow changes are even more complex and depend not only on the duration and extent of ischemia but also on the presence or absence of local recirculation disturbances (no-reflow phe-

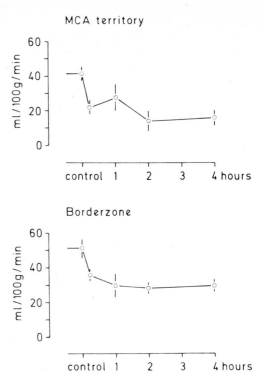

Fig. 4.3 Measurement of cortical blood flow in the center and in the border zone of the middle cerebral artery territory following transorbital occlusion of this vessel. Note that there is no significant progression of ischemia in the border zone.

nomenon, Ames et al, 1968). In general, ischemia is followed by a phase of reactive hyperemia which, however, may be reduced or abolished by local recirculation disturbances (Crockard et al, 1976). Since the latter depend on various systemic factors such as blood viscosity, local perfusion pressure, brain edema and intravascular coagulation, a considerable individual variability exists. According to Crockard et al (1976), reactive hyperemia and hyperoxia were present in 20 per cent, hyperoxia without hyperemia occurred also in 20 per cent, and in the remaining 60 per cent neither flow nor oxygen pressure returned to normal within 40 min after release of the clamp. Despite the slow restoration of flow, functional recovery may return after considerable periods of ischemia. Under favorable conditions, full neurological recovery has been observed after middle cerebral artery occlusion for up to four hours (Crowell et al, 1970, Dodson et al, 1975a, Shima et al, 1979), and neuronal function may even improve after 24 hours when the development of edema can be reduced or prevented (Waltz, 1976). Therapeutic possibilities to ameliorate flow disturbances, both after reversible or permanent middle cerebral artery occlusion, are described below.

Flow regulation. In the center of the ischemic territory, regulation of blood flow is severely disturbed. *CO₂ reactivity* is diminished, abolished or even reversed, i.e., blood flow may decrease with increasing arterial $P\text{co}_2$ (Symon, 1970, Waltz, 1970). This paradoxical CO_2 response is presumably due to intracerebral steal phenomena because vasodilation in the healthy brain causes an increase of blood flow in the non-ischemic areas and, in consequence, a reduced blood supply to the ischemic brain regions.

Autoregulation of blood flow to changes in blood pressure is generally also abolished (Waltz, 1968, Symon et al, 1973, 1976). Occasionally blood flow falls with decreasing blood pressure but does not rise with increasing pressure (Waltz, 1968). There are two explanations for this phenomenon. When local blood perfusion pressure is near the lower limit of the autoregulatory capacity, vessels are maximally dilated and a decrease of pressure cannot be compensated by a further reduction of vascular resistance. An increase of blood pressure, on the other hand, may shift the local perfusion pressure into the autoregulatory range, causing an appropriate vasoconstriction for maintenance of blood flow. Similarly, a slight decrease of vascular tone, e.g., by sympathectomy, may cause failure of autoregulation under threshold conditions (Zervas et al, 1976). An alternative explanation is 'false autoregulation' (Miller et al, 1975). In the presence of edema, an increase in blood pressure is associated with an increase in local tissue pressure, resulting in little improvement of the actual tissue perfusion pressure. Failure of autoregulation can be demonstrated in such instances by dehydrating the brain in order to reduce brain edema.

The disturbance of flow regulation seems to be a function of the severity of ischemia. Autoregulation begins to fail at flow values of about 40 per cent; CO_2 reactivity is more resistant and fails only at lower flow levels (Symon et al, 1976). For this reason a dissociation may be observed between abolished autoregulation and preserved CO_2 reactivity in the peripheral regions of an infarct.

Ischemic disturbances of flow regulation are, in general, longlasting. CO_2 reactivity does not recover earlier than 5 to 12 days after middle cerebral artery occlusion (Waltz, 1979), and autoregulation may still be abolished after as long as three years (Symon et al, 1975).

Following middle cerebral artery occlusion flow changes have also been described in the *opposite non-ischemic hemisphere*. Generally, a decrease of flow has been observed but occasionally flow increased (Waltz, 1967; Ginsberg et al, 1977; Reivich et al, 1978). The decrease has been explained by transcallosal functional suppression (*diaschisis*, in the sense of von Monakow, 1914) associated with a coupled reduction of both brain metabolism and blood flow. However, this finding is not consistent and has not been confirmed in our series of experiments in which animals anesthetized by either barbiturate or halothane did not exhibit such behavior during the initial four hours of vascular occlusion (Hossmann & Schuier, 1980). The occasional increase of flow in the opposite hemisphere is difficult to explain and may be related to reverse steal effects induced by the sudden reduction in the size of the vascular bed following middle cerebral artery occlusion. However, other general physiological effects may also be involved.

Functional sequelae

In awake cats or monkeys, *neurological symptoms* develop gradually rather than abruptly after middle cerebral artery occlusion (Hayakawa & Waltz, 1975b, Little, 1977). After a few seconds to one minute, circling movement toward the side of the occluded middle cerebral artery begins, accompanied or followed by forced ambulation, tonic deviation of the head and neck toward the ischemic hemisphere, weakness of opposite limb and an apathetic or akinetic state which lasts for several hours. General symptoms such as collapse are absent, nor is there generalized seizure activity as in gerbils following carotid occlusion (Cohn, 1979).

In anesthetized animals the early functional deficits are generally assessed by electrophysiological recording. The *electroencephalogram,* after a free interval of a few seconds, is initially activated and

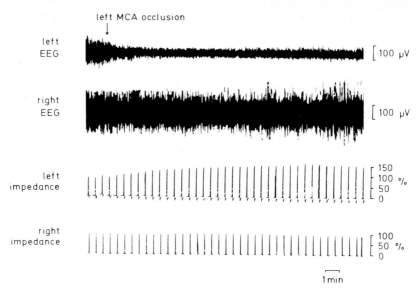

Fig. 4.4 Recording of the EEG and of cortical impedance following occlusion of the left middle cerebral artery in cat. Note the rapid suppression of the EEG and the increase of ipsilateral impedance as a consequence of extracellular volume shrinkage (from Hossmann & Schuier, 1979b).

then rapidly decreases in amplitude (Fig. 4.4). The early activation correlates with a transient increase in unit activity (Heiss et al, 1976a). During the initial few hours of middle cerebral artery occlusion, suppression of the electroencephalogram affects both the fast and the slow frequency components, i.e., the electroencephalogram decreases in amplitude but does not slow down (Hossmann & Schuier, 1980). Only after several hours a slow wave focus appears which apparently is associated with the development of vasogenic brain edema (see below).

A shift in the *cortical steady potential* occurs after one to three minutes when ischemia includes the grey matter and after about five minutes when only deeper structures are involved (Heilbrun & Goldring, 1968). The cortical steady potential, which in the healthy animal ranges between 1–5 mV, suddenly shifts toward negativity, presumably as a consequence of cell membrane depolarization. This shift has been related to the development of irreversible ischemic brain damage (*terminal depolarization*) because a close correlation has been observed between its appearance and the development of neurological deficits (Anthony et al, 1963). More recent observations, however, indicate that the shift is not an indicator of irreversibility

because full neurological recovery has been observed after periods of ischemia which by far exceed the interval following which terminal depolarization occurs (Hossmann, 1971).

Terminal depolarization is accompanied by other electrophysiological events which presumably are also related to cell membrane depolarization: a sudden increase in cortical impedance, and the release of intracellular potassium into the extracellular space. *Cortical impedance* rises by more than 100 per cent during the first hour of ischemia, indicating an increase of cell volume at the expense of the extracellular space (Branston et al, 1978, Hossmann & Schuier, 1979b, see Fig. 4.4). Using the Maxwell approach, the changes in the volume of the extracellular space can be calculated quantitatively (Hossmann, 1977). Within five minutes, it decreases from 20 to 15 per cent, and within the first hour further to about 12 vol. per cent (Hossmann & Schuier, 1979b, Fig. 4.5). *Extracellular potassium* sharply rises after a few minutes from about 3 meq/l to 30–80 meq/l (Branston et al, 1977). The peak value of extracellular potassium depends on two factors: intracellular release, and clearance into the blood and surrounding brain tissue. In complete ischemia, it may rise up to 100 meq/l (Vyskocil et al, 1972), but this value is rarely

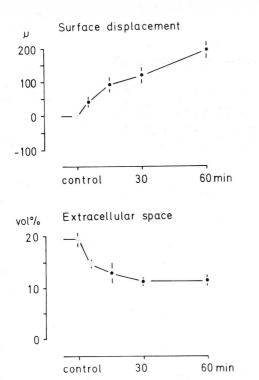

Fig. 4.5 Relationship between ischemic brain swelling and narrowing of the extracellular space following middle cerebral artery occlusion in cats. Brain swelling was assessed by recording the displacement of the cortical surface in respect to the calvarium, and extracellular space by impedance measurement (from Schuier & Hossmann, 1980).

reached in experimental infarcts because even under unfavorable conditions some remaining blood flow persists.

It has been stressed by several authors that the various electrophysiological signs of ischemia are *threshold* dependent, and therefore occur at different densities of flow reduction in graded ischemia (Symon et al, 1977). The most sensitive is the EEG which begins to flatten at flow values which are only slightly below normal and becomes isoelectric when blood flow decreases below 15 ml/100 g/min (Morawetz et al, 1979). The amplitude reduction is linear to the flow decrease, indicating that with increasing density of ischemia an increasing portion of the neuropil is involved (Hossmann & Schuier, 1980, Fig. 4.6). Evoked potentials begin to decrease at flow values below 20 ml/100 g/min, and are completely suppressed below 15 ml/100 g/min (Branston et al, 1974, 1977). Cortical unit activity ceases at about 18 ml/100 g/min (Heiss et

al, 1976a), impedance begins to rise between 6–9 ml/100 g/min (Branston et al, 1978), and extracellular potassium below 8–10 ml/100 g/min (Branston et al, 1974, Strong et al, 1977, Astrup et al, 1977). A disturbance of net water and electrolyte content of the brain appears at flow values below 10–15 ml/100 g/min (Hossmann & Schuier, 1979a, b, Symon et al, 1979), see Fig. 4.6. These thresholds are remarkably similar in different species and under different anesthetic drugs, indicating that basic mechanisms are involved. It is interesting to note that both the electroencephalogram and evoked potentials are completely suppressed at flow values which are definitely above the threshold of cell membrane depolarisation. Thus, a penumbra (Astrup et al, 1977) exists between functional and structural neuronal damage which may explain that in regional ischemia — in contrast to global ischemia — functional recovery may be possible after as long as 24 hours, provided blood flow remains above the threshold for structural integrity.

Ischemic brain edema

Experimental middle cerebral artery occlusion is accompanied by a rapid development of brain edema. From a pathophysiological standpoint, two phases can be distinguished: an early (cytotoxic) type of edema, followed by a delayed (vasogenic) phase. This two-stage pathogenesis is different from other types of edema and justifies the introduction of a separate category of ischemic brain edema. Excellent reviews have been published recently by Katzman et al (1977) and Klatzo (1979).

Early (cytotoxic) phase of ischemic brain edema. Brain edema by definition is an increase in water content of the brain tissue. As has been described above, disturbances of water homeostasis are threshold-dependent and appear at flow rates between 10–15 ml/100 g/min. Ischemic brain edema, in consequence, develops only when this degree of ischemia is reached (critical ischemia, Hossmann & Schuier, 1979a, b). The following observations refer to experiments in which blood flow decreased below this threshold.

Development of ischemic brain edema is a surprisingly rapid process. Already one minute

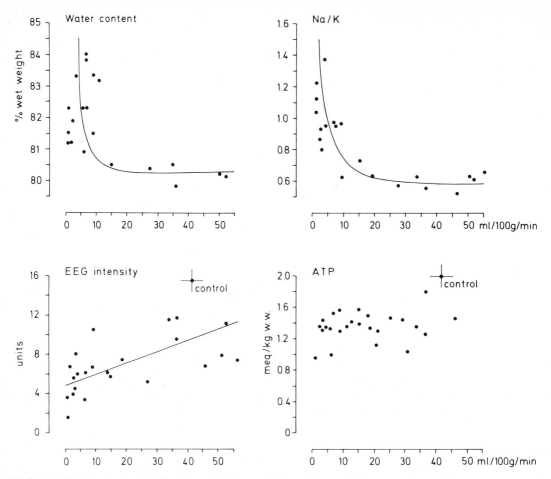

Fig. 4.6 Relationship between cortical blood flow in the center of the middle cerebral artery territory and water content, the ratio of cortical sodium/potassium content, the intensity of the EEG and the ATP content. There is a definite threshold relationship between blood flow, water content and ion homeostasis, but not between blood flow and EEG or ATP content (from Hossmann & Schuier, 1980).

after MCA occlusion, an early swelling of the brain can be detected by sensitive volume gauges (Fig. 4.5), and after a few hours (two hours in our series, three hours in experiments performed by Watanabe et al, 1977b) water content of the *grey matter* is significantly increased (Fig. 4.7). The early onset of brain swelling presumably is partly due to an increase of blood volume in the territory of the middle cerebral artery because the decrease in local blood perfusion pressure evokes an autoregulatory dilation of the vasculature. However, this is not the sole reason because there is evidence of a rapid intracerebral disturbance of water homeostasis, as demonstrated by the changes in cortical impedance (see above). Calculation of the extracellular volume

fraction by impedance reveals an inverse relationship between extracellular space and brain swelling (Fig. 4.5). This suggests a predominantly intracellular accumulation of edema fluid (Schuier & Hossmann, 1980).

Water uptake is closely associated with a disturbance of ion homeostasis. Inhibition of the energy-dependent ion exchange pumps causes an equilibration of transmembrane ion concentrations with loss of brain tissue potassium and increase of sodium (Bremer et al, 1978, Schuier & Hossmann, 1980). The inverse changes of these two cations result in a steep increase of the sodium/potassium ratio which, as a sensitive indicator of ischemic cell damage, is significantly

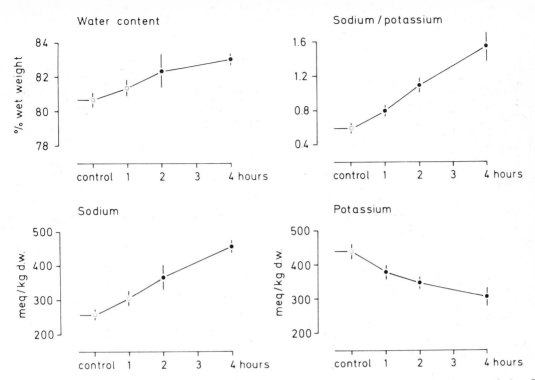

Fig. 4.7 Changes in water and electrolyte content of the cerebral cortex of cat following middle cerebral artery occlusion. Only those animals were evaluated in which blood flow decreased below the critical threshold for induction of brain edema. Note the gradual deterioration of water and ion homeostasis during the initial four hours of ischemia (from Schuier & Hossmann, 1980).

increased already one hour after middle cerebral artery occlusion (Fig. 4.7).

Edema formation in the *white matter* is more variable and less prominent than in the grey matter (Watanabe et al, 1977b, Hossmann & Schuier, 1979a, b, Symon et al, 1979). The reason is presumably the fact that the flow threshold for induction of edema in the white matter is lower than that of the grey matter and therefore rarely attained under usual experimental conditions.

Water accumulation during the early phase of ischemia results from two different processes: an increase of tissue *osmolality* in the ischemic territory — presumably due to the accumulation of lactic acid and the release of ions from intracellular binding sites — and a decrease of *extracellular sodium* activity after depolarization of cell membranes. These changes cause osmotic and ionic concentration gradients between blood and brain which are equilibrated by a shift of water and sodium from the blood into the brain and a release of potassium from the brain into the blood (Schuier

& Hossmann, 1980). Regional ischemia is rarely complete and for this reason the gradients are equilibrated at the same rate as they build up because the remaining blood supply provides the necessary reservoir of fluid and electrolytes. In order to estimate the actual osmotic and ionic capacity of the ischemic brain, blood flow must be stopped completely. When this is done, tissue osmolality during one hour increases by about 50 mosmol and extracellular sodium decreases by 60 meq/l (Hossmann, 1976). Shifts of this order of magnitude easily explain the actually observed changes in water and electrolyte content of the ischemic brain.

Cell swelling associated with the development of cytotoxic edema is of critical importance for the manifestation of brain infarcts. Swelling affects predominantly the perivascular astroglial cells and, therefore, may cause compression of the microcirculation (Little et al, 1976). Edema, in consequence, aggravates the primary ischemic impact and eventually may lead to complete cessation of blood flow. This process explains why in animals with flow reduction to below the threshold of edema formation, ischemia was progressive whereas in others with a lesser reduction of flow, blood flow remained stable or even gradually improved (Hossmann & Schuier, 1979a).

Delayed (vasogenic) phase of ischemic edema. When occlusion of the middle cerebral artery exceeds a certain duration, the blood-brain barrier may become permeable to circulating macromolecules. The delay of the breakdown of the barrier depends on the duration of ischemia. After permanent middle cerebral artery occlusion, barrier damage appears after three to six hours (Olsson et al, 1971; Kamijyo et al, 1977) see Fig. 4.8. When

the ischemic process. The breakdown of the barrier results in the development of (vasogenic) edema, which slowly accumulates not only in the ischemic territory but also in the surrounding brain tissue (Fig. 4.8). Edema spreads mainly into the white matter where it reaches a maximum after four to seven days (O'Brien et al, 1974). At that time white matter water content may be as high as 80 per cent, corresponding to a volume increase of 60 per cent. This degree of edema may damage the brain in two different ways: by increasing intracranial pressure and by causing mass shifts (Hayakawa & Waltz, 1975a, Tulleken et al, 1974). Local tissue pressure in the ischemic territory may rise to 80 mmHg as compared to 15 mmHg on the opposite side

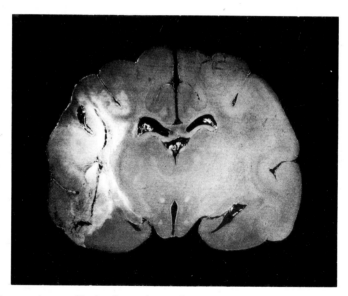

Fig. 4.8 Development of vasogenic type of brain edema 6 hours after middle cerebral artery occlusion in cat. Exudation of serum proteins is traced by a specific immunofluorescence technique.

ischemia is of shorter duration, the interval increases and may be as long as 20 hours (maturation phenomenon, Ito et al, 1976). In all likelihood, the breakdown of the blood-brain barrier is an indicator of irreversible ischemic tissue damage and not a symptom of ischemia *per se* (Shibata et al, 1974, Watanabe et al, 1977b). This is the reason that in reversible or noncritical ischemia, the barrier may remain intact.

Although barrier damage is a consequence of tissue necrosis rather than an accompaniment of ischemia, it nevertheless influences the sequelae of

(O'Brien & Waltz, 1973a). This may lead to a further decrease of blood flow in non-critical ischemic brain regions and thus may enhance and enlarge the primary ischemic territory. By causing mass shifts, edema furthermore may evoke transtentorial or even cisternal herniations with fatal compressions of the brain stem. Ng & Nimmannitya (1970) in fact observed a transtentorial prolapse in 78 per cent of all patients with severe brain swelling following stroke. Treatment of the vasogenic component of ischemic edema, therefore, may improve the final outcome of stroke even although it may be without influence on the degree of ischemic tissue necrosis.

Biochemical observations

The reduction of blood flow in the territory of the occluded middle cerebral artery results in a decrease of regional oxygen availability and, in consequence, a disturbance of the *cerebral redox state*. This is most dramatically demonstrated by continuous recording of cortical NADH fluorescence, using an *in vivo* spectrofluometer (Sundt & Anderson, 1975, Ginsberg et al, 1976). NADH sharply increases and already reaches a peak value 30 to 70 seconds after middle cerebral artery occlusion. Thereafter it again decreases, presumably because of the development of collateral flow to the ischemic territory, and because of reduced oxygen demands of the tissue after suppression of electrocortical activity (cortical shutdown, Bito & Myers, 1972). The final increase of NADH depends on the actual flow rate in the ischemic territory: the lower the flow, the higher the NADH concentration (Ginsberg et al, 1976). It increases with increasing blood pressure but does not change at varying Pco_2 levels (Sundt et al, 1976), apparently because both autoregulation and CO_2 reactivity of blood flow are abolished (see above).

The reduced oxygenation of the tissue is accompanied by a disturbance of the *energy-producing metabolism*. The yield of energy-rich phosphate bindings per mol glucose is 38 mol. P under aerobic, but only two mol P under anerobic conditions. Glycolysis, in consequence, is stimulated, glucose, creatine phosphate and ATP decline and lactate rises to more than 25 μmol/g (Michenfelder & Sundt, 1971, Sundt & Michenfelder, 1972, Schuier & Hossmann, 1980, Fig. 4.9). In contrast to complete ischemia, where ATP is completely used up within a few minutes, a certain basal level of 30 per cent or more is maintained for periods up to three hours or longer (Sundt & Michenfelder, 1972, Held et al, 1975, Yamamoto et al, 1979, Schuier & Hossmann, 1980). The delayed breakdown of the energy metabolism apparently is the reason that the revival time of the brain after MCA occlusion is considerably longer than after total circulatory arrest. This is also reflected by the second messenger cAMP beginning

to decrease only after one to three hours (Flamm et al, 1978b) in contrast to its rapid alteration in complete ischemia.

Recently, several *regional biochemical approaches* have become available which allow the qualitative and quantitative assessment of various metabolic parameters in intact brain slices, and thus provide the possibility to correlate precisely the biochemical changes with the morphological substrate. The slices are obtained by cutting the brain in a cryostat following *in situ* freezing with liquid nitrogen.

Regional glucose consumption can be measured using the autoradiographic deoxyglucose method (Sokoloff et al, 1977). In the center of the infarct, metabolic rate of glucose is reduced or abolished, but there are patchy areas of enhanced glucose consumption in the periphery, probably as the consequence of increased glycolytic rate in anaerobic borderzones (Ginsberg et al, 1977, Welsh et al, 1977, 1980). Interestingly, a slight decrease of CMR glucose has also been observed in the opposite hemisphere. This has been interpreted as a metabolic indicator of diaschisis (Ginsberg et al, 1977).

For the assessment of the distribution of substrates of the energy-producing metabolism, various techniques have been described. *Regional NADH concentration* is measured by illuminating a frozen brain section with ultraviolet light and recording the resulting NADH fluorescence on photographic film (Welsh et al, 1977). *Regional ATP content* can be recorded by the bioluminescent technique, described by Kogure and Alonso (1978), and *regional glucose content* by the bioluminescent technique of Paschen et al (1980). When these techniques are applied to adjacent cryostat sections of the same brain, significant differences in the distribution of the various substrates of energy-producing metabolism appear which had not been realized before using conventional tissue sampling techniques (Fig. 4.10A & B). We have recently performed such a study in cats following MCA occlusion at varying blood pressure levels (Paschen et al, 1980). The sizes of the infarcts were inversely related to the blood pressure, and varied from minor involvement of the basal ganglia at normotension to infarction of the total supplying territory of the middle cerebral artery at severe hypotension. In the center of the infarcts, NADH fluorescence was increased and

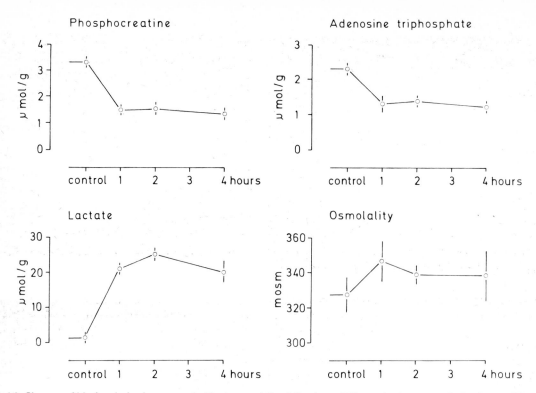

Fig. 4.9 Changes of biochemical substrates and of brain osmolality following middle cerebral artery occlusion in cats. Note the relatively high level of phosphocreatine and adenosine triphosphate during the initial four hours after vascular occlusion (from Hossmann & Schuier, 1979b).

both ATP and glucose depleted. However, there were consistent differences in the regional distribution of these substrates. The region in which NADH fluorescence increased was always smaller than that in which ATP decreased, which in turn covered a smaller region than that in which glucose was depleted. This indicates that the redox state of the brain is disturbed at an appreciably higher degree of ischemia than that necessary for depletion of primary and secondary energy reserves.

The failure of energy-producing metabolism necessarily results in a disturbance of all energetic metabolic and catabolic processes. Most of these processes have been investigated under experimental conditions other than middle cerebral artery occlusion and will not be discussed here (for reference see Siesjö, 1978). Using the middle cerebral artery occlusion model the following observations were made. *Ribosomal disaggregation* occurred after 1.5 to 4.5 hours of ischemia (Little et al, 1974b), resulting presumably in an inhibition of protein synthesis. It is interesting to note that

following complete cerebro-circulatory arrest, ribosomal disaggregation occurred during post-ischemic recirculation and not during ischemia itself (Kleihues & Hossmann, 1971). The disaggregation after middle cerebral artery occlusion, therefore, may be related to the interaction of a remaining (trickling) blood flow with the ischemic brain tissue.

Neuro-transmitter metabolism has been studied by several authors but the results are controversial (Zervas et al, 1974, Cohen et al, 1975, Bowen et al, 1976, Goodhart et al, 1977). The only consistent finding is a substantial decrease of

Fig. 4.10 Regional distribution of NADH fluorescence, glucose and ATP bioluminescence 30 min after middle cerebral artery occlusion of cats. (a) At normal blood pressure; (b) during induced hypotension. The biochemical changes are much more wide-spread during hypotension. In both experiments, the increase in NADH fluorescence is restricted to a smaller region than the regional changes of ATP and glucose. This indicates that the ischemic threshold for disturbance of cerebral redox state is lower than that for the preservation of ATP and glucose stores (from Paschen et al, 1981).

NADH fluorescence

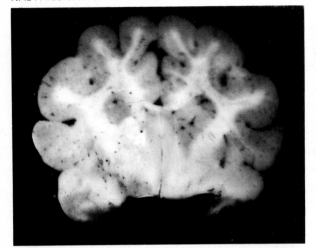

NADH fluorescence

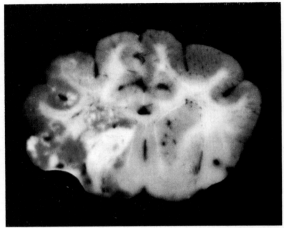

ATP bioluminescence

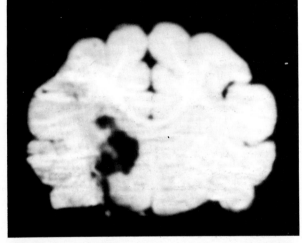

ATP bioluminescence

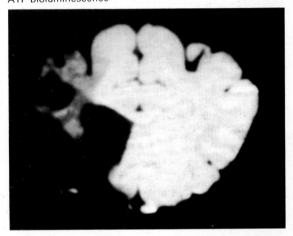

Glucose bioluminescence

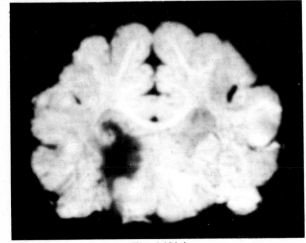

Glucose bioluminescence

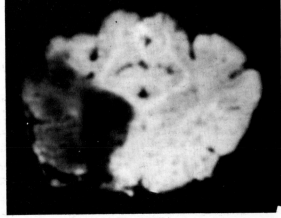

Fig. 4.10(a)   **Fig. 4.10(b)**

dopamine, which is most pronounced in those regions in which the density of dopaminergic neurons is highest (Zervas et al, 1974). Noradren-aline, in contrast, correlates only loosely with the severity of brain ischemia (Cohen et al, 1975): it usually decreases after 1 to 7 days, but sometimes it remains unchanged or even increases, and the concentration seems also to depend on the ma-nipulation of the middle cerebral artery during surgical exposure. These observations suggest that middle cerebral artery occlusion has a more pronounced effect on dopaminergic than on nor-adrenergic neurons.

A much disputed question is the significance of *free radical reactions* on tissue damage after middle cerebral artery occlusion. Flamm et al (1978a) observed a 65 per cent decrease of ascorbic acid after 24 hours of ischemia. This decrease was attributed to the appearance of free radical reac-tions because ascorbic acid is a naturally occurring antioxidant. Since, in the absence of antioxidants, free radicals cause a variety of pathobiochemical changes such as peroxidation of phospholipids, damage of mitochondrial and other cytoplasmic membranes will result. This concept is of interest and may explain the putative protective effect of barbiturates during ischemia (see below) because certain barbiturates are free radical scavengers. However, there are also arguments against such a mechanism (Rehncrona et al, 1980), and the role of free radical damage must still be considered as highly speculative.

Neuropathology

Ischemic morphological alterations, even of the most subtle degree, appear after much longer intervals following middle cerebral artery occlusion than physiological or biochemical disturbances. The interval between the onset of ischemia and the appearance of morphological changes is called 'manifestation time'. It depends on the type of morphological change and may vary considerably using different methods of morphological investigation.

The earliest alterations are multifocal and appear after 15 min in the cortex (Garcia et al, 1977). They consist of a swelling of neuronal mitochon-dria, of neurites and perivascular astrocytes in the periphery of the supplying territory of the middle cerebral artery. During the subsequent two to three hours a gradual condensation of neuronal cyto-plasm with eosinophilic staining, nuclear pyknosis and angularity of the cell body develops, leading to the well-known phenomenon of Spielmayer's ischemic cell change (Crowell et al, 1970; Garcia & Kamijyo, 1974; Little et al, 1974; Dodson et al, 1977; Garcia et al, 1977). The condensation of cytoplasma should not be confused with artefactual dark neurons of Cammermeyer (1961) and, there-fore, should be evaluated only in optimally fixed material and with caution.

During the early phase of ischemia, mitochon-dria of astrocytes remain intact and capillaries, oligodendroglial cells and myelin sheaths are undamaged (Garcia et al, 1977). In the pericytes of the vasculature, lysosomes accumulate (Dodson et al, 1976a) but in the neurons these cell organelles remain normal (Little et al, 1974a). The remark-able inverse volume change of neurons and astro-cytes indicates that fluid shifts occur between these two compartments and that these shifts are more complex than might appear from the global changes in brain water content described above.

The earliest histochemical damage becomes apparent after 12 hours (McDonald et al, 1972). Esterases, oxidoreductases, acid and alkaline phos-phatases, cytochrome-oxidase and other enzymes begin to either increase or decrease. The changes are relatively slow and significant alterations are not observed earlier than one day after the onset of middle cerebral artery occlusion.

At this time the outlining of the infarcted territory is easily recognized by histological stain-ing. All cell elements stain significantly less with anilin stains, and the infarcts, therefore, are distinctly demarcated from the more deeply stained normal tissue. After three to four days inflamma-tory changes appear, consisting of infiltration of lymphocytes, leucocytes and macrophages into the infarcted territory, and after 10 days massive resorption of the necrotic tissue is present (Garcia, 1975). It has been noted that phagocytosis is almost exclusively by blood-borne cells and that local pericytes do not participate in this process (Dodson et al, 1976a).

The *localization* of the histological lesions de-pends on the severity of ischemia. At relatively high flow rates, only basal ganglia and the capsula interna are involved, but increasing portions of the cortical grey matter are affected with increasing density of ischemia (Dodson et al, 1976b). Since animals with severe ischemia rarely survive, damage in chronic experiments is generally restricted to circumscribed subcortical regions (Brierley & Symon, 1977).

Several attempts have been made to determine quantitatively the critical flow threshold below which tissue necrosis develops. Morawetz et al (1978) and Tamura & Sano (1979) measured flow values below 12 to 15 ml/100 g/min in irreversibly damaged tissue, i.e., a value which is close to the threshold of cell membrane depolarization (see above). This suggests that a prolonged state of cell membrane depolarization is not compatible with cell survival. However, the topical correlation between ischemia and tissue destruction is not absolute. When blood flow is assessed on histological sections using quantitative autoradiography, focal areas of hypo- and hyperemia are present in necrotic regions, indicating that blood flow in the ischemic territory is highly inhomogeneous (Yamaguchi et al, 1971b).

The *reversibility* of histological changes has been studied using reversible middle cerebral artery occlusion for periods up to 24 hours (Crowell et al, 1970; Dodson et al, 1975a; Kamijyo et al, 1977; Tamura & Sano, 1979). Within the initial two hours, irreversible changes are absent or sparse, after four hours mild, and only after more than six hours severe. This sequel correlates closely with the development of reperfusion disturbances (no-reflow) and vasogenic edema. However, there is no direct topical relationship between neuronal damage and capillary obstruction, indicating that both edema and microcirculatory disturbances are an accompaniment but not the reason for irreversible tissue destruction (Garcia et al, 1971; Little et al, 1976).

Therapy

An amelioration of brain damage following middle cerebral artery occlusion has been attempted in different ways: by improving blood flow, by decreasing the substrate demands of the ischemic brain and by treating side effects which are triggered by the ischemic impact and which further complicate the pathological process. A great variety of procedures has been tested in the past but none of these has yet provided a major breakthrough in the treatment of cerebral infarcts. (See Fig. 4.11)

Improvement of flow. The most direct way for improving flow is *removal of the circulatory obstruction.* Under experimental conditions, this is easily achieved by releasing the vessel clip and evidence has been provided that this results in a significant amelioration or even prevention of infarcts after ischemic periods of four hours or longer (Crowell et al, 1970; Dodson et al, 1975a; Kamijyo et al, 1977). A clinically more relevant procedure is surgical removal of a previously injected embolus. Using microsurgical techniques and with the necessary technical skill, infarcts have been prevented by embolectomy within the same interval (Dujovny et al, 1976; Okada et al, 1979; Diaz et al, 1979). An alternative procedure is the establishment of intra/extracerebral anastomoses. Probably because of the less efficient recirculation, the results are quite different: even after four hours of ischemia, and more so after 24 hours, a dramatic exacerbation of the infarct occurred, accompanied by massive hemorrhages and a definite deterioration of the neurological state (Diaz et al, 1979).

Pharmacological *vasodilation* for improving collateral blood supply to the middle cerebral artery territory has been extensively studied. Papaverin, aminophylline, ergotamine, hexobendine, prostacyclin, the calcium antagonist nimodipine, and numerous other vasodilating agents have been tested but none of these resulted in a consistent improvement of blood flow (Neumann et al, 1970; Regli et al, 1971a, c; Blöink et al, 1979). The reason presumably is that these compounds reduce the vascular resistance in the non-ischemic healthy brain tissue but not in the ischemic territory because in this region vessels are already dilated. The consequence is *intracerebral steal* with little improvement of flow in the ischemic territory. A selective dilatation of pial anastomoses without dilatation of intracerebral arteries has been attempted by sympathectomy (Blöink et al, 1979). However, this approach also did not improve blood flow.

Several authors have tried to increase the local blood perfusion pressure in the ischemic territory by either *hypercapnia* (Shalit et al, 1967; Symon et al, 1971; Yamaguchi et al, 1971a, Harrington et al, 1972) or *hypocapnia* (Soloway et al, 1971; Battistini et al, 1971; Harrington & Di Chiro, 1973): hypercapnia for improving collateralization of the infarct, and hypocapnia under the assumption that vasoconstriction in the non-ischemic brain tissue might improve the blood supply to the ischemic territory by *reverse steal*. The results were unsatisfactory. In fact, some authors noted that infarcts were smallest when CO_2 was kept as close as possible to the normal level without any deviation toward hypo- or hypercapnia (Harrington & Di Chiro, 1973).

The loss of autoregulation in the ischemic territory suggests that flow improvement should be possible by *increasing blood pressure*. Hope et al (1977), observed an amelioration of neurological function by induced hypertension but there was also evidence of an aggravation of vasogenic brain edema when blood pressure was increased (Fenske et al, 1978). In a recent series of experiments, we noticed little improvement of micropressure in small pial arteries during induced hypertension, presumably because of an autoregulatory vasoconstriction of the supplying collateral channels which, in contrast to the ischemic vessels, still respond to blood pressure changes (Matsuoka et al, in preparation). This explains why in these experiments blood flow did not increase significantly during hypertension.

Hemodilution improves blood flow more consistently. Isovolemic infusion of dextran, albumin or even saline resulted in a significant increase in blood circulation (Sundt & Waltz, 1967; Crowell & Olsson, 1972; Blöink et al, 1979). However, it should be remembered that the flow increase is only temporary (Sundt & Waltz, 1967), and that hemodilution decreases the oxygen binding capacity of the blood. This may be the reason why hemodilution did not prevent the development of ischemic brain edema (Blöink et al, 1979). The use of low viscosity oxygen carriers such as fluorocarbons, however, may be of interest for improving oxygen availability. (See Fig. 4.11)

An indirect approach for ameliorating tissue perfusion is *treatment of ischemic brain edema*. As has been described above, the early *cytotoxic type* of edema may cause microcirculatory compression by swollen perivascular astrocytes and the late vasogenic type of edema may reduce tissue perfusion pressure by local or global increase of intracranial pressure. The early cytotoxic type of edema can be treated by *osmotherapy*, using glycerol, sorbitol or mannitol (Dodson et al, 1975b, Little & O'Shaughnessy, 1979, Blöink et al, 1979, Bremer et al, 1980). Improvement of flow, however, is only temporary, and there is no influence on the electrolyte shifts associated with this type of edema. Acetazolamide should not be used for preventing water uptake because this results in a definite increase in the size of the infarcts (Regli et al, 1971b; Bremer et al, 1980). Treatment of the late *vasogenic type* of edema has been attempted using *corticosteroids*. Some authors observed a certain improvement of edema (Anderson & Cranford, 1978; Fenske et al, 1979; Bremer et al, 1980) but others denied an ameliorating effect (Donley & Sundt, 1973; Lee et al, 1974; de la Torre & Surgeon, 1976; Little, 1978). There is probably no influence on the infarct itself because the loss of tissue potassium, which is a sensitive indicator of tissue necrosis, is not affected by this treatment (Fenske et al., 1979).

Metabolic inhibition. Substrate requirements of the ischemic brain may be reduced by two different mechanisms: indirectly by inhibiting functional activity and directly by inhibiting metabolic pathways.

Inhibition of functional activity has been attempted using various central nervous system depressant agents, such as anti-epileptic drugs or anesthetics. The most widely used anesthetics are *barbiturates*. Smith & coworkers showed in 1974 that barbiturates decrease significantly the size of infarcts in dogs following middle cerebral artery occlusion, a finding which has been later confirmed by numerous authors in various animal species and under different experimental conditons (Moseley et al, 1975; Hoff et al, 1975; Corkill et al, 1976; Molinari et al, 1976; Simeone et al, 1979). However, there are other results which suggest that the barbiturate effect is not as clear-cut as it might appear (Hayakawa & Waltz, 1975c; Blöink et al, 1979). A major problem is the depression induced by barbiturates in the general cardio-respiratory state (Corkill et al, 1978, Weidler et al., 1979, Yamamoto et al, 1979) and in one series of

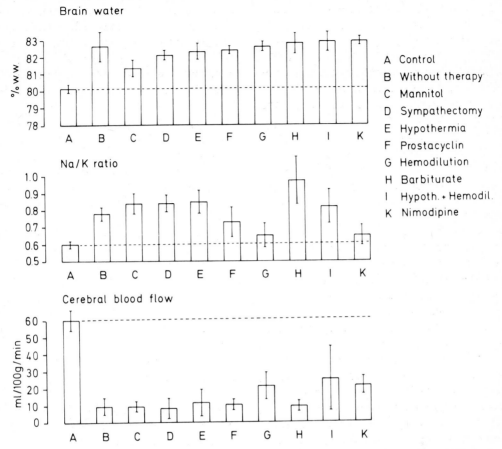

Brain water

Na/K ratio

Cerebral blood flow

A Control
B Without therapy
C Mannitol
D Sympathectomy
E Hypothermia
F Prostacyclin
G Hemodilution
H Barbiturate
I Hypoth. + Hemodil.
K Nimodipine

Fig. 4.11 Effect of various therapeutic procedures on water and electrolyte homeostasis two hours after middle cerebral artery occlusion in cats. Therapy was induced 15 min after the onset of ischemia. Note the slight improvement of brain edema by mannitol, and the improvement of ion disturbance by hemodilution and the calcium antagonist nimodipine. Barbiturates, in contrast, lead to a further aggravation of the ischemic electrolyte shifts.

experiments barbiturates decreased the size of the infarcts, but increased mortality because of cardiac insufficiency (Black et al, 1978).

It is interesting to note that barbiturates improve the outcome of small infarcts more than that of large ones. This apparently is the reason for the better results obtained in primates than in lower animal species (Michenfelder & Milde, 1975), because the relative size of the middle cerebral artery territory decreases with increasing brain volume (Waltz, 1979).

There are indications that the therapeutic effect of barbiturates is not solely due to metabolic inhibition. Other factors such as free radical scavenging (Flamm et al, 1977), reverse steal due to vasoconstriction in the healthy hemisphere

(Feustel et al, 1980), decrease of edema formation (Simeone et al, 1979), improvement of micro-circulation (Black et al, 1979) and decrease of intracranial hypertension (Shapiro et al, 1974) may also play a role. A further elucidation of the barbiturate effect may open other ways for therapeutic intervention. (See Fig. 4.11)

In contrast to the indirect action of anesthetics, a direct reduction of metabolic activity can be achieved by *hypothermia*. According to Van t'Hoff's rule the speed of chemical reactions decreases by 50 per cent when temperature decreases by 10° C. This beneficial effect is reduced or even abolished by a concomitant cold-induced increase in blood viscosity and a decrease in blood perfusion pressure. Ischemic brain damage, therefore, is little influenced by this approach (Simeone et al, 1979; Blöink et al, 1979). See Fig. 4.11.

A recent promising development is therapy of infarcts by so-called 'anti-anoxic' drugs which improve mitochondrial efficiency. During ischemia phospholipid degradation may lead to a disturbance of the permeability of mitochondrial membranes. This results in disturbances of calcium equilibrium and may cause a partial uncoupling of mitochondrial oxidative phosphorylation (Rehncrona et al, 1979). There are indications that certain drugs such as midafenone, or chlorpromazine are able positively to influence this process, and that this may lead to a better use of reduced oxygen supply (Tamura et al, 1979; Farber, 1979).

Treatment of side effects. The influence of cerebral infarcts on the function of peripheral organs is well known to clinicians, but has been little investigated under experimental conditions. One of the most important complications is the development of neurogenic pulmonary edema which is characterized by a disturbance of pulmonary gas exchange and arterial hypoxemia (Cohen & Abraham, 1976). Careful monitoring and adjustment of blood gases and the acid/base state of the blood is a prerequisite for preventing progression of tissue hypoxemia. Intravascular coagulation, stress ulcers and other neurogenic complications are nonspecific reactions following any kind of brain lesion but should also be considered, particularly when experimental infarcts are studied under chronic conditions.

OTHER EXPERIMENTAL STROKE MODELS

Carotid ligation in the gerbil

Beside middle cerebral artery occlusion, the most frequently used experimental stroke model is ligation of the carotid artery in the Mongolian gerbil (*meriones unguiculatus*, Levine & Payan, 1966; Kahn, 1972; Wexler, 1972). In the gerbil, in contrast to most other mammals, the circle of Willis is incomplete because the posterior communicating artery is absent (Berry et al, 1975). Ligation of a common carotid artery, therefore, results in ipsilateral hemispheric ischemia, the degree of which depends on the efficiency of collateral blood supply via the anterior communi-

cating artery. Since the size of this vessel differs considerably from animal to animal, the severity of ischemia varies accordingly. The incidence of stroke ('symptom-positive animals') ranges between 20 per cent (Harrison et al, 1973) and 60 per cent (Levine & Payan, 1966). It can be raised to 70 per cent by additional ligation of the contralateral external carotid artery because this reduces collateral blood supply from the opposite side (Bosma et al, 1981). However, even with this modification the variability of degree and size of the infarcts is considerable and large numbers of animals have to be used in order to obtain statistically relevant data.

Another methodological problem is the fact that gerbils frequently develop seizures after vascular occlusion, and that some of the observed changes may be due to this side effect rather than to ischemia *per se* (Cohn, 1979; Brown et al, 1979). Despite these restrictions, carotid ligation in gerbils has become a most useful experimental stroke model which in many respects resembles closely middle cerebral artery occlusion in higher mammals. Examples are the critical blood flow threshold of about 20 ml/100 g/min for production of neurological symptoms (Nakai et al, 1977), delayed post-ischemic hypoperfusion (Levy et al, 1979), the relationship between ischemia and disturbances of carbohydrate or protein metabolism (Mrsulja et al, 1975; Yanagihara, 1978; Paschen et al, 1980), and the disturbances in catecholamine and neurotransmitter metabolism (Lavyne et al, 1975; Mrsulja et al, 1976; Welch et al, 1977). The development of ischemic brain edema is also similar to that after middle cerebral artery occlusion (Harrison et al, 1973; Westergaard et al, 1976; Ito et al, 1979), and the morphological changes do not differ substantially from those observed in other stroke models (Ito et al, 1975; Levy et al, 1975; Bubis et al, 1976). The gerbil stroke model, in consequence, is a useful and reliable experimental procedure for the study of regional ischemic brain lesions which, in many instances, is of equal value to the middle cerebral artery occlusion technique.

Anoxic-ischemic encephalopathy

With the exception of gerbils, experimental occlusion of the carotid artery does not produce infarcts because the circle of Willis provides an adequate blood supply to the brain by the non-occluded contralateral carotid artery and the vertebral arteries. However, critical unilateral anoxia-ischemia is achieved when ligation of a carotid artery is combined with repeated episodes of anoxia. This procedure has been described by Levine (1960), and formerly has been frequently used for the production of cerebral infarction in rats. It is evident that the combination of anoxia and mild ischemia is a badly defined experimental procedure. Since the introduction of the gerbil stroke model, anoxic-ischemic encephalopathy is only rarely used in experimental ischemia research.

Macroembolism

Several authors have tried to occlude an intra-cranial artery by macroembolism in order to avoid craniectomy and traumatization of the brain during exposure of the artery. Successful occlusions of the main stem or branches of the middle cerebral or basilar arteries have been achieved in various animal species by embolism with silicon cylinders (Molinari, 1970; Turner, 1975; Watanabe et al, 1977; Oki et al, 1979) or homologous blood clots (Hill et al, 1955). The disadvantage of the method, as compared to vascular ligation under visual control, is the greater variability because the final location of the embolus is not predictable. A direct correlation of results obtained in different animals is therefore practically impossible. However, with the newly developed techniques for simultaneous assessment of blood flow, metabolism and bio-chemical substrates in brain sections (see above), a correlation of the various parameters in the same animal is possible. Using such an approach, the variability of the resulting infarcts may be an advantage because it allows the analysis of a greater variety of vascular occlusions than can be achieved by the usual occlusion techniques.

Microembolism

In most ischemic stroke models, one major supply-ing vessel is occluded. In microembolism, in contrast, numerous small vessels are blocked by arterial injection of microspheres (Kogure et al, 1974), air bubbles (de la Torre et al, 1962) or sub-strates which produce platelet aggregates (Fieschi

et al, 1975; Furlow & Bass, 1976). The result is a complex pathophysiological situation because oc-clusion of a number of small vessels is accompanied by reactive hyperemia in the surrounding non-occluded ones. Global flow, therefore, may be reduced, decreased or increased, depending on the number and size of microemboli. Another problem is the effect of microembolism on the blood-brain barrier. Following occlusion of a large vessel such as the middle cerebral artery, the blood-brain barrier breaks down after an interval of three to six hours (Olsson et al, 1971; Kamijyo et al, 1977). Microembolism, in contrast, causes an almost immediate breakdown of the blood-brain barrier (Schuier et al, 1978). The consequence is a rapid development of vasogenic brain edema, which is complicated by a cytotoxic type of edema, either primarily because of ischemia or secondarily because of intracranial hypertension. This ex-tremely complex situation makes it difficult to differentiate between the pathophysiological ef-fects induced by ischemia and edema, and therefore almost precludes its use for either pathophysiol-ogical or pharmacological studies. When reversible microembolism is produced with air bubbles or platelet aggregates, this technique may be of use for producing transient ischemic attacks. Its appli-cation to the study of ischemic stroke, however, is not recommended.

Stroke-prone spontaneously hypertensive rats

One of the major disadvantages of most experi-mental stroke models is the fact that cerebro-vascular occlusion is produced in animals with normal undamaged vasculature. The general hemodynamic situation, therefore, is not readily comparable with that encountered under clinical conditions, in which always some degree of vascular disease is present. One of the most promising experimental models to mimic the clinical situ-ation more closely is a stroke-prone strain of spontaneously hypertensive rats (Okamoto et al, 1974). This strain exhibits spontaneously stroke-like symptoms in about 60 per cent of female and 80 per cent of male hypertensive rats. The vascular alterations and the predilection of cerebrovascular lesions resemble the ones observed in man and the risk factors also seem to be similar in both species

(Yamori et al, 1976). Stroke-prone spontaneously hypertensive rats, therefore, are particularly suited for the study of preventive therapeutic approaches. On the other hand, the investigation of the pathophysiology or biochemistry of stroke itself is of lesser importance because the onset of stroke is not foreseeable and the individual variability is greater than in any other stroke model.

Miscellaneous procedures

Other experimental approaches which occasionally have been used for the production of stroke include carotid artery ligation in hypertensive rats (Choki et al, 1977), extracranial occlusion of the internal maxillary artery in the goat (Miletich et al, 1975), occlusion of the common carotid artery after ligation of the anterior and posterior cerebral arteries in the monkey (West & Matsen, 1972), or occlusion of small pial arteries in the rabbit (Ross Russell, 1971). Although relevant observations have been made using these techniques, they have not found general application in ischemia research. From an experimental standpoint this is certainly justified because the comparison and interpretation of the results obtained in different laboratories are much easier when standardized experimental models are used, such as the middle cerebral artery occlusion in cats and monkeys or the carotid artery occlusion in gerbils. However, it should be considered that these models do not represent the whole variety of cerebrovascular lesions observed in man. The development and use of other stroke models is certainly warranted.

REFERENCES

Abraham J, Ott E O, Aoyagi M, Tagashira Y, Achari A N, Meyer J S 1975 Regional cerebral blood flow changes after bilateral external carotid artery ligation in acute experimental infarction. Journal of Neurology, Neurosurgery and Psychiatry 38:78–88

Ames III A, Wright R L, Kowada M, Thurston J M, Majno G 1968 Cerebral ischemia. II. The no-reflow phenomenon. American Journal of Pathology 52:437–453

Anderson D C, Cranford R E 1979 Corticosteroids in ischemic stroke. Stroke 10:68–71

Anthony L U, Goldring S, O'Leary J L, Schwartz H G 1963 Experimental cerebrovascular occlusion in dog. Archives of Neurology 8:515–527

Astrup J, Symon L, Branston N M, Lassen N A 1977 Cortical evoked potential and extracellular K+ and H+ at critical levels of brain ischemia. Stroke 8:51–57

Battistini N, Casacchia M, Fieschi C, Nardini M, Passero S 1971 Treatment of experimental cerebral infarction with passive hyperventilation. In: Ross Russell R W (ed) Brain and blood flow, Pitman, London, p 102–106

Berry K, Wisniewski H M, Svarzbein L, Baez S 1975 On the relationship of brain vasculature to production of neurological deficit and morphological changes following acute unilateral common carotid artery ligation in gerbils. Journal of the Neurological Sciences 25:75–92

Bito L Z, Myers R E 1972 On the physiological response of the cerebral cortex to acute stress (reversible asphyxia). Journal of Physiology (London) 221:349–370

Black K L, Weidler D J, Jallad N S, Sodeman T M, Abrams G D 1978 Delayed pentobarbital therapy of acute focal cerebral ischemia. Stroke 9:245–249

Black K L, Weidler D J, Randall O S 1979 Improved cerebral microcirculation in focal cerebral ischemia after treatment with pentobarbital. Clinical Research 27:A 714

Blair R D G, Waltz A G 1970 Regional cerebral blood flow during acute ischemia: Correlation of autoradiographic measurements with observations of cortical microcirculation. Neurology 20:802–808

Blöink M, Hossmann V, Hossmann K-A 1979 Treatment of experimental infarcts following middle cerebral artery occlusion in cats. In: Bès A, Géraud G (eds) Circulation cérébrale, Excerpta Medica, Toulouse, p 85–87

Bosma H-J, Paschen W, Hossmann K-A 1981 Cerebral ischemia in gerbils using a modified vascular occlusion model. Excerpta Medica. In: Meyer J S et al (eds) Cerebral vascular disease 3. Excerpta Medica, Amsterdam, Oxford, Princeton, p 280–285

Bowen D M, Goodhardt M J, Strong A J, Smith C B, White P, Branston N M, Symon L, Davison A N 1976 Biochemical indices of brain structure, function and hypoxia in cortex from baboons with middle cerebral occlusion. Brain Research 117:503–507

Brandt L, Andersson K-E, Edvinsson L, Hindfelt B, Ljunggren B, McKenzie E, Tamura A, Teasdale G 1980 Effects of perivascular microapplication of nifedipine on cat pial arteriolar and venular caliber. In: Betz E et al. (eds) Pathophysiology and pharmacotherapy of cerebrovascular disorders, G. Witzstrock Verlag, Baden-Baden, Köln, New York, p 19–23

Branston N M, Strong A J, Symon L 1977 Extracellular potassium activity, evoked potential and tissue blood flow. Journal of the Neurological Sciences 32:305–321

Branston N M, Strong A J, Symon L 1978 Impedance related to local blood flow in cerebral cortex. Journal of Physiology (London) 275:81P–82P

Branston N M, Symon L, Crockard H A, Pasztor E 1974 Relationship between the cortical evoked potential and local cortical blood flow following middle cerebral artery occlusion in the baboon. Experimental Neurology 45:195–208

Bremer A M, Yamada K, West C R 1978 Experimental regional cerebral ischemia in the middle cerebral artery territory in primates. Stroke 9:387–391

Bremer A M, Yamada K, West C R 1980 Ischemic cerebral edema in primates: Effects of acetazolamide, phenytoin, sorbitol, dexamethasone, and methylprednisolone on brain water and electrolytes. Neurosurgery 6:149–154

Brierley J B, Symon L 1977 The extent of infarcts in baboon brains three years after division of the middle cerebral artery. Neuropathology Applied Neurobiology 3:217–218

Brown A W, Levy D E, Kublik M, Harrow J, Plum F, Brierley J B 1979 Selective chromatolysis of neurons in the gerbil brain: A possible consequence of 'epileptic' activity produced by common carotid artery occlusion. Annals of Neurology 5:127–138

Bubis J J, Fujimoto T, Ito U, Mrsulja B J, Spatz M, Klatzo I 1976 Experimental cerebral ischemia in Mongolian gerbils. V. Ultrastructural changes in H_3 sector of the hippocampus. Acta Neuropathologica 36:285–294

Cammermeyer J 1961 The importance of avoiding 'dark' neurons in experimental neuropathology. Acta Neuropathologica 1:245–270

Choki J I, Yamaguchi T, Takeya Y, Morotomi Y, Omae T 1977 Effect of carotid artery ligation on regional cerebral blood flow in normotensive and spontaneously hypertensive rats. Stroke 8:374–379

Cohen J A, Abraham E 1976 Neurogenic pulmonary edema. A sequela of non-hemorrhagic cerebrovascular accidents. Angiology 27:280–292

Cohen H P, Waltz A G, Jacobson R L 1975 Catecholamine content of cerebral tissue after occlusion or manipulation of middle cerebral artery in cats. Journal of Neurosurgery 43:32–36

Cohn R 1979 Convulsive activity in gerbils subjected to cerebral ischemia. Experimental Neurology 65:391–397

Corkill G, Chikovani O K, McLeish I, McDonald L W, Youmans J R 1976 Timing of pentobarbital administration for brain protection in experimental stroke. Surgical Neurology 5:147–149

Corkill G, Sivalingam S, Reitan J A, Gilroy B A, Helphrey M G 1978 Dose dependency of the post-insult protective effect of pentobarbital in the canine experimental stroke model. Stroke 9:10–12

Crockard H A, Symon L, Branston N M, Juhasz J 1976 Changes in regional cortical tissue oxygen tension and cerebral blood flow during temporary middle cerebral artery occlusion in baboons. Journal of the Neurological Sciences 27:29–44

Crowell R M, Olsson Y 1972 Impaired microvascular filling after focal cerebral ischemia in the monkey: Modification by treatment. Neurology 22:500–504

Crowell R M, Olsson Y, Klatzo I, Ommaya A 1970 Temporary occlusion of the middle cerebral artery in the monkey: Clinical and pathological observations. Stroke 1:439–448

Denny-Brown D, Meyer J S 1957 The cerebral collateral circulation. 2. Production of cerebral infarction by ischemic anoxia and its reversibility in early stages. Neurology 7:567–579

Diaz F G, Mastri A R, Ausman J I, Chou S N 1979 Acute cerebral revascularization after regional cerebral ischemia in the dog. Part 2: Clinicopathological correlation. Journal of Neurosurgery 51:644–653

Dodson R F, Miyakawa Y, Wai-Fong Chu L, Ishihara N, Naritomi H, Hsu M C Deshmukh V D 1977 An ultrastructural assessment of an embolic method of producing cerebral ischemia. Stroke 8:337–341

Dodson R F, Tagashira Y, Kawamura Y, Wai-Fong Chu L 1975a Morphological responses of cerebral tissues to temporary ischemia. Canadian Journal of Neurological Sciences 2:173–177

Dodson R F, Tagashira Y, Wai-Fong Chu L 1975b The effects of glycerol on cerebral ultrastructure following experimentally induced cerebral ischemia. Journal of the Neurological Sciences 26:235–243

Dodson R F, Tagashira Y, Wai-Fong Chu L 1976a Acute pericytic response to cerebral ischemia. Journal of the Neurological Sciences 29:9–16

Dodson R F, Tagashira Y, Wai-Fong Chu L 1976b Acute ultrastructural changes in the middle cerebral artery due to the injury and ischemia of surgical clamping. Canadian Journal of Neurological Sciences 3:23–27

Donley R F, Sundt T M, Jr 1973 The effect of dexamethasone on the edema of focal cerebral ischemia. Stroke 4:148–155

Donley R F, Sundt T M, Anderson R E, Sharbrough F W 1975 Blood flow measurements and the 'look through' artifact in focal cerebral ischemia. Stroke 6:121–131

Dujovny M, Osgood C P, Barrionuevo P, Hellstrom R, Maroon J 1976 Experimental middle cerebral artery microsurgical embolectomy. Acta Neurochirurgica 35:91–96

Farber J L 1979 The pathogenesis of irreversible, ischemic cell injury. Journal of Molecular and Cellular Cardiology 11:21

Fenske A, Fischer M, Regli F, Hase U 1979 The response of focal ischemic cerebral edema to dexamethasone. Journal of Neurology 220:199–209

Fenske A, Kohl J, Regli F, Reulen H J 1978 The effect of arterial hypertension on focal ischemic edema. Journal of Neurology 219:241–251

Feustel P J, Ingvar M C, Severinghaus J W 1980 The effect of barbiturates on cerebral oxygen availability (aO_2) and local blood flow (1CBF) during middle cerebral artery occlusion (MCAO). Federation Proceedings: Federation of American Societies for Experimental Biology 39;383

Fieschi C, Battistini N, Volante F, Zanette E, Weber G, Passero S 1975 Animal model of TIA: An experimental study with intracarotid ADP infusion in rabbits. Stroke 6:617–621

Fisk J R, Bender M, Owens G 1969 Experimental cerebrovascular occlusion. New technic for evaluation. New York State Journal of Medicine 69:537–541

Flamm E S, Demopoulos H B, Seligman M L, Poser R, Ransohoff J 1978a Free radicals in cerebral ischemia. Stroke 9:445–447

Flamm E S, Demopoulos H B, Seligman M L, Ransohoff J 1977 Possible molecular mechanisms of barbiturate-mediated protection in regional cerebral ischemia. Acta Neurologica Scandinavica (Supplement 64) 56:150–151

Flamm E S, Schiffer J, Viau A T, Naftchi N E 1978b Alterations of cyclic AMP in cerebral ischemia. Stroke 9:400–402

Furlow T W, Bass N H 1976 Arachidonate-induced cerebrovascular occlusion in the rat. Neurology 26:297–304

Garcia J H 1975 The neuropathology of stroke. Human Pathology 6:583–598

Garcia J H, Cox J V, Hudgins W R 1971 Ultrastructure of the microvasculature in experimental cerebral infarction. Acta Neuropathologica 18:273–285

Garcia J H, Kalimo H, Kamijyo Y, Trump B F 1977 Cellular events during partial cerebral ischemia. I. Electron microscopy of feline cerebral cortex after middle-cerebral-artery occlusion. Virchows Archiv; B:Cell Pathology (Berlin) 25:191–206

Garcia J H, Kamijyo Y 1974 Cerebral infarction. Evolution of histopathological changes after occlusion of a middle cerebral artery in primates. Journal of Neuropathology and Experimental Neurology 33:408–421

Ginsberg M D, Reivich M, Frinak S, Harbig K 1976 Pyridine nucleotide redox state and blood flow of the cerebral cortex following middle cerebral artery occlusion in the cat. Stroke 7:125–131

Ginsberg M D, Reivich M, Giandomenico A, Greenberg J H 1977 Local glucose utilization in acute focal cerebral ischemia: Local dysmetabolism and diaschisis. Neurology 27:1042–1048

Goodhardt M J, Strong A J, Bowen D M, White P, Branston N M, Symon L, Davison A N 1977 The effects of middle-cerebral-artery occlusion on neurotransmitter metabolism in baboons. Biochemical Society Transactions 5:160–163

Habermehl K H 1973 Zur Topographie der Gehirngefäße des Hundes. Anatomy, Histology, Embryology 2:327–353

Hallenbeck J M, Furlow T W 1979 Prostaglandin I$_2$ and indomethacin prevent impairment of post-ischemic brain reperfusion in the dog. Stroke 10:629–637

Hanson E J, Anderson R E, Sundt T M 1975 Comparison of [85]krypton and [133]Xenon cerebral blood flow measurements before, during, and following focal, incomplete ischemia in the squirrel monkey. Circulation Research 36:18–26

Harrington T, Di Chiro G 1973 Effect of hypocarbia and hypercarbia in experimental brain infarction. A microangiographic study in the monkey. Neurology 23:294–299

Harrington T, Major M, Ommaya A K, Di Chiro G 1972 Oxygen availability in ischemic brain following hypocarbia and hypercarbia, polarographical depth electrode recordings in evolving and completed experimental stroke in the monkey. Stroke 3:692–701

Harrison M J G, Brownbill D, Lewis P D, Ross R, Russell R W 1973 Cerebral edema following carotid artery ligation in the gerbil. Archives of Neurology 28;389–391

Hayakawa T, Waltz A G 1975a Changes of epidural pressures after experimental occlusion of one middle cerebral artery in cats. Journal of the Neurological Sciences 26:319–333

Hayakawa T, Waltz A G 1975b Immediate effects of cerebral ischemia: Evolution and resolution of neurological deficits after experimental occlusion of one middle cerebral artery in conscious cats. Stroke 6:321–327

Hayakawa T, Waltz A G 1975c Intracranial pressure, blood pressure, and pulse rate after occlusion of a middle cerebral artery in cats. Journal of Neurosurgery 43:399–407

Heilbrun M P, Goldring S 1968 Steady potential and pathologic correlates of cerebrovascular occlusion of dog. Archives of Neurology 19:410–420

Heiss W-D, Hayakawa T, Waltz A G 1976a Cortical neuronal function during ischemia. Effects of occlusion of one middle cerebral artery on single-unit activity in cats. Archives of Neurology 33:813–820

Heiss W-D, Hayakawa T, Waltz A G 1976b Patterns of changes of blood flow and relationships to infarction in experimental cerebral ischemia. Stroke 7:454–459

Held K, Jacobsen O, Kraft K, Berghoff W 1975 Regional cerebral metabolism in experimental brain infarction. In: Langfitt T W, McHenry L C, Jr, Reivich M, Wollman H (eds) Cerebral circulation and metabolism, Springer, New York, Heidelberg, Berlin, p 82–84

Hill N C, Millikan C H, Wakim K G, Sayre G P 1955 Studies in cerebrovascular disease. Experimental production of cerebral infarction by intracarotid injection of homologous blood clot. Mayo Clinic Proceedings 30:625–633

Høedt-Rasmussen K, Sveinsdottir E, Lassen N A 1966 Regional cerebral blood flow in man determined by intra-arterial injection of radioactive inert gas. Circulation Research 18:237–247

Hoff J T, Smith A L, Hankinson H L, Nielsen S L 1975 Barbiturate protection from cerebral infarction in primates. Stroke 6:28–33

Hope D T, Branston N M, Symon L 1977 Restoration of neurological function with induced hypertension in acute experimental cerebral ischaemia. Acta Neurologica Scandinavica (Supplement 64) 56:506–507

Hossmann K-A 1971 Cortical steady potential, impedance and excitability changes during and after total ischemia of cat brain. Experimental Neurology 32:163–175

Hossmann K-A 1976 Development and resolution of ischemic brain swelling. In: Pappius H, Feindel W (eds) Dynamics of brain edema, Springer, Berlin, Heidelberg, New York, p 219–227

Hossmann K-A, Schuier F J 1979a Metabolic (cytotoxic) type of brain edema following middle cerebral artery occlusion in cats. In: Price T R, Nelson E (eds) Cerebrovascular diseases, Raven Press, New York, p 141–165

Hossmann K-A, Schuier F J 1979b Pathophysiology of stroke edema. In: Zülch K J et al. (eds) Brain and heart infarct II, Springer, Berlin, Heidelberg, New York p 119–129

Hossmann K-A, Schuier F J 1980 Experimental brain infarcts in cats. I. Pathophysiological observations. Stroke, 11: 583–582

Hudgins W R, Garcia J H 1970 Transorbital approach to the middle cerebral artery of the squirrel monkey: A technique for experimental cerebral infarction applicable to ultrastructural studies. Stroke 1:107–111

Ingvar D H, Lassen N A 1962 Regional blood flow of the cerebral cortex determined by krypton[85]. Acta Physiologica Scandinavica 54:325–338

Ito U, Go K G, Walker J T, Spatz M, Klatzo I 1976 Experimental cerebral ischemia in Mongolian gerbils. 3. Behavior of blood-brain barrier. Acta Neuropathologica 34:1–6

Ito U, Ohno K, Nakamura R, Suganuma F, Inaba Y 1979 Brain edema during ischemia and after restoration of blood flow. Measurement of water, sodium, potassium content and plasma protein permeability. Stroke 10:542–547

Ito U, Spatz M, Walker J T Jr, Klatzo I 1975 Experimental cerebral ischemia in Mongolian gerbils. 1. Light microscopic observations. Acta Neuropathologica 32:209–223

Kahn K 1972 The natural course of experimental cerebral infarction in the gerbil. Neurology 22:510–515

Kamijyo Y, Garcia J H 1975 Carotid arterial supply of the feline brain. Applications to the study of regional cerebral ischemia. Stroke 6:361–369

Kamijyo Y, Garcia J H, Cooper J 1977 Temporary regional cerebral ischemia in the cat. A model of hemorrhagic and subcortical infarction. Journal of Neuropathology and Experimental Neurology 36:338–350

Katzman R, Clasen R, Klatzo I, Meyer J S, Pappius H M, Waltz A G 1977 Report of joint committee for stroke resources. 4. Brain edema in stroke. Stroke 8:512–540

Klatzo I 1979 Cerebral oedema and ischaemia. In: Smith

W T, Cavanagh J B (eds) Recent advances in neuropathology, Churchill Livingstone, Edinburgh p 27–39

Kleihues P, Hossmann K-A 1971 Protein synthesis in the cat brain after prolonged cerebral ischemia. Brain Research 35:409–418

Kogure K, Alonso O F 1978 A pictorial representation of endogenous brain ATP by a bioluminescent method. Brain Research 154:273–284

Kogure K, Busto R, Scheinberg P, Reinmuth O M 1974 Energy metabolites and water content in rat brain during the early stage of development of cerebral infarction. Brain 97:103–114

Lavyne M H, Moskowitz M A, Larin F, Zervas N T, Wurtman R J 1975 Brain H³-catecholamine metabolism in experimental cerebral ischemia. Neurology 25:483–485

Lee M C, Mastri A R, Waltz A G, Loewenson R B 1974 Ineffectiveness of dexamethasone for treatment of experimental cerebral infarction. Stroke 5:216–218

Levine S 1960 Anoxic-ischemic encephalopathy in rats. American Journal of Pathology 36:1–17

Levine S, Payan H 1966 Effects of ischemia and other procedures on the brain and retina of the gerbil (Meriones unguiculatus). Experimental Neurology 16:255–262

Levy D E, Brierley J B, Plum F 1975 Ischaemic brain damage in the gerbil in the absence of 'no-reflow'. Journal of Neurology, Neurosurgery and Psychiatry 38;1197–1205

Levy D E, Van Uitert R L, Pike C L 1979 Delayed postischemic hypoperfusion: A potentially damaging consequence of stroke. Neurology 29:1245–1252

Little J R 1977 Implanted device for middle cerebral artery occlusion in conscious cats. Stroke 8:258–260

Little J R 1978 Modification of acute focal ischemia by treatment with mannitol and high dose dexamethasone. Journal of Neurosurgery 49:517–524

Little J R, Kerr, F W L, Sundt T M Jr 1974a The role of lysosomes in production of ischemic nerve cell changes. Archives of Neurology 30:448–455

Little J R, Kerr F W L, Sundt T M Jr 1976 Microcirculatory obstruction in focal cerebral ischemia: An electron microscopic investigation in monkeys. Stroke 7:25–30

Little J R, Sundt T M, Kerr F W L 1974b Neuronal alterations in developing cortical infarction. An experimental study in monkeys. Journal of Neurosurgery 39:186–198

Little J R, O'Shaughnessy D 1979 Treatment of acute focal ischemia with continuous CSF drainage and mannitol. Stroke 10:446–450

MacDonald V D, Sundt T M, Winkelmann R K 1972 Histochemical studies in the zone of ischemia following middle cerebral artery occlusion in cats. Journal of Neurosurgery 37:45–54

Meyer J S, Denny-Brown D 1957 The cerebral collateral circulation 1. Factors influencing collateral blood flow. Neurology 7:447–458

Meyer J S, Fukuuchi Y, Kanda T, Shimazu K, Hashi K 1972 Regional cerebral blood flow measured by intracarotid injection of hydrogen. Comparison of regional vasomotor capacitance from cerebral infarction versus compression. Neurology 22:571–584

Michenfelder J D, Milde J H 1975 Influence of anesthetics on metabolic, functional and pathological responses to regional cerebral ischemia. Stroke 6:405–410

Michenfelder J D, Sundt T M Jr 1971 Cerebral ATP and lactate levels in the squirrel monkey following occlusion of the middle cerebral artery. Stroke 2:319–326

Miletich D J, Ivankovic A D, Albrecht R F, Toyooka E T 1975 Cerebral hemodynamics following internal maxillary artery ligation in the goat. Journal of Applied Physiology 38:942–945

Miller J D, Garibi J, North J B, Teasdale G M 1975 Effects of increased arterial pressure on blood flow in the damaged brain. Journal of Neurology, Neurosurgery and Psychiatry 38:657–665

Molinari G F 1970 Experimental cerebral infarction. I. Selective segmental occlusion of intracranial arteries in the dog. Stroke 1:224–231

Molinari G F, Moseley J I, Laurent J P 1974 Segmental middle cerebral artery occlusion in primates: An experimental method requiring minimal surgery and anesthesia. Stroke 5:334–339

Molinari G F, Oakley J C, Laurent J P 1976 The pathophysiology of barbiturate protection in focal ischemia. Stroke 7:3–4

Monakow von C 1914 Die Lokalisation im Grosshirn und der Abbau der Funktion durch kortikale Herde. J F Bergmann Verlag, Wiesbaden

Morawetz R B, Crowell R H, De Girolami U, Marcoux F W, Jones T H, Halsey J H 1979 Regional cerebral blood flow thresholds during cerebral ischemia. Federation Proceedings: Federation of American Societies for Experimental Biology 38:2493–2494

Morawetz R B, De Girolami U, Ojemann R G, Marcoux F W, Crowell R M 1978 Cerebral blood flow determined by hydrogen clearance during middle cerebral artery occlusion in unanesthetized monkeys. Stroke 9:143–149

Moseley J I, Laurent J P, Molinari G F 1975 Barbiturate attenuation of the clinical course and pathologic lesions in a primate stroke model. Neurology 25:870–874

Mrsulja B B, Mrsulja B J, Ito U, Walker J T, Spatz M, Klatzo I 1975 Experimental cerebral ischemia in Mongolian gerbils. 2. Changes in carbohydrates. Acta Neuropathologica 33:91–103

Mrsulja B B, Mrsulja B J, Spatz M, Ito U, Walker J T, Klatzo I 1976 Experimental cerebral ischemia in Mongolian gerbils. 4. Behavior of biogenic amines. Acta Neuropathologica 36:1–8

Nakai K, Welch K M A, Meyer J S 1977 Critical cerebral blood flow for production of hemiparesis after unilateral carotid occlusion in the gerbil. Journal of Neurology, Neurosurgery and Pschychiatry 40:595–599

Neumann L, Betz E, Benzing H 1970 Wirkung einer Unterbindung der Arteria cerebri media auf Durchblutung, Sauerstoffdruck und Säure-Basen-Haushalt in deren Versorgungsgebiet. Internationale Zeitschrift für angewandte Physiologie 29:29–43

Ng L K Y, Nimmannitya J 1970 Massive cerebral infarction with severe brain swelling: A clinicopathological study. Stroke 1:158–163

O'Brien M D, Jordan M M, Waltz A G 1974 Ischemic cerebral edema and the blood-brain barrier. Distributions of pertechnetate, albumin, sodium, and antipyrine in brains of cats after occlusion of the middle cerebral artery. Archives of Neurology 30:461–465

O'Brien M D, Waltz A G 1973a Intracranial pressure gradients caused by experimental cerebral ischemia and edema. Stroke 4:694–698

O'Brien M D, Waltz A G 1973b Transorbital approach for occluding the middle cerebral artery without craniectomy. Stroke 4:201–206

O'Brien M D, Waltz A G, Jordan M M 1974 Ischemic cerebral edema. Distribution of water in brains of cats after occlusion of the middle cerebral artery. Archives of Neurology 30:456–460

Okada Y, Shima T, Yamamoto M, Uozumi T, Kawasaki T 1979 Experimental middle cerebral artery embolization and embolectomy. Acta Neurochirurgica Supplement 28:222–225

Okamoto K, Yamori Y, Nagaoka A 1974 Establishment of the stroke-prone spontaneously hypertensive rat (SHR). Circulation Research (Supplement 1) 34, 35:143–153

Oki S, Shima T, Okada Y, Ishikawa S, Uozumi T 1979 Experimental infarction of the brain stem. Acta Neurologica Scandinavica (Supplement 72) 60:314–315

Olsson Y, Crowell R M, Klatzo I 1971 The blood-brain barrier to protein tracers in focal cerebral ischemia and infarction caused by occlusion of the middle cerebral artery. Acta Neuropathologica 18:89–102

Paschen W, Bosma H-J, Hossmann K-A 1980 Evaluation of ischemic brain lesions in Mongolian gerbils by regional enzymatic techniques. Hoppe-Seyler's Zeitschrift für Physiologische Chemie 361:312

Paschen W, Matsuoka Y, Niebuhr I, Hossmann K-A 1981 Regional biochemistry of the energy-producing metabolism of the cat brain following middle cerebral artery occlusion. In: Cervos-Navarro J, Fritschka E (eds) Cerebral microcirculation and metabolism, Raven Press, New York, p 337–342

Paschen W, Niebuhr I, Hossmann K-A A bioluminescence method for the demonstration of regional glucose distribution in brain slices. Journal of Neurochemistry 36:513–517

Pasztor E, Symon L, Dorsch N W, Branston N M 1973 The hydrogen clearance method in assessment of blood flow in cortex, white matter and deep nuclei of baboons. Stroke 4:556–567

Petersen J N, Evans J P 1937 The anatomical end results of cerebral arterial occlusion. Transactions of the American Neurological Association 63:88–93

Prosenz P 1971 The cerebral hyperperfusion syndrome. Experimental investigations on its circulatory mechanisms and its metabolic effects. Verlag Brüder Hollinek, Wien

Rasmussen T Harvey J 1951 Occlusion of the middle cerebral artery. Archives of Neurology and Psychiatry 66:20

Regli F, Yamaguchi T, Waltz A G 1971a Cerebral circulation. Effects of vasodilating drugs on blood flow and the microvasculature of ischemic and nonischemic cerebral cortex. Archives of Neurology 24:467–474

Regli F, Yamaguchi T, Waltz A G 1971b Effects of acetazolamide on cerebral ischemia and infarction after experimental occlusion of middle cerebral artery. Stroke 2:456–460

Regli F, Yamaguchi T, Waltz A G 1971c Responses of surface arteries and blood flow of ischemic and nonischemic cerebral cortex to aminophylline, ergotamine tartrate, and acetazolamide. Stroke 2:461–470

Rehncrona S, Folbergrova J, Smith D S, Siesjö B K 1980 Influence of complete and pronounced incomplete cerebral ischemia and subsequent recirculation on cortical concentrations of oxidized and reduced glutathione in the rat. Journal of Neurochemistry 34:477–486

Rehncrona S, Mela L, Siesjö B K 1979 Recovery of brain mitochondrial function in the rat after complete and incomplete cerebral ischemia. Stroke 10:437–446

Reivich M, Ginsberg M, Slater R, Jones S, Kovach A, Greenberg J, Goldberg H 1978 Alterations in regional cerebral hemodynamics and metabolism produced by focal cerebral ischemia. European Neurology (Supplement 1) 17:9–16

Ross Russell R W 1971 The reactivity of the pial circulation of the rabbit to hypercapnia and the effect of vascular occlusion. Brain 94:623–634

Rudolph A M, Heymann M A 1967 The circulation of the fetus in utero: Methods for studying distribution of blood flow, cardiac output and organ blood flow. Circulation Research 21:163–184

Sakurada O, Kennedy C, Jehle J, Brown J D, Carbin G L, Sokoloff L 1978 Measurement of local cerebral blood flow with iodo [^{14}C] antipyrine. American Journal of Physiology 234:H59–H66

Schuier F J, Vise M, Hossmann K-A, Zülch K J 1978 Cerebral microembolization. II. Morphological studies. Archives of Neurology 35:264–270

Schuier F J, Hossmann K-A 1980 Experimental brain infarcts in cats. 2. Ischemic brain edema. Stroke 11:593–601

Shalit M N, Reinmuth O M, Scheinberg P 1967 Some hemodynamic aspects of regional brain ischemia. Transactions of the American Neurological Association 92:75–78

Shapiro H M, Wyte St R, Loeser J 1974 Barbiturate-augmented hypothermia for reduction of persistent intracranial hypertension. Journal of Neurosurgery 40:90–100

Shibata S, Hodge C P, Pappius H M 1974 Effect of experimental ischemia on cerebral water and electrolytes. Journal of Neurosurgery 41:146–159

Shima T, Okada Y, Ishikawa S, Miyazaki M, Uozumi T 1979 Experimental embolization of the middle cerebral artery and embolectomy: A pathophysiological study. In: Lovenberg W (ed) Prophylactic approach to hypertensive diseases, Raven Press, New York, p 533–538

Siesjö B K 1978 Brain energy metabolisms. John Wiley & Sons, Chichester, New York, Brisbane, Toronto

Simeone F A, Frazer G, Lawner P 1979 Ischemic brain edema: Comparative effects of barbiturates and hypothermia. Stroke 10:8–12

Smith A L, Hoff J T, Nielsen S L, Larson C P 1974 Barbiturate protection in acute focal cerebral ischemia. Stroke 5:1–7

Sokoloff L, Reivich M, Kennedy C, Des Rosiers M H, Patlak C S, Pettigrew K D, Sakurada O, Shinohara U 1977 The (^{14}C) deoxyglucose method for the measurement of local cerebral glucose utilization: Theory, procedure, and normal values in the conscious and anesthetized albino rat. Journal of Neurochemistry 28:897–916

Soloway M, Moriarty G, Fraser J G, White R J 1971 Effect of delayed hyperventilation on experimental cerebral infarction. Neurology 21:479–485

Steen P A, Soule E H, Michenfelder J D 1979 Detrimental effect of prolonged hypothermia in cats and monkeys with and without regional cerebral ischemia. Stroke 10:522–529

Strong A J, Goodhardt M J, Branston N M, Symon L 1977 A comparison of the effects of ischaemia on tissue flow, electrical activity and extracellular potassium ion concentration in cerebral cortex of baboons. Biochemical Society Transactions 5:158–160

Sundt T M, Anderson R E 1975 Reduced nicotinamide adenine-dinucleotide fluorescence and cortical blood flow in ischemic and nonischemic squirrel monkey cortex. 1.

Animal preparation, instrumentation 1, and validity of model. Stroke 6:270–278

Sundt T M Jr, Anderson R E, Sharbrough F W 1976 Effect of hypocapnia, hypercapnia, and blood pressure on NADH fluorescence, electrical activity, and blood flow in normal and partially ischemic monkey cortex. Journal of Neurochemistry 27:1125–1133

Sundt T M Jr, Michenfelder J D 1972 Focal transient cerebral ischemia in the squirrel monkey: Effect on brain adenosine triphosphate and lactate levels with electrocorticographic and pathologic correlation. Circulation Research 30:703–712

Sundt T M Jr, Waltz A 1966 Experimental cerebral infarction: Retro-orbital, extradural approach for occluding the middle cerebral artery. Mayo Clinic Proceedings 41:159–168

Sundt T M Jr, Waltz A G 1967 Hemodilution and anticoagulation. Effects on the microvasculature and microcirculation of the cerebral cortex after arterial occlusion. Neurology 17:230–238

Symon L 1970 Regional cerebrovascular responses to acute ischaemia in normocapnia and hypercapnia: An experimental study in baboons. Journal of Neurology, Neurosurgery and Psychiatry 33:756–762

Symon L, Branston N M, Chikovani O 1979 Ischemic brain edema following middle cerebral artery occlusion in baboons: Relationship between regional cerebral water content and blood flow at 1 to 2 hours. Stroke 10:184–191

Symon L, Branston N M, Strong A J 1976 Autoregulation in acute focal ischemia. An experimental study. Stroke 7:547–554

Symon L, Crockard H A, Dorsch N W C, Branston N M, Juhasz J 1975 Local cerebral blood flow and vascular reactivity in a chronic stable stroke in baboons. Stroke 6:482–492

Symon L, Held K, Dorsch N W 1973 A study of regional autoregulation in the cerebral circulation to increased perfusion pressure in normocapnia and hypercapnia. Stroke 4:139–147

Symon L, Khodadad G, Montoya G 1971 Effect of carbon dioxide inhalation on the pattern of gaseous metabolism in ischaemic zones of the primate cortex. An experimental study of the 'intracerebral steal' phenomenon in baboons. Journal of Neurology, Neurosurgery and Psychiatry 34:481–486

Symon L, Lassen N A, Astrup J, Branston N M 1977 Thresholds of ischaemia in brain cortex. Advances in Experimental Medicine and Biology 94:775–782

Tamura A, Asano T, Sano K, Tsumagari J, Nakajima A 1979 Protection from cerebral ischemia by a new imidazole derivate (Y-9179) and pentobarbital. A comparative study in chronic middle cerebral artery occlusion in cats. Stroke 10:126–134

Tamura A, Graham D, McCulloch J, Teasdale G 198 Focal cerebral ischaemia in the rat. In: Betz E et al (eds) Pathophysiology and pharmacotherapy of cerebrovascular disorders. G Witzstrock Verlag, Baden-Baden, 172–176

Tamura A, Sano K 1979 The temporary occlusion of middle cerebral artery in cats. The correlation between the rCBF and the histological changes. No To Shinkei Brain and Nerve Tokyo 31:1005–1015

Torre de la E, Meredith J, Netsky M G 1962 Cerebral air embolism in the dog. Archives of Neurology 6:307–316

Torre de la J C, Surgeon J W 1976 Dexamethasone and DMSO in experimental transorbital cerebral infarction. Stroke 7:577–583

Traupe H, Heiss W-D 1980 Perfusion patterns after MCA-occlusion of various duration. In: Betz E et al. (eds) Pathophysiology and Pharmacotherapy of Cerebrovascular Disorders. G Witzstrock Verlag, Baden-Baden, 177–181

Tulleken C A F, Meyer J S, Ott E O, Abraham J, Dodson R F 1974 Brain tissue pressure gradients in experimental infarction and space occupying lesions. Clinical Neurology and Neurosurgery 77:198–211

Turner J H 1975 Brain scan in cerebral ischemia. An experimental model in rat. Stroke 6:703–706

Vise W M, Schuier F J, Hossmann K-A, Takagi S, Zülch K J 1977 Cerebral microembolization. 1. Pathophysiological studies. Archives of Neurology 34:660–665

Vyskocil F, Kriz N, Bures J 1972 Potassium-selective microelectrodes used for measuring the extracellular brain potassium during spreading depression and anoxic depolarization in rats. Brain Research 39:255–259

Wade J G, Amtorp O, Sörensen S C 1975 No-flow state following cerebral ischemia. Role of increase in potassium concentration in brain interstitial fluid. Archives of Neurology 32:381–384

Waltz A G 1967 Cortical blood flow of opposite hemisphere after occlusion of middle cerebral artery. Transactions of the American Neurological Association 92:293–294

Waltz A G 1968 Effect of blood pressure on blood flow in ischemic and in nonischemic cerebral cortex. The phenomena of autoregulation and luxury perfusion. Neurology 18:613–621

Waltz A G 1970 Effect of Pa CO$_2$ on blood flow and microvasculature of ischemic and nonischemic cerebral cortex. Stroke 1:27–37

Waltz A G 1976 Pathophysiology of cerebral infarction. Clinical Neurosurgery 23:147–154

Waltz A G 1979 Clinical relevance of models of cerebral ischemia. Stroke 10:211–213

Waltz A G, Sundt T M Jr 1967 The microvasculature and microcirculation of the cerebral cortex after arterial occlusion. Brain 90:681–696

Watanabe O, Bremer A M, West C R 1977a Experimental regional cerebral ischemia in the middle cerebral artery territory in primates. 1. Angio-anatomy and description of an experimental model with selective embolization of the internal artery bifurcation. Stroke 8:61–70

Watanabe O, West C R, Bremer A 1977b Experimental regional cerebral ischemia in the middle cerebral artery territory in primates 1. 2. Effects on brain water and electrolytes in the early phase of MCA stroke. Stroke 8:71–76

Weber R, Furuse M, Brock M, Dietz H 1974 The single dye passage: A new technique for the study of cerebral blood flow distribution. Stroke 5:247–251

Weidler D F, Jallad N S, Black K L 1979 Critical plasma pentobarbital levels in the treatment of acute ischemic stroke. Research Communications in Chemical Pathology and Pharmacology 26:35–45

Welch K M A, Chabi E, Buckingham J, Bergin B, Achar V S, Meyer J S 1977 Catecholamine and 5-hydroxytryptamine levels in ischemic brain. Influence of parachlorophenylalanine. Stroke 8:341–346

Welch K M, Hashi K, Meyer J S 1973 Cerebrovascular response to intracarotid injection of serotonin before and after middle cerebral artery occlusion. Journal of Neurology, Neurosurgery and Psychiatry 36:724–735

Welsh F A, Greenberg J H, Jones S C, Ginsberg M D, Reivich M 1980 Correlation between glucose utilization and metabolite levels during focal ischemia in cat brain. Stroke 11:79–84

Welsh F A, O'Connor M J, Langfitt T W 1977 Regions of cerebral ischemia located by pyridine nucleotide fluorescence. Science 198:951–953

West C R, Matsen F A 1972 Effects of experimental ischemia on electrolytes of cortical cerebrospinal fluid and on brain water. Journal of Neurosurgery 36:687–699

Westergaard E, Go G, Klatzo I, Spatz M 1976 Increased permeability of cerebral vessels to horseradish peroxidase induced by ischemia in Mongolian gerbils. Acta Neuropathologica 35:307–325

Wexler B C 1972 Pathophysiological responses to acute cerebral ischemia in the gerbil. Stroke 3:71–78

Yamaguchi T, Regli F, Waltz A G 1971a Effect of PaCO$_2$ on hyperemia and ischemia in experimental cerebral infarction. Stroke 2: 139–147

Yamaguchi T, Waltz A G, Okazaki H 1971b Hyperemia and ischemia in experimental cerebral infarction: Correlation of histopathology and regional blood flow. Neurology 21:565–578

Yamamoto M, Okada Y, Shima T, Ishikawa S, Uozumi T, Yamada K, Kawasaki T 1979 Regional cerebral energy metabolism in dogs following artificial embolization of the middle cerebral artery. Acta Neurologica Scandinavica (Supplement 72) 60:48–49

Yamori Y, Horie R, Handa H, Sato M, Fukase M 1976 Pathogenetic similarity of strokes in stroke-prone spontaneously hypertensive rats and humans. Stroke 7:46–53

Yanagihara T 1978 Experimental stroke in gerbils: Effect on translation and transcription. Brain Research 158:435–444

Zervas N T, Hori H, Nagoro M, Wurtman R 1976 Neurogenic regulation of cerebral blood flow following ischemia. Stroke 7:113–118

Zervas N T, Hori H, Negora M, Wurtman R J, Larin F, Lavyne M H 1974 Reduction in brain dopamine following experimental cerebral ischemia. Nature 247:283–284

5

Cerebral blood flow and metabolism in stroke patients

Cesare Fieschi and Gian Luigi Lenzi

The last 30 years have seen a growing interest in the physiology of the cerebral blood flow (CBF) brought about by the development of new quantitative methods. This growth has gone through three phases, but latterly there has been a decline in the enthusiasm of the neurological world, mainly due to a lack of clinical application. Only very recently, a fourth phase, due to the introduction of positron emission tomography (PET), has revived the impetus of the research effort and may lead, it is hoped, to better returns in terms of clinical usefulness.

We may therefore outline the four phases:

PHASE 1, 1945–1960: invasive quantitative techniques for measurement of global CBF: the nitrous oxide method of Kety & Schmidt (1948), with its variants (Lassen & Munch, 1955).

PHASE 2, 1961–1975: invasive quantitative techniques for measurement of regional blood flow (rCBF) by intracarotid injection of radioactive inert gases (Lassen et al, 1963).

PHASE 3, 1970–1978: non-invasive quantitative techniques for measurement of rCBF by inhalation (Obrist et al, 1967) or intravenous injection of radioactive inert gases (Agnoli et al, 1968; Thomas et al, 1979).

PHASE 4, 1978 to the present: quantitative evaluation of regional CBF and cerebral metabolism of oxygen and glucose by positron emission tomography (Kuhl et al, 1977; Reivich et al, 1979; Frackowiak et al, 1980a & b).

Other non-quantitative methods of clinical interest such as sequential scintiphotography (Heiss et al, 1972), intravenous technetium angiography (Plainiol et al, 1971), intracarotid injection of radioalbumin (Fazio et al, 1963), intracarotid radioactive microsphere angiography (Blandino et

al, 1973) or intracarotid infusion of very short-lived radioactive inert gases (Fazio et al, 1977 & 1979) have also been used to study disturbances in brain perfusion in patients with pathology of the large extracranial arteries and in patients submitted to EC-IC bypass surgery.

The present chapter will be mainly devoted to studies performed on acute CVD with the 'invasive' techniques for measurement of rCBF. There is a brief introduction on the basic physiology of the cerebral circulation and its control and some additional material on studies with PET.

For a more detailed and comprehensive analysis of the physiopathology of CBF the reader is referred to reviews such as those of Sokoloff (1959), Betz (1972), Olesen (1974), Mosmans (1974) Lassen and Skinhøj (1975) and Ingvar & Lassen (1975).

THE PHYSIOLOGY OF CBF

In the last century Roy & Sherrington (1890) suggested that metabolites generated within the nervous tissue played a primary role in the regulation of the blood flow of the brain. In their view, 'acid' products due to increased neuronal metabolism in response to a functional activation led to a local vasodilatation with local increase of CBF. However, for many decades this theory found no supporters and CBF was thought to follow passively the systemic blood pressure until Kety & Schmidt (1948) indicated that CBF in fact remained constant in spite of variations in perfusion pressure.

Due to the continuous activity of neurons in the healthy brain, during sleep as well as in wakefulness, CBF has a nearly constant value of about 55 ml/100 g/min, provided the $PaCO_2$ does not vary. The concept of a constant CBF in the normal, healthy brain, although still valid as an 'average' value, has had to be modified after the introduction of techniques for regional CBF quantitation, which have shown that local increases up to 100 per cent, as well as equivalent reductions in flow, can be detected in different physiological conditions of activation or deactivation.

In this respect, the old concept of Roy & Sherrington has proved to be true. Besides, the 'function-linked' regulation is not the only regulatory mechanism of rCBF, which is in fact controlled by four major mechanisms, namely: metabolic, neurogenic autoregulation and chemical regulation.

Metabolic regulation is basically what had been observed by Roy & Sherrington: their 'acid' products are probably the H^+ and K^+ ions, released by local metabolism in direct proportion to the local function, and probably acting via Ca^{++} on the contractile state of the arteriolar smooth muscle, as described below.

By this mechanism, local CBF is continuously coupled to local metabolic demands, which depend on the local functional activity (Raichle et al, 1976).

The *neurogenic regulation* of the CBF is still under discussion. The new neurohistological techniques and the work of Edvinsson have revealed several cerebral vascular neuroeffector mechanisms. The brain's vascular bed receives a well-developed *autonomic innervation*, but its final effects on CBF are still controversial. In animals, particular brain stem regions are capable of producing large increases in CBF. The action of cerebrovascular cholinergic nerves is probably a direct vasodilatation in combination with inhibition of sympathetic vasoconstrictor adrenergic tone.

The *autoregulation* of CBF is a fundamental mechanism, which insures a constant supply of blood and substrates, within a large spectrum of perfusion pressure, to the brain. It is probably the result of a myogenic response of the smooth muscle cells of the arteriolar wall to the increase in transluminal pressure. Autoregulation implies that the cerebral vessels dilate when the pressure rises. This mechanism shows a lower limit (60 mmHg)

and an upper limit (180–200 mmHg). Outside these limits, CBF varies passively with pressure. This mechanism is frequently altered in disease.

The *chemical regulation* of CBF is based on the response of arterioles to the $PaCO_2$. CBF increases 5 per cent for each mmHg increase in $PaCO_2$ (Reivich, 1964). The CO_2 response is mediated by pH variations in the periarteriolar space, and it is influenced also by the local bicarbonate concentration. This mechanism is basically a homeostatic one: with a rise in $PaCO_2$ the flow increase allows a rapid wash-out of the metabolically produced CO_2. Therefore hypercapnia and hypocapnia exert a profound influence on CBF. In addition oxygen tension in arterial blood is able to change CBF, in particular where there is a marked arterial hypoxia (below 50 mmHg). Since at this level a progressive brain tissue lactacidosis occurs, probably the CO_2 and O_2 mechanisms are interrelated.

Principles of the rCBF method

The method for measurement of rCBF with radioactive inert gases was proposed by Lassen & Ingvar in 1961. Its principle is the assumption that the removal of a freely diffusible and inert indicator from a tissue is a function of the perfusion rate of that tissue. If one uses radioactive γ-emitting isotopes as indicators, it is then possible to record the clearance from various areas of the brain through the intact cranium by multiple detectors placed over the patient's scalp. The recording lasts from 10 to 15 min after the injection of the tracer, dissolved in physiological saline and administered as a single bolus in the internal carotid artery, during which time the patient is assumed to remain in a steady state.

The radioactive gas originally used was Krypton -85 (^{85}Kr). Its radioactive characteristics permit a good counting efficiency because of the high energy of its radiations (0.5 MeV), but the physical half-life of this isotope is rather long (10.5 years) and only 0.4 per cent of its emissions are in the form of γ-rays. Hence, if one is to record through the skull, the quantity injected must be high (3 mCi) with a radiation dose to the brain reaching 29 mrad/mCi (Høedt-Rasmussen, 1967). Because of these disadvantages investigators have turned to another radioactive inert gas, Xenon-133 (^{133}Xe).

This is also a γ-emitter (99 per cent of its incident radiations) with an energy of 0.081 MeV, permitting the administration of a lower dose with each intracarotid injection (0.5 to 1 mCi), with a radiation dose to the brain of 17 mrad/mCi injected. Its physical half-life of 5.3 days precludes long storage after preparation but reduces the hazards of contamination of the atmosphere. However, because of the low energy of its gamma radiations, its usefulness is hampered by self-absorption in the tissue, leading to a significant degree of Compton scattering which accounts for 13 to 20 per cent of the total counts picked up by the probes over the scalp (Posner, 1973). Thus, opposite any given probe, the overlapping radiation coming from adjacent regions of the brain constitutes a serious limitation for a method designed to evaluate the blood flow of circumscribed cerebral regions and for that reason the use of a more efficient radioactive tracer is preferable.

Flow is not the only variable governing the rate of removal of a tracer from brain tissue; the relative solubility of this tracer in brain and blood (brain: blood partition coefficient λ) is another important factor to be considered. In the case of Kr and Xe which are lipid soluble, the λ is above one, higher for white than for grey matter, and will vary with haematocrit or alteration in brain constituents as encountered in various types of pathology.

For a normal haematocrit and in normal brain tissue, the λ for Kr has been found to be 1.32 for white matter and 0.97 for grey matter, and for Xe, 1.57 and 0.84 respectively, with a weighted mean for whole brain of 1.11 for Kr and 1.13 for Xe (assuming a constant proportion of 60 per cent grey and 40 per cent white matter in each region to be measured). These are the standard values employed by most investigators although 'with some hesitation' (Høedt-Rasmussen, 1967).

Indicators with a partition coefficient uniformly closer to 1, such as N_2O, H_2 or water, would be more reliable and allow more precise calculations.

Eichling (1979) pointed out that it is interesting that investigators have almost exclusively relied on one set of published values of λ for Xenon in brain for over 10 years, although major difference exist with other reported values. O'Brien & Veall (1974) have demonstrated major variations of λ for different tissues, concluding that the use of normal brain: blood values for ^{133}Xe may result in substantial errors when calculating rCBF in patients with cerebral disease. In other words rCBF differences may reflect only changes in regional λ.

Mathematical processing

From the data recorded by the probes rCBF can be calculated in several ways.

Compartmental analysis. This assumes that the clearance curve is the sum of two monoexponential components (Lassen et al, 1963) and is based on the existence of two compartments in brain, white and grey matter, whose relative flows are known from autoradiographic studies to differ by a factor of four (Freygang & Sokoloff, 1959). By this approach the regional flow value for any given area of the brain is obtained from the biexponential analysis of the corresponding clearance curve as follows:

$$F_{bc} \text{ ml/100 g/min} = (F_g \times W_g + F_w \times W_w)/W_g + W_w$$

where F_{bc} represents the rCBF, F_g and W_g represent the flow and the relative weight of the rapidly perfused compartment, i.e., the grey matter (frequently referred to as the 'fast phase' or the 'cortical flow') while F_w and W_w represent the flow and the relative weight of the slowly perfused compartment, i.e., the white matter ('slow phase'). Although this bicompartmental analysis can provide the investigator with useful information, its results must be interpreted with caution; the weights of the two components vary in the same individual according to functional activity, the administration of sedative drugs, or the presence of pathology (Wilkinson & Browne, 1970). The 'fast phase' and 'slow phase' should thus be interpreted more on a physiological than an anatomical basis.

In our own control series of 10 subjects without central nervous system diseases (mean age of 52 years), we obtained with this analysis the following values which are comparable to those reported in the literature for similar age groups: mean rCBF $= 44.7 \pm 6.2$; $F_g = 78.2 \pm 18.3$; $F_w = 20.8 \pm 2.7$; $W_g = 43$ per cent ± 6.3; at a mean arterial PCO_2 of 41.6 vol per cent (see Table 5.1).

Stochastic analysis, or 'height-over-area-equation' (Zierler, 1965), gives values for rCBF without compartmental estimates. It is based on the assumption that in any region with a perfusion of f, the mean transit time $\bar{t}$ of a tracer with a distribution volume of V is equal to:

$$\bar{t} = V/f \qquad (1)$$

If perfusion is expressed as flow per 100 g of tissue, as such:

$$F = f/W \times 100 \qquad (2)$$

where W represents the weight of the tissue in grams, then equation (1) can be rewritten as follows:

$$\bar{t} = \frac{V}{W} \times \frac{100}{F} \qquad (3)$$

or

$$F = \frac{V}{W} \times \frac{100}{\bar{t}} \qquad (4)$$

Since $\bar{t}$ corresponds to the total area (A) under the clearance curve over the maximum height (H) reached by this curve, equation (4) will finally become:

$$F_{10} = \frac{V}{W} \times \frac{H}{A} \times 100 \qquad (5)$$

where F_{10} (flow for a 10 min recording) represents the rCBF expressed in ml per 100 g of brain tissue per minute and (V/W) represents the distribution volume of the tracer per unit weight of tissue, that is weighted λ which is assumed, as for the bicompartmental analysis, to be a known constant.

Since, as stated above, the latter can vary and should be determined for any given condition, the stochastic analysis has essentially the same limitations as the bicompartmental approach without giving as detailed information. For practical purposes rCBF values obtained with either method are fairly similar, as computed from six data groups:
$\triangle F_{BC} - F_{10} = 0.2$ per cent, NS (see Table 5.1).

With the *initial slope analysis* or two minute-flow index, introduced by Høedt-Rasmussen in 1967, rCBF is calculated from the slope of the initial part of the clearance curve regarded as monoexponential for the first one or two minutes of the recording. One then corrects for the λ of the grey matter only, since it is assumed that during this early phase the bulk of the counts are coming from this compartment.

Despite understandable theoretical objections and a systematic difference between rCBF values obtained from the initial slope, F (init) and those calculated by the other types of analysis, as computed from four data-groups ΔF (init) $- F_{10} = 17$ per cent, $p < 0.05$ (see Table 5.1). The short duration of recording required and the rapid analysis of data possible without a computer has rendered the use of this simplified approach very popular for clinical purposes. Its results, however, should be regarded as a relative 'index' of cerebral perfusion rather than as an absolute flow value.

One major theoretical objection to the rCBF methods, whatever mode of calculation is used, involves recirculation and extracerebral contami-

Table 5.1 Mean rCBF values found in awake conscious control subjects without demonstrable organic brain disease

| Author | No. patients | No. probes | Mean age | Tracer | Compartmental analysis | | | | Stochastic analysis F_{10} | Initial slope F (init.) | $P_a co_2$ mmHg |
					F_g	F_w	$W_{g\%}$	F_{BC}			
Lassen et al (1963)	6-Hosp.	2	45	^{85}-Kr				$60 + 13$			
Ingvar & Lassen (1965)	7-Normal	4	21–47	^{85}-Kr	80 ± 11	21 ± 3	$49 + 4$	50	50 ± 5	55 ± 6	38.6
Fieschi et al (1966)	10-Hosp.	4	52	^{85}-Kr	78 ± 18	21 ± 3	43 ± 6	45 ± 6	42 ± 5		41.6 (vol %)
Hoedt-Rasmussen (1967)	9-Hosp.	1		^{85}-Kr	81 ± 6	23 ± 4	48 ± 5	50	50 ± 8		40
Zingesser et al (1968)	10-Normal	4	33	^{133}-Xe				54 ± 6			
McHenry et al (1969)	5-Hosp.	8		^{133}-Xe	77 ± 6	22 ± 1	54 ± 6	52 ± 3	54 ± 3		39
Wilkinson et al (1969)	10-Hosp.	16	46	^{133}-Xe	87 ± 17	22 ± 4	46 ± 5	51 ± 9	53 ± 6	60 ± 14	45
Olesen et al (1971)	8-Hosp.	35	52	^{133}-Xe					50 ± 5	64 ± 9	41
Svemdottir et al (1971)	11-Hosp.	32	38	^{133}-Xe	84 ± 12	22 ± 3	50 ± 7	53	51 ± 5	60 ± 10	39
				Mean	81	22	48	52	50	60	

nation. In fact, the entire amount of gas washed out from the brain is not cleared completely in a single passage through the lungs; this is especially true in patients with impaired ventilation: perfusion ratio. There will thus be, during the course of the study, a reintroduction of gas to the brain from the systemic circulation as well as contamination of the regional fields by radiations coming from the slowly perfused extracranial tissue (8–10 cc/min) by way of the external carotid artery. These two factors both act to blunt the initial slope of the clearance curves (Figs 5.1A and B).

Normal values

We have collected the mean rCBF values obtained under local anaesthesia in control subjects by various authors (Table 5.1). Some of these measurements were done in healthy volunteers, but for the most part they were simultaneous with cerebral angiography in patients hospitalized for neurological investigation but in whom no overt organic brain pathology could be demonstrated.

Though one cannot strictly equate mean rCBF with hemispheric CBF measured by the Kety-Schmidt method or its variants, it is interesting to note that the former is of the same order of magnitude as the latter for which we have reproduced some of the published results for healthy subjects (Table 5.2). No formal comparison

Table 5.2 Mean global CBF (GCBF) values obtained in normal individuals with the Kety-Schmidt method or its variants

Author	No. patients	Tracer	GCBF
Kety & Schmidt (1948)	14-Normal	N_2O	54
Lassen & Munck (1955)	20-Normal	^{85}Kr	52
Lassen et al (1960)	11-Normal	N_2O	50
Lewis et al (1960)	9-Normal	N_2O	57
		Mean:	53

has been attempted here in view of the differences in age, technique, and clinical conditions between the various data-groups involved.

It can also be noticed that the bicompartmental analysis of rCBF has yielded, in man, a ratio of F_w to F_g close to that obtained in laboratory animals by autoradiographic technique, e.g. Freygang & Sokoloff (1959) found in cats a ratio of 1/4.3 and Reivich et al (1969) reported a ratio of 1/4.5 in cats.

In the case of rCBF this ratio lies between 1/3.5 and 1/4, though the variation in the relative weight of the grey and white compartments puts emphasis on the functional nature of these 'compartments'.

The CBF shows an age-related dependence, with a progressive decline in cerebral circulation (and metabolism as well) throughout the lifespan, from childhood to senescence. The CBF decay is not linear, and little difference appears to exist between normal volunteers of 30 or 60 years of age.

Reproducibility and regional variations. The CBF landscape

In order to assess the clinical reliability and limitations of such a method, various authors (Lassen et al, 1963; Ingvar & Lassen, 1965; Agnoli et al, 1968; McHenry et al, 1969; Wilkinson et al, 1969) have studied its reproducibility and defined its *measurement error*, accounted for by methodological inaccuracies as well as normal physiological variations bound to occur during the procedure; these two factors cannot be separated experimentally. This *measurement error* is expressed as the coefficient of variation of the differences between two consecutive measurements done in the same subjects under similar conditions, and varies according to the author, *from four to nine per cent* (see Table 5.3).

The reproducibility of the rCBF method can be considered as good, provided enough time elapses between two consecutive injections of the tracer to permit its complete washout from the tissue and a return of the counts to background level. Indeed, there exists no significant difference in mean hemispheric rCBF obtained from two subsequent measurements except in the case of Wilkinson et al (1969) who found a nine per cent lower value for the second study (p < 0.02), a difference which cannot be explained by changes in $PaCO_2$, by variations in perfusion pressure or by too short a lag between tracer injections.

Paulson (1970) has proposed that the mean of the coefficients of variation (CV) be determined individually in each subject of a control series studied under normal physiological conditions; accordingly, in any patient and in any region where the rCBF varies more than CV ± 2 s.d. from the mean hemisphere rCBF, it may reasonably be

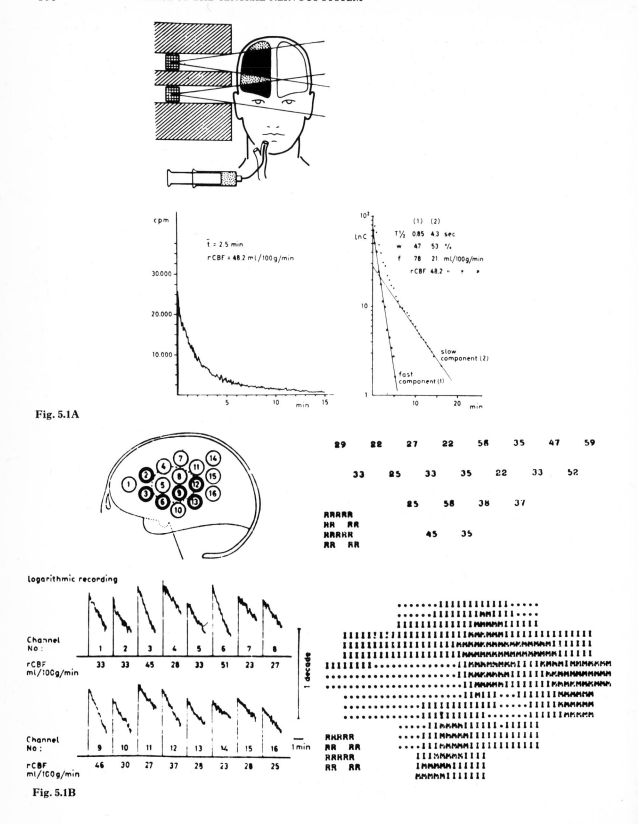

Fig. 5.1A

Fig. 5.1B

Table 5.3 Measurement error of the rCBF method: coefficient of variation of the differences between two subsequent measurements done in similar conditions

Author	Total no. of probes	Lag between meas. (min)	Tracer	Type of analysis	F_1	F_2	$\triangle F_{2-1}\%$	s.d. of differences	Meas. errors (coef. var.) %	P_aCO_2 %
Lassen et al (1963)	19	20	[85]-Kr	Biocomp.	43	40	−7, NS	2.6 pr[a]	6	
Ingvar & Lassen (1965)	28	20	[85]-Kir	Stoc.-10[1]	50	49.5	−1	4.4 pr[a]	9	49.8–49.5
Høedt-Basmussen (1967)	8	15	[85]-Kr	Stoc.−10[1]	38	37	−3, NS	1.8 pr[a]	5	38.4–38.4
Fieschi, et al (1969)	70	>30	[85]-Kr	Biocomp.	45.4	45.6	+0.5	3.5 pr[a]	8	
McHenry et al (1969)	80	25	[133]-Xe	Stock.−10[1]	34	33.5	−1.5, NS	1.25 pa[b]	4	35–35
Wilkinson et al (1969)	80	30	[133]-Xe	Biocomp.	53	48	−9, p<0.02	1.75 pa[b]	4	42.4–43.2

assumed that there is a 'regional or focal disturbance in flow' at the <0.05 level of certainty. From the information available in the literature (Table 5.4) a limit of 20 per cent has been used in our analysis of the case records reported in the section on mathematical processing (see above) to identify regions with focal flow disturbances, although some authors have accepted lesser changes when observed in a number of adjacent regions.

The multi-detector devices for measuring rCBF by intracarotid injection of Xenon-133 mainly quantify cortical rCBF, as outlined above. Besides these pitfalls, they may be utilized to study the function of different cortical regions, as indirectly judged from its rCBF level.

CBF in resting, awake, subjects shows a typical 'landscape' (Ingvar & Lassen, 1975) with peaks and valleys which deviate ±20–30 per cent from

Fig. 5.1A *(Top)*: Registration of the clearance curve of [85]Kr injected into the internal carotid artery. *(Bottom left)*: Actual recording of a clearance curve. Regional blood flow can be calculated from the mean transit time t̄ (t = area/height of the curve) on the basis of the equation:

$$\frac{1}{\bar{t}} = \frac{F}{V^{85}Kr} = \frac{F}{\lambda W} \times 100$$

where F = rCBF (ml/100 g/min); $V^{85}Kr$ = volume of distribution of [85]Kr; λ = mean partition coefficient of [85]Kr (1.09); W = unit weight of the brain (1 g). *(Bottom right)*: Semilogarithmic plot of the clearance curve. Two exponential components are evident, showing the blood flow rates of the fast (f_1) and the slow (f_2) compartments and their relative weights (w_1 and $^1w_2$). Compartmental analysis is based on the following equations:

$$C(t) = I_1 e^{-k_1 t} + I_2 e^{-k_2 t}$$

where C = recorded radioactivity; I_1 and I_2 = intercepts with the y axis of the fast and the slow components; K_1 and K_2 = slopes of the fast and the slow components.

$$rCBF = \frac{I_1 \lambda_1 K_1 + I_2^* \lambda_2 K_2}{I_1 + I_2^*} \times 100 \ (ml/100 \ g/min)$$

where λ_1 (0.95) and λ_2 (1.30) = partition coefficients of [85]Kr for the fast and the slow components; I_2^* = intercept of the slow component corrected for the short injection time and partition coefficient

$$I_2^* = I_2 \frac{\lambda_1 K_2}{\lambda_2 K_2}$$

$$W_1\% = \frac{I_1}{I_1 + I_2^*} \times 100; \qquad W_2\% = \frac{I_2}{I_1 + I_2^*} \times 100$$

$$f_1 = K_1 \lambda_1 \times 100; \qquad f_2 = K_2 \lambda_2 \times 100 \ (ml/100 \ g/min)$$

Fig. 5.1B *(Left)*: rCBF measured with ^{133}Xe in 16 regions. The evaluation of the curves is limited to the initial two minutes. *(Right)*: Further reduction of the size of probes allows rCBF to be measured in up to 35 regions. Use of a small digital computer on-line gives the rCBF values per unit time (numbers in the left upper part of the figure = rCBF in ml/100 g/min) along with a graphical representation of the regions with increased (MM) and decreased (...) blood flow. The symbol R indicates that the right hemisphere has been explored. (Courtesy of Dr N. A. Lassen.)

Table 5.4 Regional variability of rCBF as determined from the individual coefficients of variations obtained from a control series.

Author	No. of patients	No. of probes per patient	Tracer	Type of analysis	$F \pm s.d.$	Mean coef. variation $\pm$ s.d.	Limit: C.V. $\pm$ 2 s.d.
Ingvar (1965)	7-Normal	4	[133]-Xe	Stoc.-10	49.8 $\pm$ 5.4	11[a]	
Høedt-Rasmussen et al (1967)	7-Hosp.	16	[133]-Xe	Stoc.-10		9.3[b] $\pm$ 2.5	14
Zingesser et al (1968)	10-Normal	4	[133]-Xe	Bicomp.	53.4	11.1[b] $\pm$ 3.4	18
Agnoli et al (1968)	15-Hosp.	4–5	[85]-Kr	Bicomp.	45.4 $\pm$ 7.3	16[a]	
Jaffe et al (1970)	5-Hosp.	8	[133]-Xe	Stoc.-10	54 $\pm$ 5.9	11[a]	
Paulson (1970)	11-Hosp.	16	[133]-Xe	Stoc.-10		8.5[b] $\pm$ 1.6	12
				F(init.)		10.6[b] $\pm$ 2.6	16
Olesen et al (1971)	8-Hosp.	35	[133]-Xe	F(init.)	64 $\pm$ 9	8.2[b] $\pm$ 1.2	11

[a] Mean coefficient of variation obtained from pooled probe values.
[b] Mean coefficient of variation obtained from individual C.V. for each patient.

the mean flow level of the investigated cerebral hemisphere, with high flows in premotor and frontal regions and low flows in temporal and parietal regions. Obviously only regions supplied by carotid circulation may be assessed, but in very recent years the studies from the Scandinavian groups on functional activation of rCBF have produced stimulating results, only briefly summarized here (see Ingvar, 1975–1979).

In general, a stimulation, be it a rhythmic hand movement, a tactile stimulation or an auditory stimulation, activates its corresponding cerebral region, with regional increases as high as 60–80 per cent above the mean hemisphere flow. Furthermore, purely mental tasks activate particular cerebral regions. The largest amount of 'brain work' during conscious perception is carried out by premotor and frontal cortex, which are responsible for the programming and planning of motor reactions and behaviour in general.

As outlined by Ingvar (1979) 'the activation of the primary pathways corresponds to the reception of the afferent impulses' and 'the general increase in activation is related to the perception' of the sensory stimuli.

It is interesting that not only voluntary motor activity, but also the intention to perform a voluntary movement or the concept of a movement increases rCBF, in particular in the frontal lobes and also in temporal regions, where it is supposed that memory engrams are localized (Ingvar & Philipson, 1977). These observations have also been confirmed at the metabolic level with different techniques (Raichle et al, 1976; Phelps et al, 1980).

OTHER TECHNIQUES FOR QUANTITATIVE rCBF

Xenon-133 inhalation method

This technique is based on the same principle as the original Kety-Schmidt method, i.e., measurement of cerebral uptake and clearance of an inert diffusible gas administered by inhalation. The method, first introduced by Veall & Mallett (1966) and further developed by Obrist et al (1967), consists of a brief inhalation of ^{133}Xe with extracranial monitoring of its subsequent clearance for a period of 10 to 15 minutes.

The detectors utilized for this technique are larger than those employed for the intracarotid approach, measuring 2.5 cm in diameter. These dimensions produce a field of view 10 cm in diameter at mid-hemisphere.

The clearance curves are subjected to a bicompartmental analysis, using isotope concentration in the end-expired air to correct for recirculation of the indicator.

Two clearance rates are obtained, a faster clearing compartment, considered to be the grey matter, and a slower clearing compartment, representing white matter and the external carotid territory (scalp and skull). The main advantage of this approach is its non-invasiveness, but several pitfalls appear to restrict its reliability and applications. Detectors must be wider in order to achieve sufficient statistics, thus leading to a decrease in regionality. Recirculation correction is not easy or strictly accurate and particularly in patients with pulmonary pathology this may be the cause of large errors. Extracranial contamination is heavy. The variability in normal volunteers ranges from between ± 13 per cent and ± 22 per cent (data from Obrist et al, 1975 and from Wang and Busse, 1975). Furthermore we should recall that the energy of the photons emitted by ^{133}Xe causes only a 60 per cent detection at 1 cm depth of tissue (that is nearly scalp plus skull) and a 40 per cent detection of the activity at 3 cm depth. This indicates that extracerebral activity contributes 1.5 times to the recorded statistics in respect to the cortical activity.

In conclusion, the ^{133}Xe inhalation method may be considered a good approximation in very experienced hands but with limitations still to be fully understood, especially in pathological conditions. The data from Obrist et al (1975) and Wang and Busse (1975) indicate a fast component rCBF of 66.4 ± 8.7 ml/100 g/min for normal young people.

Xenon-133 intravenous method

This method has been proposed by Agnoli et al (1969) and by Austin et al (1972) and it has recently experienced revived utilization by Thomas et al (1979). In fact, intravenous injection of ^{133}Xe avoids heavy contamination of the air sinuses and the correction for recirculation is described as easier.

The technique of Thomas et al (1979) involves an i.v. injection of 5–7 mCi of ^{133}Xe in 5 ml of saline. The clearance of the isotope from the skull is monitored by six external detectors, 25 mm in diameter. A seventh detector monitors the exhaled ^{133}Xe, which is equivalent to the end-tidal ^{133}Xe and therefore approximates to the arterial ^{133}Xe content in patients with normal lungs. The expired ^{133}Xe curve is utilized for correcting the clearance curves recorded from the skull, which are subjected to a bi-compartmental analysis in order to obtain the fast-clearing component. The analysis is basically that used by Obrist.

Thomas et al (1979) have shown a good correlation between CBF values obtained with the intravenous technique and those obtained in the same patients with the intracarotid approach. In six patients CBF (i.v.) was 49.9 ± 20.0 and CBF (i.c.) was 50.3 ± 18.9, with a mean difference of

0.42 ± 4.4. The main criticism regarding this study is the surprisingly large s.d. in both the techniques.

A similar approach, utilized by Meric et al (1979), indicates the main source of error as being the difficulty of defining the precise instant when clearance begins.

Emission tomography methods

These very recent techniques may be divided into two major groups: (a) single photon emission tomography; (b) positron emission tomography.

Emission computerized tomography (ECT), while exploiting the same basic principles of image reconstruction, differs from X-ray transmission computerized tomography in the type of information obtained and the experimental method used. In ECT, a radioactive tracer of a biological process is measured in terms of activity, time and location, after its introduction into the body by intravenous injection, oral ingestion or by inhalation.

The first approach, single photon emission tomography, has been pioneered by Fazio et al (1977) with the continuous intracarotid infusion of ^{81}Krypton^m, a very short-lived isotope ($T1/2 = 13$ s). The rapid radioactive decay of this gas, relative to the perfusion turnover rate per unit volume, results in a brain concentration at equilibrium much lower than that in the carotid inflow. Under these conditions, equilibrium of the isotope in the brain depends on the balance between arrival of ^{81}Kr^m and radioactive decay, since the contribution of ^{81}Kr^m washout to this process is relatively small. The brain signal is more dependent on perfusion than on washout, therefore the images at equilibrium recorded during continuous intracarotid infusion of ^{81}Kr^m reflect the regional arrival of the gas, i.e., regional CBF.

The use of a rotating gamma camera as a recording device during this procedure allows tomographic sections to be obtained (Fazio et al, 1979).

A similar approach has also been employed by Uemura et al (1979). The major drawbacks of this technique are its invasiveness and the impossibility, so far, to quantitate rCBF, but this approach is very suitable for dynamic studies, due to the short half-life of the indicator.

The second approach, Positron Emission Tomography (PET), has recently opened a completely new and exciting field, particularly for the possible quantitation of both rCBF and rCMR for glucose or oxygen. This technique exploits the property of positron emitting isotopes of annihilation by producing two gamma-rays travelling in opposite directions at approximately 180° to one another. These gamma-rays can be detected by paired, opposed scintillators set to record an event only if both detectors sense annihilation photons simultaneously (Phelps et al, 1978).

Furthermore the most suitable biological tracers are positron emitters, (^{15}O, ^{11}C, ^{13}N, etc.), thus allowing direct labelling of physiological substrates. Unfortunately, these isotopes, due to their short half-life, can only be used in the vicinity of a particle accelerator such as a cyclotron, thus making PET a major economic investment.

Three major techniques for CBF assessment have been employed: Ter-Pogossian et al (1971) and later Raichle et al (1976) have both used intracarotid injection of labelled water ($H_2{}^{15}O$), in conjunction with quantitation of $CMRO_2$ obtained by injecting labelled oxyhemoglobin. This group have used both single detectors and a positron emission tomograph. Kuhl and co-workers utilize $^{13}NH_3$ as CBF indicators, but their studies have focused more on rCMRGlc quantitation obtained with i.v. injection of ^{18}F-2-Fluoro-2-deoxy-D-glucose (Phelps et al, 1979).

Jones et al (1976) have developed the technique of continuous inhalation of labelled oxygen (^{15}O) and labelled carbon dioxide ($C^{15}O_2$) to quantitate $rCMRO_2$ and rCBF. This technique is currently utilized by other groups (Baron et al, 1978; Ackermann et al, 1980) and has recently received a conclusive refinement for its application to a PET device (Frackowiak et al, 1980a & b).

Recent reviews on PET give further details (Raichle, 1979; Lenzi et al, 1981). Results on cerebral metabolism will be summarized in a separate paragraph in this chapter.

Reactivity of the cerebral vascular bed

We have already briefly summarized the capability of the cerebral vascular bed to autoregulate to pressure and its sensitivity to CO_2. The former plays a protective role in that, within certain limits, it maintains the overall cerebral perfusion constant in the face of abrupt changes in perfusion pressure induced by alterations in arterial, venous, or intracranial pressure; the latter permits fine adjustment of the local blood supply to local metabolic needs and functional activity of the tissue. Reviews of the physiology of cerebral circulation such as those of Reivich (1969), Betz (1972), Fieschi & Bozzao (1972a) and Purves (1972), discuss in detail the function of local myogenic reactivity and the role of the autonomic nervous system in the vasomotor responses of the cerebral vessels. These studies emphasize the predominant role of local metabolic signals (CO_2, H^+, K^+, and to a lesser extent O_2), in modulating the tone of the smooth muscle of the cerebral arterioles, although neurogenic factors are probably also involved, especially when acute and marked changes in perfusion pressure are taking place.

These normal vasomotor responses can be impaired to various degrees in pathological states, and this impairment may be the only local vascular disturbance detectable. Investigators have designed simple clinical tests to evaluate the reactivity of the cerebral vascular bed after induced changes in systemic arterial pressure (SAP) or $PaCO_2$. To test the integrity of *autoregulation*, a controlled rise in SAP is induced with an intravenous drip-infusion of angiotensin II or a controlled hypotension with a short-acting ganglion blocking agent, such as tripmetaphon, while maintaining $PaCO_2$ unchanged. The administration of these drugs must be adjusted to keep the SAP 25 to 30 mmHg above or below the patient's baseline pressure which will determine the choice of the drug to be used: the usual rates are approximately 1 λ/min for angiotensin and 5 mg/min for tripmetaphon. The entire duration of the test can be kept within 20 minutes if the initial slope analysis is used to calculate rCBF. Normally, rCBF should not be affected by these induced changes in SAP and should remain constant, within the experimental error of the method. But in interpreting this test, one must be aware that autoregulation operates within certain limits (60–160 mmHg) which may vary according to age, baseline SAP, and $PaCO_2$ (Fig. 5.2). Below 60 mm and above 160 mm of Hg, brain perfusion will passively follow perfusion

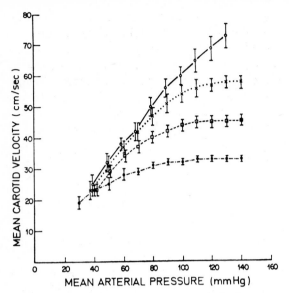

Fig. 5.2 Autoregulation: lowest curve was obtained on room air with the three succeeding ones obtained on 6, 9, and 12 per cent CO_2, respectively. (From Raichle and Stone (1971–1972) In European Neurology, p. 3, fig. 1.)

pressure; this may lead in the former case to cerebral ischaemia and in the latter to vasogenic oedema and hypertensive encephalopathy — the 'break-through phenomenon' (Lassen & Agnoli, 1972; Strandgaard et al, 1974).

To test CO_2 *reactivity* it is usually easier, in most clinical circumstances, to induce hypercapnia by inhalation of 5 per cent CO_2 in air administered through a facial mask for 20 minutes (10 min to reach equilibrium and from 2 to 10 min to record the clearance curve). In young, cooperative subjects and in comatose patients passively ventilated, one can instead induce hypocapnia by hyperventilation. The response of the cerebral vascular bed to CO_2 is complex, but in physiological conditions and for a $PaCO_2$ varying from 25 to 60 mm Hg, brain perfusion is practically linear with $PaCO_2$, with a positive slope in the normal conscious man of 1.34 to 2.17 ml/100 g/min per mmHg of $PaCO_2$ (Grubb et al, 1974). But since CO_2 also tends to influence SAP, the interpretation of this test can become rather difficult in cases where autoregulation is also impaired, for instance in ischaemic areas (Waltz, 1968) or at high levels of $PaCO_2$ (Harper, 1965; Raichle & Stone, 1971). In fact the loss of autoregulation will also allow for an increase

in CBF when SAP increases and may prevent the differentiation of the specific effect of CO_2 on the vascular bed. To minimize the possible role of SAP, some investigators have used variation in cerebrovascular conductance ($CVC = \triangle F/SAP$) to evaluate the alterations of vasomotor reactivity to CO_2 (Ackerman et al, 1973).

For practical purposes, in normal individuals breathing 5 per cent CO_2 in air, the rCBF is usually increased by 20 per cent or more, but in acute brain lesions such as trauma, intracerebral haemorrhage, ischaemia or certain metabolic encephalopathies, vessels can show variable degrees of 'vasoparalysis' to CO_2. Paradoxical reactions secondary to vasoparalysis may then take place in the damaged regions such as a regional reduction in flow during hypercapnia ('steal phenomenon') or a regional augmentation during hypocapnia ('counter-steal phenomenon') (Lassen & Palvölgyi, 1968).

Practical considerations of methodology

In closing this section on methodology, we would like to emphasize a few practical points we believe essential for a meaningful interpretation of the results. First, it is important that the patient remains immobile during the recording of the clearance curve and that the position of the external probes stays unchanged for a much longer period, if one wishes to perform repeated measurements to compare accurately the regional values, for instance, after infusion of a vasoactive drug. Ideally, the type of collimation used and the position of the probes on the scalp should be carefully standardized to facilitate comparison of the values obtained by different investigators using this technique.

It is also essential that haematocrit, SAP, and P_aCO_2 be monitored during the procedure since CBF may be affected by any of these three variables. Blood viscosity has been shown to influence brain perfusion in patients with long-standing polycythemia (Kety, 1950) or experimentally, in dogs, in which haematocrit was decreased by replacing blood with plasma or dextran (Haggendal & Norback, 1966).

These observations have been recently confirmed by Thomas et al (1977) and Humphrey et al (1980), showing a significant inverse relationship between CBF and haematocrit and between CBF and blood viscosity.

We have already mentioned the importance of SAP and P_aCO_2; the ideal situation is one where both parameters remain fairly constant while spontaneous changes in rCBF are induced by drugs acting directly on the cerebrovascular bed. Only P_aCO_2 should change when reactivity to CO_2 is being tested, and only SAP when testing autoregulation. However precise the recording and analysis of the clearance curve and however numerous the probes, the complexity of the method makes us have reservations on the use of such a technique for clinical purposes, notwithstanding the valuable physiological, pharmacological and pathophysiological information it has helped to gather. We might add that this technique is not entirely without risk, although the severity and frequency of its complications are lower than reported for carotid angiography, provided that one follows the recommendations formulated by Ingvar & Lassen (1973) and by Mosmans (1974).

It follows that rCBF studies by direct puncture of the carotid artery or preferably by selective catheterization of the vessel should always be performed in conjunction with an angiographic study, save in very specific instances where it can be of direct potential benefit to the patient. We still share the following view expressed by Mosmans (1974) in his review:

At the present stage the rCBF studies do not appear to contribute sufficiently to establish diagnosis and/or to localize cerebral lesions to justify introduction as a routine method of investigation in clinical neurology. This opinion is also motivated by the fact that the investigation involves the catheterization of the internal carotid artery, so that a well trained multidisciplinary team and expensive equipment are required.

The relative decline of clinical studies performed with the intracarotid approach and the development of non-invasive methods stress this point even more.

The recent introduction of the PET techniques is probably destined to enlarge greatly the field of study, due to its relative non-invasiveness and also to the simultaneous quantitation of circulatory and metabolic parameters.

RESULTS OBTAINED IN CEREBROVASCULAR DISEASES (CVD)

The following observations on rCBF in stroke and focal vascular disease are derived from a comprehensive analysis of data published by four different groups of investigators: 1. Paulson (1970); Paulson et al (1970); Skinhøj et al (1970). 2. McHenry et al (1972). 3. Agnoli et al (1968); Fieschi et al (1969). 4. Ackerman et al (1973); Iliff et al (1974).

Global hemispheric changes

Following an ischaemic lesion in the territory of the internal carotid artery, the involved hemisphere, as might be expected, shows a lower mean rCBF than that of control subjects without organic brain disease. This is true for brain softening (BS) as well as brain haemorrhage (BH), and an analysis of variance has shown that the difference between the controls and the stroke patients is significant (Table 5.5). Indeed this reduction was noted in all case records for F(init) as well as for F_{10} and F_{BC}.

Table 5.5 Mean rCBF values in brain softenings, intracerebral haemorrhages, and transient ischaemic attacks as computed from data published by four groups of investigators

	No. of cases	rCBF (init.)	No. of cases	rCBF^{10BC}
Brain softenings	40	44.6 ± 16.8	85	37.8 ± 19.2
TIA	30	52.2 ± 12.7	29	46.0 ± 14.7
Brain haemorrhage			7	32.4 ± 11.3
Controls (see Table 5.1)		55–64		42–54

Similar results had been found previously by Fieschi & Bozzao (1972b), who reported that the rCBF in 50 of their patients with cerebral ischaemic disease was significantly lower than that of controls, mainly due to a decrease in fast flow, in spite of a slightly higher P_aCO_2 (Table 5.6). These authors also showed that in cases where rCBF declined to levels of 20 ml/100 g/min or less, the clearance curve tended to become mono-exponential: a true 'fast-phase' had practically disappeared. It seems from other observations (Høedt-Rasmussen & Skinhøj, 1964; Meyer et al, 1970) that this reduction in flow is not necessarily confined to the hemisphere ipsilateral to the lesion, but can also involve the contralateral undamaged hemisphere

Table 5.6 Mean rCBF in control subjects and in patients with cerebral ischaemic lesions (from Fieschi and Bozzao, Progress in Brain Research, Vol. 35, p. 388, table 2)

		Compartmental analysis				P_aCO_2 (Vol. %)
		f_1-Grey (ml/100 g/min)	f_2-White (ml/100 g/min)	W_1%	F	
Normals	$\bar{x}$	78.2	20.8	43.0	44.7	41.6
	s.d.	18.3	2.7	6.3	6.2	
Cerebral lesions	$\bar{x}$	51.4	15.8	40.8	30.2	44.8
	s.d.	14.4	4.3	9.0	8.4	
% reduction from controls		34.0[a]	24.0[a]	5.0	32.0[a]	(+3.2 vol. %)

[a] $p < 0.01$.

in what has been referred to as transneural diaschisis.

Slater et al (1977) have studied this phenomenon with the ^{133}Xe inhalation technique, showing a significant blood flow decrease (over 15 per cent) in the non-affected hemisphere, with a maximum depression occurring about one week after the stroke. Reivich et al (1978) underline the fact that 'diaschisis is not a phenomenon that reaches its peak at the onset of a stroke, but is a process that increases during the first week after stroke'.

The results summarized above are by no means specific for stroke since rCBF has been found similarly affected in other types of pathology, such as tumours (Cronquist & Agee, 1968) or head injuries (Fieschi et al, 1972b). Moreover one does not know if these diffuse alterations in rCBF are directly related to the stroke or can be partly accounted for by pre-existing vascular disease (Sokoloff, 1961). Our analysis indicates that in CVD there exists a correlation between the underlying vascular pathology and the magnitude of the rCBF reduction as demonstrated by the grouping of patients with stroke according to the presence or absence of an occlusion of the middle cerebral artery (MCA) or some of its major collaterals (Table 5.7). There is a significant difference in mean rCBF between these two groups of patients, though one must also be aware of other factors that may reduce perfusion after total occlusion of a major intracerebral vessel. These include ischaemic brain oedema and a decrease in brain metabolism which accompanies any of the marked impairments in the level of consciousness produced by a stroke. This correlation is also underlined by the significant difference in mean rCBF existing between

Table 5.7 Difference in mean hemispheric rCBF between cases with and without MCA occlusion[a]

	No. of cases	rCBF (init.)	2 $CBF^{10}BC$
MCA occlusion	38	30.2 ± 8.9	31.5 ± 6.9
No occlusion	68	47.3 ± 12.7	40.4 ± 10.1
Difference (%)		+56.5[b]	+28.0[b]

[a] Occlusion of main trunk or of some of its major branches as seen by angiography.
[b] $p < 0.01$.

patients with stroke and those with transient ischaemic attacks (TIA) studied at various times after the episode. It appears that the cerebrovascular bed in TIA is still capable of compensating for local reductions in perfusion (Table 5.5).

Lastly, the data of Prosenz et al (1972) on hemispheric blood flow measured by ^{133}Xe clearance and a scintillation gamma camera can also be interpreted similarly. These authors reported that among their 23 patients with ischaemic CVD studied in the subacute phase (two weeks to three months after the attack) who had no impairment of consciousness at the time of the measurement and who eventually survived, those with the greatest neurologic deficit had the lowest blood flow.

Regional changes in flow

There are two types of circumscribed disturbance in brain perfusion that can be observed in stroke: regional ischaemia and regional hyperaemia, often called 'luxury perfusion'. The recognition of these alterations in flow is the major contribution of the rCBF method to the understanding of the physiopathology of cerebrovascular diseases.

The so-called 'luxury perfusion syndrome', an

expression coined by Lassen (1966), corresponds to the angiographic findings of capillary blush and early filling of veins (Cronquist & Laroche, 1967) and to the venous congestion sometimes seen on the surface of the cortex by neurosurgeons, i.e. 'the red veins syndrome' of Feindell & Perot (1965). Localized reactive hyperaemia is not peculiar to CVD and has been noticed in post-traumatic (Reivitch et al, 1969) and post-epileptic states (Penfield, 1938). It is the consequence of lactic acidosis in or around hypoxic tissues provoking a localized dilatation of the arteriolar bed by a direct effect on the vessel walls (Michenfelder & Sundt, 1971). The significance to the brain of reactive hyperaemia is still unclear, but it probably indicates that the reactivity of the vessels to the chemical environment is still present. In fact, it appears to be in excess of the tissue metabolic activity inasmuch as O_2 extraction in such regions is frequently reduced below control levels (Symon, 1971).

Recent measurements of both circulatory and metabolic parameters in acute stroke have enlarged the concept to include 'relative luxury perfusion', where there is a decrease in oxygen or glucose uptake larger than the decrease in rCBF (Frackowiak et al, 1980).

It is clear that therapeutic measures aimed at increasing blood flow, such as the administration of CO_2 or induction of hypertension in cases with impaired autoregulation, would be of doubtful value to these regions at that stage.

Regional ischaemia and regional hyperaemia are usually superimposed on a more diffuse hemispheric disturbance in flow and both may present simultaneously in different areas of the same hemisphere, sometimes with hyperaemic foci of various sizes bordering a central nucleus of ischaemia. These hyperemic borders have been referred by Reivich et al (1977) to a hypermetabolism around the lesion, in particular for glucose. In contrast, the evaluation of oxygen metabolism (Fig. 5.3) rarely shows this hypermetabolic ring (Baron et al, 1978; Castaigne et al, 1980, Frackowiak et al, 1980).

We remind the reader that we have adopted a variation in rCBF of ± 20 per cent from the hemisphere mean as an indication of the presence of a regional disturbance in perfusion. Data

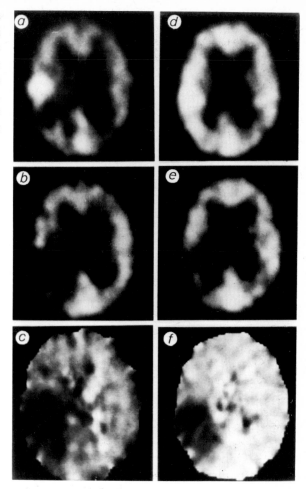

Fig. 5.3 Tomographies of a patient presenting with a left hemisphere thromboembolic stroke. All the scans were taken at the OM lim + 6 cms. Scans a, b, c were taken 4 days after the stroke, scans d, e, f, 18 days after the stroke. Scans a, d represent the cerebral distribution of the rCBF; scans b–e the cerebral distribution of $rCMRO_2$; scans c, f the cerebral distribution of rOER.

Note the hyperaemia in the border of the lesion in the acute phase (a), the huge depression of the oxygen extraction (c).

Two weeks after the first oxygen-15-PET examination, there was a complete recovery of rCBF, with luxury perfusion in the affected region (d), but without recovery of $CMRO_2$ (e) and OER (f). (From Lenzi et al, 1980)

collected from works quoted previously have been recalculated and reclassified accordingly. We are aware that these stringent criteria certainly lead to an underestimation of the number of regions with focal disturbances.

In spite of this, the proportion of patients with regional CBF disturbances in the i.c. [133]Xe study is seen to be high in the early phase of a stroke and

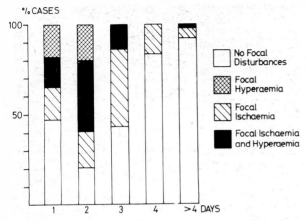

Fig. 5.4 Incidence of regional disturbances in flow in patients with stroke, as computed from case records included in Table 5.5.

tends to drop drastically after the first three days: this is especially true for focal hyperaemia (Fig. 5.4). Therefore it seems reasonable to conclude that these regional haemodynamic changes are directly related to stroke.

In fact, the clinical correlation between impaired neurological function and location of rCBF disturbances is high (Wong et al, 1973). There is also a relationship, as shown by Heiss (1979), between rCBF values within the lesion and the severity of neurological symptoms, and between rCBF and prognosis for clinical recovery. The rCBF of the group with complete disappearance of neurological symptoms was significantly different from rCBF in all other groups: 33.4 ± 3.5 ml/100 g/min in comparison to a critical value of 28 ml/100 g/min below which morphological infarction occurs and functional recovery is thus impossible.

These data have confirmed the clinico-pathological study of Agnoli et al (1970) and the previous study of Marshall (1972), which concluded that 'the agreement (between regional changes in perfusion and clinical localization) for hemiparesis, hemisensory loss and expressive dysphasia was high, while that for hemianopia was less good, presumably because this sign may arise as a result of a lesion at a number of sites'.

Regional disturbances of vascular reactivity

As we have seen, the normal vasomotor responses of the cerebrovascular bed can be altered after a stroke; these alterations can be circumscribed or diffuse, simultaneous or dissociated; e.g., when autoregulatory mechanisms are impaired, the brain is no longer protected against changes in perfusion pressure and CBF passively follows SAP.

At times, impairment in autoregulation may lead to paradoxical reactions, e.g., a decrease in rCBF during hypotension. This phenomenon could be the consequence of concomitant changes in the extravascular pressure of greater magnitude than the changes in SAP (Fieschi et al, 1972); the variation in extravascular pressure will thus neutralize or reverse the effect of SAP on perfusion pressure in these vascular beds where autoregulation is lost ('false' autoregulation).

When the reactivity to CO_2 is altered, the local circulation will no longer be regulated by the local metabolic needs of the tissues. Here also paradoxical responses can be encountered. Thus, during hypercarbia, rCBF may be decreased, rather than increased, in the diseased areas: this phenomenon is referred to as the 'intracerebral steal' (Lassen & Palvölgyi, 1968). Conversely, rCBF may be increased during hypocarbia in these same areas: this is known as the 'intracerebral counter-steal' (Pistolese et al, 1972). The 'intracerebral steal' would be accounted for by a redistribution of blood from the region with impaired reactivity to regions around the lesion which still react normally to CO_2 by vasodilatation, thus creating a pressure gradient between non-reacting and reacting regions in favour of the latter. The 'counter-steal' is explained by a similar mechanism operating in the opposite direction. These alterations in vasoreactivity can be demonstrated by the clinical tests already described.

As a threshold for impaired autoregulation, we have adopted the criterion of Fieschi et al (1969), i.e., a variation in rCBF of ± 16 per cent from baseline after infusion of angiotensin or tripmetaphon. This value of 16 per cent corresponds to the mean difference in flow between the baseline and post-infusion measurements ± 2 s.d., over the mean rCBF for the baseline measurement, or twice the measurement error (see Table 5.3). Impaired CO_2 reactivity has been defined as an increase in rCBF of less than 20 per cent during 5 per cent CO_2 inhalation, or decreases in rCBF of less than 20 per cent during a hyperventilation which lowers the P_aCO_2 by at least 5 mmHg. Our analysis has shown that CO_2 reactivity is impaired in approximately 45 per cent of cases after a stroke but that it is rapidly regained after the first three days (Fig. 5.5). During this early phase, paradoxical responses are frequent. Autoregulation, on the other hand, is altered in 75 per cent of patients but here again it improves markedly three days after the stroke (Fig. 5.6). Therefore from a haemodynamic standpoint, the acute phase lasts usually no longer than three or four days.

These results, however, are to be interpreted cautiously because they are dependent to a large extent on the ability of the regional method to depict localized and subtle alterations in flow. In this respect, the experimental findings of Symon & Brierly (1975) are worth mentioning. These authors measured cortical blood flow with hydrogen clearance in eight monkeys, three years after ligation of the MCA. They found that even if the mean regional flow in the infarcted zone was normal (48 ml/100 g/min), it was unevenly distributed; some regions of the infarct had a perfusion as low as 21 ml/100 g/min, others as high as 89 ml/100 g/min. Moreover, even after three years, the CO_2 reactivity of the vascular bed remained impaired while autoregulation, preserved at the periphery of the infarct, was abolished in its centre.

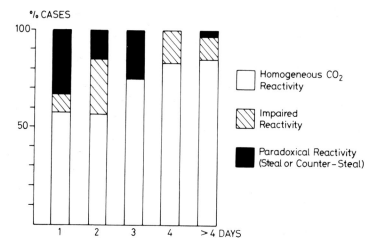

Fig. 5.5 Incidence of abnormal reactivity to CO_2 in patients with stroke (data from same sources as for Fig. 5.4).

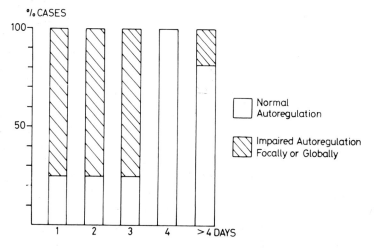

Fig. 5.6 Incidence of impaired autoregulation in patients with stroke (data from same sources as for Fig. 5.4).

However, no paradoxical reactions were encountered.

rCBF and arterial occlusion

Frequently in stroke, no vascular abnormalities are seen on angiography, yet rCBF measurements will often indicate the presence of focal haemodynamic changes in the involved hemisphere. One would therefore expect to find more pronounced focal rCBF abnormalities in cases where an occlusion of the MCA or its branches can be demonstrated angiographically. In the case records we have analyzed, 40 per cent of the patients with stroke showed such an occlusion. Although those with and without occlusion had a comparable proportion of focal abnormalities when studied in the acute phase (62 per cent and 55 per cent, respectively), in the group with occlusion there was a higher prevalence of ischaemic foci (56 per cent vs. 33 per cent), while hyperaemic foci were present in both groups in 43 per cent of the cases (Fig. 5.7).

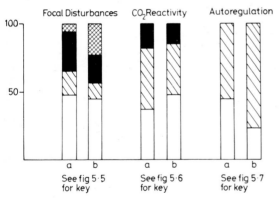

a. Patients with MCA occlusion

b. Patients without occlusion

Fig. 5.7 Incidence of foci of hyperaemia and ischaemia, and of disturbances of autoregulation and CO_2 reactivity in the acute phase (three days) of ischaemic strokes with and without MCA occlusion.

Moreover, as previously shown in Table 5.7, the mean hemispheric rCBF in cases without occlusion was 28 per cent higher than that for cases with occlusion. These differences in the mean hemispheric rCBF as well as in the pattern of the regional disturbances support the view that there are two distinct types of haemodynamic disturbance.

Patients with and without occlusion showed a high proportion of impaired and/or paradoxical responses to CO_2 as well as (though not always associated with) a frequent loss of autoregulation, the latter being found in 60 per cent of cases with occlusion and 86 per cent of cases without occlusion. Some patients without occlusion displayed a paradoxical or 'false' autoregulation in the involved region. The frequent loss of autoregulation stresses the fact that patients with acute stroke require careful monitoring of their blood pressure in the hours following the ictus. In those without demonstrable arterial occlusion, in which the perfusion pressure in the infarcted zones is less likely to be reduced, any rise in SAP should be prevented in order to forestall the development of vasogenic oedema, whereas in patients with occlusion, any fall in SAP should be corrected to avert further extension of ischaemia.

rCBF measurements in transient ischaemic attacks

In transient ischaemic attacks, clinical symptoms, although transient, usually last longer than focal ischaemia since time must be allowed for recovery of tissue function. During the recovery phase, focal haemodynamic abnormalities with various degrees of vasoparalysis may persist and continue after ischaemia has disappeared and neurological function has been regained. The duration and degree of these focal disturbances are related to the severity of the insult, and the recording of such disturbances may help in establishing the period during which patients remain at risk after an episode of TIA.

In a study of 12 such patients, Skinhøj et al (1970) were able to show definite disturbances of the rCBF and of its regulation for up to one day following the attack, but not for longer. Similar disturbances were encountered for up to four days in 12 cases with 'minor apoplectic attacks', though we feel these cases should rather be considered as completed strokes. In another study, Rees et al (1971) observed focal disturbances in 7 out of 10 patients with TIA studied by compartmental analysis 8 to 90 days after the last clinical episode. These consisted of changes in the fast phase flow (F_g), the slow phase flow (F_w), or the weight of the fast compartment (W_g) and were sometimes

Table 5.8 rCBF abnormalities coinciding with the site of the lesion as clinically determined in patients with completed stroke. (From Marshall (1972) Sixth Salzburg Conference, p. 71.)

Clinical defect	History		Physical examination	
	No. of cases	Per cent coinciding	No. of cases	Per cent. coinciding
Paresis	22	73	20	85
Sensory loss	9	78	11	82
Expressive dysphasia	11	82	6	83
Receptive dysphasia	2	0	2	0
Hemianopia	9	56	11	73

limited to a single region. These results, at variance with those of Skinhøj, are interpreted by the authors as an indication that following a clinical TIA there may remain a small 'silent' brain infarction. It may also indicate that bicompartmental analysis is more suitable for depicting subtle changes in regional perfusion. As far as the cerebral vasoreactivity is concerned, both reports agree that it remains normal between attacks, a result which tends to discount the 'haemodynamic' hypothesis, according to which TIAs occur most frequently in areas with marginal perfusion where the local reactivity of the vascular bed is altered (Denny-Brown, 1960).

Because of these limited abnormalities, the mean rCBF measured after an episode of TIA remains in the normal range and is significantly higher ($+17$ ml/100 g/min — bicompartmental analysis — or $+48$ per cent, $p < 0.001$) than that found in completed strokes, as computed from 29 of the cases of TIA reported in the case records surveyed for which the F_{BC} was available (Table 5.5). It is probable that rCBF values in TIA would have been lower had they been obtained during the attack itself.

The 'haemodynamic' hypothesis has recently been revived by the observation of a chronic 'misery perfusion' in patients who had repetitive TIAs of the same cerebral territory over two months prior to the study (Lenzi et al, 1977 & 1978) and in recent cerebral infarction (Castaigne et al, 1980).

rCBF in arterial hypertension

Patients with arterial hypertension but without cerebral symptoms show normal rCBF values.

This means that autoregulation is preserved; however Strandgaard et al have shown that the limits of autoregulation are modified in severe chronic hypertension. In particular, the lower limit of autoregulation, which is normally 60–70 mmHg, may be as high as 110–130 mmHg. Therefore symptoms of cerebral ischemia may appear at higher levels than normally; i.e. the so-called 'ischaemic threshold' is raised. The cerebral symptoms characteristic of malignant hypertension (hypertensive encephalopathy) are probably related to the 'break through' of cerebral autoregulation at its upper limit, with an overdistension of vessel walls and vasogenic oedema. It is thus of fundamental importance to decrease the blood pressure in these patients. Also, in patients with a cerebrovascular accident accompanied by a severe hypertensive crisis, the lowering of blood pressure may lead to an improvement in the focal neurological signs (Meyer et al, 1967). Furthermore, the 'break through' of autoregulation at its upper limits produces an increase of the intracranial pressure, mainly because of the vasogenic oedema due to the transudation of fluid out of the thin-walled cerebral arterioles.

It has long been known that when intracranial pressure is increased the CBF is decreased. Osmotic agents such as mannitol (Johnston et al, 1972) and glycerol (Antonini et al, 1977) which lower intracranial pressure may increase CBF and also improve clinical symptoms.

rCBF measurements in normal pressure hydrocephalus

Though this condition is not related directly to CVD, it is useful to mention briefly some of the findings obtained with ^{133}Xe clearance in normal pressure hydrocephalus (NPH) since they suggest that a haemodynamic derangement may be an important component of this syndrome.

According to Mathew (1974), rCBF was focally reduced in 15 patients with NPH, particularly in the areas supplied by the anterior cerebral artery. When restudied after the operation 'patients with higher preoperative rCBF and higher degrees of increase in rCBF after lowering CSF pressure (via a lumbar puncture) appear to improve better with CSF shunting', while patients with lower preoperative rCBF and lesser changes in perfusion after removal of CSF responded poorly to treatment.

The results obtained by Salmon & Timperman (1971) are somewhat different. In a limited series of patients with post-traumatic encephalopathy these authors could find no correlation between preoperative rCBF and clinical improvement after shunting. Their results suggest, however, as in the previous case, that the degree of clinical improvement could be linked to the haemodynamic effects of the shunt, since the only patients to benefit from the operation were those who showed after the procedure an increase in mean rCBF (especially those with a marked increase in W_g). In the light of these results, further rCBF studies in this condition may be of interest.

rCBF in diabetes

Dandona et al (1978) have demonstrated that the reactivity of cerebral blood vessels in diabetic patients is altered, whilst the mean CBF was not different from a control, age-matched population. These findings indicate that diabetics have a diminished cerebrovascular reserve and are thus at increased risk of cerebrovascular disease, being less able to compensate when necessary by increasing CBF. Diabetes is known to be a risk factor for cerebrovascular diseases and these data may indicate the underlying abnormality.

rCBF in subarachnoid haemorrhage (SAH)

The reports on rCBF and on metabolism in SAH are scanty and often contradictory, particularly in relation to medical treatment and to surgical aspects, such as the timing of operation (James, 1968; Ferguson et al, 1972; Symon et al, 1972; Bergvall et al, 1973).

In general, an impairment of rCBF and $rCMRO_2$ is found both locally, in the ipsilateral hemisphere and in the entire brain, whether the study is performed before or after the surgery. More severely ill patients, with or without evidence of vasospasm, show the more severe impairment of CBF.

The correlation between neurological deficit and focal ischaemia was 'roughly' present for Heilbrun et al (1972), present only in the severely ill patients

in a percentage larger than 50 per cent for Grubb et al (1977) and 'fairly good' for Ishii (1979).

Three major points seem fairly well established:

a. there is a direct relationship between the decrease in CBF and the clinical grade of the neurological deficit;
b. a poor outcome can be expected in patients with impairment of autoregulation;
c. vasospasm has an important influence on the morbidity and mortality of patients with SAH.

In addition, vasospasm seems to induce an increase of cerebral blood volume (CBV) (Grubb et al, 1977). The decrease of CBF and $CMRO_2$ and the increase in CBV depends on the degree of vasospasm. Ishii (1979) emphasizes that a preoperative mean CBF greater than 30 ml/100 gm/min indicated a good prognosis, and that surgery should be delayed in patients with impaired vascular reactivity. Further confirmation of these conclusions is needed.

Studies of cerebral metabolism and blood flow in CVD

The recent development of techniques for emission tomography has produced some initial reports on rCBF and rCMR for oxygen or glucose in CVD.

The field has been pioneered by the St. Louis group, which utilized for their first studies, external signal detectors for the intracarotid injected oxygen-15 (Ter-Pogossian et al, 1970; Carter et al, 1972). Single cases were reported in 1978 by Kuhl et al, with $^{13}NH_3$ as an indicator for CBF and ^{18}F-DOG as an indicator for CMRGlc. In their series of ten stroke patients they showed 'focal inhomogeneities and mismatching of the two tracers used, reflecting uncoupling of the usual perfusion-metabolism relationship'. In addition, they reported 'focal reactive zones of increased glucose utilization at the periphery of some early infarcts, possibly due to an increase in the rate of anaerobic glucose metabolism in the hypoxic but still perfused border zones'. The larger report from the same group (Kuhl et al, 1980) on the same patients, stresses the point that the metabolic uptake is a more sensitive indicator of cerebral dysfunction than rCBF or CT scanning.

The uncoupling between flow and metabolism, in situations ranging from luxury perfusion to the critical perfusion or to post-ischaemic hypermetabolism, is one of the main reasons for the interest in these new techniques.

This uncoupling was demonstrated in chronic CVD by Lenzi et al (1978) with the oxygen-15 inhalation technique. In TIA they found regions of low flow relative to metabolism ('misery perfusion') whereas in completed stroke a 'luxury perfusion' condition prevails.

Baron et al (1978; 1980) have found a normal oxygen extraction ratio in brain infarcts over 30 days old, both rCBF and rCMRO$_2$ being depressed to an equal extent in the lesion. Recent infarcts tend to show a decreased oxygen extraction, local flow being high in relation to the reduced oxygen utilization. These authors underline the inconsistency and heterogeneity of CBF in recent cerebral infarction and almost invariably they found profound disturbances of the oxygen extraction. A series of acute ischaemic CVA has recently been reported by the Hammersmith group (Lenzi et al, 1980; Frackowiak et al, 1980). CMRO$_2$ appears to be always decreased within the infarcted areas, while CBF was decreased, normal, or increased. The oxygen extraction ratio is always depressed acutely within the lesion. Regions distant from the site of an acute infarction and also in the contralateral hemisphere were often affected by a consistent decrease in both CMRO$_2$ and CBF in a coupled fashion (i.e., with normal extraction ratio). In addition, the cerebellar hemisphere contralateral to the side of cerebral lesion showed a decrease in both rCBF and rCMRO$_2$. The overall reduction in CMRO$_2$ shows a close correlation with the level of consciousness in these patients.

In the subacute phase (seven days after the onset of symptoms) regional CBF had consistently returned to normal. The rCMRO$_2$ remained depressed in patients with no clinical recovery, but tended to return to normal in patients with clinical improvement. In contrast with the studies utilizing ^{18}F-DOG as the metabolic indicator, the group working with oxygen-15 seldom observed post-ischaemic hypermetabolism. This fact may be due to the different metabolic uptakes of glucose and oxygen in post-anoxic states.

From the initial reports, it seems that the metabolic parameters do correlate better with clinical state and outcome than does CBF.

THERAPEUTIC APPLICATIONS

Effect of drugs on rCBF in CVD

Regional blood flow studies have shown that the effect of most drugs on the normal cerebral vascular tree is homogeneous and have added little to our knowledge of the pharmacology of cerebral circulation since the comprehensive review by Sokoloff (1959).

Drugs acting on CBF may be classified, following Carpi (1973), into five major groups:

a. drugs derived from biological molecules with vasomotor activity, e.g., adrenaline, acetylcholine, histamine, dopamine;

b. drugs acting on smooth muscle receptors on peripheral vessels, e.g., nitrites, xanthine, papaverine;

c. drugs acting on metabolic and functional activity of the nervous tissue, e.g., barbiturates, amphetamines;

d. drugs acting on physico-chemical characteristics of the blood, e.g., osmotic agents, dextran;

e. drugs with vasoactive properties.

Noradrenaline, angiotensin, and other hypertensive agents act on the cerebral circulation through an increase in systemic blood pressure, since their direct action on cerebral vessels is negligible at concentrations sufficient to act upon the peripheral vascular tree (Olesen, 1972). These drugs induce a very slight cerebral vasoconstriction and can thus be safely used to increase cerebral perfusion when SAP is reduced below the threshold level for autoregulation or when autoregulation is impaired. The sympathomimetic drug, tinofedrine, seems to be capable of directly increasing CBF (Merory et al, 1978) by 28 per cent in acute administration to patients with multi-infarct dementia. In spite of some limited successes (Farhat & Schneider, 1967), the beneficial effect of such a treatment in CVD remains to be proven. It seems clear that the increase in perfusion pressure above the upper threshold level is counter-productive as it favours the development of brain oedema, especially in infarcted areas (Lassen & Agnoli, 1972).

Similarly, many systemic vasodilators exert no direct effect on the cerebral blood vessels and act only on cerebral perfusion when autoregulation is abolished, through changes in systemic pressure. This is true for ganglionic-blocking agents and the majority of the peripheral vasodilators (Heiss et al, 1970).

In fact, a careful assessment of the action on CBF of drugs such as dihydroergotoxine (Heiss, 1973; 1979), nicergoline (Iliff et al, 1977), and dihydroergocristine shows a moderate increase only in a small percentage of patients.

The xanthine derivatives induce cerebral vaso-constriction, thus reducing mean and regional CBF. However, in an ischaemic region this response is often impaired, thus leading to a beneficial counter-steal phenomenon. Other drugs have similar actions, such as serotonin (Deshmukh & Harper, 1973) and prostaglandin F2α (Yamamoto et al, 1972), though this last drug may act on cerebral oxygen consumption rather than on vascular smooth muscle (Pickard, 1973).

Papaverine still remains the prototype of drugs acting on vascular smooth muscle and has a vasodilatory effect on the cerebral vascular tree. Unfortunately, its action is very short-lasting and often impaired in cerebral regions affected by CVD. A similar vasodilatatory property has been demonstrated for cyclandelate and bencyclan. However, there is poor correlation between increased rCBF and clinical improvement.

Unfortunately studies on cerebral metabolism and blood flow which also include careful clinical observations are so far lacking. In fact, the clinical usefulness in CVD of drugs actively dilating cerebral vessels or producing a local increase of CBF in an ischaemic region through a counter-steal phenomenon, remains controversial since it has never been clearly demonstrated that such an increase will modify the disease process.

There has been recent interest in drugs acting on the metabolic and functional activity of the nervous tissue, mainly because of experimental evidence that barbiturates given after global brain ischaemia lessen the eventual degree of dysfunction.

Safar et al (1979) have utilized high-dose barbiturate loading in patients after cardiac arrest, and suggest that there is an ameliorating effect on brain damage. Other experimental data have not substantiated this claim in global or in regional brain ischaemia (Black et al, 1978), though the reduction of $CMRO_2$ is theoretically useful. The same uncertainty persists on the role of drugs decreasing cerebral metabolism, such as gamma-hydroxybutyrate and gamma-butyrolactone (MacMillan, 1980).

Hyperosmolar agents by intravenous infusion have been used in the acute phase of stroke by Ott et al (1974). The infusion is usually followed by a significant increase in rCBF in infarcted areas; this increase is presumed to be secondary to reduction in local oedema in the early phase of an infarct and to the subsequent reduction in capillary resistance. These agents thus act indirectly via perfusion pressure rather than directly on the vessel wall. The increase in perfusion brought about by hyperosmolar agents is not necessarily beneficial, since the lesion may already be irreversible and blood flow in those areas may be higher than metabolic requirements.

In an attempt to restore the impaired microcirculation in the ischaemic area, low molecular weight dextran has been utilized by Gilroy et al (1969), Gottstein et al (1976) and Matthews et al (1976). Gottstein (1969) has demonstrated a 40 per cent increase in CBF, but the clinical correlates of this effect are still uncertain. Furthermore, Heiss et al (1971) found only a very slight CBF increase after dextran.

The final group collects together drugs with miscellaneous properties, such as vincamine derivatives, naftidrofurile and piribedil. Many of these drugs are recommended in chronic CVD but have not been studied in acute stroke with measurements of blood flow.

From this brief review, it appears that, as stated by Matthews (1978), 'no specific method of treatment that has been efficiently evaluated has been convincingly shown to be of benefit' and that 'experimental studies in man and animals have greatly advanced knowledge of the events leading to cerebral infarction and of its effects, but have thrown little light on the mechanism of recovery'. In fact, well-conducted trials of the effect of drugs on rCBF (and on $rCMRO_2$ and rCMRGlc as well) in CVD are few in number and often contradictory.

We strongly suggest that centres with PET facilities should initiate such trials, in order to evaluate the many therapeutic approaches to CVD in a rational manner.

rCBF measurements as a safeguard during carotid surgery

During carotid endarterectomy for the prophylactic treatment of cerebral vascular disease, the artery needs to be temporarily occluded below the lesion. Since the use of an external shunt to protect the brain during the period of occlusion presents its own difficulties and cannot always be used efficiently, a reduction of cerebral blood flow during the period of carotid clamping is to be expected. The duration and degree of this reduction is obviously critical but cannot be predicted beforehand. Therefore tests have been devised to evaluate the level to which rCBF will be reduced by clamping. If the level is too low, special procedures have to be employed during endarterectomy, or surgery avoided, because of the high risk of permanent ischaemic complications that may follow.

Several procedures have been proposed in order to screen patients before surgery: percutaneous digital compression under EEG control, Doppler examination of blood flow through the ophthalmic arteries, evaluation of CBF with the atraumatic ^{133}Xe inhalation technique during carotid compression. All these may be useful in detecting those patients in whom surgery would be dangerous. EC-IC bypass may be indicated in these patients *prior* to endarterectomy. The monitoring of CBF is also relevant *during* surgery.

One of the proposed tests, performed under anaesthesia immediately before the endarterectomy, consists in the total clamping, for two minutes, of the internal carotid artery above the stenosis. The ipsilateral rCBF F(init) is measured before and during the test (Pistolese et al, 1971). In a study conducted with one detector (Jennett et al, 1966), it was reported that if the CBF of the homolateral hemisphere is reduced by more than 25 per cent from the pre-clamping value, the probability of neurological damage following the

endarterectomy is high. Evidently, this threshold is likely to vary with the length of the carotid clamping, since a given reduction in perfusion considered safe for a short period of clamping may become dangerous if the interruption of flow is prolonged. Because the time factor is difficult to assess in advance, a strict limit must be put on the critical rCBF level in order to avoid permanent cerebral ischaemia if the endarterectomy should last beyond the usual 10 to 20 minutes. This critical threshold is now put at 30 ml/100 g/min in normocapnic patients. Below this level the incidence of ischaemic complications increases significantly. Thus if the rCBF should fall below 30 ml/100 g/min during the test, it is felt that the operation should not be attempted unless a better perfusion is achieved, either by external shunts and/or by induced rises in the arterial pressure, a measure that should increase flow in regions where autoregulation is abolished. An elevation of arterial pressure by 20 to 30 mmHg with pressor amines has proved helpful in keeping blood flow above the safety limit in six out of eight cases reported by Pistolese et al (1971), and has permitted the operation to be performed successfully. If that measure fails, only then should a shunt be attempted or other means to reduce complications be tried, such as deep barbiturate anaesthesia, hypothermia or hyperbaric oxygen (Jennett et al, 1969), or the operation cancelled.

We would suggest, in conclusion, that the best safeguard against complications produced by ischaemia due to carotid clamping consists in the monitoring of rCBF and arterial pressure above the stenosis (stump pressure) during an occlusion test of two minutes, to be repeated with moderate increments in SAP if flow in any region is below the critical threshold of 30 ml/100 g/min. This constitutes, in our opinion, one of the most valuable clinical applications of the rCBF method.

rCBF measurements for the EC-IC bypass surgery

This new surgical approach to the treatment of CVD has been favourably received by a large number of neurosurgeons. It has been recommended for patients without a severe neurological deficit and with ipsilateral carotid or MCA occlusion. The typical patient is therefore neurologically intact but has had TIAs in a particular carotid territory, on which the angiography has demonstrated severe stenosis or occlusion unsuitable for direct surgery.

In these cases such an intervention is appropriate, and an increase in rCBF has been demonstrated. Meric et al (1980) have demonstrated a significant increase in CBF in six out of 12 cases, with a fairly satisfactory relationship between clinical and circulatory improvements.

However, it has to be shown that such cases would have suffered a worse outcome without surgery, and an international research effort is now under way to establish this point.

The strict indications outlined by Reichman have themselves often been 'bypassed' and not infrequently patients with a severe established neurological deficit have been submitted to this type of surgery.

In 1978, it was pointed out the need for assessment of both perfusion and metabolism before and after surgery. It has to be emphasized again that to increase rCBF to a region of morphological damage and decreased oxygen utilization is obviously useless. Probably the rCBF evaluation alone will be sufficient only when CT and neurological examination indicate that no structural damage has occurred or that there is a real risk of a further and more destructive stroke.

We are convinced that the most relevant parameter to be evaluated is the regional extraction of oxygen (or glucose). It is in those patients with critical under perfusion that EC-IC bypass surgery is likely to be most rewarding. This view is substantiated by more recent reports by Baron et al (1980), Ross et al (1980) and Hungerbuhler et al (1980).

CONCLUSIONS

The Kety-Schmidt method for measurement of global CBF led to a greater understanding of the physiological and pharmacological mechanisms acting upon the cerebral vasculature. More recently, rCBF determinations with radioactive inert gases have added to our knowledge by introducing newer concepts of pathophysiological and clinical importance such as the recognition that alterations in brain perfusion could be limited to circumscribed areas of brain, as illustrated by the luxury perfusion syndrome and the local vasoparalysis of the post-hypoxic and ischaemic brain. Some of these new findings, such as the existence of the steal and counter-steal or the notion that a false autoregulation due to vasogenic oedema could take place during marked increases in SAP, have influenced our therapeutic approach to stroke.

These observations have stressed the importance of SAP for the regulation of brain perfusion in the acutely damaged brain where the vascular network will react passively to changes in transmural pressure. Therefore the control of blood pressure as well as the prevention of brain oedema seems of prime importance in any attempt to restore CBF in the acute phase of a stroke, or as a preventive measure during carotid surgery.

Yet, in spite of the impact these new notions have had on our understanding of brain infarction, the rCBF technique has not been widely used for patient care. It is too complex to be employed routinely despite the specific information it can provide, and improved methodology remains a main objective for the future in order to increase its usefulness. Requirements could be summarised as follows: the development, for clinical application, of noninvasive and reliable methods for measurement of rCBF and local or regional energy metabolism, and of techniques for assessing the state of the microcirculation. These may help us to understand the mechanisms leading to uneven distribution of flow in ischaemic brain and, in some regions, to the 'no reflow' phenomena, the immediate correction of which could possibly lead to more rapid resolution of ischaemia.

Until then, and apart from its usefulness as a research tool in clinical physiology and pharmacology, the major practical application of the rCBF method will remain confined to specific diagnostic problems such as those discussed: the preoperative monitoring of patients undergoing carotid surgery, perhaps the evaluation of the potential benefits to be expected of a ventriculoatrial shunt in normal pressure hydrocephalus, the indication for EC-IC bypass surgery in patients with ipsilateral carotid occlusion and the clinical evaluation of patients with organic dementias in diagnostic and therapeutic studies.

It is hoped that methodological developments will permit a reorientation of efforts in this field, moving towards more basic considerations, and will further justify the interest already shown by many in the regional approach to cerebral blood flow.

REFERENCES

Ackerman R H, Subramanyam R, Correia J A, Alpert N M, Taveras J M 1980 Positron imaging of cerebral blood flow during continuous inhalation of $C^{15}O_2$. Stroke 11:45–49

Ackermann R H et al 1973 The relationship of the CO_2 reactivity of cerebral vessels to blood pressure and mean resting blood flow. Neurology 23:21

Agnoli A, Fieschi C, Bozzao L, Battistini N, Prencipe M 1968 Autoregulation of cerebral blood flow. Studies during induced hypertension in normal subjects and in patients with cerebrovascular disease. Circulation 38:800

Agnoli A, Fieschi C, Prencipe M, Battistini N, Bozzao L 1970 Relationship between regional haemodynamics in acute cerebrovascular lesions and clinico-pathological aspects. In: Meyer J S et al (eds) Research on the cerebral circulation, Fourth International Salzburg Conference: Charles C Thomas, Springfield

Agnoli A, Prencipe M, Priori A M, Bozzao L, Fieschi C 1969 Measurements of rCBF intravenous injection of ^{133}Xe. A comparative study with the intra-arterial injection method. In: Brock M et al (eds) Cerebral blood flow, Springer-Verlag, Berlin

Antonini F M et al 1977 Effects of intravenous infusion of glycerol on regional cerebral blood flow in cerebral infarction. Gerontology 23:376–380

Austin G, Horn N, Rouhe S, Hayward W 1972 Description and early results of an intravenous radioisotope technique for measuring regional cerebral blood flow in man. European Neurology 8:43–51

Baron J C, Bousser M G, Comar D, Kellershohn C 1980 Human hemispheric infarcts studied by positron emission tomography and the 15-oxygen continuous inhalation technique. In: Salomon G, Caille J (eds) Computerized tomography, Springer-Verlag pp 231–237

Baron J C et al 1978 Etude tomographique chez l'homme du debit sanguin et de la consommation d'oxygene du cerveau par inhalation continue d'oxygene-15. Revue Neurologique 134:545–556

Bergvall U, Steiner L, Forster D M C 1973 Early pattern of cerebral circulatory disturbances following subarachnoid haemorrhage. Neuroradiology 5:24–32

Betz E 1972 Cerebral blood flow: its measurement and regulation. Physiological Reviews 52:595

Blandino G, Bonanno N, Conforti P, Meduri M 1973 A comparison of standard carotidography, hemispheric scintigraphy (with MAAI-131) and regional blood flow measurements (with ^{133}Xe) in brain vascular patients. Journal of Nuclear Biology and Medicine 17:58

Carpi A 1973 The pharmacology of cerebral circulation. In: International Encyclopedia of Pharmacology and Therapeutics, Pergamon Press, Oxford

Carter C C, Eichling J O, Davis D O, Ter-Pogossian M M 1972 Correlation of regional cerebral blood flow with regional oxygen uptake using ^{15}O method. Neurology 22:755–762

Castaigne P, Baron J C, Bousser M G, Comar D, Kellershohn C 1980 Positron emission tomography in human

hemispheric infarction: a study with ^{15}O continuous inhalation technique. In: Bes A, Géraud G (eds) Cerebral circulation and neurotransmitters, Excerpta Medica p 29–36

Collice M, Fazio F, Fieschi C, Arena O 1979 Tridimensional assessment of regional cerebral perfusion in patients treated by extracranial-intracranial (EC-IC) anastomosis. Acta Neurologica Scandinavica 60:494–495 (Suppl. 72)

Cronquist S, Agee F 1968 Regional cerebral blood flow in intracranial tumours. Acta radiologica (diagnosis) 7:393

Cronquist S, Laroche F 1967 Transitory hyperaemia in focal cerebral vascular lesions studied by angiography and regional blood flow measurements. British Journal of Radiology 40:270

Dandona P, James I M, Newbury P A, Woollard M L, Beckett A G 1978 Cerebral blood flow in diabetes mellitus: evidence of abnormal cerebrovascular reactivity. British Medical Journal 2:325–326

Denny-Brown D 1960 Recurrent cerebrovascular episodes. Archives of Neurology 2:194

Deshmukh V D, Harper A M 1973 The effect of serotonin on cerebral and extracerebral blood flow with possible implications in migraine. Acta Neurologica Scandinavica 49:649

Eichling J 1979 Non-invasive methods of measuring regional cerebral blood flow. In: Price T R, Nelson E (eds) Cerebrovascular disease, Raven Press, New York p 51–56

Farhat S M, Schneider R C 1967 Observations on the effect of systemic blood pressure on intracranial circulation in patients with cerebrovascular insufficiency. Journal of Neurosurgery 27:441

Fazio C, Fieschi C, Agnoli A 1963 Direct common carotid injection of radioisotopes for the evaluation of cerebral circulatory disturbances. Neurology 13:561–574

Fazio F, Nardini M, Fieschi C, Forli C 1977 Assessment of regional blood flow by continuous carotid infusion of Krypton-81 m. Journal of Nuclear Medicine 18:962–966

Fazio F, Fieschi C, Nardini M, Collice M, Possa M 1979 Assessment of regional cerebral blood flow by continuous carotid infusion of Krypton-81 m and emission computerized tomography. Acta Neurologica Scandinavica 60:192–193 (suppl 72)

Feindel W, Perot P 1965 Red cerebral veins: a report on arteriovenous shunts in tumours and cerebral scars. Journal of Neurosurgery 22:315

Ferguson G G, Harper A M, Fitch W 1972 Cerebral blood flow measurements after spontaneous subarachnoid haemorrhage. European Neurology 8:15–22

Fieschi C 1980 Cerebral blood flow and energy metabolism in vascular insufficiency. Editorial. Stroke 11:431–432

Fieschi C, Bozzao L 1972a The physiology of cerebral circulation: Pharmacology of the cerebral circulation. In: International encyclopedia of pharmacology and therapeutics, Pergamon, London

Fieschi C, Bozzao L 1972b Clinical aspects of regional blood flow. In: Meyer J S, Schade J P (eds) Progress in brain research, Elsevier, Amsterdam, London, New York

Fieschi C, Lenzi G L 1979 CBF for the evaluation of the effects of drugs in chronic cerebrovascular insufficiency. In : Tognoni G, Garattini S (eds) Drug treatment and prevention in cerebrovascular disorders, Elsevier, Amsterdam, London, New York, p 13–21

Fieschi C, Agnoli A, Prencipe M, Battistini N, Bozzao L, Nardini M 1969 Impairment of the regional vasomotor response of cerebral vessels to hypercarbia in vascular diseases. European Neurology 2 : 13

Frackowiak R S J, Jones T, Lenzi G L, Heather J D 1980b Regional cerebral oxygen utilization and blood flow in normal man using oxygen-15 and positron emission tomography. Acta Neurologica Scandinavica (in press)

Frackowiak R S J, Lenzi G L, Jones T, Heather J D 1980a The quantitative measurement of regional cerebral blood flow and oxygen metabolism in man using oxygen-15 and positron emission tomography : theory, procedure and normal values. Journal Computer Assisted Tomography 4 : 727–736

Freygang W H, Sokoloff L 1959 Quantitative measurement of regional circulation in the central nervous system by the use of radioactive inert gas. In : Advances in biological and medical physics, Academic Press, London

Grubb R L, Raichle M E, Eichling J O, Gado M H 1976 Effects of subarachnoid hemorrhage on cerebral blood volume, blood flow and oxygen utilization in humans. Journal of Neurosurgery 46 : 446–453

Grubb R L, Raichle M E, Eichling J O, Ter-Pogossian M M 1974 The effects of changes in $P_a CO_2$ on cerebral blood volume, blood flow, and vascular mean transit time. Stroke 5 : 630–639

Haggendal E, Norback B 1966 Effect of viscosity on cerebral blood flow. Acta Chirurgica Scandinavica (suppl 364) 13

Harper A M 1965 The inter-relationship between $P_a CO_2$ and blood pressure in the regulation of blood flow through the cerebral cortex. Journal of Neurology, Neurosurgery and Psychiatry 28 : 449

Heilbrun M P, Olesen J, Lassen N A 1972 Regional cerebral blood flow studies in subarachnoid hemorrhage. Journal of Neurosurgery 37 : 36–44

Heiss W D 1973 Drug effects on regional cerebral blood flow. Journal of the Neurological Sciences 19 : 461

Heiss W D 1979 Relationship of cerebral blood flow to neurological deficit and to long-term prognosis of stroke. In : Zülch K J, Kaufmann W, Hossmann K A, Hossmann V (eds) Brain and heart infarct II, Springer-Verlag, Berlin, p 280–292

Heiss W D, Prosenz P, Gloning K, Tschabitscher H 1970 Regional and total cerebral blood flow under vasodilating drugs. In : Ross Russell R W (ed) Brain and blood flow, Pitman, London, p 270

Heiss W D, Prosenz P, Roszucky A 1972 Technical considerations in the use of a gamma 1600-channel analyser system for the measurement of regional cerebral blood flow. Journal of Nuclear Medicine 13 : 534

Høedt-Rasmussen K 1967 Regional cerebral blood flow : the intra-arterial injection method. Acta Neurologica Scandinavica 43 : 1 (Suppl. 27)

Høedt-Rasmussen K, Skinhøj E 1964 Transneural depression of the cerebral hemispheric metabolism in man. Acta Neurologica Scandinavica 40 : 41

Humphrey P R D et al 1980 Viscosity, cerebral blood flow and haematocrit in patients with paraproteinaemia. Acta Neurologica Scandinavica 59 :

Iliff L D, DuBoulay G H, Marshall J, Ross Russell R W, Symon L 1977 Effect of nicergoline on cerebral blood flow. Journal of Neurology, Neurosurgery and Psychiatry 40 : 746

Iliff L D, Zilkha E, DuBoulay G H, Marshall J, Ross Russell R W, Symon L 1974 Cerebrovascular CO_2 reactivity of the fast and slow clearing compartments. Stroke 5 : 607

Ingvar D H 1965 Normal values of rCBF in man, including flow and weight estimates of grey and white matter. Acta Neurologica Scandinavica 41 : 72 (Suppl. 14)

Ingvar D H 1975 Patterns of brain activity revealed by measurements of regional cerebral blood flow. In : Benzon A (ed) Symposium VIII, Brain work, Munksgaard, Copenhagen p 397–413

Ingvar D H 1979 'Hyperfrontal' distribution of the cerebral grey matter flow in resting wakefulness ; on the functional anatomy of the conscious state. Acta Neurologica Scandinavica 60 : 12–25

Ingvar D H, Lassen N A 1965 Methods for cerebral blood flow measurements in man. British Journal of Anesthesia 37 : 216

Ingvar D H, Lassen N A 1973 Cerebral complications following measurement of rCBF with intra-arterial 133-Xenon injection method. Stroke 4 : 658

Ingvar D H, Lassen N A (eds) 1975, Brain work, Munksgaard, Copenhagen

Ingvar D H, Philipson L 1977 Distribution of cerebral blood flow in the dominant hemisphere during motor ideation and motor performance. Annals of Neurology 2 : 230–237

Ishii Ryo J 1979 Regional cerebral blood flow in patients with matured intracranial aneurysms. Journal of Neurosurgery 50 : 587–594

Jaffe M E, McHenry L C, Goldberg H I 1970 Regional cerebral blood flow measurement with small probes. II. Application of the method. Neurology 20 : 225

James I M 1968 Changes in cerebral blood flow and in systemic arterial pressure following spontaneous subarachnoid haemorrhage. Clinical Science 35 : 11–22

Johnston I H, Paterson A, Harper A, Jennet W B 1972 The effect of mannitol on intracranial pressure and cerebral blood flow. In : Brock, Dietz (eds) 'Intracranial pressure' Springer, Berlin pp 176–180

Jones T, Chesler D A, Ter-Pogossian M M 1976 The continuous inhalation of oxygen-15 for assessing regional oxygen extraction in the brain of man. British Journal of Radiology 49 : 339–343

Kety S S 1950 Circulation and metabolism of the human brain in health and disease. American Journal of Medicine 8 : 205

Kety S S, Schmidt C F 1948 The nitrous oxide method for the quantitative determination of cerebral blood flow in man : theory, procedure and normal values. Journal of Clinical Investigation 27 : 476–483

Kuhl D E, Phelps M E, Hoffman E J, Robinson G D, MacDonald N S 1977 Initial clinical experience with 18-F-2-Fluoro-2-Deoxy-D-Glucose for determination of local cerebral glucose utilization by emission computed tomography. Acta Neurologica Scandinavica 56 : 192–193 (Suppl 64)

Kuhl D E, Phelps M E, Kowell A P, Metter E J, Selin C, Winter J 1980 Effects of stroke on local cerebral metabolism and perfusion : mapping by emission computed tomography of 18-FDG and $^{13}NH_3$. Annals of Neurology 8 : 47–60

Lassen N A 1966 The luxury perfusion syndrome and its possible relation to acute metabolic acidosis localised within the brain. Lancet ii 1113–1115

Lassen N A, Agnoli A 1972 The upper limit of autoregulation of cerebral blood flow. On the pathogenesis of hypertensive encephalopathy. Scandinavian Journal of Clinical and Laboratory Investigations 30 : 113

Lassen N A, Munch O 1955 The cerebral blood flow in man determined by the use of radioactive Krypton. Acta Physiologica Scandinavica 33 : 30

Lassen N A, Palvölgyi R 1968 Cerebral steal during hypercapnea and the inverse reaction during hypocapnia observed by the 133-Xenon technique in man. Scandinavian Journal of Clinical and Laboratory Investigation 22 (Suppl 102)

Lassen N A, Skinhøj E 1975 Regional cerebral circulation in man and its regulation. In : Williams D (ed) Modern trends in neurology — 6 Butterworths, England p 59–82

Lassen N A et al 1963 Regional cerebral blood flow in man determined by Krypton-85. Neurology 13 : 719

Lenzi G L, Jones T, Frackowiak R S J 1981 Positron emission tomography : state of the art in neurology. Advances in Nuclear Medicine (in press)

Lenzi G L, Frackowiak R S J, Heather J D, Buckingham P S, Jones T 1980 Metabolic and circulatory aspects of the acute stroke. XXXVIII International congress of physiological sciences ; satellite symposium on cerebrovascular disease, Tubingen 1980

Lenzi G L, Jones T, McKenzie C G, Moss S 1977 Regional studies of oxygen uptake and blood flow in chronic cerebrovascular disorders using the oxygen inhalation technique. In : Meyer J S, Lechner H, Reivich M (eds) Cerebral vascular disease, Excerpta Medica p 187–190

Lenzi G L, Jones T, McKenzie C G, Buckingham P D, Clark J C, Moss S 1978 Study of regional cerebral metabolism and blood flow relationships in man using the method of continuously inhaling oxygen-15 and oxygen-15 labelled carbon dioxide. Journal of Neurology, Neurosurgery and Psychiatry 41 : 1–10

Marshall J 1972 The evaluation and prognosis of acute cerebrovascular insufficiency as determined by rCBF analysis. In : Meyer J S et al (eds) Sixth Salzburg conference on cerebrovascular diseases, Thieme, Stuttgart

Mathew N T 1974 The importance of CSF pressure regional CBF dysautoregulation in the pathogenesis of normal pressure hydrocephalus. Intracranial pressure II. In : Lundberg N et al (eds) Proceedings of the Second international symposium on intracranial pressure, Springer-Verlag, Berlin

McHenry L C, Jaffe M E, Goldberg H I 1969 Regional Cerebral blood flow measurements with small probes. I. Evaluation of the method. Neurology 19 : 1198

McHenry L C, Goldberg H I, Jaffe M E, Kenton E J, West J W, Cooper E S 1972 Regional cerebral blood flow : response to carbon dioxide in cerebrovascular disease. Archives of Neurology 27 : 403

Meric P, Seylaz J, Correze J-L, Luft A, Mamo H 1979 Measurement of regional cerebral blood flow by intra-venous injection of ^{133}Xe. Medical Progress through Technology 6 : 53–63

Merory J et al 1978 Effect of tinofedrine (Homburg D8955) on cerebral blood flow in multi-infarct dementia. Journal of Neurology, Neurosurgery and Psychiatry 41 : 900–902

Meyer J S, Shinohara Y, Kanda T 1970 Diaschisis resulting from acute unilateral cerebral infarction. Archives of Neurology 23 : 241–247

Michenfelder J D, Sundt T M 1971 Cerebral ATP and lactate levels in the squirrel monkey following occlusion of the middle cerebral cortex. Stroke 2 : 319

Mosmans P C M 1974 Regional cerebral blood flow in neurological patients : clinical significance and correlation with EEG. Van Gorcum, Assen

O'Brien M D, Veall N 1974 Partition coefficients between various brain tumours and blood for ^{133}Xe. Physics in Medicine and Biology 19 : 472

Obrist W D, Thompson H K, Herschel King C, Shan Wang H 1967 Determination of regional cerebral blood flow by inhalation of ^{133}Xe. Circulation Research 20 : 124

Obrist W D, Thompson H K Jr, Shan Wang H, Wilkinson W D 1975 Regional cerebral blood flow estimated by ^{133}Xenon inhalation. Stroke 6 : 245–256

Olesen J 1972 The effect of intracarotid epinephrine, nor-epinephrine and angiotensin on the regional cerebral blood flow in man. Neurology 22 : 978

Olesen J 1974 Cerebral blood flow : methods for measurement, regulation effects of drugs and changes in disease, Fadls Forlag, Copenhagen

Olesen J, Paulson O B, Lassen N A 1971 Regional cerebral blood flow in man determined by the initial slope of the clearance of intra-arterially injected ^{133}Xe. Stroke 2 : 519

Paulson O B 1970 Regional Cerebral blood flow in apoplexy due to occlusion of the middle artery. Neurology 20 : 63–77

Paulson O B, Lassen N A, Skinhøj E 1970 Regional cerebral blood flow in apoplexy without arterial cerebral occlusion. Neurology 20 : 125–138

Penfield W 1938 The circulation of the epileptic brain. Research Publication of the Association for Research in Nervous and Mental Diseases 18 : 605

Phelps M E, Hoffman E J, Huang S C, Kuhl D E 1978 ECAT, a new computerized tomographic imaging system for positron emitting radiopharmaceuticals. Journal of Nuclear Medicine 19 : 635–647

Phelps M E, Huang S C, Hoffman E J, Selin C, Sokoloff L, Kuhl D E 1979 Tomographic measurement of local cerebral glucose metabolic rate in humans with (F-18)-2-Fluoro-2-deoxy-D-glucose : validation of the method. Annals of Neurology 6 : 371–388

Pickard J D 1973 The mechanism of action of prostaglandin F2α on cerebral blood flow in the baboon. Journal of Physiology 234 : 46

Pistolese G R et al 1971 Effects of hypercapnia on the cerebral blood flow during the clamping of the carotid arteries on surgical management of cerebrovascular insufficiency. Neurology 21 : 95–100

Planiol T, Floyrac R, Itti R, Rouzaud M, Degiovanni E, Gories P 1971 La gamma-angio-encephalographie dans l'insuffisance circulatoire cerebrale. Revue Neurologique 125 : 56

Posner J B 1973 Newer techniques of cerebral blood flow measurements. Sixth conference on cerebrovascular diseases Princeton 1972 Grune and Stratton, New York

Prosenz P, Chimani N, Heiss W D, Kothbauer P, Tschbitscher H, Sollner E 1972 Prognosis of brain infarction based on blood flow measurements by means of the Xenon clearance method. European Neurology 8 : 124

Purves M J 1972 The physiology of the cerebral circulation. Monographs of the Physiological Society 28 Cambridge University Press

Raichle M E 1979 Cerebral hemodynamic, metabolic and biochemical studies using positron emission tomography. In: Baillière J B (ed) Cerebrovascular Disease Second Conference Salpêtrière p 161–183

Raichle M E, Stone H L 1971 Cerebral blood flow autoregulation and graded hypercapnia. European Neurology 6:1

Raichle M E, Grubb R L, Gado M H, Eichling J O, Ter-Pogossian M M 1976 Correlation between regional blood flow and oxidative metabolism. Archives of Neurology 33:523–526

Rees J E, DuBoulay E P G H, Bull J W D, Marshall J, Russell R W R, Symon L 1971 Persistence of disturbance of regional cerebral blood flow after transient ischaemic attacks. In: Pitman (ed) Brain and blood flow, London

Reivich M 1964 Arterial pCO_2 and cerebral haemodynamics. American Journal of Physiology 206:25

Reivich M 1969 Regulation of the cerebral circulation. In: (eds) 'Clinical Neurosurgery, William and Wilkins, Baltimore

Reivich M, Marshall W J S, Kassell N 1969 Loss of autoregulation produced by cerebral trauma. In: Brock M et al (eds) 'Cerebral blood flow', Springer-Verlag, Berlin

Reivich M et al 1978 Alterations in regional cerebral hemodynamics and metabolism produced by focal cerebral ischaemia. European Neurology 17:9–16 (Suppl 1)

Reivich M et al 1979 The 18-F-Fluorodeoxyglucose method for the measurement of local cerebral glucose utilization in man. Circulation Research 44:127–137

Roy C S, Sherrington M B 1890 On the regulation of the blood supply of the brain. Journal of Physiology 11:85–108

Salmon J H, Timperman A L 1971 Cerebral blood flow in post-traumatic encephalopathy. The effect of ventriculo-atrial shunt. Neurology 21:33

Skinhøj J E, Høedt-Rasmussen K, Paulson O B, Lassen N A 1970 Regional cerebral blood flow and its autoregulation in patients with transient local cerebral ischaemic attacks. Neurology 20:485

Slater R, Reivich M, Goldberg H, Banka R, Greenberg J 1977 Diaschisis with cerebral infarction. Stroke 8:684–690

Sokoloff L 1959 The action of drugs on the cerebral circulation. Pharmacological Reviews 11:1

Sokoloff L 1961 Aspects of cerebral circulatory physiology of relevance to cerebrovascular disease. Neurology 11:34

Strandgaard S, MacKenzie E T, Sengupta D, Rowan J O, Lassen N A, Harper M 1974 Upper limit of autoregulation of cerebral blood flow in the baboon. Circulation Research 18:435

Symon L 1971 Hyperemia in the cerebral circulation. In: Ross Russell R W (ed) Brain and blood flow, Pitman, London

Symon L, Brierly J B 1975 Morphological changes in cerebral blood vessels in chronic ischaemic infarction; functional changes obtained by hydrogen clearance. Stroke

Symon L, Ackerman R, Bull J W D 1972 The use of the Xenon clearance in subarachnoid hemorrhage. Post-operative studies with clinical angiographic correlation. European Neurology 8:8–14

Ter-Pogossian M M, Eichling J O, Davis D O, Welch M J 1970 The measure in vivo of regional cerebral oxygen utilization by means of oxyhemoglobin labelled with radioactive oxygen-15. Journal of Clinical Investigation 49:381–391

Ter-Pogossian M M, Eichling J O, Davis D O, Welch M J, Metzger J 1969 The determination of regional cerebral blood flow by means of water labelled with radioactive oxygen-15. Radiology 93:31–40

Thomas D J et al 1979 An intravenous [133]Xenon clearance technique for measuring cerebral blood flow. Journal of the Neurological Sciences 40:53–63

Thomas D J et al 1977 Effect of haematocrit on cerebral blood flow in man. Lancet 2:941–943

Uemura K et al 1979 Three dimensional imaging of regional brain circulation using radionuclide computed tomography and continuous infusion of Kripton-81 m. Acta Neurologica Scandinavica 60:190–191 (suppl 72)

Veall N, Mallett B L 1966 Regional cerebral blood flow determination by ^{133}Xe inhalation and external recording. The effect of arterial recirculation. Clinical Sciences 30:353–369

Waltz A G 1968 Experimental cerebral ischaemia: effects on cortical microvasculature and blood flow. Scandinavian Journal of Clinical and Laboratory Investigation 22 (Suppl 102)

Wang H S, Busse E W 1975 In: Harper A M, Jennett W B, Miller J D, Rowan J O (eds) Blood flow and metabolism in the brain, Churchill Livingstone, Edinburgh, p 817–818

Wilkinson I M S, Browne D R G 1970 The influence of anesthesia and of arterial hypocapnia on regional blood flow in the normal human cerebral hemisphere. British Journal of Anesthesiology 42:472

Wilkinson I M S, Bull J W D, DuBoulay G H, Marshall J, Ross Russell R W, Symon L 1969 Regional cerebral blood flow in the normal cerebral hemisphere. Journal of Neurology, Neurosurgery and Psychiatry 32:367–8

Wong E, Bull J W D, DuBoulay G H, Marshall J, Ross Russell R W, Symon L 1973 Regional cerebral blood flow in completed strokes and transient ischaemic attacks: a clinical correlation. Neurology 23:949–952

Yamamoto Y L, Feindel W, Wolfe L S, Katoh H, Hodge C P 1972 Experimental vasoconstriction of cerebral arteries by prostaglandin. Journal of Neurosurgery 37:385

Zierler K L 1965 Equations for measuring blood flow by external monitoring of radioisotopes. Circulation Research 16:309

Zingesser L H, Schechter M M, Dexter J, Katzman R, Scheinberg L C 1968 On the significance of spasm associated with rupture of a cerebral aneurysm. Archives of Neurology 18:520

6

Ischaemic cerebral oedema

M. D. O'Brien

The definition of cerebral oedema is a relative increase in the water content of the brain and this may be either in the intracellular or extracellular compartments or both. The amount of oedema, determined experimentally, is usually expressed as a per cent reduction in dry weight, or as an increase in the percentage difference between wet and dry weights. Cerebral oedema may also be determined indirectly by changes in specific gravity. There are two other causes of brain swelling, vascular congestion and hydrocephalus; these are not due to oedema but may be confused with it. The early literature distinguished between brain swelling or dry oedema (Hirnschwelling) and brain oedema or wet oedema (Hirondem), according to the appearance of the cut surface of the brain (Reichardt, 1904). It is now possible to explain these differences by a consideration of the possible changes in each of the four intracranial fluid compartments.

The intracranial fluid compartments

The four intracranial fluid compartments are intravascular, intracellular, extracellular and cerebrospinal fluid (Fig. 6.1). The first three of these compartments are separated by membrane barriers, which maintain their interior milieu; the extracellular space and the cerebrospinal fluid are in continuity. The blood-brain barrier has many functions, but as far as oedema formation is concerned this discussion will be limited to the transendothelial resistance to water diffusion and the passage of macromolecules as well as to the state of the endothelial tight junctions. Other properties of the blood-brain barrier, such as active and facilitated transport, will not be discussed although these properties play an important part in the passage of osmotically effective molecules, such as the sugars.

Water is freely diffusible between all these

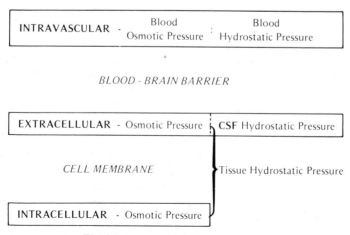

Fig. 6.1 Intracranial fluid compartments.

compartments and its movement is entirely passive following osmotic and hydrostatic pressure gradients. The rate of equilibration depends on the hydraulic conductivity of the various membranes and this is much less for the blood-brain barrier than in other vascular beds. The amount of oedema formation depends on the tissue compliance, which is a composite of the compliance of all the compartments. White matter tissue compliance is much greater than that of grey matter and this difference is the reason why white matter usually becomes much more oedematous and why this is more extensive than in the overlying cortex.

The blood hydrostatic pressure is the source of all intracranial hydrostatic pressures and is the principal driving force in the formation of oedema. The intra and extracellular hydrostatic pressures can be considered together as the tissue hydrostatic pressure, although these two compartments may alter volume separately under differing osmotic pressures. If the hydrostatic pressure is zero, it is possible to have a shift of water from the extracellular space to the intracellular space due to membrane failure, without an increase in total brain tissue water and this of course, is not cerebral oedema.

These fluid compartments are all interdependent but it is convenient to consider the factors which alter the volume of each compartment separately.

1. *The intravascular compartment.* Brain swelling due to vascular congestion occurs when cerebral blood vessels are fully dilated by anoxia or hypercapnia, provided that there is adequate input under sufficient pressure to distend small blood vessels and this may require some elevation in blood pressure. This is the first stage of high altitude 'cerebral oedema'. Initially this is brain swelling due to vascular congestion because of the anoxic stimulus combined with an elevation of blood pressure with exertion. In experimental animals considerable congestion can be achieved with anoxia or hypercapnia alone, the endothelial cells are relatively resistant to hypoxia and tight junctions are preserved. In experimental animals it is almost impossible to produce oedema by anoxia alone because cardiac problems supervene. Venous hypertension leads to vascular congestion but not to oedema unless the blood brain barrier is damaged (Cuypers et al, 1976).

2. *The extracellular compartment.* Brain swelling due to extracellular oedema has been called 'vasogenic oedema' (Klatzo, 1976) and corresponds to wet oedema since the cut surface of the brain oozes oedema fluid. It can be conveniently divided into oedema with an intact blood-brain barrier and oedema with a damaged blood-brain barrier.

Oedema with an intact blood-brain barrier is an ultrafiltration of plasma and may occur with a moderate or slow rise of blood pressure into a dilated or disautoregulated vascular bed; it is the next stage after vascular congestion. It can be produced quite easily in experimental animals by a rise in blood pressure with hypercapnia (Meinig, et al, 1972) or following the application of pressure to the cortex to produce loss of autoregulation. This is one of the mechanisms of oedema formation around cerebral tumours and, together with vascular congestion, is the principal cause of rapid swelling of the brain which may follow the surgical removal of a large intracranial mass, such as a meningioma. If the blood-brain barrier is damaged, the next stage in severity, there is protein extravasation and osmotic extracellular oedema in addition to the hydrostatic oedema. Hypertensive encephalopathy is a good clinical example. It may be produced experimentally with a rapid rise in blood pressure alone or at lower levels of blood pressure with loss of autoregulation (Johansson, 1976). It may also be induced by trauma, either by pressure or by freezing.

Extracellular oedema spreads extensively through white matter by bulk flow along hydrostatic pressure gradients and not by diffusion, since it has been shown that substances with different diffusion coefficients travel at the same speed and further than they would by diffusion alone (Reulen, 1976). The oedema fluid eventually reaches the CSF with which it is in continuity, so that CSF pressure has some effect on oedema resolution. Some oedema fluid is cleared by absorption into the blood vessels.

It is possible to have the blood-brain barrier open to macromolecules without the formation of oedema and this has been demonstrated following infusions of hypertonic solutions. It was postulated that the hypertonic solution caused shrinkage of the endothelial cells and opening of tight junctions (Rapoport et al, 1971); the finding of horseradish peroxidase in the tight junctions was said to support this view (Klatzo, 1972). However, the tight junctions have never been observed to open and it now seems clear endothelial cells merely become more permeable to macromolecules, which traverse the cells by pinocytosis (Rapoport, 1976a, Nag et al, 1977, Petito, 1979). It is possible that oedema does not develop because the osmotic gradient is not sufficiently altered by the extravasation of protein in the presence of a hyperosmolar vascular compartment, but the relationship between extracellular protein and osmolarity is not linear and there may well be a threshold before significant oedema can develop (Rapoport, 1976b). This dissociation between macromolecule extravasation and oedema formation occurs in stroke (O'Brien et al, 1974) and epileptic seizures, where the seizure-induced hypertension causes most of the damage to the blood-brain barrier and enhanced micropinocytosis (Petito et al, 1976).

Experiments to investigate the relationship of macromolecule extravasation and oedema formation are complicated by the technical difficulties of obtaining very accurate measurements of small changes in water content, whereas very small amounts of protein tracer, suitably labelled, can be measured with great accuracy. Very small percentage changes in water content may however result in relatively large volumetric and pressure changes, for example a 2.5 per cent increase in water content may quadruple the intracranial pressure (Rosomoff & Zugibe, 1963).

3. *The intracellular compartment.* This has been called 'metabolic' or 'cyotoxic' oedema. It is caused by anything which damages cell metabolism, particularly the sodium pump mechanism, producing a change in the osmotic balance across the cell membrane. This type of oedema corresponds to the dry oedematous brain because the oedema is contained in the cells and the cut surface of the brain is not unduly wet. It can be produced experimentally with a wide range of poisons such as cyanide and hexachlorophene and by specific sodium pump inhibitors such as ouabain (Tanaka et al, 1977). Direct traumatic damage to the cell, including the cold injury, also results in destruction of cell membranes.

A combination of intracellular and extracellular oedema is produced by reducing the osmotic pressure of the blood with infusions of distilled water or by dialysis. Such osmotic oedema must be rather rare in clinical practice, but it may occur in patients with diabetes if the blood sugar falls precipitously from high levels.

4. *The cerebrospinal fluid compartment.* The CSF hydrostatic pressure is one determinant of the overall cerebral perfusion pressure and it is a measure of the average tissue and venous pressures. It is not as important as it may seem because focal cerebral oedema may alter the local perfusion pressure without significant change in the CSF pressure. This phenomenon has even been demonstrated with generalised oedema associated with triethyl tin poisoning and with water intoxication, but these experiments show that oedema alone does not reduce blood flow to critical levels without a rise in intracranial pressure. (Meinig et al, 1973, Marshall et al 1976a).

The effect of oedema on cerebral function

Obviously, in metabolic oedema, function is impaired at the outset since the oedema is due to cellular malfunction; but extracellular or vasogenic oedema appears to have remarkably little effect on cell function as shown by electrical activity and evoked responses until blood flow falls to critical levels (Marshall et al, 1976b). This is shown clinically in patients with benign intracranial hypertension, who may remain quite alert despite considerable cerebral oedema. Focal cerebral oedema may be more serious with the production of a rapidly expanding mass effect and intracranial herniation. In one series (Plum, 1961) cerebral swelling contributed to or caused deterioration or death in 20 per cent of 106 stroke patients.

Ischaemic cerebral oedema

It is possible for ischaemia to produce all the forms of brain swelling and oedema that have been discussed. Intravascular congestion and an ultrafiltrate oedema with an intact blood-brain barrier requires an increase in the hydrostatic pressure to capillaries through disautoregulated and maximally dilated arteries and arterioles. This may occur in stroke if the collateral circulation is exceptionally good or if an embolus impacts, fragments and moves off, leaving a patent vessel to feed the distal disautoregulated vascular bed which is then exposed to systemic pressures. Transient episodes of local perfusion failure due to a fall in systemic pressure could produce the same circumstances. However, these mechanisms are not likely to be very important in most patients with stroke, where oedema formation is largely due to ischaemic cell damage, with failure of the sodium pump, together with damage to the blood-brain barrier with protein extravasation; that is, a combination of metabolic and vasogenic oedema.

The degree of ischaemia is not homogeneous throughout an infarct; furthermore, the development of an infarct is a rapidly evolving situation with different parts of the lesion developing at different rates. All the various mechanisms of oedema formation may occur in stroke and this will vary not only throughout the lesion but also with time.

The important factors which determine the formation of ischaemic cerebral oedema are the rate of development, the duration and the depth of ischaemia and the extent to which the systemic blood pressure is transmitted to the infarct. In addition, there are the secondary effects of the ischaemic process on hydrostatic and osmotic pressures of each fluid compartment and the feedback effect these changes have on blood flow and intracranial pressure.

If ischaemia is absolute and the blood flow zero, electrical activity of the neurones stops in a few seconds, followed by failure of the sodium pump and glucose depletion. Intracellular oedema, mostly derived from the extracellular space, is evident after a few minutes and there is a massive rise in lactate. Up to this stage the process is potentially reversible, but thereafter a stepwise sequence of organelle failure occurs as thresholds for survival are reached and passed. The preservation of some circulation would prolong this sequence and provided that the blood hydrostatic pressure remains low in the infarct, the blood-brain barrier remains intact and there is virtually no leak of protein.

However, ishaemia is usually less than complete. Symon (1967) has reported blood pressures of between 25 and 40 per cent of normal in the vascular bed distal to a proximal middle cerebral artery occlusion in monkeys and flows down to 25 per cent of normal in this model (Symon et al, 1974). Autoradiographic blood flow studies in experimental animals have also shown flows which range from zero to near normal values in the territory of an occluded vessel. Some blood flow, therefore, usually exists which slows down the development of the infarct and the process may be arrested at any stage. The depth of ischaemia is very important and may be quite critical. Shibata et al (1974) showed no change in the electrolyte or water content of the brain following middle cerebral artery occlusion in dogs, but when the ischaemic insult was increased by reducing the blood pressure, oedema and infarction resulted. The brain can survive mild ischaemia for some time but it is intolerant of profound ischaemia for even short periods, so that the depth of ischaemia is more critical than its duration (Symon et al, 1979). Other animal experiments have shown that the presence or absence of venous obstruction is an important factor (Hossman & Oleson, 1970), since recovery is poorest and damage greatest if both arteries and veins are occluded at the same time. The situation is better if the veins are left unobstructed and better still if the brain is perfused with saline during the arterial occlusion. These experiments imply that both stasis and accumulation of metabolites are important factors in ischaemic damage.

Whether or not the blood-brain barrier opens to macromolecules depends on the blood hydrostatic pressure at capillary level as well as the duration and depth of ischaemia. With no pressure and no flow there is no protein extravasation, partly because the distending pressure is zero and partly because of a squeeze on the extracellular space and capillaries by swollen glia (Reulen 1976), which may increase resistance to macromolecule extravasation and also reduces the spread of extracellular oedema. Little (1976) has shown that the swelling of astrocytic foot processes occurs initially near blood vessels and spreads from there; this suggests that the fluid is derived from the vascular compartment. With some hydrostatic pressure and sufficient ischaemia, the blood-brain barrier opens eventually, but only after an interval of some hours. The duration for which the barrier remains open is variable and also depends on the duration and depth of ischaemia and local hydrostatic pressure.

Seigel et al (1972), using micro-emboli in rats, showed a big shift of sodium at four hours but the blood-brain barrier did not open until 8–16 hours. Klatzo (1972) using bilateral carotid occlusion in gerbils found the blood-brain barrier open at 24 hours after 30 minutes of occlusion in 50 per cent of animals, whereas if the occlusion was prolonged to 6 hours, the barrier was open 60 minutes in all animals. Harrison et al (1975) using the same gerbil model, found that the oedema was maximal at 8 hours but that the blood-brain barrier did not open until 18–24 hours. Garcia et al (1979) found peak oedema levels at 4 days in rhesus monkeys following middle cerebral artery occlusion with greatest blood-brain barrier breakdown at 7–10 days. Petito (1979) using the Levine rat model, showed a leak of horseradish peroxidase at one minute and thirty minutes by a process of increased pinocytosis. Evans blue leakage did not occur until one and a half and two hours, and was then associated with necrotic vessel walls. This process almost certainly depends on adequate perfusion pressure and would account for the early if less obvious increase in extracellular oedema despite a blood-brain barrier intact against large molecules.

Hossman (1976) found that after one hour of total ischaemia in cats the extracellular space diminished from 18.9 volumes per cent to 8.5 volumes per cent (Fig. 6.2), while the total water content and intracranial pressure remained unchanged. This indicated a shift of water from the extracellular to the intracellular space. There was no increase in the water content of the brain because there was no input. Following reperfusion there was rapid increase in the extracellular fluid and a corresponding rise in intracranial pressure and water content of the brain; the resulting state being a combination of extracellular and intracellular oedema. Ito et al (1979) have shown in gerbils that if there is a restoration of flow after less than an hour of ischaemia, the water content is reduced, whereas if the restoration is delayed until about three hours, there is a massive rise in water content demonstrating that damage to the blood-brain barrier occurs between these times in this model. Symon (1979) found that reperfusion after 30 minutes of middle cerebral artery occlusion in monkeys was not associated with any significant

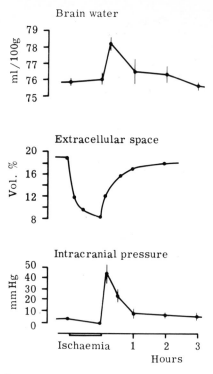

Fig. 6.2 Reduction in extracellular space without a change in intracranial pressure or the formation of oedema after one hour of total ischaemia in cats. Reperfusion restores the extracellular volume and causes a marked rise in intracranial pressure and considerable oedema. (from Hossmann (1976), Development and resolution of ischaemic brain swelling. In: Dynamics of brain oedema. Springer Verlag, Berlin p 219–227. Reproduced by kind permission of the author).

increase in water content, whereas reperfusion after 90 minutes occlusion was associated with an increase in water content where the reperfusion had occurred, although this was very patchy with much of the territory affected by the no-reflow phenomenon.

O'Brien et al (1974) studied the distribution of water in the brains of cats from 4 hours to 20 days after occlusion of the middle cerebral artery. (Fig. 6.3). In this model the water content reached a maximum at two days and was always greater in infarcted brain and less in ischaemic areas, but it also affected the opposite hemisphere (diaschisis). This might be due to a compression oedema since in this model quite high pressure differences can be recorded epidurally (O'Brien & Waltz, 1973). At the same time blood-brain barrier function was studied with ^{99}technetium^m pertechnetate and ^{131}I-labelled albumin (O'Brien et al, 1974). The

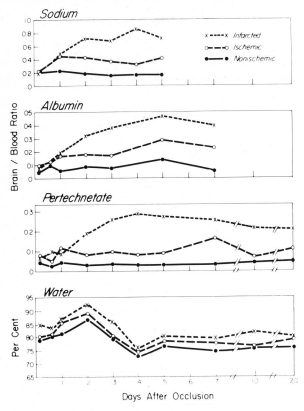

Fig. 6.3 Distribution of water, technetium pertechnetate, albumin and sodium after occlusion of the middle cerebral artery in cats. (from O'Brien et al (1974). Ischaemic cerebral oedema and the blood-brain barrier. Archives of Neurology 30:461–465).

greatest extravasation of these tracers did not occur until three or four days after infarction and remained high for the duration of the study. Comparison of the extravasation of these tracers to water showed continued high levels of the tracer long after the water level had returned to normal. This is in accord with the clinical experience that oedema is maximal between one and three days after a stroke, whereas the technetium pertechnetate brain scan may not reach the maximum lesion to background ratio until seven to ten days.

It seems clear, therefore, that the sequence of events in the formation of oedema due to cerebral ischaemia is as follows: firstly, there is a shift of water from the extracellular to the intracellular space, which occurs with even slight ischaemia, and some extracellular oedema may occur, probably associated with increased pinocytosis if local

perfusion pressure is adequate. Only later does the blood-brain barrier open to macromolecules if the ischaemia is sufficient to cause cellular disruption and this depends principally on the blood hydrostatic pressure at capillary level. It is not clear why the oedema is maximal at two days and then improves, not apparently following the subsequent breakdown of the blood-brain barrier. It may be that the perfusion pressure is inadequate in the infarcted area and that the osmotic effect is insufficient.

Clinical evaluation

It is not possible to determine clinically the contribution of oedema to the neurological deficit. Computerised tomography has now made this possible. An average reduction of 10 Hounsfield units was found at the time of maximal swelling following an infarct in one series (Clasen et al, 1979) and this corresponds to a six per cent increase in water content. The calculation of water content from the CT scan in the chronic state after infarct is complicated by the loss of lipid which occurs at this stage.

Treatment

The widely discrepant experimental and clinical reports of various treatment methods using different agents and experimental models is probably due to the varying degrees of ischaemia, its duration, the availability of a collateral circulation and the hydrostatic pressure in the infarct. In addition there are species differences in brain volume, including the relative amounts of grey and white matter, anatomical variations in the cerebral circulation and species variation in response to drugs. Most of the experimental models of cerebral oedema are not appropriate to the study of ischaemic oedema. This applies to triethyl tin and hexachlorophene poisoning, osmotic oedema, micro-embolisation, hydrophillic seeds, mechanical trauma and pressure from balloons. The cold injury produces a clear reproducible lesion, which mimics ischaemic oedema pathologically with both intracellular and extracellular fluid accumulation, but the local haemodynamic aspects are very different from most strokes because unlike the cold injury lesion, an infarct is usually protected from the systemic pressure.

Great caution must therefore be exercised in drawing parallels between most of the animal experimental studies reported about different treatment methods to patients with stroke. The treatment of ischaemic cerebral oedema is based on the various ways in which the fluid content of the different compartments can be modified. In practice, only the vascular compartment hydrostatic and osmotic pressures can be altered directly but such changes may secondarily affect the other intracranial fluid compartments. The vascular hydrostatic pressure can be changed by alterations in blood pressure or by alteration in vessel calibre. The vascular osmotic pressure can be altered by infusion of hypertonic solutions. The CSF hydrostatic pressure can be lowered by drainage, but this is not relevant to ischaemic oedema and would probably increase extracellular oedema by increasing the hydrostatic pressure gradient. Finally, it may be possible to mitigate the effects of ischaemia on membrane barriers, particularly the blood-brain barrier, since there are a number of drugs which alter the properties of membranes, particularly steroids. Barbiturates (Michenfelder et al, 1976, Simeone et al, 1979, Lawner et al, 1979, Marshall, 1980) may have an effect both on cellular metabolism as well as cell membranes.

Hydrostatic pressures

The effect of changes in systemic pressure depends almost entirely on the extent to which this is transmitted to the capillaries. If the major arterial supply to an infarcted region is occluded, then the blood supply to the infarct is from the collateral circulation and, at least in the acute stage, the flow will be pressure dependent because the arterioles will be maximally dilated by the anoxic-ischaemic stimulus. Symon et al (1976) have shown that the loss of autoregulation is proportional to the degree of ischaemia, particularly for falls in blood pressure. They found that autoregulation was partly preserved when the post-occlusion flow was greater than 40 per cent of normal, but absent when the flow was less than 20 per cent. Under these circumstances an increase in pressure causes an

increase in flow and this has been shown in patients (Goldberg et al, 1977).

Conversely, and perhaps more critically and clinically important, is that a reduction in pressure causes a fall in flow. If the collateral circulation has to travel a considerable distance, as would occur in bilateral carotid occlusion, there may be autoregulation against a rise in systemic pressure in responsive vessels too distant from the infarct to be affected by it and this considerably reduces the perfusion pressure within the ischaemic/infarcted area. If the main arterial supply to the infarct is patent or if the collateral supply is exceptionally good, particularly with small lesions, the situation is rather different. This is becuase the infarcted area is then exposed to systemic pressures and an increase in blood pressure will tend to open the blood-brain barrier early and drive the formation of extracellular oedema. This has been studied extensively in animals with two basic types of experimental model. In cold injury, the lesion is exposed to systemic pressures from the start (Fig. 6.4). Klatzo et al (1967), showed that by increasing

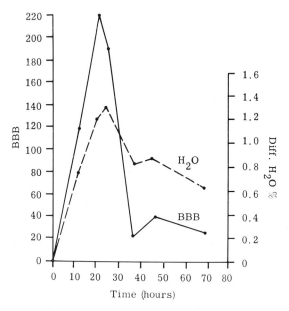

Fig. 6.4 Time course of blood brain barrier disturbance to ^{125}I-diiodo fluorescine and oedema formation in the cortex of rabbits after cold injury (from Hermann et al 1972). Influence of dexamethasone on water content, blood brain barrier and glucose metabolism in cold injury oedema. In: Steroids and brain oedema. Springer Verlag, Berlin, p 77–85. (Reproduced by kind permission of the authors).

the blood pressure in cats with the cold injury to 200 mm Hg, oedema reached the levels in two hours that would normally take six hours to achieve in normotensive animals; lowering the blood pressure inhibited oedema formation. The other principal experimental model is the use of temporary arterial clips which are then removed after varying intervals of time, so that exposure to arterial pressure occurs after infarction. In these circumstances a rise in blood pressure may increase the flow; however, false autoregulation may also occur, i.e., a rise in pressure that is not accompanied by a rise in flow in a disautoregulated vascular bed. This is due to an increase in oedema caused by the rise in pressure, which squeezes the capillaries, thereby preventing dilatation and an increase in blood flow (Miller et al, 1976). This phenomenon may occur without a comparable rise in intracranial pressure. Grote & Schubert (1977) have shown that cold induced oedema can prevent subsequent dilation by anoxia and Frei et al (1973) have shown that reactive hyperaemia only occurs in non-oedematous brain. A linear inverse relationship has been found between cerebral blood flow and water content in the brain adjacent to cerebral tumours, showing the effect of focal oedema, (Reulen et al, 1972). These observations suggest that it is the local tissue hydrostatic pressure which determines the local perfusion pressure and not the average

intracranial pressure; i.e., there may be local squeeze on small vessels without a rise in intracranial pressure.

Fluctuations in blood pressure may be even more harmful as has been demonstrated by Matakas et al (1972) in monkeys. Extracellular oedema was induced by balloon compression. Subsequent to release, the intracranial pressure rose to a level which depended on the systemic blood pressure. The blood pressure was then increased with norepinephrine, the perfusion increased and the cerebral blood flow increased, but so did the oedema and the intracranial pressure. When the effect of the norepinephrine wore off, the blood pressure fell but the intracranial pressure fell proportionately less. For example, a blood pressure change of 100 to 150 mm Hg and back to 100 was accompanied by an intracranial pressure change of 60 to 90 and then back only to 80. This effect was repeated with each rise in blood pressure until the intracranial pressure was the same as the systemic pressure and the perfusion pressure zero. The clinical correlation and possible consequences of this in hypertensive stroke patients with poor blood pressure control are obvious. A reduction in blood pressure might retard the formation of oedema and this has been shown to occur with the cold injury and is likely to occur in patients if the lesion is exposed to systemic arterial pressure, but since flow in disautoregulated vascular beds is pressure dependent, a reduction in pressure could well have a critical effect on cellular metabolism. Astrup et al (1977) have shown that evoked responses cease at flow rates below 15–20 ml per 100 g per minute and disruption of cell membranes with potassium flux occurs at around 6 ml per 100 g per minute. Symon et al (1978) have shown that the biggest shift of water occurs at the higher blood flow threshold and not at the level of cellular disruption. Since the optimal perfusion pressure requirements are likely to vary considerably in different parts of an infarct and at different stages, it is obvious that no general advice can be given about the control of blood pressure except perhaps to avoid extremes.

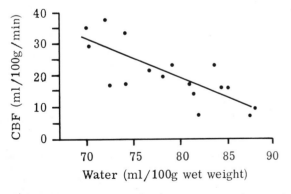

Fig. 6.5 Relation between regional water content and regional cerebral blood flow in cerebral oedema adjacent to brain tumours (cortex and white matter, r = 0.79) (from Reulen et al, 1972). The effect of dexamethasone on water, electrolyte content and on regional cerebral blood flow in perifocal brain oedema in man. In: Steroids and brain oedema. Springer Verlag, Berlin p 241. (Reproduced by kind permission of the authors).

The effect of alteration in vessel calibre

The principal effect of alteration in P_{CO_2} is on the size of vascular compartment. Hypercapnia produces cerebral vasocongestion in normal brain by dilatation of responsive arteries and this would certainly lead to an increase in brain swelling, partly from the vasocongestion and partly from the transmission of higher hydrostatic pressures to small vessels. Hypocapnia causes marked vasoconstriction of responsive vessels and, although some CO_2 responsiveness is preserved in most infarcts, it would have little effect on blood vessels dilated by an anoxic-ischaemic stimulus. However, hypocapnia is probably the quickest method of producing a rapid reduction in intracranial pressure and may prevent intracranial herniation with a large infarct, but it is necessarily a short term procedure and is unlikely to be of long term benefit.

Alteration in blood osmolality

Osmotic agents can only reduce the tissue water content of perfused brain. They only work if the endothelial and cell membranes are intact, and, therefore, reduce the water content of normal brain and have a beneficial effect on the oedema induced by triethyl tin and in osmotic oedema, but they are much less effective in ischaemic oedema. If, however, a large infarct is producing a mass effect and there is significant extracellular oedema in normal surrounding brain due to disautroregulation or in areas of ischaemia but not infaction, then osmotic agents would have some effect. Blood flow might also be improved by an effect on the swelling of perivascular astrocytic foot processes if perfusion was adequate (Little, 1976), since this is a very early change in ichsaemia (Garcia & Kamijyo, 1974). A similar response is produced by forced diuresis, although some of the agents used, such as furozamide (Reed, 1969) or acetazolomide (Reed, 1968) also reduce CSF formation and this may have a beneficial effect in reducing intracranial pressure and improving oedema resolution. In order to avoid rebound effects, it is better to use osmotic agents which remain in the vascular compartment.

There are theoretical reasons for avoiding vigorous use of osmotic agents and hyperventilation in acute strokes because of the much greater affect of these procedures on normal brain whose shrinkage might allow expansion of the lesion, so that any failure to maintain the osmotic effect or vasoconstriction might result in a rebound rise in intracranial pressure.

Possible effects of drugs on the blood-brain barrier

Steroids probably produce their protective effect on cell membranes by an intercalation with the unsaturated fatty acid chain tails, which tends to stabilise the membrane and perhaps make it less susceptible to a wide variety of insults, including mechanical damage, ischemia and the effect of free radicals, (Demopoulos et al, 1972, Ortega et al, 1972, Butterfield & McGraw, 1978, Flamm et al, 1978). A free radical is any substance with a lone electron in its outer orbit. Free radical production occurs spontaneously in lipids in the presence of oxygen and is controlled by a number of processes, including antioxidants; both the water soluble antioxidants (ascorbic acid) and the lipid soluble (the tocopherols) have a marked quenching effect on free radicals. Unsaturated long chain fatty acids are the most susceptible to free radical damage and nerve tissue and membranes contain large amounts of these lipids, but it is not known how much of the damage to cell membranes in ischaemia is due to the action of free radicals.

It is possible that steroids may prevent or stop free radical reactions by quenching as well as protecting membranes by an intercalation in fatty acid chains. If this is how steroids produce their effect in cerebral oedema, they would have no effect on the initial intracellular swelling in ischaemia and it would be surprising if they were effective in the subsequent extracellular oedema, because intercalation cannot occur if a membrane is severely damaged. In addition, the speed of events following infarction would overwhelm the possible effect of steroids. These factors probably explain the widely discrepant reports of the effects of steroids in ischaemic oedema. Numerous experiments have shown a protective effect if the steroids are given before the onset of ischaemia. Other experiments have shown a reduced mortality in a variety of stroke models but little or no effect on less severe infarcts. This is in accord with clinical experience and is in marked contrast to the dramatic effect of steroids on the oedema associated with space occupying lesions and experimentally induced cold lesions. The oedema associated with tumours is principally extracellular and is partly due to loss of autregulation in the surrounding brain subjected to the pressure of an expanding lesion and where the hydrostatic pressure is transmitted normally to the arterioles, and partly to the spread of oedema formed in the lesion (Blasberg et al, 1979). This type of oedema responds very well to steroids, probably because of the relatively slow progression of the lesion which allows the intercalation of steroids into the preserved blood-brain barrier membranes with stabilisation and restoration of barrier function. When stroke produces large focal lesions and a mass effect, steroids may be effective in reducing the pressure induced extracellular oedema in surrounding brain rather than by an effect on ischaemic cerebral oedema. Yamaguchi et al (1976) showed that cerebral oedema produced by bilateral carotid ligation in rats was not affected by steroids, but that steroids had a beneficial effect on the oedema associated with the extravasation of Evans blue dye following disautoregulation induced by pressure.

The evidence suggests, therefore, that steroids are effective in vasogenic oedema but not in metabolic oedema and it is the latter which is the principal problem in the early stages of an infarct. Vasogenic oedema may become an important factor later, at a time when there is damage to the blood-brain barrier but steroids could not be expected to have much effect in this situation.

Acknowledgement

This chapter was originally published as 'Ischaemic Cerebral Oedema — a review' by O'Brien M.D. Stroke 10:623–628 and is reproduced by permission of the American Heart Association, Inc.

REFERENCES

Astrup J, Symon L, Branston N M, Lassen N A 1977 Cortical evoked potential and extracellular K+ and H+ at critical levels of brain ischaemia. Stroke 8:51–57

Blasberg R G, Gazendam J, Patlak C S, Fenstermacher J D 1980 Quantitative autoradiographic studies of brain edema and a comparison of multi-isotope autoradiographic techniques. Advances in Neurology 28:255–270

Branston N M, Bell B A, Hunstock A, Symon L 1980 Time and flow as factors in the formation of postichemic edema in primate cortex. Advances in Neurology 28:291–298

Butterfield J D, McGraw C P 1978 Free radical pathology. Stroke 9:443–445

Clasen R A, Huckman M S, von Roenn K A, Pandolfi S, Laing I 1979 Cerebral edema in strokes, a correlative CT study. 1st International Ernst Reuter Symposium on Brain Edema. Berlin. In press

Cuypers J, Matakas F, Potolicchio S J Jnr 1976 Effect of central venous pressure on brain tissue pressure and brain volume. Journal of Neurosurgery 45:89–94

Demopoulos H B, Miluy P, Kakari S, Ransohoff J 1972 Molecular aspects of membrane structure in cerebral edema. In: Reulen H J, Schurmann K (eds) Steroids and Brain Edema. Springer-Verlag, New York p 29–55

Flamm E S, Demopoulos H B, Seligman M L, Poser R G, Ransohoff J 1978 Free radicals in cerebral ischemia. Stroke 9:445–447

Frei H J, Wallenfang T H, Poll W, Reulen H J, Schubert R, Brock M 1973 Regional cerebral blood flow and regional metabolism in cold induced edema. Acta neurochirurgica. (Wein) 29:15–28

Garcia J H, Kamijyo Y 1974 Cerebral infarction: evolution of histopathological changes after occlusion of a middle cerebral artery in primates. Journal of Neuropathology and Experimental Neurology. 33:408–421

Garcia J H, Conger K A, Morawetz R, Halsey J H Jr 1980 Postischemic brain edema: quantitation and evolution. Advances in Neurology 28:147–169

Goldberg H I, Banka R S, Reivich M 1977 Effect on regional cerebral blood flow in ischemic stroke of vasopressor therapy. Stroke 8:6

Grote J, Schubert R 1977 The effect of brain edema on cortical oxygen supply during arterial normoxia and arterial hypoxia. Bibl. Anat. 15 part 1:335–358

Harrison M J, Arnold J, Sedal L, Ross Russell R W 1975 Ischemic swelling of cerebral hemisphere in the Gerbil. Journal of Neurology, Neurosurgery & Psychiatry 38:1194–1196

Hossman K A 1976 Development and resolution of ischemic brain swelling. In: Pappius H M, Feindel W (eds) Dynamics of brain edema Springer-Verlag, New York p 219–227

Hossman K A, Oleson Y 1970 Suppression and recovery of humoral function in transient cerebral ischemia. Brain Research 22:313–325

Ito U, Ohno K, Nakamura R, Suganuma F, Inaba Y 1979 Brain edema during ischemia and after restoration of blood flow. Stroke 10:542–547

Johansson B B 1976 Water content of rat brain in acute arterial hypertension. In: Pappius H M, Feindel W (eds) Dynamics of brain edema. Springer-Verlag, New York p 28–31

Klatzo I 1967 Neropathological aspects of brain oedema. Journal of Neuropathology and Experimental Neurology 26:1–14

Klatzo I 1972 Pathophysiological aspects of brain edema. In: Reulen H J, Schurmann K (eds) Steroids and brain oedema. Springer-Verlag, Heidelberg p 1–8

Klatzo I, Wisniewski H, Steinwall D, Streicher E 1967 Dynamics of cold injury edema. In: Klatzo I, Seitelberger F (eds) Brain edema. Springer-Heidelberg p 554–563

Lawner P, Laurent J, Simeone F, Fink E, Ruben E 1979 Alteration of ischemic brain edema by pentobarbital after carotid ligation in the gerbil. Stroke 10:644–647

Little J R 1976 Microvascular alterations and edema in focal cerebral ischemia. In: Pappius H M, Feindel W (eds) Dynamics of brain edema. Springer-Verlag, New York p 256–243

Marshall L F 1980 Treatment of brain swelling and brain edema in man. Advances in Neurology 28:459–469

Marshall L F, Bruce D A, Graham D I, Langfitt J R 1976a Triethyl tin induced cerebral edema. In: Pappius H M, Feindel W (eds) Dynamics of brain edema. Springer-Verlag, New York 83–86

Marshall L F, Bruce D A, Graham D I, Langfitt J W 1976b Alterations in behaviour, brain electrical activity, cerebral blood flow and intracranial pressure produced by treithyl tin sulphate induced cerebral edema. Stroke 7:21–25

Matakas F, Waechter R von, Eibs G 1972 Relation between cerebral perfusion pressure and arterial pressure in brain edema. Lancet 1:684

Meinig G, Reulen H J, Hadjidimos A, Siemon C, Bartko D, Schurmann K 1972 Induction of filtration oedema by extreme reduction of cerebrovascular resistance associated with hypertension. European Neurology 8:97–103

Meinig G, Reulen H J, Magawly C 1973 Regional cerebral blood flow and cerebral perfusion pressure in global brain oedema induced by water intoxication. Acta Neurochirurgica (Wein) 29:1–13

Michenfelder J D, Milde J H, Sundt T M Jnr 1976 Cerebral protection of barbiturate anaesthesia: use of the middle cerebral artery occlusion in Java monkeys. Archives of Neurology 33:345–350

Miller J D, Reilly P L Farrar J K, Rowan J O 1976 Cerebrovascular reactivity related to focal brain edema in the primate. In: Pappius H M, Feindel W (eds) Dynamics of brain edema. Springer-Verlag, New York p 68–76

Nag S, Robertson D M, Dinsdale H B 1977 Cerebral cortical changes in acute experimental hypertension. Laboratory Investigation 36:150–161

O'Brien M D, Waltz A G 1973 Intracranial pressure gradients caused by experimental cerebral ischemia and edema. Stroke 4:694–698

O'Brien M D, Waltz A G, Jordan M M 1974 Ischemic cerebral edema. Archives of Neurology 30:456–460

O'Brien M D, Jordan M M, Waltz A G 1974 Ischemic cerebral edema and the blood brain barrier. Archives of Neurology 30:461–465

Ortega B D, Demopoulos H B, Ransohoff J 1972 The effect of antioxidants on experimental cold induced cerebral oedema. In: Reulen H J, Schurmann K (eds) Steroids and brain edema. Springer-Verlag, New York p 167–175

Petito C K 1979 Early and late mechanisms of increased vascular permeability following experimental cerebral infarction. Journal of Neuropathology and Experimental Neurology

Petito C K, Schafer J A, Plum F 1976 The blood brain barrier in experimental seizures. In: Pappius H M, Feindel W (eds) Dynamics of brain edema. Springer-Verlag, New York p 38–42

Plum F 1961 Brain swelling and edema in cerebrovascular disease. ARNMD 41:318–348

Rapoport S I 1976a In: Pappius H M, Feindel W (eds) Dynamics of Brain Oedema. Springer-Verlag, New York p 382 (discussion)

Rapoport S I 1976b Blood brain barrier in physiology and medicine, Raven Press, New York

Rapoport S I, Hori M, Klatzo I 1971 Reversible osmotic opening of the blood brain barrier. Science 173:1026–1028

Reed D J 1968 The effects of acetazolamide on pentobarbital sleep time and CSF flow in rats. Archives Int. Pharmocodynamics 171:206–215

Reed D J 1969 The effect of furosamide on CSF flow in rabbits. Archives Int. Pharmocodynamics 178:324–330

Reichardt M 1904/5 Zur Entsenhung des Hirndrucks. Dtsch. Zschr. Nervenhk 28:306

Reulen H K 1976 Vasogenic brain oedema. British Journal of Anaesthesia 48:721–752

Reulen H J, Hadjidimos A, Schurmann K 1972 The effect of Dexamethasone on water and electrolyte content and on rCBF in perifocal brain edema in man. In: Reulen H J, Schurmann K (eds) Steroids and brain edema. Springer-Verlag, New York p 239–252

Rosomoff H L, Zugibe F T 1963 Distribution of intracranial contents in experimental oedema. Archives of Neurology 9:26–34

Seigel B A, Meidinger R, Elliott A J, Studer R, Curtis C, Morgan J, Potchen E J 1972 Experimental cerebral microembolism — multiple tracer assessment of cerebral edema. Archives of Neurology 26:73–77

Shibata S, Hodge C, Pappius H M 1974 The effect of cerebral ischemia on cerebral water and electrolytes. Journal of Neurosurgery 41:146–159

Simeone F A, Frazer G, Lawner P 1979 Ischemic brain edema, comparative effects of barbiturates and hypothermia. Stroke 10:8–12

Sutton L N, Bruce D A, Welsh F A, Jaddi J L 1980 Metabolic and electrophysiologic consequence of vasogenic edema. Advances in Neurology 28:241–254

Symon L 1967 A comparative study of middle cerebral pressure in dogs and macaques. Journal of Physiology 191:449–465

Symon L, Branston N M, Chikovani O 1979 Ischemic cerebral edema following middle cerebral artery occlusion in baboons — relationships between regional cerebral water content and blood flow at 1 to 2 hours. Stroke 10:184–191

Symon L, Branston N M, Strong A J 1976 Autoregulation in acute focal ischemia. Stroke 7:547–554

Symon L, Pasztor E, Branston N M 1974 The distribution and density of reduced cerebral blood flow following acute middle cerebral artery occlusion. An experimental study by the technique of hydrogen clearance in baboons. Stroke 5:355–364

Tanaka R, Tanimura K, Veki K 1977 Ultrastructural and biochemical studies on Ouabain induced oedematous brain. Acta neuropathologica (Berlin) 37:95–100

Yamagushi M, Shirakata S, Yamasaki S, Matasomoto S 1976 Ischemic brain edema and compression brain edema — water content, blood brain barrier and circulation. Stroke 7:77–83

7

Coma in ischemic cerebral vascular disease

John J. Caronna

Altered consciousness occurs in ischemic cerebro-vascular disease to the extent that the pathological process, directly or indirectly, involves the brainstem reticular formation. Acute coma accompanies bilateral brainstem infarction involving the para-median reticular formation of the diencephalon, midbrain or pons. Coma is seldom the initial sign of uncomplicated infarction of the cerebral hemispheres but may develop several days later when cerebral edema increases the bulk of a large infarct and leads to transtentorial herniation. Similarly, delayed coma follows swelling of an infarcted cerebellar hemisphere when compression of the underlying brainstem interferes with the functioning of the ascending reticular activating system.

Before considering the pathophysiology of coma in ischemic stroke it is necessary to review the anatomical substrate of normal consciousness.

Regulation of consciousness

The human nervous system undergoes daily cycles of sleep and wakefulness characterized by striking changes in sensitivity to environmental stimuli and in motor activity. These global changes in level of consciousness depend upon a brainstem regulatory mechanism, the ascending reticular activating system (ARAS) (Moruzzi & Magoun, 1949).

Anatomically, the ARAS consists of the para-median regions of the tegmentum of the midbrain and pons not associated with cranial nerves or specific ascending or descending pathways. Included in the ARAS are the functionally related medial, intralaminar and reticular nuclei of the thalamus. By its location, the ARAS has access to incoming sensory information and widespread connections to cortical and subcortical motor systems.

Normal consciousness has two basic aspects: arousal and awareness. Mutually sustaining areas of both the ARAS and the cerebral hemispheres are required to maintain full consciousness.

Arousal is a crude function, which is simply wakefulness, and reflects activation of the ARAS by somatosensory stimuli or by internal motivational systems such as hunger. Natural sensory stimuli activate not only specific sensory relays to cortical sensory areas appropriate to the stimulus modality, but also the nonspecific projection system (ARAS) which produces cortical arousal. Clinically, arousal is indicated by eye opening either in response to stimulation or spontaneously. In some cases, (see below) arousal can occur in spite of complete destruction of the hemispheres (Brierley et al, 1971).

Awareness is manifested by cognition of self and environment, and implies functioning cerebral hemispheres.

Coma and stupor

Coma is a pathological state in which neither arousal nor awareness is present. The comatose patient maintains a sleeplike unresponsiveness from which he cannot be aroused. Eye opening does not occur even in response to noxious stimuli, no comprehensible speech is produced and the extremities move neither to commands nor appropriately to localize or ward off noxious stimuli (Bates et al, 1977). Nonpurposive, stereotyped, reflex movements such as flexor (decorticate) or extensor (decerebrate) posturing may be present. Stupor resembles coma except that the patient can be aroused if strong external stimulation is applied (Plum & Posner, 1980).

Pathophysiology of coma in cerebral infarction

Cerebral infarctions causing coma may be divided into three pathophysiological categories: discrete supratentorial lesions, discrete infratentorial lesions and diffuse bilateral lesions.

A unilateral supratentorial lesion does not cause coma until brain swelling with herniation impairs function either of the opposite hemisphere, or more frequently, of the rostral brainstem.

Discrete structural lesions in the tegmentum of the rostral brainstem make arousal impossible by interrupting impulses from the ARAS to the hemispheres.

Acute lesions producing diffuse bilateral impairment of the cerebral hemispheres, but not the brainstem, usually lead to a transient comatose state. For example, in some cases of anoxic-ischemic injury due to the cardiac arrest both hemispheres are severely damaged but the brainstem is preserved. After a period of coma lasting hours to days, wakefulness returns without evidence of purposive behavior or cognition. This functionally decorticate state of eyes-open unconsciousness is distinct from coma and has been termed the 'vegetative state' (Jennett & Plum, 1972).

Coma due to global ischemia and diffuse hemisphere dysfunction will be considered separately under cardiac arrest (see below).

Discrete supratentorial and infratentorial infarcts leading to coma will be discussed in terms of the pathophysiology of coma described above.

1. SUPRATENTORIAL INFARCTION

The extent of cerebral edema after ischemic infarction is approximately proportional to the amount of brain infarcted (Plum et al, 1963). If brain injury is negligible, the degree of brain swelling will be correspondingly small. By contrast, if virtually all of the cortex and subcortex of one hemisphere is infarcted, the resulting brain swelling may be great enough to cause herniation of the hemisphere beyond the confines of the supratentorial compartment.

Devastating supratentorial infarction usually follows sudden occlusion of the internal carotid or of the stem of the middle cerebral artery (MCA). The area infarcted often is the entire cortical and subcortical distribution of the MCA. Cortical branches of the MCA supply all the motor and sensory cortex controlling the face, hand and arm, and the expressive speech area (Broca's area) of the dominant hemisphere (superior division of MCA), as well as part of the visual radiation and macular cortex at the tip of the occipital lobe, and the receptive speech area (Wernicke's area) of the dominant hemisphere (inferior division of the MCA). Subcortical or lenticulostriate branches of the most proximal portion or stem of the MCA supply the basal ganglia and motor fibers from the face, hand, arm *and* leg in the genu and posterior limb of the internal capsule (Mohr et al, 1980).

A. The clinical syndrome of proximal MCA occlusion

The presence of paralysis of the face, arm *and* leg as part of the syndrome of hemisphere infarction is characteristic of proximal MCA occlusion. Infarction of the cortex supplied by the superior and inferior divisions of the MCA results in a contralateral hemiplegia involving the face, hand and arm, sparing the leg. There is a hemisensory deficit, a homonymous hemianopsia, and if the dominant hemisphere is affected, total (expressive and receptive) aphasia. Infarction of motor fibers of the internal capsule supplied by the lenticulostriate branches of the proximal MCA leads to a contralateral hemiplegia including paralysis of the lower extremity.

Consciousness and brainstem functions are preserved initially but decline when herniation of the infarcted hemisphere occurs. Clinically, two syndromes of herniation associated with supratentorial lesions are recognized.

Central downward transtentorial herniation

Large hemisphere infarcts may act like deep midline masses to displace the diencephalon caudally through the tentorial incisura. Failure of the

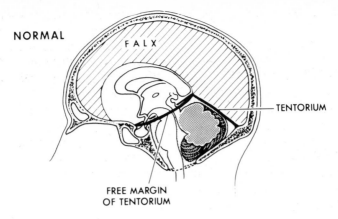

Fig. 7.1 Normal brainstem.

rostral brainstem and then the pons and medulla follows in an orderly, rostral-caudal progression (McNealy & Plum, 1962). Central herniation in its initial stages produces symmetrical signs which may be mistaken for metabolic encephalopathy. Clinically, the first signs reflect failure of the diencephalon: reduced consciousness; pupils small, 1 to 3 mm with preserved reaction to light (central type of Horner's syndrome); bilateral signs of corticospinal and extrapyramidal tract dysfunction, paratonic rigidity, grasp reflexes, decorticate posturing; and periodic respirations. At this state rostral-caudal deterioration is potentially reversible, although no uniformly effective therapy to reduce the cerebral edema of infarction exists. When signs of midbrain failure appear (fixed, dilated or mid-dilated pupils; decerebrate rigidity), it is likely that distortion and compression have led to brainstem infarction, and irreversible coma.

Herniation of the temporal lobe (uncal herniation syndrome)

Hemisphere swelling may displace the temporal lobe uncus medially over the edge of the tentorial incisura and compress the third cranial nerve, the adjacent midbrain and the posterior cerebral artery (Jefferson, 1938). The earliest sign of uncal herniation is ipsilateral pupillary dilatation with a preserved or sluggish light reaction. As the uncus continues to compress the midbrain, the patient becomes deeply comatose and manifests an ipsilateral third nerve palsy and contralateral decerebrate

posturing. Bilateral decerebrate rigidity develops when the contralateral cerebral peduncle is compressed against the tentorial edge opposite to the side of herniation. Beyond this point, brainstem dysfunction will progress in a manner clinically indistinguishable from that caused by central herniation.

Clinical course of transtentorial herniation

At postmortem examination, patients dying within a week after massive hemispheric infarction have considerable brain swelling with hemispheral shift across the midline. Usually transtentorial herniation accounts for total brainstem failure. Studies of pathologic material indicate that the swelling reaches a maximum within two to four days and

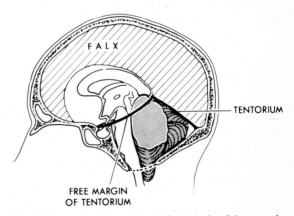

Fig. 7.2 Brainstem compression with upward and downward herniation.

then gradually resolves (Shaw et al, 1959). The time course of acute clinical deterioration and death or recovery after massive stroke usually parallels the temporal profile of edema accumulation and resolution.

Clinical observations suggest that cerebral edema causes worsening of signs and a decline in level of consciousness in about one-fifth of cases of acute massive supratentorial infarction. Plum (1966) reported that 14 of 106 patients with large cerebral hemispheric ischemic strokes developed gradual worsening into stupor and then coma with clinical signs of progressive rostral-caudal deterioration due to transtentorial herniation. Twelve of the 14 patients in coma had clinical signs of symmetrical brainstem dysfunction typical of the central transtentorial type. Unilateral pupillary dilatation due to uncal herniation and ipsilateral third cranial nerve compression were observed only twice in Plum's series but have been observed more frequently by others. Eight of the 14 patients died. In each, postmortem examination confirmed the presence of cerebral hemispheric edema and secondary transtentorial herniation. In an autopsy study of 353 patients dying with acute supratentorial ischemic strokes, Ng & Nimmannitya (1970) similarly noted in 47 (13 percent) that edema and transtentorial herniation were the predominant or major contributing causes of death.

B. Prognosis in acute massive supratentorial infarction

In general, survival is better after ischemic stroke than after either subarachnoid hemorrhage or intracerebral hemorrhage. Coma, however, implies a poor prognosis in any disease causing structural brain damage (Plum & Posner, 1980).

In a series of 500 patients in nontraumatic coma, we found that outcome at one year was related mainly to early clinical signs of neurologic damage and, to a lesser degree, to the cause of coma (Levy et al, 1981). Patients with subarachnoid hemorrhage and other cerebrovascular disorders, both ischemic and hemorrhagic, had the worst outcome; those with global ischemia due to cardiac arrest, intermediate; and those with hepatic encephalopathy and miscellaneous metabolic causes of coma, the best. Out of 143 patients with ischemic or hemorrhagic stroke, excluding subarachnoid hem-

orrhage, 74 percent never recovered from coma and only eight percent achieved an independent life. The remainder required chronic hospitalization because of the vegetative state (5 percent) or severe disability (13 percent).

Plum (1966) noted that approximately one-half of patients who developed progressive rostral-caudal deterioration after ischemic stroke went on to die. Patients who died developed fixed, unreactive pupils and other signs of midbrain compression. By contrast, patients whose signs of progressive brainstem dysfunction halted at the diencephalic level, and who retained pupillary light reflexes, made a slow recovery and survived.

In our prospective study of 143 comatose patients with cerebrovascular disease, we found that the best level of neurological recovery at one year correlated strongly with the severity of clinical dysfunction observed during the first days of coma (Levy et al, 1981). At admission to the study (usually within 6 to 12 hours after the onset of coma), absence of pupillary light reflexes, corneal reflexes, oculovestibular responses to icewater, or oculocephalic responses (doll's eyes) were each associated with less than a five percent chance of attaining independent function. At this early point, no single clinical variable identified patients destined to do well.

By the end of the first day, absent corneal reflexes precluded a satisfactory recovery and the absence of pupillary light reactions was an almost equally unfavorable sign. Absent caloric or doll's-eye responses and the lack of any motor response to noxious stimuli were also unfavourable. At three days no patient recovered consciousness who still lacked pupillary light reflexes, corneal reflexes or motor responses. On the other hand, at one day and three days, survival was achieved by most patients who either opened their eyes in response to noise, or obeyed commands, or spoke any words. Functional recovery in such patients, however, always was poor because of the severity of their residual motor and sensory deficits.

2. OTHER SUPRATENTORIAL STROKES CAUSING COMA
A. Cerebral embolism

Acute cerebral embolism is sometimes regarded as

a potential cause of coma even in the absence of transtentorial herniation (Wells, 1959). The experience of most physicians is that unconsciousness is uncommon with unilateral embolism even when there is acute massive cerebral infarction (Fisher, 1961; Carter, 1964). Nevertheless, cases of stupor or coma after hemispheral cerebral embolism have been described. In a few instances, the clinical picture may reflect the fact that the embolus has lodged opposite a previously damaged hemisphere, or that dissemination of embolic material has caused bilateral cerebral abnormalities or has directly affected the rostral brainstem reticulum. Large emboli occluding the proximal middle cerebral artery and causing extensive unilateral infarction may be associated with widespread and bilateral physiologic inhibition of neural and vascular function, a process known as *diaschisis*. In some cases the contralateral inhibition of neural function is mediated via the electrophysiologic effects of epileptiform discharges (Schwartz et al, 1973).

B. Bilateral thalamic infarction (the mesencephalic artery syndrome)

A rare syndrome of acute coma followed by permanent defects in arousal and cognition accompanies bilateral infarctions involving the medial portions of the thalamus and the adjacent paramedian mesencephalic region. (Mills & Swanson, 1978; Segarra, 1970).

The syndrome results from ischemia in the distribution of that thalamo-subthalamic perforating arteries that arise from the proximal posterior cerebral artery. At its apex the basilar artery divides into two posterior cerebral arteries which course supratentorially to ramify over the temporal and occipital lobes. Branches from the mesencephalic artery, (the proximal part of the PCA between its origin at the bifurcation of the basilar and its junction with the posterior communicating artery) supply the red nucleus, subthalamic nucleus, substantia nigra, medial portion of the cerebral peduncle, oculomotor nucleus, midbrain reticular formation, medial longitudinal fasciculus, medial lemniscus, medial thalamus, lateral geniculate body, quadrigeminal plate and pineal gland (Caplan, 1980).

Patients with restricted thalamic infarction without midbrain injury have an abrupt onset of coma without other signs of brainstem dysfunction. Most have signs of bilateral corticospinal tract dysfunction. Depending on the extent of the infarct, coma gives way within several days, either to a hypokinetic, apathetic state of consciousness with profound disturbances of memory and cognitive function, or to a semi-vegetative state of wakefulness with even less evidence of cognition (akinetic mutism).

Bilateral paramedian thalamic infarction sparing the mesencephalon produces few or no characteristic clinical signs during coma, but when wakefulness reappears, a loss of voluntary upward gaze and sometimes downward gaze can be appreciated (Mills & Swanson, 1978). At this stage infarction of the thalamus sometimes can be identified by CT scanning.

3. SUBTENTORIAL INFARCTIONS CAUSING COMA

Two kinds of posterior fossa strokes cause coma: those located within the brainstem that destroy the paramedian midbrain pontine reticular formation and its associated pathways, and those located in the cerebellum that secondarily compress the brainstem reticular formation (Plum & Posner, 1980).

A. Ischemic brainstem stroke

General features

The diagnosis of acute brainstem infarction usually can be made from the fact that signs of brainstem damage accompany or precede the onset of coma. The ARAS in the midbrain and pons lies close to nuclei and pathways influencing pupillary size and reactivity, reflex eye movements, and other major functions, so that brainstem strokes can often be precisely localized anatomically by the clinical findings. For example, at the midbrain level centrally placed infarcts interrupt the pathway for the pupillary light reflex. The resulting coma is accompanied by dilated or mid-dilated pupils that are unreactive to light. The pupil may assume an eccentric position in the iris, a phenomenon called corectopia (Selhorst et al, 1976). Infarcts at the level of the pons spare the oculomotor nuclei but interrupt the ocular sympathetic pathways and the medial longitudinal fasciculus. Coma due to pontine infarction is characterized by small reactive pupils, and absent reflex lateral eye movements (Kubik & Adams, 1946).

Specific syndromes: occlusion of the basilar artery

Occlusion of the basilar is a serious event that often is incompatible with survival. Occlusion of one vertebral artery when the other is patent causes the relatively benign syndrome of lateral medullary infarction (Fisher et al, 1961). Obstruction of flow in both vertebral arteries or in a lone, unpaired vertebral artery, produces a syndrome similar to basilar artery occlusion.

The clinical features of basilar artery occlusion differ depending upon whether the cause of occlusion is embolism or thrombosis *in situ*. Embolism tends to involve the distal portion of the basilar artery. By contrast, atheromatous occlusion affects the proximal and midportions of the vessel (Kubik & Adams, 1946).

Emboli small enough to pass through the vertebral arteries into the larger basilar artery usually will be arrested at the top of the basilar artery at its bifurcation into the posterior cerebral arteries. Loss of consciousness occurs immediately because of obstruction of the blood supply to the mesencephalic ARAS. Unilateral or bilateral third cranial nerve palsies are characteristic. Hemiplegia or quadriplegia with decerebrate or decorticate posturing occur. In this type of coma, unequal pupils both fixed to light and bilateral corticospinal tract dysfunction resemble and may be confused with midbrain failure caused by transtentorial uncal herniation. A history of vertebrobasilar TIAs, or the observation that coma came on suddenly accompanied by bilateral oculomotor dysfunction from its onset, serve to distinguish acute brainstem dysfunction from slowly evolving brainstem compression due to herniation.

Smaller emboli which occlude the rostral basilar artery only transiently before fragmenting and passing into one or both posterior cerebral arteries either may not result in permanent neurological deficits or may produce infarction of portions of the midbrain, thalamus and of the temporal and occipital lobes.

Thrombosis *in situ* occurs in the proximal and midportions of the basilar artery. Pontine infarction due to basilar thrombosis is associated with unilateral or bilateral damage to the sixth cranial nerve or nucleus. Horizontal eye movements are impaired but vertical nystagmus and ocular bobbing may be present. The pupils are constricted and may be pinpoint, but remain reactive to light. Hemiplegia or quadriplegia are usual.

In unconscious patients the syndrome of basilar occlusion may be confused with pontine hemorrhage. A CT brain scan serves to differentiate between ischemic infarction and hematoma.

Coma due to occlusion of the basilar artery carries a poor prognosis for survival. In some cases the basis pontis is permanently injured but not the tegmentum of the brainstem. Such patients regain consciousness if they have lost it, but remain quadriplegic. The term 'locked-in' has been applied to this de-efferented state (Plum & Posner, 1980). Locked-in patients may be able to signify that they are conscious by blinking to command (Karp & Hurtig, 1974). In patients who lack any clinical signs of consciousness, a conventional EEG with stimulation and/or cortical evoked responses may be needed to distinguish the locked-in state from coma or the vegetative state (Hawkes & Bryan-Smyth, 1974).

4. ACUTE CEREBELLAR INFARCTION

General features of cerebellar herniation syndromes causing coma

Direct compression of the brainstem. When a cerebellar infarct increases in size due to edematous swelling, the underlying pons and medulla are compressed against the clivus (Giroux & Leger, 1962; Dinsdale, 1964). The fourth ventricle is distorted and obstructive hydrocephalus may occur. Brainstem infarction and hemorrhage may be a late and fatal result of compression of the vessels on the ventral surface of the brainstem (Cuneo et al, 1979).

Downward tonsillar herniation. As the mass effect increases, tonsillar herniation often occurs, which produces compression of the medulla and seals the inferior outlet of the posterior fossa. Resultant obstructive hydrocephalus exerts a downward force at the tentorial incisura that opposes any upward movement of the cerebellum. Rapid descent of the cerebellar tonsils and impaction of the medulla causes sudden apnea and circulatory collapse.

Upward transtentorial herniation. If tonsillar herniation is not fatal, increasing pressure in the posterior fossa causes upward herniation into and through the incisura. Displacement of the cerebellum through the tentorial incisura is more likely to occur (1) when the mass originates near the incisura, e.g., in the cerebellar vermis, (2) when drainage of the lateral ventricles relieves obstructive hydrocephalus and reduces pressure above, and (3) when the tentorial incisural opening is large (Sunderland, 1958).

As upward herniation develops, the displaced cerebellar vermis distorts the midbrain and cerebral aqueduct and buckles the quadrigeminal plate so that the inferior colliculi fold under the superior colliculi and together both structures shift upward beneath the splenium of the corpus callosum. Herniation of the vermis through the incisura displaces Galen's vein upward against the splenium and the unyielding free edge of the falx. Acute compression of Galen's vein may produce hemorrhagic infarction in the diencephalon and the adjacent subcortical white matter if venous collateral channels fail. Hemispheric branches of the superior cerebellar arteries may be compressed by upward herniation of the cerebellum against the free edge of the tentorium, just as the posterior cerebral arteries that travel just above the tentorial edge are compressed in downward transtentorial herniation of the uncus. In some cases, this results in further infarction of the cerebellar hemispheres.

In a recent review of the literature we found 39 cases of upward herniation confirmed by postmortem examination (Cuneo et al, 1979). A cerebellar lesion caused upward herniation most frequently (65 percent) and was most often a hemorrhage (10 cases). Upward herniation followed cerebellar infarction in five patients. Lesions in the cerebellopontine angle (13 percent), in the pons (11 percent) and in the fourth ventricle (11 percent) were also associated with upward herniation.

Clinical syndrome of cerebellar infarction

The symptoms of cerebellar infarction in conscious patients are consistent and resemble those of cerebellar hemorrhage. Common complaints include difficulty standing and walking, headache, nausea, vomiting, dizziness, clumsiness and slurred speech. The onset of symptoms is abrupt in one-third of patients. With progression of infarction or swelling, the majority of patients develop a lateral gaze palsy or nystagmus toward the side of infarction. Facial palsies are common but dysfunction of other cranial nerves, and corticospinal and sensory defects typically are absent unless lateral medullary infarction has occurred coincident with cerebellar infarction (Duncan et al, 1975). As edema develops around the infarct, hydrocephalus and impaired cognitive function or depressed consciousness appear.

Diagnosis. An expanding cerebellar mass produces a characteristic syndrome of coma, small reactive pupils, abnormal doll's eye and ice water caloric responses and corticospinal tract dysfunction. These initial signs of pontine compression are followed by signs of midbrain dysfunction as already described above for transtentorial herniation. It is the gradual caudal to rostral progression of brainstem dysfunction which identifies the cause of coma as cerebellar herniation.

Examination of the posterior fossa by CT scanning reveals a large area of decreased density. The development of hydrocephalus usually can be detected on CT scan. If a CT scan is not available, vertebral angiography may be helpful in the diagnosis but the procedure is time-consuming and the results are often ambiguous. Lumbar puncture is unhelpful diagnostically and may hasten the process of herniation. Small infarctions of the cerebellum do not cause coma and can be managed without surgery. When an extensive cerebellar infarction is recognized surgical exploration of the posterior fossa and resection of the necrotic cerebellar tissue usually is required. Some patients may stabilize after ventricular decompression to relieve hydrocephalus. Nevertheless, ventricular drainage increases the risk of upward herniation. Surgical mortality is 50 percent if the patient is operated upon while still conscious, but approaches 80 percent if the patient becomes comatose or stuporose (Greenberg et al, 1979).

Prognosis. Death from tonsillar herniation and cardiorespiratory failure is a frequent outcome of massive, untreated cerebellar infarction. Sypert & Alvord (1975) reported 28 fatal cases of cerebellar infarction: 15 patients died in the first 12 hours of coma. The mortality rate for the first 48 hours was 15 percent and death occurred within three to six days after the development of symptoms. Not all cases of extensive cerebellar infarction are fatal and patients who remain conscious one week after the onset of symptoms are unlikely to deteriorate from brain swelling or to require surgical decompression of the posterior fossa.

5. BRAINSTEM STROKES SPARING CONSCIOUSNESS

Unilateral and laterally placed infarcts

Brainstem infarcts which spare the pontine mid-brain reticular formation may destroy a remarkable amount of brain without causing coma (Plum & Posner, 1980). Unconsciousness does not occur with uncomplicated infarction of the dorsolateral area of the rostral brainstem or of the paramedian medullary reticular formation.

For example, the most frequently encountered brainstem stroke is unilateral infarction of the dorsolateral medulla, the lateral medullary or Wallenberg syndrome. Although the area infarcted is supplied by the posterior inferior cerebellar artery (PICA), the syndrome most frequently results from vertebral artery occlusion (Fisher et al, 1961). The structures supplied by the PICA include the lateral tegmentum of the medulla and portions of the cerebellum. When occlusion of the vertebral artery leads to infarction of the entire half of the medulla, the medial tegmentum and medullary pyramid are involved. Coma does not occur from unilateral or even from bilateral lesions limited to the medullary tegmentum since the ARAS is preserved.

Lacunar infarctions

Lacunar infarctions are among the most common of all cerebrovascular lesions. Occurring in 19 percent of the Harvard Cooperative Series (Mohr et al, 1978) and roughly 10 percent of autopsied brains, they are often multiple with an average of three per brain; in some cases there are 15 or more (Fisher, 1969). Lacunes represent healed ischemic infarctions, minute cavities ranging in size from 0.5 to 15.0 mm in diameter; most are 2 to 4 mm in diameter. They occur most commonly in the deep nuclei of the brain (putamen, 37 percent; thalamus, 14 percent; caudate, 10 percent). They occur in lesser numbers in the deep cerebral white matter, the anterior limb of the internal capsule, and the cerebellum (Fisher, 1965). They are characteristic of hypertensive cerebrovascular disease (Cuneo & Caronna, 1977).

Coma is not a part of any lacunar stroke syndromes. In fact, because of their small size and location in relatively silent areas of the brain, many lacunar infarctions are not recognized clinically.

6. GLOBAL ISCHEMIA (ISCHEMIC-ANOXIA)

In previous sections we discussed the effects of localized ischemia consequent on thrombotic or embolic occlusion of a cerebral artery. The result of localized ischemia is focal cerebral infarction or stroke. By contrast, generalized brain ischemia is most commonly a consequence of systemic circulatory collapse due to cardiac arrhythmia or standstill, and the result is a spectrum of multifocal neurological disorders (Caronna, 1979).

Neuropathological features of global ischemia

Neuropathological lesions usually can be grouped into one of several categories, although there may be overlap in individual cases.

A. Focal CNS injury

1. Injury to neurons in vulnerable areas. In cases of brief ischemia cell death is limited to those neurons most sensitive to anoxia. The neurons of the hippocampus and cerebellum are the cells most frequently damaged in anoxia (Brierley, 1971). Such hippocampal and cerebellar lesions may be responsible for amnesia and ataxia after cardiac arrest, but often produce no clinical deficits (Finkelstein & Caronna, 1978).

2. Anoxic leukoencephalopathy. Focal injury of cerebral white matter, often of delayed onset, has been reported following all types of ischemic-anoxic insults. The pathological lesions primarily are restricted to the deep white matter of the parietal and occipital lobes.

The clinical syndrome of anoxic leukoencephalopathy is distinctive: days to weeks after apparent recovery from global ischemia, patients suffer progressive neurological deterioration and either die or remain comatose. Delayed anoxic deterioration follows no more than two out of each thousand cardiac arrests and is not predictable by the type of ischemic-anoxic insult or the preceding clinical course (Ginsberg, 1979).

3. Infarction in borderzones. A period of circulatory arrest preceded or followed by appreciable periods of hypotension often leads to ischemic alterations concentrated in the borderzones between major cerebral arteries. Borderzone infarcts occur in the cerebral cortex. Ischemic necrosis following profound hypotension is most severe in the parieto-occipital regions where the territories of the anterior, middle and posterior cerebral arteries meet. The cerebral cortex commonly is affected bilaterally, or unilaterally if there is atherosclerotic compromise of the vessels to one hemisphere (Brierley, 1973).

Cortical borderzone infarcts often are hemorrhagic because of reperfusion when blood pressure is restored. Borderzone infarction and diffuse cortical necrosis may coexist.

Within the spinal cord there are borderzones between the anterior spinal artery and the segmental arteries from the aorta. Severe hypotension or disruption of the segmental arteries causes infarction of the spinal cord in the thoraco-cervical and the lower thoraco-lumbar regions. The thoracic cord usually is involved at the borderzone between the anterior spinal artery and the artery of Adamkewicz (Silver & Buxton, 1974).

The borderzone hypothesis best explains the focal neurological deficits observed in patients resuscitated after cardiac arrest. However, the topography and severity of cerebral infarcts cannot be predicted from clinical estimates of the efficacy or duration of resuscitative efforts.

B. Diffuse CNS injury

Prolonged cardiac arrest causes widespread death of neurons. Certain groups of neurons are vulnerable to even moderate degrees of anoxia: pyramidal cells in Sommer's sector of the hippocampus, Purkinje cells of the cerebellum and pyramidal cells of the third and fifth layers of the cerebral cortex. More severe degrees of anoxia affect neurons in the amygdala, lateral putamen, caudate, lateral geniculate, thalamus, substantia nigra, and inferior colliculi. Hypothalamic neurons usually are spared. Profound anoxia affects even the brainstem nuclei including the locus ceruleus, the vestibular, trigeminal, dorsal vagal and hypoglossal nuclei, as well as pontine neurons. By contrast, the medullary olives and the cuneatus and gracilis nuclei are resistant to anoxic ischemic injury in adults, but are more vulnerable in children.

Neurological outcomes after global ischemia

Cardiac arrest may be considered as causing both metabolic and structural damage to the central nervous system. Patients with brief episodes of systemic circulatory arrest who suffer milder degrees of cerebral ischemia-anoxia demonstrate the clinical features of a reversible metabolic encephalopathy. Coma, if present, lasts only a few hours, usually less than twelve. On awakening, these patients do not demonstrate focal, motor, sensory or intellectual deficits but may be transiently confused or amnestic for hours to days (Table 7.1, A). Recovery is rapid and complete, so that these patients usually can resume their previous occupations (good recovery). Rarely patients suffer delayed neurological deterioration.

Patients with more severe or prolonged systemic ischemic-anoxia suffer stroke-like infarcts in specific areas of the brain. Patients in this group (Table 7.1, B) are usually in coma for at least 12 hours and, upon regaining consciousness, manifest lasting focal or multifocal motor, sensory and intellectual deficits. Recovery occurs slowly over

Table 7.1 Neurological syndromes following global ischemia

A. *Coma < 12 hours*
   Pathology: No damage or scattered ischemic neurons
   Clinical: Transient confusion often followed by anterograde amnesia
   Outcome: Rapid, complete recovery; delayed deterioration (rare)

B. *Coma > 12 hours*
   1. Cerebral syndrome
   Pathology: Focal or multifocal infarcts of cortex, especially in boundary zones
   Clinical: Amnesia
            Dementia
            Bibrachial or quadriparesis
            Cortical blindness, visual agnosia
            Also may occur: seizures, myoclonus (acute state); Ataxia, intention myoclonus, Parkinsonism (chronic stage)
   Outcome: Slow, often incomplete, recovery

   2. Spinal cord syndrome (may occur in isolation or accompany cerebral syndrome)
   Pathology: Focal or multifocal infarcts of spinal cord, especially in the lower thoracic boundary zone
   Clinical: Flaccid paralysis of lower limbs
            Urinary retention
            Loss of pain and temperature sense
            Preserved touch and position sense
            Also may occur: Bowel infarction due to non-occlusive intestinal ischemia
   Outcome: No or incomplete recovery

C. *No recovery of consciousness*
   1. Destruction of hemispheres alone
   Pathology: Laminar necrosis of cortex (neocortical death)
   Clinical: Vegetative state (awake but unaware)
   Outcome: Prolonged survival in vegetative state

   2. Brain death
   Pathology: Necrosis of cortex + Brainstem ± Spinal cord
   Clinical: No evidence of cortical activity, no brainstem reflexes, reflexes of purely spinal origin may persist
   Outcome: Systemic death within days

weeks to months and often is incomplete (moderate or severe disability).

Among the focal signs manifest in this group of patients are partial or complete cortical blindness, bibrachial paresis, and quadriparesis. Cortical blindness is usually transient and probably results from disproportionate ischemia in the arterial borderzones of both occipital lobes. Bilateral infarction of the cerebral motor cortex in the borderzone between the anterior and middle cerebral arteries may be responsible for the bibrachial paresis sparing the face and legs which is seen following cardiac arrest.

The spinal cord is more resistant to transient ischemia than more rostral parts of the central nervous system. Nevertheless, cases of spinal cord infarction, without evidence of cerebral injury, occur (Table 7.1, B). Necrosis of the central structures of the spinal cord can occur in critical borderzones at the periphery of the territory supplied by a main contributory vessel.

A third group of resuscitated patients (Table 7.1, C), with more widespread destruction of brain, remain hospitalized in a vegetative state (VS) or die a neurological death. Some patients with severe irreversible brain damage who survive for more than a few days regain eye opening, sleep-wake cycles, spontaneous roving eye movements and other reflex activities at brainstem and spinal cord level but remain in a functionally decorticate state of wakefulness without awareness (Jennett & Plum, 1972). This vegetative state is distinct from the sleep-like condition of coma. In certain extreme cases, prolonged survival for weeks or months in a vegetative state has been associated with an iso-electric EEG. Detailed neuropathological analysis of two such cases indicated that the hemispheres had been destroyed while certain brainstem and spinal structures remained intact. This neuropathological condition has been termed neocortical or cerebral death (Brierley et al, 1971) and must be distinguished from *total* cerebral *and* brainstem destruction (Brain Death). In our experience, neocortical death has occurred most often in cases of cardiac arrest superimposed upon a cerebral hypermetabolic state induced by generalized motor seizures.

TREATMENT OF ISCHEMIC-ANOXIC COMA

The clinical management of patients in coma following cardiac arrest involves the prevention of cerebral injury. Adequate cerebral circulation should be restored immediately by the elimination of cardiac dysrhythmias, the maintenance of an effective systemic blood pressure and the correction of acid-base and electrolyte abnormalities. If either medullary depression or injury to the chest wall prevents adequate ventilation, a mechanical ventilator must be employed. In spontaneously breathing patients an increased concentration of inspired oxygen can be administered to deliver increased amounts of oxygen on a cellular level. Beyond these basic measures to restore homeostasis, no other uniformly satisfactory methods of treatment have been found.

Prognosis based on clinical findings

As part of an international study to define more accurately the clinical features that predict outcome in coma (Levy et al, 1981) we performed neurological examinations on 210 patients in coma caused by cardiac arrest (150), respiratory arrest (22), or profound hypotension (38) and followed them for one year. Patients entered in the study were resuscitated by standard means and all were in coma (see definition above) for at least six hours after resuscitation.

Only 12 percent achieved independence in daily life (good outcome) within the first year; the remainder either died while still in coma (58 percent), never improved beyond the vegetative state (20 percent), or regained consciousness but remained severely disabled (10 percent).

Analysis of early clinical signs permitted separation of patients into groups with a relatively good or a poor prognosis. At admission, the absence of any two: pupillary constriction to light, corneal reflexes, or motor responses identified 66 poor prognosis patients, only one of whom subsequently improved even to a level of severe disability. The presence of any motor response to noxious stimulation in the remaining patients identified 99 subjects, 22 of whom achieved a good outcome. At one day after the onset of coma, the absence of any two: spontaneous eye movements (either roving or orienting), pupillary light reflexes, or corneal responses, identified 39 poor prognosis patients, none of whom ever regained consciousness. By contrast, the presence of any motor response, normal spontaneous eye movements, or normal doll's eye or caloric responses in the remaining patients identified 93 subjects, 24 of whom achieved a good outcome.

The trends which have emerged from this study suggest that repeated clinical observations of coma after global ischemia will permit neurological outcome to be predicted with a high degree of probability. Furthermore, recovery from ischemic-anoxic coma depends strongly on the degree of brain damage as reflected by early clinical signs of brain function. Future therapeutic trials in cardiac arrest, therefore, should stratify patients accordingly.

Brain death, cerebral death and irreversible coma

In recent years the rapid development of intensive-care techniques has focused attention on the questions of what criteria should be applied to pronounce death in patients in whom respiration and circulation are maintained artificially. The medical profession as a whole has accepted, in such cases, a 'brain-centered' definition of death in place of the traditional 'heart and lung' formulation. There is general agreement among physicians, and, to a lesser degree, among the general population, that brain death is an appropriate determinant of death of a human being, and that, once this has occurred, further artificial support is fruitless and should be withdrawn. The concept of brain death poses moral and ethical problems as well as biological ones. For the physician, however, the main, immediate problem is whether he can accurately distinguish brain dead subjects without any possibility of recovery, from other comatose patients who have a chance of even partial recovery.

Brain death, cerebral death and irreversible coma: definitions

Brain death means irreversible cessation of all functioning of the entire brain, including both cerebral hemispheres and the brainstem. In other words in brain death no neurological functions exist above the cervical spinal cord (Plum & Posner, 1980).

The key point is the definition of the term 'functioning' or 'functions'. The functions of an organ are those specific, purposeful activities which are unique to that organ. For example, the function of the heart is to pump blood, the function of the lungs is to conduct gaseous exchange. The brain, the most complex organ in the human body, has many functions, all determined at a clinical level, not at a cellular, biochemical, microscopic or electrical level. Therefore, the intention of the brain death definition is to designate the medical determination of death at the clinical level according to accepted medical criteria. The fact that there may be some brain cells still metabolically active is conceptually, practically and legally irrelevant to the clinical determination of brain death.

The term 'cerebral death' should not be used when brain death is meant. Cerebral death denotes destruction of the hemispheres with preservation of brainstem reflexes. The terms 'persistent vegetative state' and 'neocortical death' (see above) have been applied respectively to the clinical and pathological features of this entity.

A diagnosis of brain death is biologically not necessarily the same thing as a diagnosis of irreversible coma, and the two terms are not interchangeable. Some patients in irreversible coma are brain dead, a far greater number are irreversibly unconscious because of permanent and severe brain damage but retain a fragment of neurological function such as pupillary reaction to light or cerebral electrical activity (EEG). Unlike brain death, in which both the cerebral hemispheres and brainstem are destroyed, the pathology of irreversible coma often is limited to the cerebral hemispheres or to focal areas of the brainstem. Destruction of both cerebral hemispheres permanently eliminates cognition but permits a vegetative survival which may be prolonged for months or years (Levy et al, 1978). Destruction of the brainstem reticular formation which has an indispensible 'pacemaker' role in maintaining wakefulness results in a permanent sleep-like state.

Any discussion of the question of when to switch off the ventilator must keep these three concepts, brain death, cerebral or neocortical death, and irreversible coma, separate.

Clinical criteria of brain death

Several committees and reviewers have proposed clinical criteria for brain death (see Plum & Posner 1980 for review). Representative criteria are outlined in Table 7.2. In essence, brain death is diagnosed when there is no discernible evidence of either cerebral hemispheral or brainstem function for an extended period, usually 12 hours or more, and when the loss of brain function is the result of structural and not of reversible metabolic disease

Table 7.2 Brain death criteria

Determination of Brain Death shall be made in accordance with the mandatory criteria listed below. All observations, tests and findings shall be recorded in the patient's chart. Supplementary criteria may be used at the physician's discretion.

Mandatory criteria

1. *Coma of established cause*
   a. No potentially anesthetizing amounts of either toxins or therapeutic drugs can be present; hypothermia below 30°C or other physiological abnormalities must be corrected to the extent medically possible.
   b. Irreversible structural disease or a known and irreversible endogenous metabolic cause due to organ failure must be present.
   c. A twelve-hour period of no brain function must have elapsed.

2. *No cerebral function*
   No behavioral or reflex response involving structures above the cervical spinal cord can be elicited by noxious stimuli delivered anywhere in the body.

3. *No brainstem reflexes*
   a. The pupils must be fixed to light.
   b. No corneal reflexes can be present.
   c. There must be no response to icewater calorics (50 ml. in each ear).
   d. No spontaneous respirations must occur during apneic oxygenation for a period sufficient to maximally stimulate breathing.

NOTE: The circulation may be intact and purely spinal cord reflexes may be retained.

Supplementary criteria

The twelve hours period of observation may be shortened to as little as six hours in cases of established irreversible structural damage provided that the mandatory clinical criteria are confirmed by one or more of the supplementary criteria.

1. An EEG for 30 minutes at maximal gain reflects absence of cerebral electrical activity
2. Brainstem auditory or short latency somatic evoked responses reflect absence of function in vital brainstem structures.
3. No cerebral circulation present on angiographic examination.

or depression by drugs. The clinical examination for brain death includes attention to cerebral hemisphere function and brainstem reflexes, as well as laboratory tests as discussed below.

Coma of established cause

The cerebral lesion must be structural, bearing in mind that an initially metabolic insult such as occurs in massive liver necrosis, prolonged hypoglycemia or anoxia, also can lead to irreversible structural damage. Any possibility that the patient has suffered from drug poisoning or that hypothermia or an electrolyte abnormality is contributing to the depth of coma must be excluded by appropriate tests.

The patient should have no clinical evidence of cerebral function or brainstem reflexes for a period of at least 12 hours with no demonstrable improvement whatsoever. This period of observation must be extended to 24 or more hours, or until negative toxicology screen results are obtained, if drug overdosage is a possibility. The period of observation may be shortened to as little as six hours if, for example, a competent neurosurgeon explores a head wound and finds the brain transected, or if one or more of the supplementary tests (Table 7.2) confirms the absence of cerebral circulation and/or electrical activity.

No cerebral function

The patient's supraorbital ridges, sternum and each extremity should be vigorously stimulated. There must be no appropriate response to stimulation, in that the patient must not rouse, groan, grimace, withdraw the head or limbs from an applied stimulus, or attempt to push away the examiner's hand. Reflex responses such as decerebrate extension or decorticate flexion of the limbs, which are mediated by subcortical but supraspinal cord pathways must be absent. The spinal cord may be intact, therefore rudimentary reflex responses such as muscle stretch reflexes, plantar responses, plantar withdrawal (triple flexion), abdominal reflexes and tonic neck reflexes, all of which depend upon functions of the spinal cord, may be preserved.

No brainstem reflexes

The pupils must be fixed to light stimulation. The pupils may be either widely dilated (as may happen when a dopamine infusion is necessary to maintain the circulation) or mid-dilated, but stimulation with an intensely bright light must fail to yield any evidence of pupillary constriction.

The corneal blink reflex must be absent when the tip of a cotton-wool applicator is applied to either cornea.

The oculocephalic (doll's eye) and *oculovestibular* (ice water caloric) responses both must be absent. The oculovestibular response is elicited by irrigating each tympanic membrane with 50 ml of ice water for 30 to 45 seconds, and observing whether there is any movement of the eyes toward the side of the tympanic irrigation. There should be no ocular movement during three minutes of observation after ice water has been injected.

The patient must be apneic and not recover spontaneous ventilatory function after the respirator has been turned off to allow arterial PCO_2 ($PaCO_2$) to attain a level high enough to maximally stimulate respiratory drive. Evidence indicates that the threshold for respiratory stimulation may approach a $PaCO_2$ of 60 mm Hg in patients with brain damage and that the rate of rise of $PaCO_2$ during respiratory arrest is approximately 3 mm Hg/min. The duration of respiratory arrest needed to allow $PaCO_2$ to reach or exceed 60 mm Hg is not constant and will vary depending on the level of $PaCO_2$ prior to the onset of apnea. Therefore, to confirm absolute apnea, blood gas monitoring is required to verify either normocapnia prior to beginning apnea for ten minutes, or if a patient is hypocapnic, $PaCO_2$ in excess of 60 mm Hg at the end of apnea. No absolute period of apnea sufficient to establish brain death can be recommended in the absence of blood gas determinations (Schafer & Caronna, 1978).

The respirator should be disconnected according to the following procedure. All patients are mechanically ventilated with 100 percent oxygen for 10 minutes before the start of apnea. The electrocardiogram is monitored continuously and the blood pressure measured intermittently before and during apnea. An arterial sample is drawn and analyzed for pH, PaO_2 and $PaCO_2$ before beginning apnea so that hypoxemia may be detected. Caution is advised when hypoxemia exists in individuals being mechanically ventilated with high concentrations of oxygen since apnea may worsen this abnormality. The respiratory then is disconnected and 100 percent oxygen at a rate of 6 l/min is administered via endotracheal tube. The reservoir bag must be observed for signs of spontaneous respiratory activity. Arterial blood samples for pH, PaO_2 and $PaCO_2$ should be drawn at the end of 10 minutes, or more in apneic patients.

Patients who breathe should be replaced on mechanical ventilation.

The *circulation* may still be functioning normally. If all the above criteria are met, the presence of a normal blood pressure does not indicate a recoverable brain.

When the above conditions have been fulfilled two physicians can certify that death has occurred.

The clinical diagnosis of brain death generally is not difficult, nor likely to be in error, if the criteria outlined in Table 7.2 are rigorously followed. The validity of the clinical criteria for diagnosing brain death (independent of supplementary tests) has been confirmed by several published series both in the U.S.A. and the U.K. (see Jennett et al, 1981 for review). Nevertheless, recovery after supposed brain death has been alleged in patients who were thought to be brain dead but, in fact, were not. Review of such cases has revealed that in each instance the clinical criteria were not satisfied. There has not been, so far as we know, a single reported case in which the criteria of brain death were met and yet the patient survived.

In our own series of 500 patients in coma, not due to trauma or drug intoxications, there were 14 patients who met the clinical criteria for brain death (Levy et al, 1981). In no case was ventilation discontinued yet all suffered cardiac arrest within hours to 28 days after the diagnosis.

Supplementary tests

It is our view that the clinical criteria are reliable and so conservative that, when properly applied, they will never lead to the diagnosis of death in a patient who might survive. Therefore, there is no need for confirmatory tests when all the clinical conditions for diagnosis of brain death have been fulfilled. Nevertheless, the diagnosis of brain death carries a heavy responsibility and some medical centres have found it useful to employ supplementary tests to provide verifiable support to the clinical evaluation or to shorten the period of observation.

Although brain death is a common occurrence and has gained wide acceptance among physicians, many laymen, and indeed some physicians, are not fully confident about the accuracy of the diagnosis of brain death. This anxiety can only be dispelled by continued examinations and discussion by members of the fields of medicine, law, philosophy and theology, on the questions generated by new medical technologies.

Acknowledgements

Supported by contract NS-42328 and grant NS-03346 from the National Institute of Neurological and Communicative Disorders and Stroke, of the United States Public Health Service.

REFERENCES

Bates D, et al 1977 A prospective study of nontraumatic coma: methods and results in 310 patients. Annals of Neurology 2:211–220

Brierley J B 1971 The neuropathological sequelae of profound hypoxia. In: Brierley J B, Meldrum B S (eds.) Brain hypoxia. William Heinemann Ltd, London. p 147–151

Brierley J B 1973 Pathology of cerebral ischemia. In: McDowell F H, Brennan R W (eds.) Cerebral vascular diseases, Eighth Conference. Grune & Stratton, New York. p 59–75

Brierley J B, Adams J H, Graham D I, Simpson J A 1971 Neocortical death after cardiac arrest, Lancet 2:560–565

Caplan L R 1980 Top of the basilar syndrome. Neurology 30:72–79

Caronna J J 1979 Diagnosis, prognosis and treatment of hypoxic coma. In: Fahn S, Davis J N, Rowland L P (eds.) Advances in neurology volume 26. Raven Press, New York. p 1–19

Carter A B 1964 Cerebral infarction. Pergamon Press, Oxford

Cuneo R A, Caronna J J 1977 The neurologic complications of hypertension. Medical Clinics of North America 61, No. 3:565–580

Cuneo R A, Caronna J J, Pitts L, Townsend J, Winestock D P 1979 Upward transtentorial herniation. Archives of Neurology 36:618–623

Dinsdale H B 1964 Spontaneous hemorrhage in the posterior fossa. Archives of Neurology 10:200–217

Duncan G W, Parker S W, Fisher C M 1975 Acute cerebellar infarction in the PICA territory. Archives of Neurology 32:364

Finkelstein S, Caronna J J 1978 Amnestic syndrome following cardiac arrest. Neurology 28:389

Fisher C M 1961 Clinical syndromes in cerebral artery occlusion. In: Fields W S (ed) Pathogenesis and treatment of cerebrovascular disease, Charles C Thomas, Springfield, Illinois. p 151–181

Fisher C M 1965 Lacunes: Small, deep cerebral infarcts. Neurology 15:744–784

Fisher C M 1969 The arterial lesions underlying lacunes. Acta Neuropathologica 12:1–15

Fisher C M, Karnes W, Kubik C 1961 Lateral medullary infarction, the pattern of vascular occlusion. Journal of Neuropathology and Experimental Neurology 20:323–379

Ginsberg M D 1979 Delayed neurological deterioration following hypoxia. In: Fahn S, Davis J N, Rowland L P (eds.) Advances in neurology volume 26. Raven Press, New York. p 21–47

Giroux J C, Leger J L 1962 Hematomas of the posterior fossa: a report of three cases. Canadian Medical Association Journal 87:59–61

Greenberg J, Skubick D, Shenkin H 1979 Acute hydrocephalus in cerebellar infarct and hemorrhage. Neurology 29:409

Hawkes C H, Bryan-Smyth L 1974 The electroencephalogram in the locked-in syndrome. Neurology 24:1015–1018

Jefferson G 1938 The tentorial pressure cone. Archives of Neurology and Psychiatry 40:857–876

Jennett W B, Plum F 1972 The persistent vegetative state: A syndrome in search of a name. Lancet 1:734–737

Jennett B, Gleave J, Wilson P 1981 Brain death in three neuro-surgical units. British Medical Journal 282:533–539

Karp J S, Hurtig H I 1974 Locked-in state with bilateral midbrain infarcts. Archives of Neurology 30:176–178

Kubik C S, Adams R D 1946 Occlusion of the basilar artery—a clinical and pathological study. Brain 69:6–121

Levy D E, Knill-Jones R P, Plum F 1978 The vegetative state and its prognosis following nontraumatic coma. Annals of the New York Academy of Science 315:293–306

Levy D E, Bates D, Caronna J J et al 1981 Prognosis in nontraumatic coma. Annals of Internal Medicine 94:293–301

McNealy D E, Plum F 1962 Brainstem dysfunction with supratentorial mass lesions. Archives of Neurology 7:10–32

Mills R P, Swanson P D 1978 Vertical oculomotor apraxia and memory loss. Annals of Neurology 4:149–153

Mohr J P, et al 1978 The Harvard Cooperative Stroke Registry: a prospective registry. Neurology 28:754–762

Mohr J P, Fisher C M, Adams R D 1980 Cerebrovascular Diseases. In: Isselbacher K J, Adams R D, Braunwald E, Petersdord R G, Wilson J D (eds.) Harrison's principles of internal medicine, 9th edn. McGraw-Hill, New York. ch. 365, p 1911–1915

Moruzzi G, Magoun H W 1949 Brainstem reticular formation and activation of the EEG. Electroencephalography and Clinical Neurophysiology 1:455–473

Ng LKY, Nimmanitya J 1970 Massive cerebral infarction with severe brain swelling. Stroke 1:158–163

Plum F 1966 Brain swelling and edema in cerebral vascular disease. Research Publications Association for Research in Nervous and Mental Diseases 41:318–348

Plum F, Posner J B, Alvord E C 1963 Edema and necrosis in experimental cerebral infarction. Archives of Neurology 9:563–570

Plum F, Posner J B 1980 The diagnosis of stupor and coma edition 3, Davis, Philadelphia

Schaefer J A, Caronna J J 1978 Duration of apnea needed to confirm brain death. Neurology 28:661–666

Schwart M S, Prior P F, Scott D F 1973 The occurrence and evolution in the EEG of a lateralized periodic phenomenon. Brain 96:613–622

Segarra J M 1970 Cerebral vascular disease and behavior. I. The syndrome of the mesencephalic artery (basilar artery bifurcation). Archives of Neurology 22:408–418

Selhorst J, Hoyt W, Feinsod M, Hosobuchi Y 1976 Midbrain corectopia. Archives of Neurology 33:193–195

Shaw C M, Alvord E C Jr., Berry R G 1959 Swelling of the brain following ischemic infarction with arterial occlusion. Archives of Neurology 1:167–177

Silver J R, Buxton P H 1974 Spinal stroke. Brain 97:539–550

Sunderland S 1958 The tentorial notch and complications produced by herniations of the brain through that aperture. British Journal of Surgery 45:422–438

Sypert G W, Alvord E C 1975 Cerebral infarction: A clinicopathological study. Archives of Neurology 32:357–363

Wells C E 1959 Cerebral embolism. Archives of Neurology and Psychiatry 81:667–677

8

The investigation of strokes

Michael J. G. Harrison

This chapter basically concerns the investigation of patients who have suffered a completed stroke although the techniques discussed are also relevant to the management of patients with transient ischaemic attack (TIAs). The management of both TIA and stroke patients is dealt with elsewhere and the choice of which investigation should be used in particular clinical circumstances is considered in those chapters.

In this account the investigation of the nature of the cerebral lesion will precede clarification of the nature of the vascular lesion.

INVESTIGATION OF THE CEREBRAL LESION

Cerebrospinal fluid (c.s.f.)

The distinction between acute cerebral haemorrhage and cerebral infarction can be made in 80 per cent of instances by examination of the c.s.f., but lumbar puncture is not without risk in patients with large hemisphere haematomas or infarcts. In the absence of computerised tomography lumbar puncture may still be useful in diagnosis.

Blood staining of the c.s.f. occurs in approximately 75 per cent of patients with haemorrhage (73 per cent Aring & Merritt 1935: 80 per cent McKissock et al 1959). Xanthochromia may develop as soon as four to six hours after bleeding and last for up to three to four weeks. Elevation of the c.s.f. pressure to over 300 mm c.s.f. may be found in some 40 per cent of fatal cases of haemorrhage (Aring & Merritt 1935).

Blood staining of the fluid is rare in cerebral infarction (1.5 per cent Aring & Merritt, 1935)

Table 8.1 Summary of investigation of the cerebral lesion

1. Distinction of stroke from non vascular causes of acute neurological deficit such as tumour, encephalitis multiple sclerosis.

Radionuclide scanning	Serial scans may be necessary
CAT scanning	to distinguish tumour
E.e.g.	Encephalitis
C.s.f.	M.S. encephalitis
Angiography	Tumour. Subdural haematoma

2. Distinction between cerebral haemorrhage and infarction
   CAT scanning
   C.s.f.
   Echoencephalography
   Angiography — aetiology of bleed

3. Distinction between deep and superficial cerebral infarction
   CAT scanning
   E.e.g.

4. Distinction between accessible and inaccessible haematomas
   CAT scanning
   Angiography

5. Detection of viable tissue in ischaemic area
   Positron scanning

but slight xanthochromia is occasionally encountered, presumably due to haemorrhagic infarction (Merritt & Fremont-Smith, 1937). Red cell counts in the c.s.f. fail to distinguish reliably between haemorrhagic and non-haemorrhagic infarction (Sornas et al, 1972). When rarely an elevated pressure is recorded in case of infarction the prognosis is usually poor (Plum, 1971).

White cell counts may be mildly elevated in infarction (6–50 cells per mm^3) but high counts are only common in septic embolism (100–4000 cells). Sornas found 66 per cent of haematomas to have a transitory rise of polymorphonuclear cells.

Serological tests are indicated in the young

stroke victim in whom meningovascular syphilis is suspected.

Examination of the c.s.f. is unlikely to be indicated in TIA patients.

Electroencephalography (e.e.g.)

Cerebral infarction involving the cerebral cortex produces an increase in theta and delta activity, frequently associated with a local reduction in alpha rhythm. These focal changes are maximal immediately after the insult and therefore are often detectable before abnormalities can be seen on isotope or computerised tomographic scans. There may be an increase in generalised slowing of the e.e.g. if oedema develops over the next three to four days (Cohn et al, 1948; Hossmann & Mies, 1980). The changes slowly resolve in weeks (Roseman et al, 1952) but are more likely to persist in cases with severe permanent neurological deficit and in patients in whom epilepsy develops. The resolution of the focal changes is of help in the differential diagnosis from tumour, but haemorrhage and infarction cannot be distinguished. A relatively normal record in a hemiplegic stroke patient suggests the possibility of a small deep lesion (Achar et al, 1966).

Brain stem infarction often produces only minor generalised slowing of the record, but may be associated with frontal intermittent delta activity or bitemporal changes (Phillips, 1964), features which are not sufficiently specific to be reliable in differential diagnosis.

Quantitative analysis of the e.e.g. has revealed that e.e.g. slowing correlates fairly well with regional reduction in blood flow (Ingvar et al, 1976). In patients with acute infarcts the local abnormalities are clearly demonstrated by the simple analysis of delta activity (Fig. 8.1). This technique also reveals that bilateral changes accompany hemisphere infarction, in keeping with the bilateral flow disturbance called diaschisis (Hossman & Mies, 1980).

E.e.g. changes are occassionaly detectable in TIA patients, probably due to the occurrence of small areas of infarction in some cases despite the brevity of the symptoms (Harrison & Marshall, 1977). E.e.g. recording may be useful in separating TIA from focal epilepsy, a distinction that can be particularly difficult when sensory symptoms predominate.

Echoencephalography

Detection of the midline echo is of limited value in cerebrovascular disease. It provides some help in the differentiation of haemorrhage and infarction on the day of the ictus since immediate midline shift usually indicates a haemorrhage (Achar et al, 1966). Extra echoes may be detectable due to subdural or intracerebral haematomas (Kanaya et al, 1968).

Isotope scans

Radioisotope scanning has the advantages of low dosage radiation, repeatability and freedom from complications. The advent of computerised tomographic scanning has improved the accuracy of localisation of areas of abnormal isotope accumulation (Ell et al, 1980).

Some 60 per cent of cerebral infarcts can be detected by scanning using single photon gamma emitters such as 99 Technetium[m] (Gado et al, 1976; Campbell et al, 1978). The classical appearance is of a wedge shaped area of uptake extending up to and including the cortex (Fig. 8.2). This configuration may help to distinguish infarction from haemorrhage and from tumour which will often present a better defined, more rounded area of uptake which often does not include the cortex (Fig. 8.3). The precise shape and site of the area of isotope concentration is better seen on computerised emission tomographic scans.

The evolution of the changes which underlie the abnormal accumulation of isotope in an infarct is also helpful in the recognition of the nature of the cerebral lesion. Scans performed within a week of onset of a non-haemorrhagic stroke are usually negative (only about 25 per cent positive). By the third week 75 per cent have a positive scan; by six weeks most such scans have faded or become normal (Tow et al, 1969). A dense uptake in the first day or two after the development of an acute hemiplegia is thus suspicious of a tumour rather than an infarct, and this suspicion would be strengthened if the uptake showed little change over the next week or two, and was more obvious

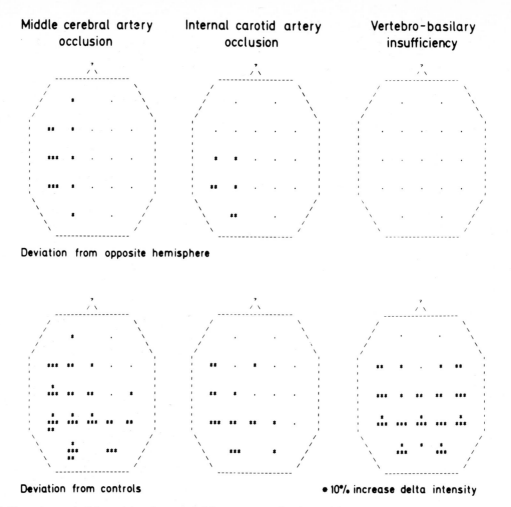

Fig. 8.1 Mean changes in delta activity of e.e.g. in 3 different groups of patients with cerebrovascular disorders. Above: side difference between 2 hemispheres. Below: difference from healthy controls. Asterisks indicate per cent changes (Hossman & Mies, 1980). Reproduced by kind permission of Dr K-A Hossman and Excerpta Medica.

at six weeks. An increase in density with a reduction in area between the first and third weeks would be more compatible with an infarct. Positive scans months after an infarct are unusual and tend to correlate with a severe persistent clinical deficit. Isotope scans can thus be used to help 'date' an infarct detected by other means.

Brain stem infarcts may sometimes be detected (44 per cent in the small series quoted by Campbell et al, 1978).

The isotope scan is a reliable way of detecting a chronic subdural haematoma which may present with an acute hemiplegia (Luxon & Harrison, 1979).

Cerebral haemorrhages may produce a positive scan. The area of increased uptake tends not to include the cortex so occasionally may be distinguishable from an infarct. It cannot be distinguished from a tumour or an abscess however.

TIA patients will not normally have a positive scan unless the diagnosis is incorrect and the underlying lesion is a tumour, subdural haematoma or arteriovenous malformation.

Computerised axial tomography (CAT transmission scanning)

Infarction may be detected as an area of low density in 50 to 75 per cent of cases (Gado et al, 1976;

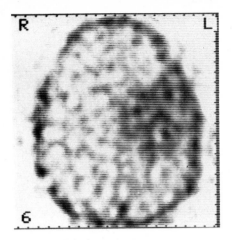

Fig. 8.2 Emission CAT scan of cerebral infarct in the middle cerebral artery territory of the left hemisphere. Wedge shaped area of increased uptake of ^{99m}Tc.

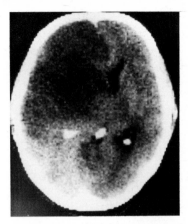

Fig. 8.4 Transmission CAT scan of recent cerebral infarct with extensive ill-defined area of low density in the left frontal region. Midline displacement of ventricles and pineal reflects the mass effect of oedematous infarct.

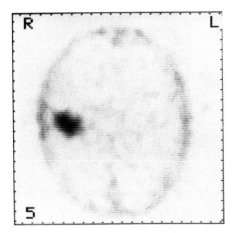

Fig. 8.3 Emission CAT scan of a cerebral metastasis in the right hemisphere. Rounded area of increased uptake deep to the cortex.

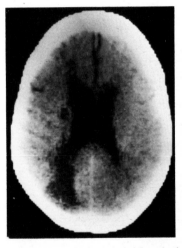

Fig. 8.5 Transmission CAT scan of old cerebral infarct posteriorly in the left hemisphere. Low density lesion well defined and associated with a dilated lateral ventricle.

Campbell et al, 1978). Normal scans may be encountered when the lesions are small and this is especially likely to be the case with brain stem infarcts. The timing of scans also has an important effect on the diagnostic yield which is at its highest 8–11 days after the ictus though many are positive at 24 hours. The area of low density is ill defined at first (Fig. 8.4) but becomes better demarcated at one to two weeks. Old infarcts appear as areas of encephalomalacia with dilatation of the ipsilateral ventricle or widening of neighbourhood sulci due to atrophy. (Fig. 8.5).

In some 5 per cent of instances the infarct is isodense and only shows up after enhancement. Enhancement by contrast media is unusual in the first week after infarction though this may occur even on day 1. The mean time to enhancement in one study of acute infarcts was 19 days (Norton et al, 1978). The pattern of enhancement may be patchy, central or peripheral. Sixty-five per cent of cases show enhancement at some stage if enough contrast material is used (Weisberg, 1980).

Interestingly, isotope uptake and enhancement do not always run in parallel though there is a correlation (Davis et al, 1977). Recently enhancement by Xenon has been studied. This has proved of value in detecting isodense subdural haematomas and may be helpful in dating infarcts seen in CAT scans since acute infarcts may show a penumbra of increased enhancement not seen round the well demarcated low density area of an old infarct. (Radue & Kendall, 1978).

Due to the presence of oedema there may be a mass effect with some shift of the midline or obliteration of ipsilateral sulci. (Figure 8.4). This is seen as soon as day 1 or 2 but is maximal over the next few days and tends to resolve by 10–20 days. A mass effect after 25 days would be most unlikely with an infarct and would be more in favour of a tumour as the cause of the neurological deficit. Tumour oedema and infarct oedema tend to give different appearances. Tumour oedema tends to outline the white matter of the hemisphere at a distance from the mass lesion and has a finger-like pattern (Fig. 8.6). Infarct oedema tends to have a

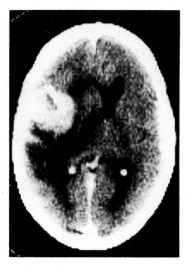

Fig. 8.6 Transmission CAT scan of cerebral metastasis with hemisphere oedema. Note different appearance of low density change due to oedema from Figure 8.4.

hemogeneous 'smudgy' appearance. This difference may reflect the difference between vasogenic and ischaemic oedema which probably also underlies its different therapeutic response to corticosteroids (O'Brien, 1979).

Lacunar infarcts due to hypertensive small vessel disease are occasionally detectable (Nelson et al, 1980), though similar clinical syndromes may

prove on scanning to be due to severe hemisphere infarction.

A normal scan at an early stage after the onset of an acute neurological deficit may be due to either lacunar infarction or to a severe hemisphere infarct, which will become detectable later.

Haemorrhagic infarcts can be difficult to detect. Patchy areas of high density within an area of mixed attenuation that has the configuration of an infarct suggest a haemorrhagic infarct, but petechial haemorrhage will be missed. Sudden deterioration in a patient with an infarct often proves to be due to secondary haemorrhage (Davis et al, 1977).

CAT scans in TIA patients may reveal small low density lesions due to the occurrence of restricted areas of infarction. The hypodense areas are usually in the basal ganglia and are reported in some 20–30 per cent of patients (Perrone et al, 1979). Unusual causes of transient neurological deficit, such as tumour, a–v malformation or subdural haematoma may be revealed.

Computerised axial tomography and radionucleide scanning are complementary in the detection of infarcts since some prove detectable by one technique and not by the other (Campbell et al, 1978). In Campbell's series 8 per cent of 141 infarcts were only detectable by CAT scans (mostly old infarcts) and 8 per cent were only detectable by isotope scans. CAT scans are more likely to be positive in the first week, and after the fourth. At the optimal time for isotope scanning (2 weeks) the yield is comparable (Davis et al, 1975).

CAT scanning has proved virtually 100 per cent accurate in detecting recent haematomas and is therefore the method of choice in distinguishing infarction and haemorrhage in the acute stroke patient. It has also revealed how often haemorrhage can cause a clinical picture indistinguishable from infarction (Harrison, 1980a), and minor clinical syndromes can be due to small haematomas (Nilsson et al, 1979). Haematomas down to 3– 5 mm in size can be detected.

Cerebral haemorrhage can be detected due to the high X-ray absorption values of blood and blood products (especially globin). Acutely (Reisner & Dal-Bianco, 1979) the scan shows an intracerebral area of high attenuation (Fig. 8.7), which fades over the coming weeks until at four to

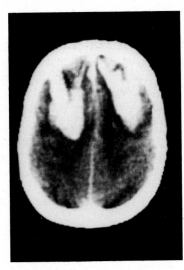

Fig. 8.7 Transmission CAT scan of bilateral frontal cerebral haemorrhage (high density areas).

six weeks a low attenuation cavity remains. The area around the acute haematoma may show low attenuation due, it is suggested, to serum expressed by the retracting clot or to a zone of ischaemic necrosis (Kendall & Radue, 1978). After three or four days a ring of enhancement may be seen together with perifocal oedema. Enhancement usually lasts only three or four weeks unless a haematoma capsule develops.

Occasionally the scan (Fig. 8.8) reveals the source of bleeding (aneurysm, arteriovenous mal-

formation, glioma). If there is no evidence of a source, especially in a normotensive subject, a repeat scan after the acute bleed has resolved may be useful, but often angiography is needed. Difficulties in interpretation arise if the scans are carried out for the first time at a stage when the haematoma has largely resolved. It may then be indistinguishable from other causes of a low density cyst-like cavity.

Further, CAT scanning of haematomas frequently provides anatomical localisation of the bleed sufficient for surgical intervention. In a series of 313 cases Fazio et al (1979) found 53 per cent to be superficial lobar haematomas almost equally distributed between frontal, parietal, temporal and occipital lobes. 44 per cent were deep. Of these, most (70 per cent) were in the region of the internal capsule. Eighteen per cent were thalamic and 11 per cent putaminal or in the external capsule. Ventricular compression was usual, displacement obvious in some 50 per cent, and ventricular bleeding present in 20–30 per cent. Deep haematomas, massive lesions and widespread ventricular spread of the blood are all adverse prognostic signs in the CAT scan (Kendall & Radue, 1978). Cerebellar and pontine haemorrhage may be difficult to distinguish clinically yet the former is surgically accessible. CAT scanning has taken the place of angiography and ventriculography in the investigation of these patients.

It has been argued (Larsen et al, 1978) that CAT scanning has added to the cost of investigation of stroke patients without clear benefit to the majority. This is a reflection of the fact that specific therapy is as yet available for only a minority of stroke victims, and the argument ignores the enormous increase in understanding of the pathophysiology of cerebral infarction that follows the ability to visualise the lesion non-invasively.

Also, although a few patients show an adverse response to the injection of contrast medium CAT scanning is less dangerous than lumbar puncture in distinguishing between haemorrhage and infarction.

Angiography

Angiography may be needed to detect the nature of the cerebral lesion if CAT scanning is unavailable

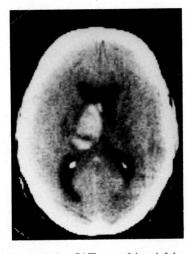

Fig. 8.8 Transmission CAT scan of deep left hemisphere haematoma (high density area). This proved to be due to bleeding into tumour.

or has given an equivocal result. An infarct may be recognised as an avascular area with or without vascular occlusion or displacement of vessels due to oedema. Delayed flow in an artery, local stasis of contrast material, loss of the normal capillary blush and early filling veins may all be seen. Areas of low flow with delayed filling or emptying of an artery are more often seen than areas of hyperaemia with early filling or shunt veins (Shah et al, 1972).

Intracerebral haemorrhage causes an avascular mass in which dye extravasation may rarely be seen (Fig. 8.9). The source of bleeding may be obvious if an aneurysm or arteriovenous malformation is revealed.

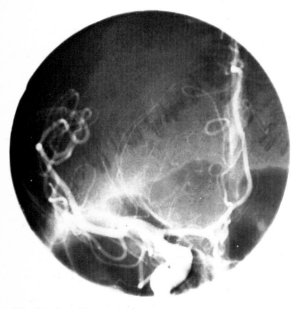

Fig. 8.9 Carotid angiogram AP view to show bowing of small vessels around a deep thalamic haemorrhage.

Tumours are detected as avascular masses or as areas of pathological circulation with stretching of surrounding vessels.

Subdural haematomas cause depression of the cortical vessels away from the vault. Oblique views may be the most useful to detect small collections.

Positron scanning

Positrons are electrons with a positive charge which combine with an electron when arrested in tissue and give rise to two high energy gamma ray photons emitted in opposite directions. There is less scatter than with the photons emitted by ^{99}Technetium^{m} and the scans using positron emitting isotopes thereby gain in depth resolution. More importantly, short-lived isotopes incorporated in metabolites such as glucose and oxygen can be used to provide imaging of regional metabolic activity. ^{18}Fluorine with a half life of two hours can be linked to glucose to monitor cerebral glucose metabolism. ^{15}Oxygen, with a two minute half life, if inhaled allows steady state measurements of regional cerebral oxygen metabolism to be made. If inhaled CO_2 is labelled with $^{15}O_2$ the scans reflect cerebral blood flow. A comparison of $^{15}O_2$ and $C^{15}O_2$ scans yields a measurement of oxygen extraction by selected areas of brain tissue and any mismatch between blood flow and metabolism can be detected.

After cerebral infarction some 75 per cent of cases show evidence of luxury perfusion with areas of relatively high blood flow (Fig. 8.10). These are believed to be areas of ischaemic damage with depressed metabolism but with loss of autoregulation and vasoparalysis due to the accumulation of ischaemic metabolites. Areas of low flow with high oxygen extraction (misery perfusion) are rare ($<$ 10%) but are of great interest since they are presumably areas of viable tissue in a state of suboptimal perfusion. Such a region could theoretically be returned to normal if flow could be increased medically or by revascularisation procedures.

$^{15}O_2$ scans may also reveal areas of depressed metabolism due to infarction which CAT scans have failed to detect (Castaigne et al, 1980).

^{18}F-Glucose scans show depressed utilisation in zones of infarction. The area of dysfunction is usually larger than that suggested by the morphometric evidence of a CAT scan. Although decreases in metabolism and perfusion are well matched in old stable infarcts there is sometimes less depression of glucose utilisation acutely, perhaps due to partial compensation by enhanced anaerobic glycolysis (Kuhl et al, 1980).

INVESTIGATION OF THE VASCULAR LESION

If the investigation of the nature of the cerebral lesion has indicated an ischaemic process, attention

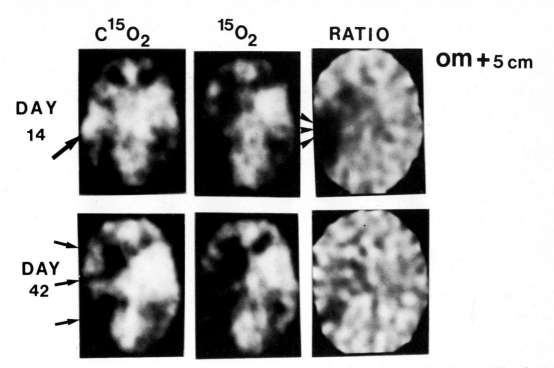

Fig. 8.10 Axial tomographic positron scans after left middle cerebral occlusion. Cuts 5 cm above the orbito-meatal line after inhalation of $C^{15}O_2$ and $^{15}O_2$ 14 days and 42 days after the stroke.

At day 14, there is an area of hyperaemia shown by high counts with the $C^{15}O_2$ scan (large arrow) at the site of low extraction shown by low counts on the $^{15}O_2$ scan. The right hand picture reflects the mismatch in the hyperaemic area between flow and oxygen extraction.

At day 42, the area of hyperaemia has given way to reduced perfusion scan and the ratio scan reflects the more normal match of flow and oxygen extraction. (Reproduced with kind permission of J. C. Baron, M. G. Bousser, D. Comar and P. Castaigne).

turns to the possible nature of the vascular pathology.

Transient ischaemic attacks are infrequently due to cardiac arrhythmias or other causes of reduced blood flow, and most frequently due to embolism (Harrison, 1974). In the carotid territory angiography reveals local disease in the internal carotid artery in some 60 per cent of cases, significantly more frequently than in control subjects (Harrison & Marshall, 1976).

Some 50 per cent of non-haemorrhagic strokes prove at autopsy to be attributable to embolism from the heart (Jorgensen & Torvik, 1966; Blackwood et al, 1969). Stroke patients therefore require careful cardiac assessment which may need to include e.e.g.s, cardiac enzyme levels and in some cases echocardiography, isotope scans for myocardial infarction and cardiac aneurysms, and Holter monitoring for dysrhythmias. Many of the remaining strokes are probably due to carotid occlusion, or to embolism from the aorta or neck vessels (Lhermitte et al, 1968).

The decision to investigate stroke victims for possibly operable stenosis of the carotid artery is a difficult one. Surgery is probably indicated for patients with transient ischaemic attacks who are found to have such a stenosis if the available vascular surgeon achieves a sufficiently low operative morbidity and mortality (Harrison, 1980b). The risks are high in patients with a recent cerebral infarct however, and it is doubtful if endarterectomy is ever indicated in such cases. The problem is most serious when a patient makes a full recovery from a completed stroke. Should surgery to prevent recurrences be considered? As the operative morbidity is probably higher in this group than in those with TIAs (Sundt et al, 1975), some would argue that operation should only be contemplated in those with a severe stenosis which is most likely to occlude (Lhermitte et al, 1968). In this case non-invasive investigation may be used to detect just such patients. If a more enthusiastic approach to endarterectomy is taken angiography will be needed more often since non-invasive tests may fail to reveal lesser degrees of atheroma that may also be the source of emboli.

The advent of the EC–IC bypass procedure has also altered the approach to the stroke patient. The procedure was devised as a way of overcoming the difficulties encountered when patients had TIAs above a carotid occlusion or in the presence of an inaccessible stenosis of the internal carotid artery or middle cerebral artery. However, the procedure was soon extended to stroke victims on the assumption that increasing the blood supply to the ischaemic hemisphere might encourage recovery of tissue rendered ischaemic but not infarcted. This policy has yet to be justified by adequate clinical trial and the morbidity of the procedure in the acute stroke patient is unacceptable. Again however, the problem arises in the patient who has recently made a good recovery — would a bypass procedure be helpful or prophylactic against recurrence?

As the non-invasive tests only detect extracranial vascular disease, angiography would be required to detect the vascular lesions that might logically be amenable to a bypass procedure.

Non-invasive tests and angiography will thus be discussed with surgical management in mind and principally in an attempt to answer the question of whether the patient who has recovered from a recent stroke or has TIAs, has an operable carotid stenosis.

Non-invasive tests of the carotid artery

Most of these tests depend on the detection of changes in flow or pressure to reveal the presence of haemodynamically significant stenosis of the carotid artery. As such they 'miss' ulcerative lesions which may be the source of mural thromboembolism without significantly encroaching on the lumen. Ultrasonic scanning and B mode imaging provide more direct visualisation of the bifurcation. (Table 8.2).

Table 8.2 Non-invasive tests of the carotid circulation (after Ackerman, 1979)

	Types of test
Pressure	Ophthalmodynamometry
Flow and/or collateral	Oculoplethysmography (Gee)
	Periorbital Doppler flow study
	Oculoplethysmography
	(Kartchner & McRae)
Turbulence anatomy	Bruit analysis
	Ultrasonic scanning
	Realtime B scan imaging

Ophthalmodynamometry

This technique depends on the assumption that raising ocular pressure until it obliterates retinal arterial pulsation will be a measure of the perfusion pressure in the ophthalmic artery, and therefore an indication of the degree of patency of the internal carotid artery. Bilateral disease confuses assessment and the method is waning in popularity.

Oculoplethysmography

Gee's method

In this method ophthalmic artery pressure is measured as ocular pulsations return when a negative pressure to the eye is slowly reduced.

Using this technique Ginsberg et al (1979) had a 93 per cent success rate with narrowing of the carotid by 60–100 per cent. Stenosis under 60 per cent did not retard the ocular pulse arrival time. Stenosis of 60 per cent, equivalent to a 80 per cent reduction in cross sectional area of the lumen, causes only a 10 mm pressure drop (de Weese et al, 1970). The method thus only reliably detects severe lesions and there are difficulties in interpretation in the presence of bilateral disease.

Kartchner & McRae's method

The pulse waveform of the two eyes is displayed simultaneously and effectively records the volume change in the eye due to pulsatile blood flow. Delay of the pulse occurs with flow reduction in the carotid artery. Again stenosis of 50 per cent will often be missed but lesions causing over 60 per cent stenosis can be picked up with a 90 per cent success rate (Kartchner & McRae, 1978).

Doppler flow studies

Flow in the supraorbital artery may be reversed after severe stenosis or occlusion of the internal carotid artery. Changes in the direction of flow in collateral arteries may be detected by a Doppler probe at rest or in response to manual compression of superficial temporal, facial and carotid arteries. A normal result is of no significance but abnormalities are encountered in 90 per cent of cases in which there is at least 75 per cent stenosis. Stenosis of the external carotid artery confuses the results and occlusion and severe stenosis give the same patterns.

Isotope angiography

Rapid sequence scinti-photography after the intravenous injection of ^{99}Technetium^m can demonstrate reduced flow on the side of a stenosed or occluded carotid artery. There are however, many false negatives (Toole et al, 1976).

Bruit analysis

The presence of a bruit over the carotid bifurcation has long been recognised as a sign of stenosis. Experimental studies have shown that a 40 per cent reduction in area of the lumen is enough to cause a bruit although the pressure gradient is insignificant. Bruits may therefore be heard over stenotic lesions that do not cause abnormalities on any of the flow or pressure-dependent tests so far discussed. Severe stenosis may however have no bruit (up to one in three according to Ackerman, 1979) and there is often no bruit with complete occlusion. Ocular bruits tend to be due to augmented flow and reflect collateral development.

The analysis of the intensity or frequency of neck bruits can be a useful adjunct to other non-invasive tests.

Ultrasonic imaging

The use of pulsed ultrasound and B mode scanning promises to overcome many of the shortcomings of other non-invasive methods. Images of the flowing column of blood (Fig. 8.11) or of the soft tissue vessel walls can be built up by the experienced

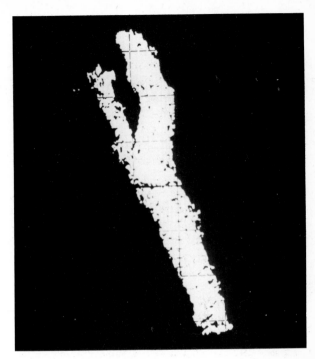

Fig. 8.11 Ultrasonic imaging of a normal carotid bifurcation. The image is built up of Doppler flow profiles and therefore represents the shape of the moving column of blood. (Illustration kindly supplied by Dr C. Warlow).

operator. Calcified plaques may distort the result and there are technical difficulties when the carotid artery divides high in the neck. The external and internal carotid artery may be confused. It may not be possible to tell a tight stenosis from a complete occlusion by imaging unless Doppler measurements of flow are carried out at the same time. As experience and equipment improve there is real hope that the detailed morphology of atheromatous disease of the carotid bifurcation may be detected and measured.

At present significant stenosis of the carotid artery can be best detected by a combination of bruit analysis, periorbital Doppler recording and oculoplethysmography. Ultrasonic imaging may take over this role in the future (Fig. 8.11) though some measure of the haemodynamic significance of the lesion is still important. If the view is taken that only severe stenotic lesions warrant endarterectomy then non-invasive investigations may well be adequate to detect the few surgical candidates. If an EC–IC bypass is to be considered or a positive surgical approach to minor degrees of athero-matous ulceration in the carotid is favoured, angiography will be necessary in all patients.

Angiography

The complications of angiography include a mortality which is under 0.5 per cent (Hass et al, 1968) and a neurological morbidity of 0.5 to 2.5 per cent. Angiography will therefore only be considered if the diagnosis of the cerebral lesion is in doubt, or if required before vascular surgery. Arch angiography is often attended by a greater risk, though if surgery is contemplated visualisation of all the major neck vessels may be mandatory. Different departments adopt different protocols to ensure adequate imaging of the carotid bifurcation, intracranial circulation and neck vessels (Kerber et al, 1978). The accuracy of angiography is good with severe disease but there are problems in the detection of minor ulcerated plaques (Croft et al, 1980). The recent development of intravenous angiography using video subtraction may allow all but the smallest extracranial lesions to be detected without the need for an arterial injection (Christenson et al, 1980).

Though the non-invasive tests already discussed are capable of detecting haemodynamically significant stenosis of the internal carotid artery in TIA patients, angiographic visualisation is needed before endarterectomy can be carried out. In a series of 211 cases of carotid territory TIAs over 50 per cent had local atheromatous disease of the bifurcation (Harrison & Marshall, 1975b). The finding of carotid stenosis was more likely in patients with a localised bruit and in those with retinal ischaemic attacks. Normal angiograms were found in 43 per cent presumably reflecting both the prevalence of more proximal sources of embolism and the difficulty of detecting minor ulcerated lesions (Croft et al, 1980).

Carotid angiography after strokes in the carotid territory reveals carotid occlusion in some 20 per cent (Fig. 8.12). Intracranial occlusions (Fig. 8.13)

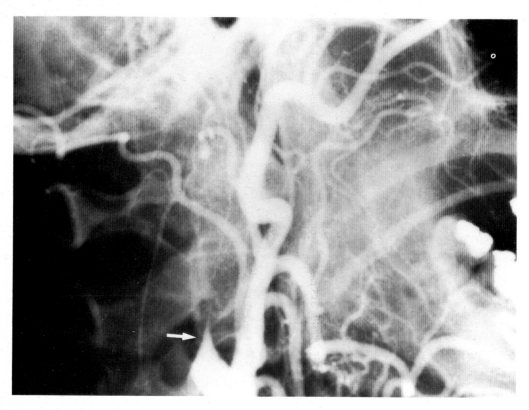

Fig. 8.12 Carotid angiogram showing occlusion of the internal carotid artery 1 cm above its origin (arrow).

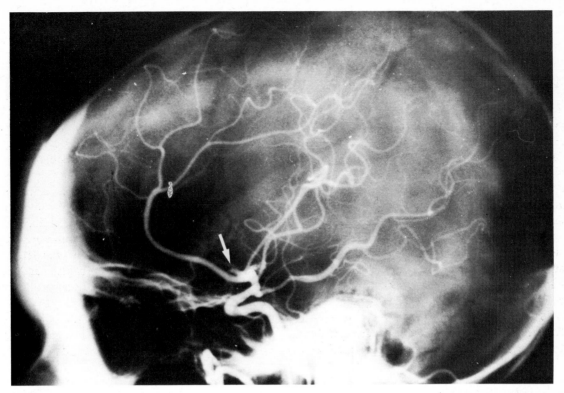

Fig. 8.13 Carotid angiogram showing occlusion of anterior branches of the middle cerebral artery at their origin (arrow). Lateral view.

are common if angiography is carried out shortly after the ictus but are less likely to be found after a delay, due to fragmentation and movement of emboli (Dalal et al, 1965; Fieschi & Bozzao, 1969). Atheromatous disease of the patent carotid artery (Figs. 8.14 & 8.15) is found in some 25 per cent of cases (Harrison & Marshall, 1975b). Angiograms are less often revealing in hypertensive stroke victims since many of the latter have small lacunar infarcts due to hypertensive small vessel disease (Harrison & Marshall, 1975b).

Surgery is rarely undertaken in the vertebro-basilar circulation and so angiography is less frequently required in the investigation of patients with TIAs or completed strokes in this territory. Persistent attacks, doubt about the cause of the clinical picture, or clinical evidence of the subclavian steal syndrome may prompt angiography. The subclavian steal syndrome is diagnosed by the evidence of stenosis of the subclavian artery with retrograde flow in the vertebral artery helping to fill the distal axillary artery. This haemodynamic

situation is not uncommon on arch angiograms in cerebrovascular disease patients (Chase & Kricheff, 1966) but if the findings are otherwise normal the prognosis is good and intervention not warranted (Fields & Lemark, 1972).

The problem of assessing which patients might be suitable for an EC–IC bypass procedure depends on demonstrating occlusion or inaccessable stenosis of the internal carotid or middle cerebral artery. (Figure 8.16). After operation a patent bypass can be demonstrated angiographically or by Doppler studies of the superficial temporal artery in about 90 per cent of patients.

The problem of deciding which patients might benefit from the bypass procedure is more difficult, and at present attempts are being made to see if the reversibility of neurological deficit in hyperbaric oxygen or after brief hypertension is predictive. Preservation of normal regional oxygen consumption in spite of a reduced regional blood flow on positron scanning might also prove a useful indication for this operation.

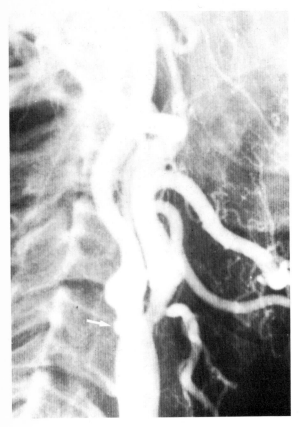

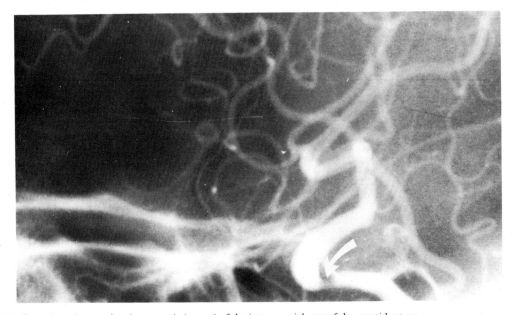

Fig. 8.15 Carotid angiogram showing severe stenosis of the internal carotid artery (arrow). The rounded filling defect immediately above the stenosis proved to be due to friable mural thrombus.

Fig. 8.14 Carotid angiogram showing atheromatous irregularity of the wall of the internal carotid artery possibly due to ulceration (arrow).

Fig. 8.16 Carotid angiogram showing stenosis (arrow) of the intra-cranial part of the carotid artery.

SUMMARY

The investigation of stroke patients has been revolutionised by the advent of computerised axial tomography (CAT Scanning). Its ability to distinguish between haemorrhage and infarction and to detect non-vascular causes of acute neurological deficits mimicking stroke has made it the investigative procedure of first choice in evolving or completed strokes. It has also advanced understanding of the evolution of tissue changes in infarction and the role of oedema.

The increased accuracy of emission computerised axial tomography has helped to preserve a role for radionuclide scanning, as it can complement information available from CAT scans, and provide additional information on the pathophysiology of infarcted tissue.

Positron scanning is now emerging as an exciting development since it provides imaging of regional cerebral metabolism. For the first time it is becoming possible to look for areas in the ischaemic brain where there is a disparity between blood flow and metabolic requirement.

Angiography remains the most reliable method of demonstrating the vascular pathology. The non-invasive tests are already helpful in the detection of haemodynamically significant stenosis of neck vessels, and new imaging techniques promise to provide an alternative to angiography in visualising the carotid bifurcation. If however, the EC–IC bypass procedure is shown to be of benefit, angiography will retain a central role in the investigation of stroke patients.

REFERENCES

Achar V S, Coe R P K, Marshall J 1966 Echoencephalography in the differential diagnosis of cerebral haemorrhage and infarction. Lancet i:161

Ackerman R H 1979 A perspective on non-invasive diagnosis of carotid disease. Neurology 29:615

Aring C D, Merritt H H 1935 Differential diagnosis between cerebral haemorrhage and cerebral thrombosis. Archives of Internal Medicine 56:435

Blackwood W, Hallpike J F, Kocen R S, Mair W G P 1969 Atheromatous disease of the carotid arterial system and embolism from the heart in cerebral infarction: a morbid anatomical study. Brain 92:897

Campbell J K, Houser O W, Stevens J C, Wahner H W, Baker H L, Folger W N 1978 Computed tomography and radionuclide imaging in the evaluation of ischaemic stroke. Radiology 126:695

Castaigne P, Baron J C, Bousser M G, Comar D, Kellersohn C 1980 Positron emission tomography in human hemispheric infarction. A study with $^{15}O_2$ continuous inhalation technique. In: Bes A, Geraude G (eds.) Cerebral circulation and neurotransmitters. Excerpta Medica p 29

Chase N E, Kricheff I I 1966 Cerebral angiography in the evaluation of the patients with cerebrovascular disease. Radiological Clinics of North America 4:131

Christenson P C, Ovitt T W, Fisher H D et al. 1980 Intravenous angiography using video subtraction. American Journal of Neuroradiology 1:379

Cohn R, Raines G N, Mulder D W, Newmann M M 1948 Cerebral vascular lesions: electroencephalographic and neuropathological correlations. Archives of Neurology and Psychiatry (Chicago) 60:163

Croft R J, Ellam L D, Harrison M J G 1980 Accuracy of carotid angiography in the assessment of atheroma of the internal carotid artery. Lancet i:997

Dalal P M, Shah P M, Sheth S C, Deshpande C K 1965 Cerebral embolism. Angiographic observations on spontaneous clot lysis. Lancet i:61

Davis K R, Taveras J M, New P F J, Schnur J A, Roberson A G 1975 Cerebral infarction diagnosis by computerised tomography. American Journal of Roentgenology 124:643

Davis K R, Ackerman R H, Kistler J P, Mohr J P 1977 Computed tomography of cerebral infarction: haemorrhagic, contrast enhancement, and time of appearance. Computerised Tomography 1:77

Ell P J, Deacon J M, Jarritt P M 1980 Atlas of computerised emission tomography. Churchill Livingstone, London

Fazio C, Bozzao L, Fantozzi L M et al 1979 The role of computerised tomography (CT) in the clarification of intracerebral haemorrhages. In: Meyer J S, Lechner H, Reivich M (eds.) Cerebral Vascular Disease 2. Excerpta Medica, Amsterdam, Oxford. p 62

Fields W S, Lemark N A 1972 Joint study of extracranial arterial occlusion VII. Subclavian steal — a review of 168 cases. Journal of the American Medical Association 222:1139

Fieschi C, Bozzao L 1969 Transient embolic occlusion of the middle cerebral and internal carotid arteries in cerebral apoplexy. Journal of Neurology, Neurosurgery and Psychiatry 32:236

Gado M H, Coleman R E, Merlis A L, Alderson P O, Lee K S 1976 Comparison of computerised tomography and radionuclide imaging in 'stroke'. Stroke 7:109

Ginsberg M D, Greenwood S A, Goldberg H I 1979 Non-invasive diagnosis of extracranial cerebrovascular disease: Oculophethysmography–phonoangiography and directional Doppler ultrasonography. Neurology 29:623

Harrison M J G 1974 Transient ischaemic attacks. In: Ledingham J G G (ed.) 10th Symposium on advanced medicine. Pitman, London. p 215

Harrison M J G 1980a Clinical distinction of cerebral haemorrhage and cerebral infarction. Postgraduate Medical Journal 56:629

Harrison M J G 1980b Surgery for ischaemic stroke. British Journal of Hospital Medicine 24:108

Harrison M J G, Marshall J 1975a Indications for angiography and surgery in carotid artery disease. British Medical Journal i:616

Harrison M J G, Marshall J 1975b The results of carotid angiography in cerebral infarction in normotensive and hypertensive subjects. Journal of Neurological Science 24:243

Harrison M J G, Marshall J 1976 Angiographic appearance of carotid bifurcation in patients with completed stroke, transient ischaemic attacks and cerebral tumour. British Medical Journal i:205

Harrison M J G, Marshall J 1977 Evidence of silent cerebral embolism in patients with amaurosis fugax. Journal of Neurology, Neurosurgery and Psychiatry 40:651

Hass W K, Fields W S, North R R, Kricheff I I, Chase N E, Bauer R B 1968 Joint study of extracranial arterial occlusion. II Angiography, techniques, sites and complications. Journal of the American Medical Association 203:961

Hossman K A, Mies G 1980 Regional EEG frequency analysis in patients with cerebrovascular disease. In: Bes A, Geraud G (eds.) Cerebral circulation and neurotransmitters. Excerpta Medica, Amsterdam, Oxford. p 67

Ingvar D H, Sjolung B, Ardo A 1976 Correlation between dominant EEG frequency, cerebral oxygen uptake and blood flow. Electroencephalography and Clinical Neurophysiology 41:268

Jorgensen L, Torvik A 1966 Ischaemic cerebrovascular diseases in an autopsy series Part I. Prevalence, location and predisposing factors in verified thromboembolic occlusions and significance in the pathogenesis of cerebral infarction. Journal of Neurological Sciences 3:490

Kartchner M M, McRae L P 1978 Clinical application of oculoplethysmography and carotid phonoangiography. In: Bernstein E F (ed.) Non-invasive techniques in vascular disease. C V Mosby St. Louis. p 201

Kanaya H, Yamasaki M, Saiki I, Furukavra K 1968 The use of echoencephalography to differentiate intracerebral haemorrhage and brain softening. Journal of Neurosurgery 28:539

Kendall B E, Radue E W 1978 Computed tomography in spontaneous intracerebral haematomas. British Journal of Radiology 51:563

Kerber C W, Cromwell L D, Drager B P, Bonk W O 1978 Cerebral ischaemia I. Current angiographic techniques complications and safety. American Journal of Roentgenology 130:1097

Kuhl D E, Engel J, Phelps M E 1980 Emission computed tomography: Application in stroke and epilepsy. In: Bes A, Geraud G (eds.) Cerebral circulation and neurotransmitters. Excerpta medica, Amsterdam, Oxford. p 37

Larsen E B, Omenn A S, Loop J W 1978 Computed tomography in patients with cerebrovascular disease: Impact of a new technology on patient care. American Journal of Roentgenology 131:35

Lhermitte F, Gautier J C, Derouesne C, Guiraud B 1968 Ischaemic accidents in the middle cerebral artery territory. Archives of Neurology 19:248

Luxon L M, Harrison M J G 1979 Chronic subdural haematoma. Quarterly Journal of Medicine 48:43

McKissock W, Richardson A, Walsh L 1959 Primary intracerebral haemorrhage. Lancet ii:683

Merritt H H, Fremont-Smith F 1937 The cerebrospinal fluid. Saunders, Philadelphia

Nelson R F, Pullicino P, Kendall B E, Marshall J 1980 Computed tomography in patients presenting with lacunar syndromes. Stroke 11:256

Nilsson B, Norrving B, Cronquist S, Muller R 1979 Diagnosis and prognosis of small intracerebral haematomas. In: Meyer J S, Lechner H, Reivich M (eds.) Cerebral vascular disease 2. Excerpta Medica Amsterdam, Oxford. p 53

Norton G A, Kishore P R S, Lin J 1978 CT contrast enhancement in cerebral infarction. American Journal of Roentgenology 131:881

O'Brien M D 1979 Ischaemic cerebral edema. A review. Stroke 10:623

Perrone P, Candelise L, Scotti G, de Grandi C, Scialfa G 1979 CT evaluation in patients with transient ischaemic attack. European Neurology 18:217

Phillips B M 1964 Temporal lobe changes associated with the syndromes of vertebrobasilar insufficiency: an electroencephalographic study. British Medical Journal ii:1104

Plum F 1971 Edema in cerebral infarction. In: Moossy J, Janeway R (eds.) Cerebral vascular diseases. Grune and Stratton. New York. p 51

Radue E W, Kendall B E 1978 Xenon enhancement in tumours and infarcts. Neuroradiology 16:224

Reisner D, Dal-Bianco P 1979 Computed tomography in intracerebral haemorrhage. In: Meyer J S, Lechner H, Reivich M (eds.) Cerebral vascular disease 2. Excerpta Medica Amsterdam, Oxford. p 66

Roseman E, Schmidt R P, Foltz E L 1952 Serial electoencephalography in vascular lesion of the brain. Neurology 2:311

Shah S, Bull J W D, du Boulay G H, Marshall J, Ross Russell R W, Symon L 1972 A comparison of rapid serial angiography and isotope clearance measurements in cerebrovascular disease. British Journal of Radiology 45:294

Sornas R, Ostlund H, Muller R 1972 Cerebrospinal fluid cytology after stroke. Archives of Neurology 26:489

Sundt T M, Sandok B A, Whisnant J P 1975 Carotid endarterectomy: complications and preoperative assessment of risk. Mayo Clinic Proceedings 50:301

Tow D E, Wagner H N, Deland F H, North W A 1969 Brain scanning in cerebral vascular disease. Journal of the American Medical Association 207:105

Weese de J A, May A G, Lipchick E O, Rob C G 1970 Anatomic and hemodynamic correlation in carotid artery stenosis. Stroke I:149

Weisberg L A 1980 Computerized tomographic enhancement patterns in cerebral infarction. Archives of Neurology 37:21

9

Clinical features of focal cerebral hemisphere infarction

John C. Meadows

Interruption of cerebral blood flow is the commonest cause of focal neurological dysfunction, and the syndromes of infarction that result provide exercises in neural and vascular anatomy. Haemorrhages may cause similar syndromes but are less common and such patients often lapse rapidly into coma which limits study of any focal deficit. The subject of cerebral haemorrhage will not be considered further here.

The size of a cerebral infarct and the syndrome that it produces depend upon many factors. Locally, these include the individual size of a particular vessel's territory, the duration of circulation arrest and the amount of collateral circulation. Individual differences in the regional localisation of higher cerebral function may also be important. Fluent aphasias, for example, do not occur in childhood; in adults, an infarct of Wernicke's area occasionally causes aphasia of conduction type rather than Wernicke's aphasia (see below); aphasia in left handers tends to be milder than in right handers, and it may occur with lesions in either hemisphere. There are probably many other examples.

Internal carotid artery occlusion

Collateral circulation is particularly important where occlusion affects the large neck vessels and where anastomoses between extracranial and intracranial vessels and through the circle of Willis may prevent any infarction at all. Because of the risk of emboli, the unoccluded but atheromatous artery commonly presents a greater risk to the brain than it does if blocked. On the other hand, internal carotid occlusion often does cause cerebral infarction. Mitchell & Schwartz (1965) in their pathological study of unselected fatal strokes, report carotid occlusion in about 20 per cent. These authors did not discuss infarct location but there may be a tendency with carotid occlusion for this to show a particular disposition for the borderzone territory between major arteries, particularly the ring of brain encircling the territory of the middle cerebral artery (Figs. 9.1, 9.5c, 9.5d). A type of asphasia associated with borderzone infarction, transcortical asphasia, may occur with carotid occlusion (Heilman et al, 1976), the characteristic feature being that the patient, though aphasic, can repeat sentences spoken to him. Preservation of peri-Sylvian structures (Wernicke's area, arcuate fasciculus, Broca's area) is held to be necessary.

Borderzone infarction in its purest and most profound form is associated with severe hypotension and is then bilateral (Romanul & Abramowicz, 1964; Adams et al, 1966). The neuropathological consequences of reduction in overall brain blood flow, according to Adams et al, depend upon the rapidity with which and the extent to which flow is reduced. These authors argue that borderzone infarction is caused by systemic hypotension that is profound in degree, and that more moderate but prolonged hypotension is responsible for the different pathological picture of diffuse cerebral neuronal loss that may occur under clinical circumstances not greatly different from those causing borderzone infarctions. Carbon monoxide poisoning may also cause typical borderzone infarction and lead, if the patient survives, to the most severe form of transcortical asphasia, isolation of the speech area (Geschwind et al, 1968).

Carotid branch occlusions

There are two branches of the internal carotid artery before it bifurcates into anterior and middle cerebral arteries.

Ophthalmic artery. Transient ischaemic attacks (amaurosis fugax) caused by emboli are common but occlusion of the ophthalmic artery at its origin is probably symptomless in most instances, because of anastomoses within the orbit. Occlusion at the origin can occur when the parent internal carotid artery is thrombosed, but persisting visual symptoms are rare. The ophthalmic artery may however remain patent, filling retrogradely on angiography, and contributes to cerebral blood flow by maintaining patency of the terminal segment of the internal carotid artery. Retrograde filling was demonstrated angiographically in 17 of 54 cases of carotid occlusion in one recent study, the figure almost doubling when assessed by directional Doppler ultrasound (Kaneda et al, 1979).

Anterior choroidal artery. This vessel supplies various important structures, including globus pallidus, parts of medical temporal lobe, of thalamus (including geniculate body) of subthalmus, of optic tract and of internal capsule, as well as the middle one-third of the cerebral peduncle (which incorporates corticospinal fibres) and substantia nigra (Stephens & Stilwell, 1969). See Fig. 9.1A. Surprisingly little deficit results from its occlusion. The artery may be spared when the internal carotid artery thromboses since it usually arises above the junction with the posterior communicating artery. It was however ligated deliberately at one time following the discovery that its accidental damage at surgery improved Parkinsonism. Although it supplies a large part of lateral geniculate body, proximal ligation caused persisting visual field defects in only one of five such cases studied by Morello & Cooper (1955), probably because of collateral anastomoses. These patients developed no other significant neurological disability though Parkinsonian rigidity and tremor did improve. This was attributed to infarction of the medial part of globus pallidus, which the authors claim is the only neural structure regularly infarcted after occlusion of anterior choroidal artery.

With distal occlusions, collateral circulation may be more limited. Infarction of lateral geniculate has been reported recently in such a case causing loss of contralateral field both superiorly and inferiorly with preservation of a horizontal band of field laterally from fixation (Frisén, 1979). The lateral choroidal (lateral posterior choroid) artery, a branch of posterior cerebral artery, also supplies lateral geniculate body, and the reverse field defect, with loss of a horizontal band of the contralateral mid-field, has been reported to accompany occlusion of this branch (Frisén et al, 1978).

The third group of vessels, reported to supply the medial part of lateral geniculate body are the several small thalmageniculate branches of posterior cerebral artery (see below).

Vertebral artery occlusion

Vertebral artery occlusion will be discussed in Chapter 7, which considers brainstem strokes.

Anterior cerebral artery occlusion

The cortical territories supplied by the three main cerebral arteries have long been known (Fig. 9.1A & B). The blood supply of other structures supplied by these vessels is summarised in Table 9.1.

Table 9.1 Subcortical structures supplied by main cerebral arteries

Anterior cerebral artery	*Posterior cerebral artery*
Anterior limb of internal capsule	Red nucleus
Inferior part of caudate nucleus	Subthalamic nucleus
Anterior column of fornix	Substantia nigra
Anterior 4/5 of corpus callosum.	Oculomotor nuclei
	Upper brainstem reticular formation
Middle cerebral artery	Superior cerebellar peduncle
(see also text on anterior choroidal a.)	Medial lemniscus
Posterior limb of internal capsule	Medial part of cerebral peduncle
Corona radiata	Quadrigeminal plate
Outer part of globus pallidus	Most of thalamus
Most of caudate nucleus	Hippocampus
Putamen.	Posterior column and crus of fornix
	Posterior 1/5 of corpus callosum

The anterior cerebral artery is the smaller of the two terminal branches of the internal carotid artery. It supplies the medial surface as well as

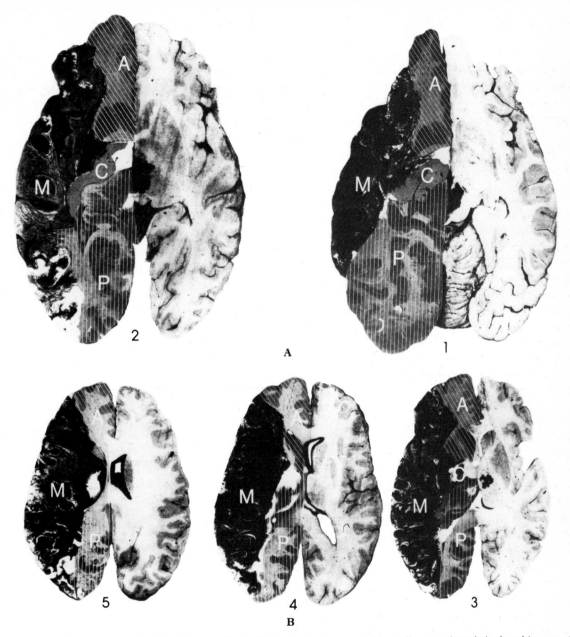

Fig. 9.1 A & B Vascular territories in the normal brain. The brain has been cut horizontally approximately in the orbito meatal plane. Successive sections from below 1–5. A—anterior cerebral territory; M—middle cerebral territory; P—posterior cerebral territory; C—anterior choroidal artery territory.

adjacent rim of lateral convexity of the entire frontal and pariental lobes, and also certain deep structures (Fig 9.1A & B). The segment proximal to the junction with anterior communicating artery is sometimes vestigial, so that one anterior cerebral artery supplies the other through the communi-cating vessel. Bilateral infarction may occasionally occur because of this, but often bilateral infarction is the result of spasm, probably propagating bilaterally, complicating subarachnoid haemor-rhage.

More commonly the anterior communicating

artery tends to protect from infarction. A patent communicating artery acts to prevent thrombus propagation occluding both the proximal and distal segments of the anterior cerebral artery, when one or other segment is initially occluded. Because of the anterior communicating artery, the proximal segment of the anterior cerebral artery can be perfused from either end; the small branches arising from it are thus in a privileged position and may escape occlusion as a consequence.

There are two groups of small branches that usually arise from the proximal segment. The inferior group, un-named, supplies optic nerve and chiasm. These vessels rarely show evidence of occlusion clinically, perhaps for the reasons just discussed, but also because they join a pial anastomosis around the optic nerve and chiasm.

The other group comprises the multiple small *medial striate arteries*, which penetrate upwards through anterior perforated substance. They supply anterior hypothalamus, part of anterior commissure, anterior columns of fornix and part of striatum. The largest branch, *Heubner's artery*, penetrates the anterior perforated substance between the medial and lateral striate arteries (the latter arising from middle cerebral artery) to supply anterior commisure, internal capsule and head of the candate nucleus. According to Stephens & Stilwell (1969) Heubner's artery does not, as is often implied, supply the cortiscospinal tract, which runs in the posterior limb of the internal capsule.

It is usually said that occlusion of Heubner's artery causes paralysis of contralateral face and upper limb (especially proximally). The author knows of no published report of proven Heubner's artery occlusion.

Occlusion of distal anterior cerebral artery beyond the junction with anterior communicating artery causes contralateral inferior crural monoplegia and cortical sensory loss. There may be some weakness of the arm, worse proximally, since the shoulder region is represented higher on the motor strip than more distal parts of the limb. It is not clear whether, in the occasional cases where there is also mild facial weakness (usually in spontaneous expression more than on command), this results from damage to frontal cortex, to basal nuclei through occlusion of deep perforating

branches of the proximal anterior cerebral artery, or to structures outside anterior cerebral territory (Fig. 9.2).

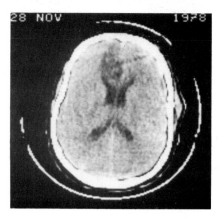

Fig. 9.2 Anterior cerebral infarction (unilateral)
 A 49-year-old man had a subarachnoid haemorrhage due to anterior cerebral aneurysm which was clipped 6 days later. He remained drowsy and mute; right hemiparesis was noted. As speech returned he was noted to be mildly aphasic. Speech and limb function recovered. He remained childish, apathetic, irritable and sexually irresponsible. Two years later there had been little improvement.

A grasp reflex and 'gegenhalten' (paratonic rigidity) may be found in the early stages of anterior cerebral artery infarction. There may be some incontinence, and a state of stupor, but once the conscious level has improved it is unusual for sphincter disturbance to continue unless frontal lobe infarction is sufficient to cause major behaviour change. The type of sphincter disturbance (sudden embarrassing incontinence often preceded by urgency) described by Andrew & Nathan (1964) may occur but seems to be commoner with tumours (Maurice-Williams 1974) than with strokes (Fig 9.3).

Extensive frontal lobe infarction especially when it affects both sides may cause a state of irritable apathy or inappropriate jocularity, with irresponsible and uninhibited behaviour which is sometimes sexually directed. Occasionally a striking confabulatory response may be seen either with (Stuss et al, 1978) or without (Kapur & Coughlan, 1970) severe amnesia. Usually there has been a subarachnoid haemorrhage from anterior communicating or anterior cerebral artery aneurysm when severe amnesia occurs (Talland et al, 1967) Ischaemic damage to the fornix, possibly through

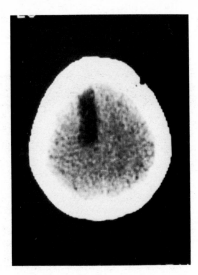

Fig. 9.3 Anterior cerebral infarction (distal territory)
A 45-year-old patient with mitral stenosis had an embolic occlusion of the left anterior cerebral artery. The right leg showed pyramidal signs and cortical sensory loss. There was transient weakness of the right arm.

occlusion of medial striate branches, may be responsible, though argument continues about the clinical significance of damage to this structure (Woolsey & Nelson, 1975) (Fig. 9.4).

Right-sided frontal damage within the territory of either anterior cerebral or middle cerebral artery may cause contralateral neglect (visual and tactile extinction, inaccurate bisection of lines, unilateral

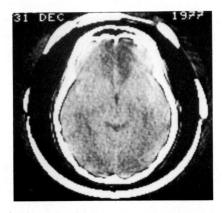

Fig. 9.4 Bilateral anterior cerebral infarction
A 37-year-old woman had a subarachnoid haemorrhage from an anterior communicating aneurysm demonstrated at angiography. Also noted was marked bilateral spasm of the subarachnoid carotid arteries. She remained stuporose responding by withdrawal to painful stimuli. She died of pulmonary complications 2 weeks later.

neglect in drawing etc.) though this is usually temporary in vascular disease (Heilman & Valenstein, 1972).

The effects of infarction of the supplementary motor area, which lies within anterior cerebral artery territory just in front of the primary motor cortex, are not accurately known but evidence is accumulating in the case of the dominant hemisphere that a form of aphasia may result. Stimulation experiments in this region are known to cause vocalisation and infarction appears to produce an initial picture of mutism, which has evolved in the cases reported through a form of transcortical motor aphasia, (very limited spontaneous speech with preserved comprehension and ability to repeat sentences spoken by the examiner), sometimes to near normality (Kyörney, 1975; Rubens, 1975; Masdeu et al, 1978). Occasional cases of anterior cerebral artery infarction have been quoted (see Rubens 1975 discussion) where aphasia is said to have approximated to Broca's type (agrammatic speech with repetition affected as severely as spontaneous speech), suggesting more inferiorly placed frontal damage. It has been suggested that deep white matter damage undercuts the cortex of the inferior part of the convexity of the frontal lobe in such cases. Occlusion of Heubner's branch has been invoked as the cause.

The other major consequence of anterior cerebral artery infarction, uncommon in well-marked form, is due to callosal damage, disconnecting parts of the two hemispheres (Geschwind & Kaplan, 1962; Rubens 1975). The most classical features comprise apraxia and agraphia of the left hand, and inability to name objects placed in the left hand.

Middle cerebral artery occlusion

The middle cerebral artery supplies most of the convexity of the cerebral hemisphere and, through penetrating branches arising at its origin, the posterior limb of the internal capsule, putamen, and parts of caudate nucleus and globus pallidus, as well as much deep white matter (see Fig. 9.1).

The penetrating branches comprise three to six *medial striate arteries* representing a continuation of those arising from the proximal anterior cerebral artery, and three to six much larger *lateral striate arteries* (Stephens & Stilwell, 1969), often called lenticulostriate arteries. Occlusion of a single penetrating artery is probably the commonest though not the only cause of pure motor hemiplegic stroke. As with other 'lacunar' (perforating artery) strokes, hypertension and intrinsic disease of the perforating artery are usually present. In a recent clinicopathological study of 11 such capsular infarcts (Fisher, 1979) most involved the posterior limb of the capsule and most (7 cases) were caused by severe atheroma involving a perforating artery; one artery was occluded by lipohyalinosis, two were patent (presumed embolic occlusion) and in one the only finding was luminal narrowing by one-third by atheroma. Pure motor hemiplegic stroke has also been reported with pontine (Fisher & Curry, 1965) and medullary (Ropper et al, 1979) lacunar infarction, and another lacunar syndrome, the dysarthria-clumsy hand syndrome, classically associated with pontine infarction (Fisher, 1967 can occur with capsular infarction (Spertell & Ransom, 1979), so the localising value of these syndromes is less precise than is sometimes supposed.

The commonest site for lacunar infarct on pathological examination is the lenticular nucleus (especially putamen), supplied by lateral striate arteries; but the clinical syndrome that results from a single lenticular lacunar infarct is uncertain. Possibly the occlusion passes unnoticed, or causes very transient hemiparesis. Bilateral and multiple lenticular infarcts may form the pathological basis of 'marche à petits pas'. Major infarction of the striatum, particularly putamen, with less involvement of descending motor pathways, seems to underlie the syndrome of post-hemiplegic athetosis in childhood (Dooling & Adams, 1975). There is initially a pure motor hemiplegia which improves to a point, but mobility is then limited by the emergence of severe athetoid movements.

Occlusion at the origin of the middle cerebral artery causes drowsiness or stupor, especially in left-sided cases (Albert et al, 1976). There is hemiplegia affecting face, arm and leg, hemianopia and cortical sensory loss. The eyes at rest tend to deviate to the side of the lesion, probably because of damage to the frontal eye field (middle frontal gyrus). Disturbances of higher cerebral function are obvious in alert patients;

aphasia is the dominant feature with left-sided infarcts and contralateral neglect with right-sided infarcts (see below).

In the few days following onset, conscious level may sometimes deteriorate because of the effects of oedema developing in relation to so large an infarct. In spite of this many patients survive. Initial flaccid hemiplegia then slowly gives place to typical spastic hemiplegia. The arm remains functionally useless but extensor tone, developing in the leg allows limited walking eventually in all but a few; these are usually left hemiplegics and an indifferent attitude may be responsible for their failure.

When the perforating branches are spared infarction is mainly cortical. The posterior limb of internal capsule, which contains the pyramidal tract (Englander et al, 1975) is not itself infarcted. Much of the cortical motor and sensory representation is destroyed but the leg and foot areas are spared. Provided subcortical infarction does not extend too deeply into corona radiata, the resulting contralateral paralysis may spare the leg (see Fig. 9.5A).

Left-sided infarction

The changes so far described do not take into account the major behavioural differences between the hemispheres. In left middle cerebral artery occlusion the clinical picture is usually characterized by profound **global aphasia.** The major areas concerned with language function are destroyed; speech may be absent at first and then is limited to no more than a few words, usually stereotyped and commonly paraphasic, spoken with effort and often out of context. Expletives may be retained. There is grossly impaired comprehension and inability to repeat material spoken by the examiner. Reading and writing is impossible. There is apraxia but testing is difficult because of the gross aphasia.

Middle cerebral artery branch occlusions fractionate this major deficit to produce various focal syndromes. Named branches are recognised arteriographically but neither their precise territories of supply nor their mode of origin from middle cerebral artery are very constant. Attempts at correlating infarcts demonstrated on isotope or

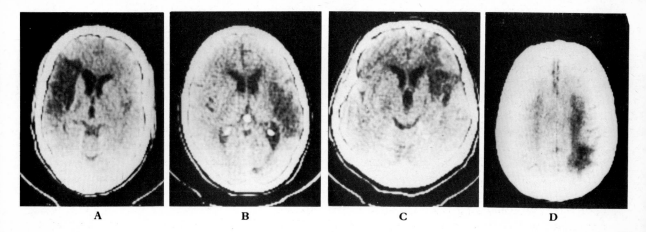

A   B   C   D

Fig. 9.5 These four scans illustrate infarction in various parts of the cortical distribution of the middle cerebral artery and its borderzone.
(A) Left middle cerebral infarction sparing basal ganglia A 46-year-old man with sudden right hemiparesis and expressive dysphasia. Right leg rapidly improved.
(B) Right parietal infarction: middle cerebral artery territory A 67-year-old man sudden onset of deadness and weakness left arm. Recent myocardial infarction. Left visual sensory inattention. Astereognosis left arm.
(C) Right middle cerebral'and borderzone infarction. A 68-year-old man with right internal carotid occlusion presented with left sided TIA progressing to left sided infarction. Leg only mildly affected. Distal weakness of arm.
(D) Right-sided middle posterior watershed infarct 78-year-old man with sudden onset of clumsiness of left arm. Complete left homonymous hemianopia. Slight weakness left arm. Cortical sensory loss; visual spatial tests abnormal.

CAT scan with named branches is not easy, nor indeed always useful.

Commonly the middle cerebral artery bifurcates in the Sylvian fissure into two main divisions, often first giving off branches to the temporal and less commonly to the frontal poles; the effects of occlusion of these polar branches is not well established.

The anterior main division branches in turn, and these vessels emerge round the frontoparietal operculum to supply frontal and anterior parietal cortex. The more or less synonymous radiological terms 'ascending frontal artery complex', 'operculofrontal group' and 'candelabra group' apply to these vessels. The posterior main division also breaks up (posterior parietal, angular and posterior temporal arteries) to supply temporal and posterior parietal cortex postero-inferior to the line of the fissure (Fig. 9.5B).

Occlusion of the anterior main division of middle cerebral artery infarcts the lower part of the convexity of the frontal lobe together with antero-inferior parietal cortex. Contralateral paralysis and cortical sensory loss affects mainly arm and face. There is Broca's aphasia (non-fluent, agrammati-

cal, effortful, dysarthric speech with inability to repeat sentences spoken by the examiner, but very little impairment of comprehension). Often there is little or no speech at first, and the characteristic aphasic type may take days or weeks to develop. In time facial weakness may sometimes be very mild indeed, in spite of almost certain infarction of the face area of Rolandic cortex. The reason for this is open to conjecture. Paralysis of the arm remains severe. Buccofacial and ideomotor apraxia of the unparalysed left limb are usual; to command the patent may be unable, for example, to protrude his tongue, suck an imaginary straw, blow out an imaginary match or imitate the use of tools such as hammer and saw (Benson & Geschwind, 1971).

Traditionally Broca's aphasia has been related to a more restricted lesion than that caused by occlusion of the anterior main division of middle cerebral artery, which destroys a large area of frontal cortex. Broca's aphasia was attributed to a lesion of Broca's area, the posterior part of the inferior frontal gyrus (Benson & Geschwind, 1971). Evidence is accumulating, however, that a larger lesion is necessary (Mohr et al, 1978). This correlates with the fact that paralysis of the arm almost always co-exists with Broca's aphasia, and indeed is a more consistent feature than facial weakness.

What deficit then results from infarction *confined* to Broca's area? This is not certain but there is some evidence that this is the condition often called aphemia (Bastian, 1887), an uncommon syndrome known to be associated with posterior inferior frontal pathology but long in search of more precise localisation. Unlike Broca's aphasia, limb paralysis in this syndrome is conspicuous by its absence or is very transient, thus according with the notion of more restricted lesion. In its severe and pure form a condition of mutism occurs, with little or no disturbance of writing. Speech slowly improves to a state of effortful but linguistically accurate speech without the agrammatism typical of Broca's aphasia. Buccofacial apraxia is usually present.

The other characteristic vascular syndrome that may arise with more posteriorly placed supra-Sylvian infarcts is that of conduction aphasia. This syndrome occurs with infarction of parietal operculum, behind Rolandic cortex. It is believed to be caused by interruption of the arcuate (superior longitudinal) fasciculus which connects Wernicke's and Broca's areas, and runs in the parietal operculum (Benson et al, 1973) but the syndrome may also occur (see below) in some cases of infarction of Wernicke's area. In conduction aphasia, fluent, paraphasic speech is accompanied by good comprehension but impaired ability to repeat words and sentences spoken by the examiner. Ideomotor apraxia is usually present. There may be contralateral cortical sensory loss or, less common, hemiparesis, though both may be absent. Occasionally too, there may be the peculiar feature of contralaterally diminished pain sensitivity, or even spontaneous pain, in lesions of the parietal operculum (Biemond, 1956; Denny-Brown & Chambers, 1958; Benson et al, 1973).

Occlusion of the posterior main division of middle cerebral artery causes aphasia, typically of Wernicke's type as its major consequence. Fluent paraphasic speech is accompanied by severe impairment of comprehension and repetition, without contralateral paralysis or sensory deficit. The lateral part of the temporal lobe which is infarcted includes Wernicke's area (posterior part of superior temporal gyrus), damage to which is believed to be

responsible for Wernicke's aphasia. Also infarcted is the angular gyrus region, but the important consequences of this (see below) may not manifest because of the aphasia (Fig. 9.5D).

Discrete infarcts destroying Wernicke's area will usually produce Wernicke's aphasia. Occasionally they will instead cause conduction aphasia (see above). It has been argued that in the latter cases *right* Wernicke's area assumes the function of comprehension but still requires to communicate with (*left*) Broca's area. The pathway by which it does so (from right to left Wernicke's area and thence forward via arcuate fasciculus) is, it is suggested, interrupted by the lesion (Benson et al, 1973). The effect, in disconnection terms, is akin to a lesion of arcuate fasciculus in the conventional model.

Rarely, another syndrome, pure word deafness, may result from infarcts close to, but sparing Wernicke's area, yet interrupting auditory input to it (Geschwind, 1965). This is discussed later.

Infarction which spares Wernicke's area but damages the angular gyrus region more posteriorly (angular artery) may cause aphasia but this is usually mild and of anomic type (fluent often circumlocutory speech due to word-finding difficulty but no paraphasia, impairment of comprehension or repetition defect). A more specific disturbance with infarcts in this region is that of alexia with agraphia (Dejerine, 1892). Gerstmann's syndrome (finger agnosia, right-left disorientation, acalculia and agraphia) may also be seen. These three syndromes may occur in relatively pure form but are more commonly combined in varying degrees. (Benson & Geschwind, 1971).

Right-sided infarction

The patient's reaction to the hemiplegia and hemisensory loss that follows major middle cerebral artery occlusions tends to be different in right-sided cases from left. The patient with a right-sided infarct has a flat, sometimes expressionless affect; he may appear indifferent to his disability and may even deny or joke about it laconically. He neglects the left side of space as well as his paralysed limbs and can even be shown to manifest neglect on the right. The indifference contrasts with the anxiety and distress that often characterises major left hemisphere strokes.

This reaction is usually attributed to right parietal damage. Yet strokes do not cause hemiplegia at all if *strictly* confined to the parietal lobe. This leads one to question traditional views about the effects of right parietal strokes. Reported cases upon which conclusions have been based in the past have been vascular lesions almost certainly extending outside parietal lobe, or tumours with distorting effects on adjacent areas, thus causing left-sided paralysis. Neglect may accompany hemiplegia resulting from infarcts localised by scanning techniques, in the right frontal lobe (Heilman & Valenstein, 1972).

What then is the result of discrete right parietal infarction? Geschwind has discussed these difficulties in the past and has reported confusional states without other obvious neurological abnormalities, in association with discrete right middle cerebral artery infarcts, some in parietal territory (Mesulam et al, 1976). It seems probable that such cases often escape correct diagnosis. The author has seen a patient with early Steele-Richardson syndrome (progressive supranuclear palsy) without clinically obvious mental change, in whom a substantial right posterior parietal infarct was seen on CAT scan. Full clinical examination failed to show any abnormality and intensive enquiry only revealed a period lasting two or three days, some six weeks earlier, when she had difficulty dressing. Dressing and telling the time, like other tasks depending upon complex constructional or spatial analysis, may be disturbed with right parietal lesions, but these do not always reach clinical notice.

Disorientation in place has also often been attributed to right parietal strokes but the author has neither seen nor read of a case where pathology has been shown to be confined to the parietal region. The classical studies of Brain (1941) Paterson & Zangwill (1944, 1945) and McFie et al (1950) led to the view that right parietal lesions cause such disorientation, although with the exception of the special type of topographical disturbance described by Brain in 1941, these authors themselves made no such claims. (Brain described a type of topographical disturbance in which massive lesions of the right parietal lobe caused inability to follow familiar routes owing to a consistent selection of right instead of left turns.)

These and later authors did show conclusively that map and plan drawing, and route finding from plans, were particularly defective in the presence of right parietal lesions. But tests such as these depend as much on constructional analysis and drawing ability — functions recognised to be disturbed by parietal lesions — as on orientation in the environment. Similar qualifications apply in the case of many tests employing mazes. The tacit assumption has prevailed that these tests explore the same mechanisms which are disturbed when patients lose their way in surroundings that should be familiar to them. There is no evidence that this is so.

Apart from the very rare type of topographical disturbance mentioned by Brain (which was seen in tumours rather than in strokes), patients who lose their way specifically are probably always suffering from 'topographical memory' loss. Where there is localisable pathology this is usually *temporal*, usually a posteriorly placed, right-sided space-occupying lesion. The odd feature is that this is not a regular association suggesting the importance of some additional factor. Possibly this additional factor in tumours is a remote contralateral effect caused by displacement and distortion, for unilateral infarcts do not cause topographical memory loss whereas bilateral infarcts sometimes do. These are in posterior cerebral artery territory and will be discussed in a later section.

Posterior cerebral artery occlusion

The two posterior cerebral arteries arise at the bifurcation of the basilar artery. In a small proportion of cases one or both arteries retain the embryonic pattern into adult life so that the vessel's major supply is via posterior communicating artery from the carotid system.

Each posterior cerebral artery supplies the occipital lobe and the medial and inferior surfaces of the temporal lobe. On its course backwards round the side of the brain stem before it reaches cerebral cortex it gives off many small branches to the upper mid-brain and posterior diencephalon, including thalmus. Some supply the mid-brain exclusively and will be considered in Chapter 7.

Others supply diencephalic structures of which thalamus is the most important.

One syndrome of thalamic infarction is the so-called thalamic syndrome of Dejerine & Roussy (1906), which is usually said to result from infarction of thalamogeniculate branches, of which there are usually three to five, (Stephens & Stilwell 1969). In this syndrome, infarction of postero-ventral nucleus of thalamus causes a hemisensory stroke. When this affects particularly spinothalamic and trigeminothalamic pathways, there often develops in time a persisting contralateral spontaneous pain, accompanied by hyperpathia, as may occur in disturbances of this pathway at other levels in the nervous system. A mild hemiparesis, which is often present at the outset, occasionally gives place to persisting athetoid posturing or tremor of the contralateral limbs. (Head & Holmes, 1920). There is also usually a hemianopia (Fig. 9.6A). Isolated infarction of the closely related subthalamus or its connections may cause hemiballismus.

The visual syndrome (Frisén et al, 1978) that may result from occlusion of lateral choroid (otherwise know as lateral posterior choroid) branch of posterior cerebral artery has been discussed in the section on anterior choroidal artery. Sometimes the vessel is duplicated right from its origin from the posterior cerebral artery (Stephens & Stilwell, 1969). Apart from supplying choroid plexus, lateral geniculate body and a part of thalamus, it also supplies crus, commissure, body and part of the anterior columns of the fornix so may possibly be important in the aetiology of some vascular cases of amnesia; if for example one lateral choroidal artery were much larger than the other and provided the exclusive supply to the commissure of the fornix, then its occlusion would damage hippocampal outflow bilaterally.

Occlusion of the basilar bifurcation usually leads to death, but blockage of perforating vessels arising from it may cause midline, butterfly-shaped infarcts involving posterior thalami and adjacent structures (Facon et al, 1958; Brain, 1958; Castaigne et al, 1962; L'Hermitte et al, 1963; Segarra, 1970). There are profound effects on cerebral function, and a somnolent form of akinetic mutism may occur. The affected patient is somnolent but rousable to an immobile mute state, yet shows no signs of major damage to descending motor

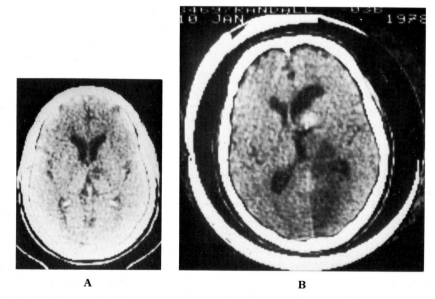

A   B

Fig. 9.6 (A) Unilateral thalamic infarction. A 72-year-old woman who developed sudden left hemianaesthesia but little weakness. Spontaneous pain and hemichorea developed week later.
(B) Posterior cerebral infarction. A 67-year-old man who had developed left hemiparesis 2 years earlier, presented with acute worsening of left sided weakness, left hemianopia and right third nerve palsy. CAT scan revealed a large aneurysm, probably arising at the junction of posterior arteries on the right, associated with infarction in the distribution of right posterior cerebral artery.

pathways. Segarra has attributed this syndrome, which may be accompanied by oculomotor disorders of varied type, to occlusion particularly of the posterior paramedian artery of Percheron, which is said to arise from the origin of one or other posterior cerebral artery and which bifurcates to supply bilaterally the posterior thalamus, rostral periventricular grey matter and reticular nuclei. If the lesion extends further forward (anterior paramedian artery of Percheron), according to Segarra dementia occurs too, as in the cases reported by Castaigne et al, 1966. Apart from the small but important brain stem/diencephalic branches the major supply of each posterior cerebral artery is to occipital and inferior temporal lobes.

The most consistent result of occlusion is a homonymous field defect, hemianopic when complete due to infarction of striate (calcarine) cortex (Fig. 9.6B). At the onset, ipsilateral headache, or pain around the eye is common. Usually the field defect is absolute and, if it does not recover in 24 hours, persists indefinitely. Similar defects may follow occlusion of the calcarine branch itself. On the other hand, infarction may sometimes be confined to calcarine cortex even when the proximal trunk is occluded, because of abundant pial anastomoses. Indeed, in rare cases there may be no clinical deficit at all with proven occlusion of the main trunk (Ross Russell, 1973) or calcarine artery (Hoyt & Newton, 1970). Infarcts affecting part of striate cortex may cause partial homonymous field defects, their pattern depending upon the well-known topographical cortical map. Such field defects are usually congruous but there are reasons for supposing that this may not always be so (see review by Meadows, 1976).

Striate cortex extends back on the medial surface of the hemisphere to the occipital lobe tip, and for a variable distance beyond on to the lateral convexity (Brindley, 1972). The posterior part of striate cortex comprises the macular representation and has a particularly abundant blood supply because of anastomoses between posterior and middle cerebral arteries. Survival of the occipital pole because of this dual supply is one reason for macular sparing in hemianopia from unilateral posterior cerebral artery occlusion. It is also responsible for the retained tunnel vision sometimes seen in bilateral posterior cerebral artery disease (see below).

Right and left-sided infarction

Hemianopia is almost always the only clinical manifestation in right-sided infarcts. In a minority of left-sided cases there is other cerebral dysfunction. The most striking syndrome is that of alexia without agraphia (pure alexia, pure word blindness).

Some reading difficulty is usual with right hemianopia owing to disturbed visual scanning, but can also be due to minor degrees of alexia without agraphia. Severe alexia without agraphia is less common and very striking.

The patient cannot read visually. He can however see the words for he can copy them slavishly. He can 'read', non-visually, words spelled aloud to him or written on the palm of the hand. When endeavouring to read visually he may succeed better with numbers or other symbols (fractions, decimals, £, % etc). He can write spontaneously but after a few moments may be unable to read back what he has written. Commonly associated is the syndrome of colour anomia, sometimes called colour agnosia. The afflicted patient has no complaint about his colour vision which can be shown to be normal. But he names colours incorrectly sometimes bizarrely, and may for example call a red item green at one time and black at another. It is interesting that a small sub-group of dyslexic boys has been recognised where colour naming is defective (Denckla, 1972).

The accepted explanation for both alexia without agraphia and this form of colour anomia is as follows. Because of left occipital infarction visual information does not reach the left hemisphere directly. It can however be transmitted from the normal right hemisphere provided that commissural fibres are intact. Information about reading and colour naming is peculiar amongst visual material (for possible reasons see Geschwind & Fusillo, 1966) in that its transmission from right to left hemisphere appears to be largely confined to the splenium of the corpus callosum. In cases of alexia without agraphia examined pathologically left occipital lobe infarction has extended forwards to destroy commissural fibres traversing the splenium.

This explanation was first proposed by Dejerine following pathological studies in two cases. The more celebrated case (Dejerine, 1892) acutely lost the ability to read, and at a much later stage suffered a second stroke that caused the loss of writing ability too. Ten days later the patient died. Post-mortem examination revealed an old infarct destroying left visual cortex and part of the splenium, preventing access of relevant visual material to the left hemisphere, according to Dejerine, and accounting for the initial pure alexia. There was a second fresh infarct in the left angular gyrus; Djerine conjectured that damage to this area, now known to be important for linguistic coding and decoding of visual symbols, was responsible for the superadded agraphia. There has been ample confirmation of these pathological findings in recent years, since Geschwind & Fusillo (1966) rekindled interest in the subject.

Two other disturbances that may be associated with left posterior cerebral artery occlusion are word-finding difficulty (anomia or nominal aphasia) and amnesia (Benson et al, 1974a). Neither is usually severe and both tend to be transient though this is not always so. The anomia is believed to be due to left inferotemporal damage, and the amnesia to infarction of hippocampus or its connections. It is often held that unilateral lesions do not cause clinical amnesia and it might be argued that in these cases there is undisclosed damage on the opposite site. This explanation is however countered by the fact that right-sided posterior cerebral artery infarction rarely if ever causes clinical amnesia.

One suggestion to account for the condition of transient global amnesia has been transient ischaemia confined to the inferotemporal region.

Bilateral cerebral infarcts

In the past, little interest has been shown in the effects of bilateral cerebral infarction. Even now it is commonplace to assume that the effect of such strokes is too complex to be worth analysis. Careful study can however throw significant light upon brain mechanisms that are bilaterally represented, where a unilateral lesion may cause little or no defect. The best known example is pseudobulbar palsy, caused by bilateral Rolandic or corticobulbar pathway infarcts, but it is in the field of higher cerebral function that bilateral infarcts may have the most striking effects.

In *anterior cerebral artery* territory, bilateral infarcts increase the behavioural changes that occur with unilateral lesions, and may be associated with much greater depression of conscious level (Nielsen & Jacobs, 1951; Barris & Schuman, 1953) even leading to death. Amnesia is more likely, but generally the effects of bilateral lesions tend to be cumulative without special features.

Within *middle cerebral artery* territory, however, there are various interesting examples of the combined effects of bilateral lesions. These include visuo-motor ataxia (associated with parieto-occipital lesions and more commonly seen with posterior cerebral artery infarcts, in which section it will be discussed), cortical deafness, some cases of pure word deafness, and rare types of aphasia.

Cortical deafness (Bramwell, 1927; Le Gros Clark & Russell, 1938; Jerger et al, 1969; Earnest et al, 1977) results from bilateral lesions of Heschl's gyrus (primary acoustic cortex) on the upper surface of the temporal lobe, or of its afferent projection. Because of bilateral projection from each ear, unilateral lesions are without effect, but bilateral lesions deprive both hemispheres of hearing and render the subject deaf, in severe cases completely.

Pure word deafness results when lesions singly or in combination spare some acoustic cortex but disconnect it from Wernicke's speech area. (Gazzaniga et al, 1973; Kanshepolsky et al, 1973). This can happen with a single critically placed left-sided subcortical infarct which destroys the auditory radiation and callosal fibres from the contralateral acoustic cortex: the left hemisphere is rendered deaf and the right hemisphere cannot transmit information to Wernicke's area which remains intact. Alternatively bilateral infarcts, one destroying acoustic cortex or radiation on the left, and the other destroying the same callosal fibres in the right hemisphere will have the same effect. The patient appears deaf to speech but not to other material, can read and in pure form has normal speech output. In practice, because of the proximity of Wernicke's area to the left-sided lesion, some degree of aphasic contamination is common.

Second-stroke aphasia. In most patients with aphasic strokes, speech improves with time. The younger the patient the better the outlook. Children in particular may regain normal language function after massive left hemisphere strokes; sometimes this happens within a matter of months suggesting prior, latent learning in the right hemisphere. In adults aphasic speech usually persists after a period of improvement. In certain cases, speech can then be shown to be arising in the right hemisphere (Kinsbourne, 1971) and a second stroke in the right hemisphere may then cause deterioration of speech.

The *posterior cerebral artery* territory provides further striking examples of the special effects that may be seen with bilateral infarcts. The common origin of the two posterior cerebral arteries from the basilar artery renders these vessels particularly liable to bilateral occlusion. When damage is severe, striate cortex may be destroyed on both sides leading to 'cortical blindness'. According to Symonds & MacKenzie (1957) this is permanent in about one quarter of cases. In a proportion there may be denial of blindness, often accompanied by confabulation; this is commoner in elderly, confused or obtunded patients. In cortical blindness the visual pathway from retina to brain stem is unaffected, and the pupillary light reflex is characteristically preserved. Direct visual connections with brain stem nuclei (then projecting via thalamus to visual association cortex) may also be responsible for the remarkable discovery in recent years that in certain cases there may be some preservation of visual function capable of influencing conscious behaviour even in the presence of a complete field loss from striate cortex destruction. The patient reported by Weiskrantz et al (1974) could for example distinguish a large ' × ' from an 'O' and detect the orientation of a rod in an area of dense field loss. Remarkable also is the fact that the patient regarded his responses as guesses and did not easily accept that he was responding accurately. How commonly this occurs in bilateral occipital lobe infarction remains to be established.

In most cases of bilateral posterior cerebral artery occlusion, however, there remains some obvious visual function, at least the ability to perceive luminous flux or movement. In many cases there is central visual sparing with good or excellent acuity and retained visual field for a few degrees around fixation because of anastomoses with middle cerebral artery branches at the occipital pole. Sometimes the preserved central field in these cases may extend as a vertical slit, either up or down from fixation, or even in both directions. When pronounced this may sometimes imply occlusion of calcarine artery itself, with collateral supply reaching upper or lower margins of striate cortex from parieto-occipital branch of posterior cerebral artery above, or the posterior temporal branch below. The striate margins represent lower and upper halves of the midline visual fields. A pathologically examined case demonstrating this is reported briefly by Meadows (1976); a stroke in this patient resulted in complete bilateral field loss except for the perimacular region and a strip of the vertical meridian above; striate cortex was destroyed bilaterally except for its inferior border.

Accompanying the visual field defects of bilateral posterior cerebral artery infarction, whether the visual loss is profound or not, it is common for there to be either confusion or amnesia or both. Confusional behaviour was emphasised first by Horenstein et al, (1967). In cases seen by the author it has usually been transient sometimes to be replaced by amnesia (retained remote memory and span of comprehension, e.g. digit span, but inability to learn new material and profound loss of recent memory). Severe amnesia may be a pronounced and persisting consequence of bilateral posterior cerebral infarcts. It has been attributed to bilateral hippocampal infarction (Glees & Griffith, 1952; Victor et al, 1961) but the view that damage to hippocampus itself is necessary has been challenged (Horel, 1978).

It is where bilateral posterior cerebral infarcts spare sufficient visual field and acuity for disturbances of higher aspects of visual function to be manifest that some of the most peculiar neurological disorders occur. Restricted inferiorly placed infarcts when situated bilaterally in the region of the occipito-temporal junction may produce the bizarre syndrome of *prosopagnosia*, the specific inability to recognise familiar faces. The prosopagnosic patient typically has no difficulty recognising everyday objects, although he may be quite unable to recognise even members of his family unless they speak, when he immediately identifies their voices. In many cases it can be shown (e.g., by the ability to match facial photographs) that facial discrimination is normal but that memory for faces is not. In the majority of such cases, there are homonymous visual field defects, almost always in the left upper quadrant and sometimes in the right upper quadrant as well. Why there should be a much higher incidence of left-sided field defects when other evidence including pathological studies indicates that bilateral lesions in the occipito-temporal region are necessary for prosopagnosia is not clear (Meadows, 1974a). There is much evidence suggesting that the right hemisphere is more important for facial recognition, but damage to both hemispheres appears to be necessary for the fully-fledged syndrome.

Topographical memory loss (loss of orientation in familiar surroundings) when due to infarction usually accompanies prosopagnosia suggesting a similar anatomical basis, but can occur independently (Whiteley & Warrington, 1978). The other but much rarer disorder that can be seen with discrete bilateral inferior occipital infarcts is a disturbance of colour vision, usually known as *acquired achromatopsia* or *cerebral colour blindness* (Meadows 1974b; Green & Lassell, 1977; Pearlman et al, 1978) The environment appears drained of colour and in severe cases the subject perceives everything in black and white.

The anatomical basis of associative *visual agnosia*, where objects are seen but not recognised (a 'percept stripped of its meaning' — Teuber, 1968) is not well established. Generally patients are elderly or have had more than one stroke. In some cases an obvious factor has been left posterior cerebral artery occlusion causing the syndrome of alexia without agraphia, as well as visual agnosia (See Geschwind, 1965; Rubens & Benson, 1971; Benson et al, 1974b). It has been argued that the lesions causing agnosia in some way separate the visual stimulus from the language area. Albert et al (1979) argue against this view on the basis of anatomical studies of a patient with multiple strokes. Bilateral loss of visuo-limbic connections was suggested as the cause in this patient. Their explanation however, does not account for other

reports in the literature of infarcts at this site causing prosopagnosia withot visual agnosia.

Visuo-motor ataxia. Bilateral superiorly placed occipital or parieto-occipital infarcts produce a disturbance of motor coordination that has been variously termed visuo-motor ataxia, optic ataxia and disturbed visual orientation. The affected patient cannot gauge visually the direction or distance of objects in space. He cannot reach out accurately for an object and walks with trepidation since he cannot orientate himself in relation to his surroundings (Holmes, 1918). Bilateral lesions are necessary for the fully developed syndrome, which is believed to be caused by a visuo-motor disconnection, and in this case there is usually disturbed visual attention, which may be to both sides so that the patient behaves as if he only notices the single object upon which his gaze is fixed. There may also be a disturbance of eye movements, a form of oculomotor apraxia. Since the parieto-occipital regions are 'watershed' or borderzone territories where arterial perfusion pressure is lowest, bilateral infarctions may be produced by episodes of systemic hypotension or may occur during cardiac surgery (Fig. 9.7) (Ross Russell & Bharucha, 1978).

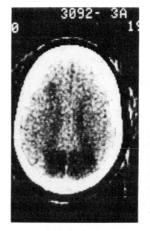
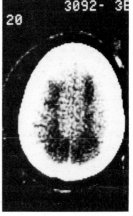

Fig. 9.7 Bilateral watershed infarction (parieto occipital) A 50-year-old patient who developed severe bilateral visual disorientation followed repeated episodes of hypotension. Loss of lower visual fields was also present.

Unilateral forms of the disorder are usually less obvious unless specifically sought. They involve one-half field; reaching with either the right or the left hand, or both may be affected within this field. Rondot et al (1977) conclude that the observed clinical variations imply the existence of both direct and crossed visuo-motor connections, the latter probably crossing corpus callosum in the splenium.

REFERENCES

Adams J H, Brierley J B, Connor R C R, Treip C S 1966 The effects of systemic hypotension upon the human brain. Clinical and neuropathological observations in eleven cases. Brain 89:235–268

Albert M L, Silverberg R, Reches A (1976) Cerebral dominance for consciousness. Archives of Neurology 33:453–454

Albert M L, Soffer D, Silverberg R, Reches A 1979 The anatomic basis of visual agnosia. Neurology 29:876–879

Andrew J, Nathan P W 1964 Lesions of the anterior frontal lobes and disturbances of micturition and defaecation. Brain 87:233–262

Barris R W, Schuman H R 1953 Bilateral anterior cingulate gyrus lesions: syndrome of the anterior cingulate gyri. Neurology 3:44–52

Bastian H C 1887 On different kinds of aphasia. British Medical Journal 2:931–936 & 985–990

Benson D F, Geschwind N 1971 The aphasias and related disturbances In: Baker A B (ed) Clinical Neurology. Harper, New York, Vol 1 p 1–25

Benson D F, Marsden C D, Meadows J C 1974a The amnesic syndrome of posterior cerebral artery thrombosis. Acta Neurologica Scandinavia 50:133–145

Benson D F, Segarra J, Albert M L 1974b Visual agnosia — prosopagnosia Archives of Neurology 30:307–310

Benson D F, Sheremata W A, Bouchard R, Segarra J M, Price D, Geschwind N 1973 Conductive aphasia. Archives of Neurology 28:339–346

Biemond A 1956 The conduction of pain above the level of the thalamus opticus. Archives of Neurology and Psychiatry 75:231–244

Brain W R 1941 Visual disorientation with special reference to lesions of the right cerebral hemisphere. Brain 64:244–272

Brain W R 1958 The physiological basis of consciousness: a critical review, Brain 81:426–455

Bramwell E 1927 A case of cortical deafness. Brain 50:579–580

Brindley G S 1972 The variability of human striate cortex. Journal of Physiology. London 225:1–3

Castaigne P, Buge A, Cambier J, Escourolle R, Brunet P, Degos J 1966 Demence Thalamique d'origine vasculaire par ramollissement bilatéral limité au territoire du pédicule rétromamillaire. Revue Neurologie 114:89–107

Castaigne P, Buge A, Escorolle R, Masson M 1962 Ramollissement pédonculaire médian, tegmento-thalamique avec ophthalmoplégie et hypersomnie. Revue Neurologique 106:357–367

Critchley M 1953 The parietal lobes. Arnold, London

Dejerine J 1892 Sur un case de cécité verbale avec agraphie, suivi d'autopsie. Mémoires de la Societe Biologique 3:197–201

Dejerine J, Roussy G 1906 Le syndrome thalamique. Revue Neurologique 1:521–532

Denckla M B 1972 Colour-naming defects in dyslexic boys. Cortex 8:164–176

Denny-Brown D, Chambers R A 1958 The parietal lobes and behaviour. Proceedings of the Association for Research in Nervous and Mental Disease 36:35–117

Dooling E C, Adams R D 1975 The pathologic anatomy of posthemiplegic athetosis. Brain 98:29–48

Earnest M P, Monroe P A, Yarnell P R 1977 Cortical deafness: demonstration of the pathologic anatomy on CT scan. Neurology 22:1172–5

Englander, R N, Netsky M G, Adelman L S 1975 Location of human pyramidal tract in the internal capsule: anatomic evidence. Neurology 25:823–826

Facon E, Steriade M, Werthein N 1958 Hypersomnie prolongée engendrée par des lesions bilatérales du système activateur medial: le syndrome thrombotique de la bifurcation du trunc basilaire. Revue Neurologique 98:117–133

Fisher C M 1967 A lacunar stroke: the dysarthria clumsy hand syndrome. Neurology 17:614–617

Fisher C M 1979 Capsular infarcts: the underlying vascular lesions. Archives of Neurology 36:65–73

Fisher C M, Curry H B 1965 Pure motor hemiplegia of vascular origin. Archives of Neurology 13:30–44

Frisén L 1979 Quadruple sectoranopia and sectorial optic atrophy: a syndrome of the distal anterior choroidal artery. Journal of Neurology Neurosurgery and Psychiatry 42:509–14

Frisén L, Holmegaard L, Rosencrantz M 1978 Sectorial optic atrophy and homonymous, horizontal sectoranopia: a lateral choroidal artery syndrome? Journal of Neurology, Neurosurgery and Psychiatry 41:374–380

Gainotti G 1972 Emotional behaviour and hemispheric side of lesion. Cortex 8:41–58

Gazzaniga M S, Glass A A, Sarno M T, Posner J B 1973 Pure word deafness and hemispheric dynamics: a case history. Cortex 9:136–143

Geschwind N 1965 Disconnexion syndromes in animals and man. Part I. Brain 88:237–294

Geschwind N, Fusillo M 1966 Color-naming defects in association with alexia. Archives of Neurology 15:137–146

Geschwind N, Kaplan E 1962 A human cerebral disconnection syndrome. Neurology 12:675–685

Geschwind N, Quadfasel F A, Segarra J M 1968 Isolation of the speech area. Neuropsychologia 6:327–340

Glees P, Griffith H 1952 Bilateral destruction of the hippocampus (Cornu Ammonis) in a case of dementia. Monatsschrift für Psychiatrie und Neurologie 123:193–204

Green G J, Lessell S 1977 Acquired cerebral dyschromatopsia. Archives of Ophthalmology 95:121–128

Head H, Holmes G 1920 In: Head H (ed) Studies in neurology. Oxford University Press p 554–560

Heilman K M, Tucker D M, Valenstein E 1976 A case of mixed transcortical aphasia with intact naming. Brain 99:415–426

Heilman K M, Valenstein E 1972 Frontal lobe neglect in man. Neurology 22:660–669

Holmes G 1918 Disturbances of visual orientation. British Journal of Ophthalmology 2:506–516

Horel J A 1978 The neuroanatomy of amnesia: a critique of the hippocampal memory hypothesis. Brain 101:403–445

Horenstein S, Chamberlain W, Conomy J 1967 Infarction of the fusiform and calcarine regions: agitated delirium and hemianopia. Transactions of the American Neurological Association 92:85–89

Hoyt W F, Newton T H 1970 Angiographic changes with occlusion of arteries that supply the visual cortex. New Zealand Medical Journal 72:310–317

Jerger J, Weikers N J, Sharbrough F W, Jerger S 1969 Bilateral lesions of the temporal lobe. Acta Oto-Laryngol. Supp. 258:1–51

Kaneda H, Irino T, Watanabe M, Kadota E, Taneda M 1979 Semiquantitative evaluation of ophthalmic collateral flow in carotid artery occlusion: ultrasonic doppler study. Journal of Neurology, Neurosurgery and Psychiatry 42:1133–1140

Kanshepolsky J, Kelley J J, Waggener J D 1973 A cortical auditory disorder: clinical, audiologic and pathologic aspects. Neurology 23:699–705

Kapur N, Coughlan A K 1980 Confabulation and frontal lobe dysfunction. Journal of Neurology, Neurosurgery and Psychiatry 43:451–463

Kinsbourne M 1971 The minor cerebral hemisphere as a source of aphasic speech. Archives of Neurology 25:302–306

Kyörney E 1975 Aphasie transcorticale et écholalie: Le problème de l'initiation de la parole. Revue Neurologique 5:347–363

Le Gros Clark W E, Russell W R 1938 Cortical deafness without aphasia. Brain 61:375–383

L'Hermitte F, Gautier J C, Marteau R, Chain E 1963 Troubles de la conscience et mutisme akinétique: étude anatomoclinique d'un ramollissement paramédian bilatéral du pédoncule cérébral et du thalamus. Revue Neurologique 109:115–131

Masdeu J C, Schoene W C, Funkenstein H 1978 Aphasia following infarction of the left supplementary motor area. Neurology 28:1220–1223

Maurice-Williams R S 1974 Micturition symptoms in frontal tumours. Journal of Neurology, Neurosurgery and Psychiatry 37:431–436

McFie J, Piercy M F, Zangwill O L 1950 Visual-spatial agnosia associated with lesions of the right cerebral hemisphere. Brain 73:167–190

Meadows J C 1974a The anatomical basis of prosopagnosia. Journal of Neurology, Neurosurgery and Psychiatry 37:489–510

Meadows J C 1974b Disturbed perception of colours in localized cerebral lesions. Brain 97:615–632

Meadows J C 1976 Disturbances of higher visual function. In: Rose F C (ed) Clinical Neurophthalmology. Chapman & Hall p 196–215

Mesulam M, Waxman S G, Geschwind N, Sabin T D 1976 Acute confusional states with right middle cerebral artery infarctions. Journal of Neurology, Neurosurgery and Psychiatry 39:84–89

Mitchell J R A, Schwartz C J 1965 Arterial disease. Blackwell, Oxford

Mohr J P, Pessin M S, Finkelstein S, Funkenstein H H, Duncan G W, Davis K R 1978 Broca aphasia. Neurology 28:311–324

Morello A, Cooper I S 1955 Visual field studies following occlusion of the anterior choroidal artery. American Journal of Ophthalmology 40:796–801

Nielsen J M, Jacobs L L 1951 Bilateral lesions of the anterior cingulate gyri. Bulletin of Los Angeles Neurology Society 16:231–234

Paterson A, Zangwill O L 1944 Disorders of visual space perception associated with lesions of the right cerebral hemisphere. Brain 47:331–358

Paterson A, Zangwill O L 1945 A case of topographical disorientation associated with unilateral cerebral lesion. Brain 68:188–212

Pearlman A L, Birch J, Meadows J C 1979 Cerebral colour blindness: an acquired defect in hue discrimination. Annals of Neurology 5:253–261

Richardson A 1976 Spotaneous intracerebral and cerebellar haemorrhage. In: Ross Russell R W (ed) Cerebral arterial disease. Churchill Livingstone, Edinburgh p 210–230

Romanul F C A, Abramowicz A 1964 Changes in brain and pial vessels in arterial border zones. Archives of Neurology 11:40–65

Rondot P, DeRecondo J, Ribadeau Dumas J L 1977 Visuomotor ataxia. Brain 100:355–376

Ropper A H, Fisher C M, Kleinman G M 1979 Pyramidal infarction in the medulla: a cause of pure motor hemiplegia sparing the face. Neurology 29:91–95

Ross Russell R W 1973 The posterior cerebral circulation. Journal of the Royal College of Physicians of London 7:331–346

Ross Russell R W, Bharucha N 1978 Recognition & prevention of borderzone cerebral ischaemia during cardiac surgery. Quarterly Journal of Medicine 47:303–23

Rubens A R 1975 Aphasia with infarction in the territory of anterior cerebral artery. Cortex 11:239–250

Rubens A L, Benson D F 1971 Associative visual agnosia. Archives of Neurology 24:305–316

Segarra J M 1970 Cerebral vascular disease and behaviour: the syndrome of the mesencephalic artery (basilar artery bifurcation). Archives of Neurology 22:408–418

Spertell R B, Ransom B R 1979 Dysarthria — clumsy hand produced by capsular infarct. Annals of Neurology 6:263–265

Stephens R B, Stilwell D L 1969 Arteries and veins of the human brain. Thomas, Springfield, Illinois.

Stuss D T, Alexander M P, Lieberman A, Levine H 1978 An extraordinary form of confabulation. Neurology 28:1166–1172

Symonds C P, MacKenzie I, 1957 Bilateral loss of vision from cerebral infarction. Brain 80:415–455

Talland G A, Sweet W H, Ballantine 1967 Amnesic syndrome with anterior communicating artery aneurysm. Journal of Nervous and Mental Diseases 145:179–192

Teuber H-L 1968 Alteration of perception and memory in man. In: Weiskrantz L (ed) Analysis of behavioural change. Harper & Row, New York

Victor M, Angerine J B, Mancall E L, Fisher C M 1961 Memory loss with lesions of the hippocampal formation. Archives of Neurology Chic. 5:244–263

Weiskrantz L, Warrington E K, Sanders M D, Marshall J 1974 Visual capacity in the hemianopic field following a restricted occipital ablation. Brain 97:709–728

Whiteley A M, Warrington E K 1978 Selective impairment of topographical memory: a single case study. Journal of Neurology, Neurosurgery and Psychiatry 41:575–578

Woolsey R M, Nelson J S 1975 Asymptomatic destruction of the fornix in man Archives of Neurology 32:566–568

10

Management of cerebral infarction

E. C. Hutchinson

Clinical and pathological studies indicate that the acute problems of cerebral infarction are concentrated in the first four weeks after the onset of symptoms. It is during this time that morbidity and mortality are determined and the important diagnostic and therapeutic problems are encountered. These are considered under two main headings; there is first a review of the limited information on mortality available in the epidemiological literature. The clinical difficulties in the initial assessment and the appropriate investigations are then briefly considered. Particular attention is paid to cerebral oedema following infarction because of the importance of secondary brain stem involvement in the acute phase of the illness. There follows a review of the different methods that have been advocated to limit the immediate effects of cerebral infarction; it concludes with the management of some complications and associated systemic disturbances which may be as important to survival as treatment of the primary lesion.

Mortality of cerebral infarction

Information on the immediate mortality of cerebral infarction cannot be precise. The two main sources of information are from epidemiological studies of unselected populations and reports derived from general hospital records. The accuracy of data from the first source is frequently questioned, and the patients studied in the second are often highly selected.

It is now traditional for clinicians to question the accuracy of the diagnosis of the cause of death in epidemiological studies. The epidemiologists reply that there is clear evidence that the gains and losses in terms of accuracy of diagnosis of cause of death will balance out if the standard of medical care and reporting are high (Acheson 1966; Kurtzke 1969). One important point established by epidemiological studies and not sufficiently emphasised in the reports on hospital patients is that cerebral infarction and cerebral haemorrhage are predominantly diseases of old age. In their studies in Oxford, Acheson & Fairbairn (1970) examined the age prevalence of cerebral vascular disease in hospital and in the general population and demonstrated clearly that the prevalence of cerebral infarction rises rapidly with increasing age. In males of the 55 to 65 age group the rate per 1000 of cerebral infarction was 1.35 whereas in the over 75 age group the rate per 1000 was 11.43.

In attributing death directly to cerebral infarction it is usual to take a period of four weeks from the acute episode. This is certainly realistic, but it obscures one important fact. Death in hemisphere infarction in the first week is usually due to massive cerebral oedema; in the next three weeks death is commonly due to systemic complications. This will be amplified later.

The mortality figures in the first four weeks given by Whisnant et al (1971) appear to be as reliable as any. Firstly, because they relate to the population of Rochester, Minnesota, where the standards of medical care available from the Mayo Clinic are excellent; secondly, the autopsy rate in the general population is high.

Using traditional clinical grounds for differentiating between cerebral haemorrhage, embolism, and thrombosis, there were 412 patients between the years 1945 and 1955 who presented with a 'cerebral thrombosis'. The death rate at the end of one month in these patients was 27 per cent. In giving these figures the authors stress the over-diagnosis of cerebral haemorrhage shown by the death certificate. The vital statistics for the United States during the period of study gave a ratio of 2.5 : 1 of cerebral haemorrhage to 'cerebral thrombosis'; in the population of Rochester over this period the same ratio was 0.15 : 1. No doubt this degree of overreporting of cerebral haemorrhage holds good for the Western world as a whole.

A 27 per cent mortality in the first month is probably a good approximation to the true figures, and this is supported by a general hospital population study where little or no selection of admissions to hospital is practised. Carter (1964), in a personally observed series of 612 patients with stroke, found that 26 per cent died within four weeks of the onset.

The clinical problem

Epidemiological studies already referred to indicate that the majority of patients who present with an acute vascular lesion of the central nervous system lasting more than 24 hours will have suffered a cerebral infarct. A precise history continues to be an important though not infallible guide to the diagnosis. For example, it is no longer believed that a study of the temporal evolution of physical signs can confidently diagnose a localised intracerebral haematoma or can differentiate between a middle cerebral artery embolus and a thrombus spreading from the internal carotid artery. Certainly a previous history of confirmed cerebral infarction, clinical evidence of extracranial arterial disease or a history of transient cerebral or retinal ischaemic attacks all provide supporting evidence for cerebral infarction, and a history of cardiac disease, particularly atrial fibrillation or recent cardiac infarction, will obviously suggest the possibility of cerebral embolus. Of major concern in the first assessment is the possibility that an apparently acute vascular lesion may be the expression of another condition requiring different treatment. Cerebral tumour and subdural haematoma are obvious examples. A previous history of headache, slight personality change or trivial head injury will suggest such a possibility.

The decision to admit a patient to hospital for treatment may be taken for several reasons but it is the severity of the neurological defect and progression or regression of signs in the first 24 hours which will dictate the degree of urgency which must be injected into the immediate management, particularly if the diagnosis is uncertain. Social problems of management at home may be a major factor in the decision as may rapid deterioration of consciousness in the face of progressive neurological signs. Occlusion of the basilar artery with quadriparesis presents a major nursing problem but this can apply with equal force to lateral medullary occlusions with dysphagia where skilled nursing in the acute phase may determine survival.

Investigations

These are designed to establish with reasonable certainty the underlying acute vascular lesion. This may not always be possible, particularly if an infarct is limited in size, but they will usually ensure there is no delay in recognising important alternative diagnoses.

Haematology. A full blood count is essential. It is usually normal at an early stage of cerebral infarction but it may provide a valuable first clue to an unsuspected diagnosis. An elevated ESR will raise the possibility of giant cell arteritis in the appropriate age group, collagen disease with 'vasculitis' or of an underlying systemic neoplasm with intracranial secondary deposits. Polycythaemia and leukaemia although rare causes of cerebral infarction can be recognised immediately. A blood film, combined with a platelet count, may be the first indication of the presence of the intravascular coagulation syndrome.

Electrocardiography. Routine e.c.g.s should be carried out in the first 24 hours as they can provide supporting evidence for pre-existing hypertension and can detect a recent transmural myocardial infarction, the possible source of a cerebral embolus.

Biochemical screen. The information obtained from biochemical screening should always be made available in the first 24 hours in major vascular lesions. A base line figure for the serum electrolytes may be useful particularly when there are progressively advancing signs. Evidence of hyperglycaemia or raised blood lipids will require further detailed investigation.

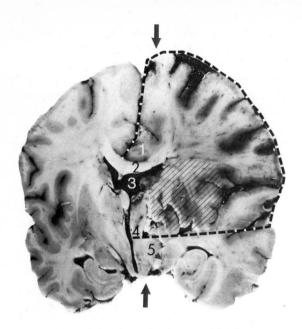

Fig. 10.1 Acute infarction and oedema resulting from internal carotid artery thrombosis spreading into anterior and middle cerebral arteries. Arrows indicate approximate position of original mid-line. Cross-hatch indicates area of encephalomalacia. Broken line indicates extent of oedema which causes: 1. Herniation of cingulate gyrus. 2. Downward displacement and rotation of corpus callosum. 3. Distortion of body of lateral ventricle. 4. Narrowing and displacement of third ventricle. 5. Herniation of uncus of temporal lobe.

Radiology. Plain X-rays of the chest and skull should be part of the routine investigations. Early inflammatory pulmonary changes can be recognised as can a primary tumour in the lung, which could alter the whole management. A detectable shift of the pineal gland in the plain films of the skull may be the first point to arouse suspicion of a mass hemisphere lesion. A hairline fracture of the skull will raise the possibility of subdural haematoma even though falls at the time of the onset of cerebral infarction commonly prove to be the cause.

C.T. scans, isotopes. C.T. scans and isotope studies make a major contribution to the diagnosis and management of cerebral infarction.

The C.T. scan will fail to demonstrate lacunar infarcts and similar small lesions in the hemispheres or the brain stem. Positive evidence of infarction, shown by areas of low attenuation, may be present within 12 hours of the onset but will commonly appear in the majority of patients within the first

week. However, it should be emphasised that in management the main value of the C.T. scan is to recognise immediately in hypertensive patients the presence of an intracerebral haematoma and to exclude such lesions as extracerebral haematoma. It is not always possible to differentiate between infarcts with oedema, cerebral tumours and inflammatory lesions but the problems can sometimes be resolved with intravenous contrast studies. In the latter case a note of caution is sounded by Pullicino & Kendall (1980) who feel that extravasation of the contrast medium may adversely affect potentially recoverable neural tissue.

In the absence of facilities for C.T. scanning isotope studies are of real value particularly when there is a possibility of an acute extracerebral haematoma over the hemispheres. The examination does not help to exclude such haematoma in the middle or posterior fossa.

Lumbar puncture. Lumbar puncture is not necessary in every patient but it may be helpful when there is doubt about the diagnosis; it should not be done if there is a clinical suspicion of a space occupying lesion or a posterior fossa lesion of any type. The changes in the cerebrospinal fluid in cerebral infarction have been detailed by Merritt & Fremont-Smith (1938) and Sornars et al, (1972). The c.s.f. pressure may be elevated in an extensive cerebral infarct, and in patients where the infarction is haemorrhagic there may be xanthochromia or free blood in the cerebrospinal fluid. The white cells can be modestly elevated but this increase usually declines during the first two weeks. In about 14 per cent of patients cerebrospinal fluid protein may show a modest elevation.

Clinical course. A combination of an accurate history and appropriate investigations will usually provide sufficient information within the first 12 hours to make a diagnosis of cerebral infarction with reasonable certainty bearing in mind that smaller hemisphere and brain stem lesions will often be a diagnosis of exclusion based on the physical signs.

Thereafter, management is based on knowledge of the possible sequence of the pathological events which may follow infarction. The most important of these to the physician is the development of oedema adjacent to the infarcted area which begins immediately after infarction and may affect the whole clinical picture within the first 24 to 48 hours.

For a further description of the causes and effects of ischaemic brain swelling see Chapter 7.

Clinical implications

The clinical relevance of brain swelling in the management of cerebral infarction is considerable. Plum & Posner (1972) in their monograph on *Stupor and Coma* divide the brain stem involvement into four stages, viz., the diencephalic stage, the mid-brain–upper pons stage, the lower pons-upper medullary stage and finally the terminal medullary stage. These stages are accompanied by pupillary and respiratory rhythm changes which are characteristic, and the elicitation of the oculocephalic and oculovestibular reflexes is useful in defining them. All stages can be observed in the progressive deterioration following massive hemisphere infarction.

In primary brain stem infarction there are disturbances of gaze which have a useful localising value when present. Fisher (1967) observed that in haemorrhage into the putamen there is a hemiparesis with the eyes deviated conjugately to the opposite side. In thalamic haemorrhages there may be a hemiparesis but the eyes are deviated downwards 'as if they were peering at the nose.' There is impairment of vertical eye movements and the pupils are 2 mm in size and unreactive. In cerebellar haemorrhage there can be forced conjugate lateral deviation of the eyes away from the side of the lesion and a paralysis of conjugate lateral gaze to the side of the lesion, or sometimes a sixth nerve palsy. There is no marked paresis of the limbs. The pupils are of average size and react normally to light.

Ocular bobbing

Ocular bobbing is a term first used by Fisher (1961) to describe a distinctive spontaneous movement of the eyes which may occur in the unconscious patient. To fulfil the criteria it is essential to demonstrate, by eliciting the oculovestibular reflex, that there is paralysis of horizontal conjugate gaze. The bobbing consists of a brisk conjugate downward jerking of the eyes followed by a slow return to the mid-position. The rate of movement

is between two and four per minute. It is a striking sign but its slow rate may make it difficult to recognise; it is by no means so rare as the literature would suggest. The importance of recognising ocular bobbing is that it is most commonly associated with intrinsic vascular lesions of the brain stem.

There is a variety of other spontaneous eye movements which have been reported in the literature in disturbances of the brain stem, cerebellum and their connections. One of these is opsoclonus, which is defined as a constant conjugate chaotic movement of the eyes. Boddie (1972) reported a patient where he observed 'ocular bobbing' change, after some weeks, to opsoclonus. The underlying lesion in the patient was probably a restricted pontine haemorrhage diagnosed on clinical grounds. He felt that ocular bobbing and opsoclonus ultimately may be shown to have a common pathophysiological basis.

Massive cerebellar infarction

Monitoring the evolving changes in neurological signs is essential in the management of posterior fossa lesions of vascular origin. In massive cerebellar infarction, although a rare event, prompt surgical treatment can result in survival with few residual signs. This is illustrated by the following case.

Case Report

Male, aged 24. Admitted 29.7.71. Discharged 20.8.71. On the morning of admission the patient complained of sudden acute vertigo and vomiting. He was unable to stand without assistance because of unsteadiness of his trunk. There was no headache immediately but on admission to hospital three hours later he complained of a right temporal headache.

On admission the blood pressure was 130/80. There were no abnormal signs on general examination. The patient was alert and speech and memory were normal. There was no neck stiffness. The only abnormality in the cranial nerves was a marked nystagmus to the right and on upward and downward gaze. The nystagmus had a rotatory component. In the limbs there was minimal bilateral ataxia but no paresis and no sensory loss. The reflexes were brisk throughout and the plantar responses were indefinite.

Investigations. C.s.f. resting pressure 120 mm of water, clear colourless fluid, acellular, protein 45 mg/100 ml, W.R. negative. Serum electrolytes, blood sugar, blood cholesterol, were all within normal limits.

The diagnosis of an intrinsic brain lesion was made, and in view of his relative youth the possibility of acute demyelination was considered.

After remaining unaltered for two days he suddenly complained of occipital headache. He was sweating profusely and his general condition deteriorated. He was drowsy but his speech was normal. The nystagmus was as noted on admission, but there was now some restriction of upward gaze. The plantar responses now showed an extensor plantar on the right but the left was still indefinite. For the first time some neck stiffness was noted. Within two hours upward gaze was further restricted and there was a divergent squint with diplopia.

In view of the signs at the onset and the clinical deterioration without obvious pyramidal weakness the diagnosis of an intrinsic brain stem lesion was abandoned and a vertebral angiogram was carried out.

This showed a large space occupying lesion in the right cerebellar hemisphere with displacement of the right superior cerebellar artery. (See Fig. 10.2)

Following angiography there was a further deterioration of consciousness and the pulse rate fell to 50 per minute. The pupils were still reacting to light. The following morning there was a further decrease in the level of consciousness but the patient still responded to commands. There was bilateral ptosis and a divergent squint. Upward movement of the eyes was now absent.

Urgent exploration of the posterior fossa was carried out by Mr. J. W. McIntosh on 2.8.71. A preliminary Myodil ventriculogram was done; this showed that the Myodil was held up in the fourth ventricle, which in its turn was displaced forward and to the left. At operation, when the dura was opened, marked swelling and herniation of the right cerebellar tonsil was noted. Soft material in the right cerebellar hemisphere was removed by suction and the tonsillar herniation through the foramen magnum was reduced. Histology showed that the softened tissue was a cerebellar infarct.

Subsequent detailed search for a possible cause of infarction failed to reveal a source of emboli or primary arterial disease.

He was discharged home 22 days after admission and had returned to work within two months. When finally reviewed on 17.4.72. he was well and working full time. No abnormal signs were detected in the central nervous system.

TREATMENT

The treatment of cerebral infarction is most usefully discussed under two headings. The first is the medical and surgical attempts to treat the infarcted brain, and the second the general medical measures which may be required in the acute phase of the illness. Attempts to minimise the disastrous effects of acute cerebral infarction may be considered under the following headings:

Control of cerebral oedema
Vasodilators
Hyperventilation
Anticoagulants
Low molecular weight dextran
Barbiturates
Surgical measures.

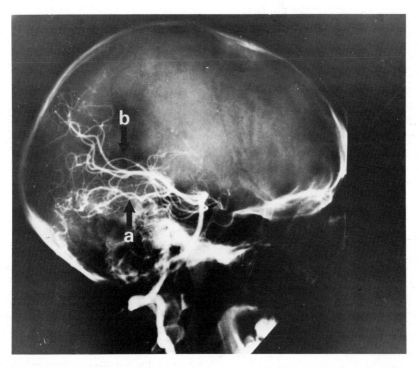

Fig. 10.2 Vertebral angiogram in massive infarct of right cerebellar hemisphere. a = Left superior cerebellar artery in normal position. b = Elevation of right superior cerebellar artery.

Cerebral oedema

Attempts to control cerebral oedema date back to the original observations of Weed & McKibben (1919) arising from their decision to observe changes in the concentration of sodium and chloride in the cerebrospinal fluid following the injection of hypertonic saline. Shortly after the intravenous injection of hypertonic sodium chloride they found that c.s.f. could not be obtained from the subarachnoid space. They immediately appreciated the significance of this observation and the results are now well known. A sustained rise in c.s.f. pressure occurred with hypotonic solutions whereas with hypertonic solutions there was an initial rise of c.s.f. pressure followed shortly by a marked fall. These observations initiated numerous attempts to control cerebral oedema over the next few decades.

Many substances attained temporary popularity but most have had the disadvantage that following the control of raised intracranial pressure there has been a 'rebound phenomenon' within a matter of hours and the c.s.f. pressure has returned to its original level or even higher. Intravenous urea remained popular for a considerable time but later it was realised that it also showed a delayed rebound phenomenon. There was also clinical evidence of toxicity of urea, particularly in high concentration, and so it lost popularity in clinical practice.

Hypertonic mannitol solution was introduced and is still useful in certain circumstances. Wise & Chater (1962) described its use in 70 patients with various intracranial lesions, and with a 20 per cent solution they found it to be an effective method for achieving temporary control of raised intracranial pressure.

For obvious reasons the majority of attempts to control cerebral oedema are carried out in patients where the oedema is secondary to tumours in the hemisphere or the posterior fossa. However, there have been studies which have attempted to influence the course of established hemisphere infarction in the acute stages with measures designed to reduce cerebral oedema. Two substances worth examining are glycerol and corticosteroids.

Glycerol

Meyer et al (1971) reported on 36 patients with acute cerebral infarction who were treated with glycerol in a dose of 1.2 g per kg of body weight every 24 hours in a 10 per cent solution of saline or in dextrose and water. Treatment was started within 72 hours of the onset. The mortality was 11 per cent and the deaths were confined to those patients who were in coma when treatment was begun. In all other patients neurological improvement was observed at the end of four days of treatment. There were no toxic side effects and it was noted that glycerol administration was associated with a fall in the c.s.f. pressure without evidence of a rebound phenomenon.

In a further report Meyer et al (1972) described the intravenous use of glycerol and its effect on hemisphere blood flow and brain metabolism in patients with an acute cerebral infarction. Seventeen patients were studied and the estimations were carried out within two weeks of the infarct in all but three patients. Arterial oxygen uptake, CO_2 tension, and pH were recorded throughout the observations and hemisphere blood flow was calculated by the hydrogen electrode technique.

During the infusion the hemisphere blood flow increased in all but one patient and a mean increase in blood flow of 8 per cent was considered to be significant. The effect on blood flow, however, was transient. The central venous pressure and the intracranial venous pressure both increased significantly during the infusion, but on completion the intracranial venous pressure fell below the pre-infusion levels.

The mean c.s.f. pressure did not change during the infusion but decreased significantly afterwards. They noted striking changes in the e.e.g during the infusion and in the majority of patients neurological function also improved. They concluded that the expansion of the perivascular space by removal of the oedema fluid within the glial cells seemed to be the primary factor in causing an increase in hemisphere blood flow.

Their conclusion was that their clinical and experimental observations gave some credence to the view that the intravenous use of glycerol was a useful form of therapy in patients with acute cerebral infarction.

Corticosteroids

The effectiveness of steroids in the control of cerebral oedema was soon appreciated. Galicich et al in 1961 reviewed the literature up to that time and described the use of dexamethasone in 14 patients with raised intracranial pressure due to tumour. They observed a dramatic improvement with relief of signs and symptoms of raised intracranial pressure. In two cases they obtained angiographic proof of decrease in the size of the intracranial mass as a result of steroids, which they felt was due to a decrease in the oedema surrounding the tumour.

Russek et al (1954) were the first to report the use of cortisone in the acute treatment of 'apoplectic stroke' in 12 patients. Three patients with cerebral haemorrhage died without benefit. In the remaining nine patients they were enthusiastic about the results. The rapid resolution of symptoms in response to steroids caused them to state that 'cortisone accomplished in one day what ordinarily might take several weeks of conservative treatment'. The dose used was 300 mg orally over 48 hours reducing to 50 mg daily at the end of the first week. Roberts (1958) considered that steroid therapy in acute and subacute vascular accidents, particularly when there was clinical evidence of brain stem involvement, made a positive contribution to treatment.

Dyken & White (1956) did not share this enthusiasm. They reported on 36 patients whom they divided into two groups according to the severity of the stroke, the age at onset and the blood pressure. Seventeen patients were treated with 300 mg of cortisone daily and 19 patients received a placebo. Thirteen deaths occurred in the treated group and 10 in the placebo group. After studying the clinical results of the survivors they detected a trend indicating that cortisone 'may be a dangerous drug to use in cerebral vascular disease'.

The experiments of Plum et al (1963) also demonstrated that steroids had little value in controlling the effects of experimental ischaemia. They gave dexamethasone to rats both before and after a controlled ischaemic insult. They found that mortality during anoxia was significantly elevated among animals treated with corticoids, and in the surviving animals treatment with steroids did not appear to have any significant effect on the clinical outcome, the extent and degree of cerebral oedema, on the cerebral electrolyte content, or on the extent of cerebral vascular damage.

The use of steroids in cerebral infarction has been re-examined in the past five years but conclusions as to their benefit are still diametrically opposed.

Patten et al (1972) carried out a double blind study on a group of patients with a sudden focal neurological deficit of less than 24 hours duration. The patients were assigned randomly to treated and control groups. Neurological examination was carried out by skilled observers at intervals over three weeks after admission and assessment was based on a scoring system. The dose of steroids was 16 mg daily of dexamethasone for 10 days followed by a gradual reduction to zero over the next week; at the conclusion of the study 17 patients had acted as controls and 14 patients were treated. The scoring system indicated that the patients treated with steroids had improved their functional status by an average of 12 per cent, whereas the placebo group had deteriorated to a similar degree. When they considered 15 patients who were severely affected by the initial infarct the benefit of steroids was, they felt, even more clearly demonstrated since the treated group improved 23 per cent, whereas the placebo group deteriorated 14 per cent. These results were statistically significant. They concluded, not unnaturally, that dexamethasone was a useful adjunct to the treatment of patients with stroke and its effect was due to controlling the amount of cerebral oedema secondary to massive cerebral infarction.

Bauer & Tellez (1973) also reported a double blind trial using dexamethasone in 50 cases with cerebral infarction. They were quite unable to detect any difference between the treated and the untreated groups. They fully appreciated the discrepancy between their findings and those of Patten et al (1972) and indicated that if there was any difference in case material between the two groups of patients then their own patients were probably more severely ill than in the trial of Patten et al (1972).

If this were true then their results might have been expected to parallel those of Patten et al (1972), who observed the best results in the most severely affected cases. No obvious reason other than unwitting case selection can be put forward to explain these widely discrepant results.

Vasodilators

The lack of agreement on the effectiveness of agents designed to reduce cerebral oedema is mirrored in the opinions expressed on the use of vasodilators. Waltz (1971) writes: 'present evidence provides no support for the use of vasodilators in the treatment of acute cerebral ischaemia'. McHenry (1972), discussing the merits of cerebral vasodilatation in cerebral infarction, wrote: 'one cannot accept the pessimism that there is no hope from more thorough evaluation and more aggressive management of the acute stroke'.

The heart of the disagreement lies in the recent advances in knowledge which have been achieved by the methods of studying regional blood flow following cerebral infarction. A detailed treatment of this topic is given in Chapter 5. It only needs to be restated briefly that following ischaemia there may be adjacent areas of vasomotor paralysis with abolition of the normal response both to CO_2 and to variations in systemic blood pressure. It has been argued that because of impaired vasomotor control, increasing the cerebral blood flow by any means may deviate blood from the ischaemic areas, achieving a result which is the reverse of that intended (intracerebral steal). The question of how serious or how frequent is this phenomenon is still debated. Cerebral vasodilatation can be induced in two ways. The first is the utilisation of the well-known response of the cerebral circulation to hypercarbia. The second is the administration by the arterial, venous or oral route of drugs capable of inducing vasodilatation.

The effect of CO_2 inhalation

The introduction by Kety & Schmidt (1945) of an ethically acceptable method of measuring the total cerebral blood flow in man was the start of unravelling the dynamic events which may follow cerebral infarction. The remarkable rapidity with which total cerebral blood flow can be restored following carotid artery occlusion was shown by the acute experiments of Shenkin et al (1951) in carotid artery occlusion carried out for intracranial

aneurysms and their observations have been expanded experimentally by Symon et al (1963) and Eklof & Schwartz (1969).

The demonstration by Kety & Schmidt (1948) that 7 per cent CO_2 in inspired air could double the cerebral blood flow inevitably led to the examination of the possibility that CO_2 may contribute to the treatment of cerebral vascular disease. It was soon shown that the response to CO_2 of the cerebral circulation affected by occlusive vascular disease is not a simple one. Fazekas & Alman (1964) in patients with angiographically proven occlusive vascular disease of the major vessels of the neck observed that there were two recognisable groups of patients. There were those who responded in a normal, or near normal, fashion to inspired CO_2 by increasing the cerebral blood flow; in other patients, apparently affected in an identical manner, there was no useful response. This observation indicated, they believed, an exhaustion of the homeostatic reserves and they concluded there was a potential danger in the use of CO_2 in cerebral vascular disease whether the disease be in the acute or chronic phase.

A clinical evaluation of the effects of 5 per cent CO_2 inhalation was carried out by Millikan (1955). Two hundred and seventy-five patients formed the basis of his observations, of whom 50 were given CO_2 and 225 were untreated. Although the design of the trial was not ideal by modern standards he could find no evidence of any benefit from the administration of CO_2.

McHenry et al (1972) carried out regional blood flow studies on normal subjects, on patients with diffuse cerebral arterial disease and on patients with known focal vascular disease which had been demonstrated by angiography. Five per cent CO_2 was administered and the effects on the regional blood flow were studied. In the normal subjects there was the anticipated increase in the cerebral blood flow. The response in diffuse cerebral vascular disease was much less, showing a mean increase of 28 per cent as compared with the normal 60 per cent. In patients with focal vascular lesions hypercarbia increased the mean cerebral blood flow but there was a less marked response in the focal areas of ischaemia. They felt that 'intracerebral steal' was a rare occurrence. For this reason they believed that the dangers of increasing cerebral blood flow by vasodilatation had been overstressed.

They did, however, conclude that on the evidence of clinical and experimental studies which had been carried out there could be no support for the view that CO_2 makes a contribution to the treatment of acute cerebral infarction. The fact that both the mean arterial pressure and cardiac output was significantly increased was, they felt, another good reason for not advocating the use of CO_2 in treatment. Few would disagree with this conclusion.

Vasodilatation by drugs

Many substances have been examined for the ability to produce cerebral vasodilatation. Papaverine is a well-established cerebral vasodilator and has been examined in some detail. Its use has been alternatively recommended and condemned and the observations on this drug illustrate well the areas of contention which apply to all vasodilator drugs acting directly on the cerebral blood vessels.

Papaverine

Jayne et al, (1952) demonstrated that intravenous papaverine hydrochloride could significantly increase cerebral blood flow in man. Using the nitrous oxide method they found a significant mean increase in flow. Since they detected no concomitant change in the mean arterial pressure or the pH of the blood they deduced that this was a direct cerebral vasodilatory effect by the drug.

Experimental evidence cited by Meyer et al (1971) indicated that oral papaverine may also be capable of increasing cerebral blood flow. In baboons, within 20 to 60 minutes after the oral administration of the drug, cerebral blood flow increased and the A-V oxygen difference decreased to a significant degree. They found no significant change in the systemic blood pressure.

The clinical use of papaverine hydrochloride in the treatment of stroke had already been reported by Meyer et al (1965). They studied a series of 66 cases, 30 of whom received intravenous papaverine and 36 acted as controls. They used a scoring system based on physical signs which they said were objective and reproducible within one point

by different observers. They monitored the cerebral arterio-venous oxygen difference and combined this with a clinical assessment of the two groups. Following papaverine they found a significant increase in the oxygen uptake of the brain and in the treated group they found a significantly greater clinical improvement than in the control group.

McHenry et al (1970) examined the effects of papaverine on regional blood flow in focal vascular disease. They examined six patients with focal cerebral vascular disease demonstrated by angiography. After basal cerebral blood flow measurements they gave 100 mg of papaverine intravenously over a 30 minute period and, 50 minutes after this, again assessed the hemisphere and regional blood flow. Before papaverine, in all six cases, the individual regional blood flow values in the area which was shown to be abnormal by angiography were all below the limits of normal as was the total hemisphere blood flow in each patient. After papaverine the mean cerebral blood flow for the whole group was increased by 18 per cent per 100 g of brain per minute, an increase which was significant. In addition to this, eight of the individual regional values for cerebral blood flow over an angiographically abnormal area also increased significantly. They emphasised that whilst they found no evidence of a decrease in flow in ischaemic areas in their patients they could not coincidentally find evidence that papaverine improved neurological function.

Olesen & Paulson (1971) studied the effects of intracarotid injection of 10 mg of papaverine on regional blood flow in 27 patients. In patients without focal flow abnormalities the regional blood flow showed a uniform increase which averaged 93 per cent. In patients with focal flow abnormalities the flow values were subnormal in the whole hemisphere and where an ischaemic focus occurred the response to papaverine was decreased, or absent. In one instance they obtained a clear-cut example of 'intracerebral steal' where a reduction of flow in the affected region was accompanied by simultaneously occurring generalised increase in flow in the rest of the brain. Examining all the experimental evidence they concluded that the existence of an 'intracerebral steal' had been convincingly demonstrated and 'that it probably occurs frequently in apoplexy after papaverine injection'. Therefore, they believed the rationale of vasodilator treatment was open to serious doubt.

Again there is the dilemma, as with agents for reducing cerebral oedema, of reconciling diametrically opposed views on the value of vasodilators in cerebral infarction. Conclusions from studies of variations in the response of the cerebral circulation in areas of focal ischaemia can only complement well designed clinical studies, they cannot replace them. At the moment the information from trials is too limited to allow useful conclusions to be drawn.

Hyperventilation and induced hypocarbia

The belief that increasing the CO_2 content in the inspired air and thus producing hypercarbia may in fact be harmful in cerebral infarction resulted in the examination of the possibility that hypocarbia induced by hyperventilation may be beneficial.

Soloway et al (1968) demonstrated that reducing the $PaCO_2$ to 25 mm restricted the area of infarction following experimental occlusion. Battistini et al (1969) showed also in experimental animals that after ischaemia hyperventilation either restored the circulation in a large part of the ischaemic area or prevented a progressive decrease in blood flow. Soloway et al (1970) on the basis of experimental data suggested that time may be all-important. In experiments where there was a delay in inducing hypocarbia for more than one hour after the occlusion a subsequent period of three to four hours of hypocarbia produced no beneficial effect on the extent of the infarct. If this observation is ultimately shown to be applicable to patients with cerebral infarction then the results may well be disappointing.

A clinical trial of hyperventilation in acute stroke has been reported by Christensen (1970). Forty two patients with an acute stroke were treated with prolonged hyperventilation; the interval between the onset and the commencement of treatment was, with few exceptions, less than 24 hours. The procedure was that the patients were ventilated through an endotracheal tube for 72 hours. The patients were randomised and in those assigned to the hypocarbic group it was aimed to obtain an $PaCO_2$ of about 25 mmHg. In the untreated group the respirator was adjusted to give an $PaCO_2$ of 40 mmHg.

When they compared patients with an occluded internal carotid artery they could find no difference between the treated and untreated group; in patients with occlusion of the middle cerebral artery they found the mortality was decreased in patients treated with hyperventilation. Among patients without evidence of arteriographic occlusion there was a reduction of the mortality but no effect on the result in terms of improved neurological function. Overall, although they emphasised that the numbers were too small for valid statistical analysis, they felt that their results suggested that hyperventilation had some beneficial effect on acute brain lesions and reduced the mortality. They admitted that the results were not impressive and did not, in their view, justify prolonged hypocarbia as a routine treatment. The treatment is difficult to perform and there are complications. Nevertheless, they felt that it was possible to select cases of stroke for treatment by induced hypocarbia; these would be the relatively young patients without cardiac or pulmonary disease and with evidence of a very recent stroke.

Anticoagulants

There is sufficient information available now on the use of anticoagulants in the management of the completed stroke due to occlusive vascular disease to refer to them only briefly. It is generally agreed that anticoagulants are contra-indicated.

Millikan (1971) discussed the use of anticoagulants in various types of occlusive cerebral vascular disease. He reviewed five contributions where the clinical condition of completed stroke was observed and where controls were compared with the treated patients. It is clear from the results obtained that there was little or no evidence that the treated group fared better than the controls in terms of recurrence of cerebral infarction; there is also the potential hazard of cerebral haemorrhage. With the growing awareness of the importance of localised intracerebral haematoma as a cause of focal cerebral vascular disease there can be little justification for treatment with anticoagulants in the acute phase of the completed stroke.

Anticoagulants may have a part to play in the

management of progressive cerebral infarction (stroke in evolution), that small minority of patients in whom neurological deficit becomes worse during a period of observation of some hours. The mechanism of progressive ischaemia is thought to be an extension or propagation of thrombus, e.g., up the internal carotid artery to involve the terminal branches. The diagnosis of progressive cerebral infarction should be made with great caution since it may resemble closely a subdural or intracerebral haematoma or even a cerebral tumour, and patients with stroke may deteriorate from extracerebral causes such as cardiac failure or hypoxia. Either the carotid or vertebrobasilar territories may be involved.

This is a difficult group of patients in which to assess the effects of anticoagulants. The degree of ultimate disability in treated and control groups has been compared (Baker et al 1962) and the proportion of patients showing progression was somewhat less in the treated group. More significantly, the death rate from cerebral infarction was also reduced by treatment (Carter, 1961). Because of the urgency of the situation the anticoagulant used is intravenous heparin for the first 48 hours (10 000 units over six hours by continuous infusion). Treatment is continued with warfarin or subcutaneous heparin (5000 units six hourly) for two weeks.

In the management of patients with recent cerebral infarction secondary to embolism from the heart, it is still common practice to use anticoagulants to lessen the risk of repeated embolism. Whisnant (1977) in a brief review of the evidence noted the absence of any conclusive proof but felt that on balance the evidence indicated some benefit to patients with mitral valve disease and atrial fibrillation. He recommended commencing anticoagulants seven days after the infarct, and most physicians would agree with this.

Low molecular weight dextran

The importance of changes in the microvasculature in determining the extent of ischaemia has been reviewed by Wells (1964). Aggregation and thrombosis of the blood components in the microcirculation and an increased viscosity due to haemoconcentration are all features which may occur. Evidence has accumulated that the use of intravenous low molecular weight dextran may be useful in combating these changes by its action in expanding plasma volume rather than by a specific effect on viscosity.

Gilroy et al (1969) reported on a clinical trial of 100 patients with acute cerebral ischaemia and infarction due to atherosclerotic thromboembolism. All patients had sustained a severe neurological deficit without improvement 24 to 72 hours before entering into the study. The patients were divided into treated and control groups on a randomised basis. Initially the treated group were given 500 ml of dextran 40 over an interval of an hour. This was followed by a slow intravenous infusion of dextran 40 at the rate of 500 ml every 12 hours. They used a scoring system already referred to (Meyer et al, 1965) and found that in the treated group there was a significant improvement in mental state and total neurological function. This improvement in the treated group was significantly better than in the untreated group. They also studied variations in platelet behaviour and demonstrated that in patients with an acute stroke platelet aggregation was increased in the venous blood. Low molecular weight dextran caused the platelet abnormality to return to normal.

Attempts to confirm the overall beneficial effect of dextran 40 have not been successful. The use of a combination of dexamethasone and dextran 40 in 40 patients was reported by Kaste et al (1976). The patients were assessed in a double-blind trial over a period of 29 days, but the authors could find no evidence of any difference in mortality or neurological disability in the treated group of patients. A report by Matthews et al (1976) showed similar results and also drew attention to a significant problem in the design of trials for the treatment of stroke. One hundred patients were included in a trial of dextran 40 and assessment after three weeks provided evidence of benefit in that patients with a severe stroke showed a significant reduction in mortality. However, this was achieved only at the cost of survival of severely disabled patients; many of these were to die in the next few months and only a few attained any independence. They naturally concluded that there was no real benefit achieved by the use of dextran 40, particularly since it was ineffective in patients who presented initially with less severe disabilities.

Barbiturates

The potential benefit of barbiturates in minimising the effects of hypoxia and ischaemia on the brain has recently attracted considerable attention. There seems to be little doubt that barbiturates will improve recovery of neurological function after cerebral ischaemia in primate animal models, (Moseley, et al 1975; Blayaert et al 1978). One problem is that it seems probable that most of the biochemical changes which follow infarction and contribute to brain damage occur in the early stages following infarction, and this will obviously restrict its use in patients who are not normally seen so early in the illness; another is that so far it is not certain whether the beneficial effects derive from a depression of oxygen usage by brain cells, reduction of blood flow or by a combination of both mechanisms. The clinical applications, therefore, are still uncertain but barbiturate therapy may have a contribution to make in the future.

Surgical treatment

There is no longer any general enthusiasm for advocating a direct surgical approach to the major neck vessels in the acute stage of cerebral infarction. Fields (1973) indicated that the mortality of such procedures was 50 per cent, which is considerably higher than the mortality for more conservative measures. This fact, combined with the development of the various imaging techniques, has also virtually removed the need for routine cerebral angiography in the acute stage of the illness.

However, developments in microsurgery have resulted in direct attempts to counter the effects of extracranial vascular occlusions. These procedures, referred to as extracranial bypass surgery, consist of establishing anastomotic communications between the branches of the external carotid artery and the intracranial circulation through the skull vault. This is usually done by anastomosing the superficial temporal artery to the middle cerebral artery, and there have been reports of establishing communications between the occipital artery and the vertebro-basilar circulation. Trials are going

forward in several centres at the moment, but it appears unlikely that such procedures will have anything more than a very restricted role in the management of acute cerebral infarction.

Neurosurgical treatment may be essential to survival in the small number of patients presenting with brain stem compression following infarcts in the posterior fossa, and an example of its value has been given in the report of a patient with massive cerebellar infarction. Treatment of hemisphere infarction by surgical decompression has been attempted but the results are discouraging. Greenwood (1968) reported on ten patients but four died, three survived with severe disability and three only were left with a 'moderate and acceptable neurological deficit'.

GENERAL MEASURES

Although the problems posed by the management of the neurological aspect of cerebral infarction are important, they must not overshadow certain aspects of general treatment which can have a major influence on the outcome. In the acute phase of the illness control of blood pressure, maintenance of fluid and electrolyte balance and the oxygen supply may be critical. The presence of diabetes mellitus or the development of epilepsy as a complication of infarction are also important.

Blood pressure

A fall in blood pressure is not a feature of uncomplicated acute cerebral infarction and the presence of hypotension should immediately prompt a search for the underlying cause. This will commonly be found to be due to myocardial infarction, pulmonary embolus, or internal bleeding. On occasions septicaemia has been recorded as the underlying cause of the hypotension (Shaw et al, 1959; Ng et al, 1970). Any of these conditions can cause hypotension which may precipitate cerebral infarction and it is rarely difficult to demonstrate its cause by routine clinical methods.

It is now believed that frequent recording of the systemic blood pressure does not make any major contribution to the assessment of brain stem ischaemia secondary to a hemisphere space occupying lesion. The classical signs of falling pulse rate and rising blood pressure are no longer regarded as reliable signs of increased intracranial pressure (Plum & Posner, 1972). In the more general context of raised intracranial pressure Miller & Adams (1972) observed that bradycardia and increased arterial tension are frequently absent even with an intracranial pressure in excess of 75 mmHg (1000 mmH$_2$O).

However, combined clinical and pathological studies have thrown some interesting light on variations of the blood pressure in association with vascular lesions. Ito et al, (1973) reported on the results of autopsies on 108 patients of whom 51 were found to have cerebral haemorrhage and 57 cerebral infarction. The vascular lesions affected the hemispheres or the brain stem but not the cerebellum. The blood pressure readings were available in all patients.

Their conclusions were quite precise. In lesions which were situated either rostral to the mid-brain or were in the medulla oblongata there was no associated elevation of the blood pressure. An elevation of the blood pressure did occur with primary pontine lesions whether they were due to haemorrhage or infarction or where cerebral haemorrhage extended into the fourth ventricle or the pons. Blood pressure elevations were more marked in tegmental pontine lesions than in lesions affecting the basilar pons. They concluded that caudal brain stem lesions, especially in the pons, had a causal role to play in blood pressure elevation following cerebral vascular accidents.

Induced hypertension

The belief that elevating the systemic arterial blood pressure — and thus altering the perfusion pressure of the brain — may be beneficial in cerebral ischaemia is not new. Shanbrom & Levy (1957), Farhat & Schneider (1967) and Wise (1970) have all published observations on its effects. Wise et al (1972) published an interesting study on the treatment of brain ischaemia with vasopressive drugs. They studied 13 consecutive normotensive patients with signs of focal brain ischaemia who were seen within four hours of the onset of the ictus. The blood pressure in these patients was elevated by drugs from a mean of 158/85 to 170/100,

and in five of these neurological function improved. Although this is a small series the case histories given are remarkable.

The first patient, a man of 54, recovered neurological function on elevation of the blood pressure from 125/80 mmHg to 170 mmHg within minutes. The neurological defect recurred no less than five times when the blood pressure was allowed to subside to its original level. Although not quite so dramatic as this, the observations in four other cases showed similar changes which would be difficult to explain by chance alone. These findings are not unexpected, for Ross Russell (1970) has demonstrated in the experimental animal that after regional occlusion the pial vessels in the ischaemic area and surrounding zones behaved passively in response to changes in blood pressure.

Management of established hypertension

A commoner clinical problem is the patient presenting with hypertension and focal neurological signs. The level of the blood pressure is of no value in differentiating between cerebral haemorrhage and cerebral infarction as the classical studies of Aring & Merritt (1935) have shown.

The clinico-pathological study of Hudson & Hylan (1958) complements this study. In 100 autopsies a well-documented clinical history of hypertension was available. They recognised a group of patients who survived cerebral haemorrhage but in only half of these was the c.s.f. bloodstained at the time of the acute episode. They rightly emphasised the considerable difficulty in differentiating between non-fatal cerebral haemorrhage and cerebral infarction.

There is evidence from pathological and clinical studies (Cole & Yates, 1967; Acheson, 1971) that a significant proportion of patients presenting with focal cerebral lesions and a diastolic blood pressure over 110 mmHg will have sustained a localised cerebral haemorrhage. On clinical grounds, however, it may be impossible to differentiate for certain between an infarct and a localised haemorrhage and, therefore, an empirical approach is necessary. The dangers of treating hypertension in the acute phase of ischaemia cerebral infarct have undoubtedly been overemphasised but they still remain. If there is evidence of focal vascular hemisphere lesion without signs of secondary brain stem involvement and if there is a history of significant, pre-existing hypertension which can be established, either from previous blood pressure readings, from e.c.g. or from radiological studies of the heart, then the blood pressure can be controlled immediately. In reducing the blood pressure experience indicates that the use of adrenergic neurone blockers, such as guanethidine or vasodilators such as hydralazine, can cause problems because of the rapidity of the fall of blood pressure. The beta-adrenergic receptor blockers, such as atenolol, given orally or by naso-gastric tube do give a more controlled fall in blood pressure and are therefore recommended. It should be emphasised that these observations apply to the management of cerebral infarction or localised intracerebral haematoma and not to 'hypertensive encephalopathy'.

Fluids and electrolytes

Disturbances of fluid and electrolyte balance must always be considered as a serious potential hazard to patients with disturbance of their conscious level (Sambrook et al, 1973). Attention to the basic principles covering the daily requirements of water (2000 to 3000 ml), sodium (80 to 120 m.Eq), potassium (60 to 90 m.Eq) and calories (2500 to 3000) will maintain a satisfactory metabolic nutritional state in the majority of patients.

It should be emphasised that the above values are basal daily metabolic requirements and do not take into account other losses of biological fluids which may occur at the time of the acute episode through vomiting or during a period of prolonged treatment. Any such losses will require to be taken into account, and careful charting of the daily intake and output (with biochemical analysis of the latter) from all sources should be established for the semicomatose or unconscious patients as soon as possible. Daily records of weight will often prove valuable in helping to assess fluid requirements. If the evidence does indicate the presence of inappropriate ADH secretion in patients with acute vascular lesions, then the patient should be given 500 ml of saline to replace the 'insensible' fluid loss plus an amount of fluid equal to the total

urine output of the previous 24 hours. The presence of unrelated lesions, such as fistulae which would increase the 'insensible' fluid loss, would require an appropriate adjustment to the 500 ml allowance.

Attention to serum and urine osmolality will aid the recognition of inappropriate ADH secretion and its differentiation from other states of hyponatraemia (Welt, et al, 1952; Cort, 1954; Taylor, 1961; El-Zayat & El-Danasoury, 1972). The clinical importance of recognising disturbances of electrolyte metabolism is emphasised when one examines the case reports of neurological abnormalities in hyponatraemia. Convulsions and drowsiness are well-recognised clinical expressions of a low serum sodium, but their occurrence without appreciation of the possible role of disturbed electrolyte levels could easily confuse the management of these patients. Epstein et al, (1961) described a 16-year-old girl who on one occasion was deeply unconscious with pin point pupils and divergent squint, neck rigidity, flaccid limbs, and bilateral extensor plantar responses. The cause was hyponatraemia and there is little doubt that such a clinical picture presenting without knowledge of the disturbance of serum electrolytes could cause considerable diagnostic confusion.

Maintaining oxygen supply

The maintenance of adequate blood oxygenation is essential in all patients in coma regardless of the cause. In the majority of patients with a restricted neurological lesion due to cerebral infarction the maintenance of an adequate airway presents no problems. If infection or pulmonary infarction develop or are superimposed on pre-existing chronic lung disease, then appropriate antibiotic therapy may be necessary.

In patients where consciousness is impaired the problems are very different. If clinical signs of hypoxia are present, then the immediate administration of 100 per cent oxygen is advisable, thereafter maintaining the arterial oxygen tension and monitoring the arterial gases where this is appropriate. The precipitating cause for the hypoxia will usually be due to one of two causes. The first is an obstructed airway, the second incipient respiratory failure due to brain stem involvement. The obstructed airway can usually be dealt with by adequate care of the upper respiratory airway maintained by simple suction. If the obstruction is in the bronchial tree then bronchoscopy may be necessary to achieve an adequate airway. It is a matter of clinical judgement whether this should be undertaken if the chances of survival are negligible.

A similar caution applies to tracheostomy. It is general experience that modern methods of resuscitation have led to a far more widespread use of intubation and tracheostomy than in the days when these procedures were reserved for upper airway obstruction. The decision to advocate tracheostomy in a patient with an extensive cerebral infarction requires justification, and the limited amount of information available on the subject would offer slender support for such action. Lancaster (1973) published the results of tracheostomy in patients with 'stroke'. Twenty-five patients were reviewed, but there were only 12 survivors from the acute stage. Of the 12 survivors eight died within 10 weeks of discharge and one within six months. All the other patients surviving required continuous nursing care. Two patients made a good recovery and indicate one of the two exceptions where assisted respiration may be justified.

These two patients presented with pontine lesions. In infarcts of the lateral medullary area some patients may appear — and are in fact — desperately ill for a period of time. Total dysphagia may render it difficult, if not impossible, to maintain adequate respiration and nutrition because of retained pharyngeal secretion; here assisted respiration by means of endotracheal intubation or tracheostomy may be justified and necessary for a time because of the remarkable capacity for recovery some of these patients show.

The other exception to the use of controlled respiration is where a trial of hyperventilation is being carried out in an attempt to influence the blood supply to the ischaemic area.

Epilepsy

The incidence of convulsions in occlusive cerebral vascular disease has been variously estimated at 7.7 per cent patients by Louis & McDowell (1967)

and 5 per cent by Moskowitz et al (1972) in the first two years of the natural history. Dodge et al (1954) as a result of a pathological study of six cases of cerebral infarction confirmed previous views that involvement of the cortex was important in the pathogenesis of epilepsy in this condition.

The figures of Aring & Merritt (1935) still appear to be as reliable as any relating to the occurrence of epilepsy in the acute phase of cerebral infarction. They observed a 6.6 per cent prevalence in pathologically proven cases of 'cerebral thrombosis'. Convulsions at the onset of cerebral haemorrhage were more than twice as frequent (14.8 per cent). The development of major convulsions in the acute stage of cerebral infarction demands treatment directed to the control of the convulsions and the maintenance of an adequate airway to avoid hypoxia. The latter has already been discussed. Anticonvulsant treatment is neither more or less difficult than in other forms of epilepsy. The intravenous use of diazepam (Valium 5 mg) is usually sufficient to achieve control. In the event of further intravenous diazepam being necessary then the modern intravenous cannulae, which permit the administration of continuous intravenous fluids and intermittent intravenous injections, are valuable.

Jacksonian epilepsy, and rarely 'epilepsia partialis continuans', may occur at the onset of an infarct. Both should be treated with routine anticonvulsants such as primidone or phenytoin as much for the comfort of the patient as anything else. The former will commonly respond briskly to treatment, the latter slowly, if at all, but will usually regress within a few days. If it does not then revision of the diagnosis will almost certainly be necessary.

Diabetes mellitus

The routine screening for diabetes mellitus should be obligatory in all forms of ischaemic vascular disease. The reported prevalence of diabetes mellitus in the general population is often an index of the degree to which the diagnosis has been pursued. The Royal College of General Practitioners' survey in 1962 reported a prevalence of 3.3 per cent in 18 532 patients. In contrast Sharp et al, (1964), in a population of 25 701, using where appropriate a battery of investigations, observed a prevalence in the population of 12 per cent.

The true frequency of diabetes mellitus in established cerebral infarction is not clearly defined. That selection of cases tends to exaggerate the prevalence of diabetes mellitus is suggested by the experience of Silverstein & Doniger (1963); in patients with arteriographic evidence of arterial occlusion a prevalence of 32 per cent was observed. In contrast Goldenberg et al (1958) in 3470 autopsies found an overall prevalence of diabetes mellitus of 7.6 per cent. There was no evidence of a higher prevalence of diabetes mellitus in patients with established cerebral vascular disease.

The age of onset of the stroke may well be important, however, for in a review by Louis & McDowell (1967) of 'young strokes' they observed a prevalence of diabetes mellitus of 42 per cent, the diabetes developing either before, during, or in the immediate follow-up period after the acute episode.

The importance of routine screening for diabetes mellitus in the acute management of established stroke is emphasised by the report of Anderson (1974). He described three patients with acute focal signs in the central nervous system presenting as emergencies. In each patient diabetes mellitus was demonstrated, and following treatment full and rapid resolution of signs occurred in two. This observation also emphasises that patients with mature onset diabetes who are admitted with cerebral infarction may require insulin and precise control of the diabetes during the acute phase of the illness.

McCurdy (1970), discussing the relatively recently recognised entity of hyperosmolar hyperglycaemic non-ketotic diabetic coma, felt that the high mortality was related not only to the absence of the classical signs of diabetic ketosis in this condition but also to the tendency to diagnose a cerebral vascular accident because of focal neurological signs and the patient's age.

The future

The undoubted advances in knowledge of the haemodynamic changes following cerebral ischaemia which have been made over the past 25 years have not been paralleled by advances in treatment. There appear to be several possible reasons for this.

One is that acute cerebral infarction, lacking the emotive appeal of cardiac infarction, has not attracted the attention it deserves as a cause of disability in the community. This may be due, in part, to lack of knowledge of the facts. If the incidence for subarachnoid haemorrhage, cerebral haemorrhage and cerebral thrombosis are considered together, then 20 per cent of attacks occur in the ages covering the working life. It is true that 40 to 50 per cent of the patients remain in hospital for more than one month but this is independent of age (Acheson & Fairbairn, 1970). There can be little justification, therefore, for regarding cerebral infarction as the province of the geriatric service alone.

A further reason which may not encourage active therapy is the understandable feeling that the majority of patients presenting with cerebral infarction are suffering from the end result of a long process of vascular degeneration. This cannot be denied. What needs to be debated is the view that there is little hope that treatment can make anything more than a marginal contribution to limiting the effects of acute cerebral infarction. It is certain that in a restricted number of infarcts in the vertebrobasilar circulation of the type already referred to it may be necessary to call on the full resources of intensive care units to achieve the best results and that these may approximate to full recovery. Such opportunities are rare. The commonest problem, both in domiciliary and hospital practice, is posed by those patients who present with limited but potentially disabling physical signs which may deteriorate or improve dramatically within the first few days after onset. The wide discrepancy between various observers on the methods of controlling such factors as cerebral oedema and intravascular stasis within and adjacent to the infarcted area of brain is an indication of our lack of knowledge. Striking progress in this field has been made and further developments may well lead to a definitive approach to treatment.

A case can be made for setting up in selected hospitals responsible for acute admissions 'stroke units' where the medical and nursing staff can develop the appropriate skills necessary to the assessment and management of a clinical problem which is frequently complex. Only then will it be possible to evaluate, in unequivocal terms, the potential lines of treatment. It may be that when a definitive assessment is available the final decision will be that the only hope lies in preventative measures such as the adequate control of hypertension and the prevention of atheroma. The evidence presently available, however, does not warrant pre-empting this conclusion by advocating a policy of therapeutic nihilism.

REFERENCES

Acheson J 1971 Factors affecting the natural history of focal cerebral vascular disease. Quarterly Journal of Medicine 40:25

Acheson R M 1966 Mortality from cerebrovascular disease in the United States. Public Health Monograph 76: 23

Acheson R M, Fairbairn A H 1970 Burden of cerebrovascular disease in the Oxford area in 1963 and 1964. British Medical Journal ii:621

Anderson J M 1974 Diabetic ketoacidosis presenting as neurosurgical emergencies. British Medical Journal iii: 22

Aring C D, Merritt H H 1935 Differential diagnosis between cerebral haemorrhage and cerebral thrombosis. A clinical and pathological study of 245 cases. Archives of Internal Medicine 56: 435

Baker R N, Broward J H, Fang H C et al 1962 Anticoagulant therapy in cerebral infarction: report of a co-operative study. Neurology (Minneapolis) 12: 823

Battistini I N, Casacchia M, Bartolini G 1969 Effects of hyperventilation on focal brain damage following middle cerebral artery occlusion. In: Cerebral blood flow. Springer Verlag, New York

Bauer R B, Tellez H 1973 Dexamethasone as treatment in cerebrovascular disease. 2. A controlled study in acute cerebral infarction. Stroke 4: 547

Blayaert A L, Nemoto E M, Safar P, Stezoski W, Mickell J J, Moossy J, Rao G P 1978 Thiopental amelioration of brain damage after global ischaemia in monkeys. Anaesthesiology 49: 390

Boddie H G 1972 Ocular bobbing and opsoclonus. Journal of Neurology, Neurosurgery and Psychiatry 35: 739

Carter A B 1961 Anticoagulant treatment in progressing stroke. British Medical Journal ii:70

Carter A B 1964 Cerebral infarction. MacMillan, New York

Christensen M S 1970 Stroke treated with prolonged hyperventilation. In: Ross Russell R W (ed), Brain and blood flow. Proceedings of the fourth international symposium on the regulation of cerebral blood flow. Pitman, London

Cole F. M, Yates P O 1967 The occurrence and significance of intracerebral micro-aneurysms. Journal of Pathology and Bacteriology 93:393

Cort J H 1954 Cerebral salt wasting. Lancet i:752

Diabetes Survey Working Party 1962 Report of a working party appointed by the Royal College of General Practitioners. British Medical Journal i:1497

Dodge P R, Richardson E P, Victor M 1954 Recurrent convulsive seizures as a sequel to cerebral infarction. A clinical and pathological study. Brain 77:610

Dyken M, White P T 1956 Evaluation of cortisone in treatment of cerebral infarction. Journal American Medical Association 162:1531

Eklof B, Schwartz S I 1969 Effects of critical stenosis of the carotid artery and compromised cephalic blood flow. Archives of Surgery 99:695

El-Zayat A, El-Danasoury M 1972 Dysnatremia and cerebrovascular accidents. Journal of Egyptian Medical Association 54:68

Epstein F H, Levitin H, Glaser G, Lavietes P 1961 Cerebral hyponatremia. New England Journal of Medicine 265:513

Farhat S M, Schneider R C 1967 Observations on the effect of systemic blood pressure on intracranial circulation in patients with cerebrovascular insufficiency. Journal of Neurosurgery 27:441

Fazekas J F, Alman W R 1964 Maximal dilatation of cerebral vessels. Archives of Neurology 11:303

Fields W S 1973 Selection of stroke patients for arterial reconstructive surgery. The American Journal of Surgery 125:527

Fisher C M 1961 Pathogenesis and treatment of cerebrovascular disease. Fields W S (ed) Thomas, Springfield, Illinois

Fisher C M 1967 Some neuro-ophthalmological observations. Journal of Neurology, Neurosurgery and Psychiatry 30:383

Galicich J H, French L A, Melby J C 1961 Use of dexamethasone in treatment of cerebral oedema associated with brain tumours. Lancet i:46

Gilroy J, Barnhart M I, Meyer J S 1969 Treatment of acute stroke with dextran 40. The Journal of the American Medical Association 210:293

Goldenberg S, Alex N, Blumenthal H T 1958 Sequelae of arteriosclerosis of the aorta and coronary arteries. A statistical study of diabetes mellitus. Diabetes 7:98

Greenwood J 1968 Acute brain infarction with high intracranial pressure: surgical indications. Johns Hopkins Medical Journal 122:254

Hudson A J, Hyland H H 1958 Hypertensive cerebrovascular disease: a clinical and pathologic review of 100 cases. Annals of Internal Medicine 49:1049

Ito A, Omae T, Katsuki S 1973 Acute changes in blood pressure following vascular diseases in the brain stem. Stroke 4:80

Jayne H W, Scheinberg P, Rich M, Belle M S 1952 The effect of intravenous papaverine hydrochloride on cerebral circulation. Journal of Clinical Investigation 31: 111

Kaste K, Fogelholm R, Waltimo O 1976 Combined dexamethasone and low molecular weight dextran in acute brain infarction: double-blind study. British Medical Journal 2:1409

Kety S S, Schmidt C F, 1945 The determination of cerebral blood flow in man by use of nitrous oxide in low concentrations. American Journal of Physiology 143: 53

Kety S S, Schmidt C F 1948 Nitrous oxide method for the quantitative determination of cerebral blood flow in man. Theory procedure and normal values. Journal of Clinical Investigation 27: 476

Kurtzke J F 1969 Epidemiology of cerebrovascular disease. Springer Verlag. New York, Berlin, Heidelberg.

Lancaster M G 1973 Tracheostomies and stroke. Stroke 4:459

Lehrich J R, Winkler G F, Ojemann R G 1970 Cerebellar infarction with brain stem compression. Diagnosis and surgical treatment. Archives of Neurology 22:490

Louis S, McDowell F 1967 Epileptic seizures in non-embolic cerebral infarction. Archives of Neurology 17:414

Matthews W B, Oxbury J M, Grainger K M R, Greenhall R C D 1976 A blind controlled trial of dextran 40 in the treatment of ischaemic stroke. Brain 99:193

McCurdy D K 1970 Hyperosmolar hyperglycemic nonketotic diabetic coma. Medical Clinics of North America 54:683

McHenry L C 1972 Cerebral vasodilator therapy in stroke. Stroke 3:686

McHenry L C, Jaffe M E, Kawamura J 1970 Effect of papaverine on regional blood flow in focal vascular disease of the brain. New England Journal of Medicine 282:1167

McHenry L C, Goldberg H I, Jaffe M E, Kenton E J, West J W, Cooper E S 1972 Regional cerebral flow. Response to carbon dioxide inhalation in cerebrovascular disease. Archives of Neurology 27:403

Merritt H H, Fremont-Smith F 1938 The cerebrospinal fluid. W B Sanders, Philadelphia

Meyer J S, Charney J Z, Rivera V M, Mathew N T 1971 Treatment with glycerol of cerebral oedema due to acute cerebral infarction. Lancet ii:993

Meyer J S, Gotoh F, Gilroy J, Nara N 1965 Improvement in brain oxygenation and clinical improvement in patients with strokes treated with papaverine hydrochloride. Journal of American Medical Association 194:109

Meyer J. S, Teraura, T, Sakamoto K, Hashi K 1971 The effect of pavabid (oral papaverine) on cerebral blood flow and metabolism in the monkey. Cardiovascular Research Centre Bulletin 9:105

Meyer J S, Fukuuchi Y, Shimazu J, Ohuchi T, Ericsson A D, 1972 Effect of intravenous infusion of glycerol on hemispheric blood flow and metabolism in patients with acute cerebral infarction. Stroke 3:168

Miller D, Adams H 1972 In: Critchley M, O'Leary J L, Jennett B (eds), Scientific foundations of neurology. Heinemann, London

Millikan C H 1955 Evaluation of carbon dioxide inhalation for acute focal cerebral infarction. Archives of Neurology and Psychiatry 73:324

Millikan C H 1971 Reassessment of anticoagulant therapy in various types of occlusive cerebrovascular disease. Stroke 2:201

Moseley J I, Laurent J P, Molinari G F, 1975 Barbiturate attenuation of the clinical course and pathologic lesions in a primate stroke model. Neurology 25:870

Moskowitz E, Lightbody F E H, Freitag N S 1972 Long term follow-up of the post-stroke patient. Archives of Physical Medicine and Rehabilitation 53:167

O'Brien M D, Waltz A G, Jordan M A 1974 Ischaemic cerebral edema. Archives of Neurology 30:456

Olesen J, Paulson O B 1971 The effect of intra-arterial papaverine on the regional cerebral blood flow in patients with stroke or intracranial tumour. Stoke 2:148

Patten B M, Mendell J, Bruun B, Curtin W, Carter S 1972 Double-blind study of the effects of dexamethasone on acute stroke. Neurology 22:377

Plum F, Alvord E C, Posner J B 1963 Effect of steroids on experimental cerebral infarction. Archives of Neurology 9:571

Plum F, Posner J B 1972 Diagnosis of stupor and coma, 2nd edn. Davis, Philadelphia

Pullicino P, Kendall B E 1980 Contrast enhancement in ischaemic lesions. Neuroradiology 19:235

Roberts H J 1958 Supportive adrenocortical steroid therapy in acute and subacute cerebrovascular accidents with particular reference to brain-stem involvement. Journal of American Geriatrics 6:686

Ross Russell R W 1970 A microangiographic study of experimental cerebral ischaemia and of the effects of blood pressure changes. In: Ross Russell R W (ed) Brain and blood flow. Proceedings of the fourth international symposium on regulation of cerebral blood flow. Pitman, London

Russek H I, Zohman B L, Russek A S 1954 Corisone in the immediate therapy of apoplectic stroke. Journal American Geriatric Society 2:216

Sambrook M A, Hutchinson E C, Aber G M 1973 Metabolic studies in subarachnoid haemorrhage and strokes — 11. Serial changes in cerebrospinal fluid and plasma urea electrolytes and osmolality. Brain 96:191

Shanbrom E, Levy L 1957 The role of systemic blood pressure in cerebral circulation in carotid and basilar artery thromboses. Clinical implications and therapeutic implications of vasopressor agents. American Journal of Medicine 23:197

Sharp C L, Butterfield W J H, Keen H 1964 Diabetes Survey in Bedford. Proceedings of the Royal Society of Medicine 57:193

Shaw C M, Alvord E C, Berry R G 1959 Swelling of the brain following ischaemic infarction with arterial occlusion. Archives of Neurology 1:161

Shenkin H A, Cabieses F, Van-Den Noordt G, Sayers P, Copperman R 1951 The hemodynamic effect of unilateral carotid ligation on the cerebral circulation of man. Journal of Neurosurgery 8:38

Silverstein A, Doniger D E 1963 Systemic and local conditions predisposing to ischaemic and occlusive cerebrovascular disease. Journal of the Mount Sinai Hospital, New York 30:435

Soloway M, Nadel W, Albin M S, White R J 1968 The effect of hyperventilation on subsequent cerebral infarction. Anesthesiology 29:975

Soloway M, Moriarty G, Fraser J G, White R J 1970 The effect of delayed hyperventilation on experimental middle cerebral artery occlusion. In: Ross Russell R W (ed) Brain and blood flow. Proceedings of the fourth international symposium on the regulation of cerebral blood flow. Pitman, London

Sornas R, Ostlund H, Muller R 1972 Cerebrospinal fluid cytology after stroke. Archives of Neurology 26:489

Symon L, Ishikawa S, Lavy S, Meyer J S 1963 Quantitative measurement of cephalic blood flow in the monkey. Journal of Neurosurgery 20:199

Taylor W H 1961 Hypernatraemia in cerebral disorders. Journal of Clinical Pathology 15:211

Waltz A G 1971 Studies of the cerebral circulation. What have they taught us about stroke? Mayo Clinic Proceedings 46:268

Weed L H, McKibben P S 1919 Pressure changes in the cerebrospinal fluid following intravenous injection of solutions of various concentrations. American Journal of Physiology 48:512

Wells R E 1964 Rheology of blood in microvasculature. New England Journal of Medicine 270:832

Welt L G, Seldin D W, Nelson W P, German W J, Peters J P 1952 Role of the central nervous system in metabolism of electrolytes and water. American Medical Association Archives of Internal Medicine 29:355

Whisnant J P, Fitzgibbons J P, Kurland L T, Sayre G P 1971 Natural history of stroke in Rochester, Minnesota, 1945 through 1954. Stroke 2:11

Whisnant J P 1977 Indications for medical and surgical therapy for ischaemic stroke. In: Thompson R A, Green J R (eds) Advances in neurology, vol 16, Raven press, New York

Wise G 1970 Vasopressor drug therapy for complications of cerebral arteriography. New England Journal of Medicine 282:610

Wise B L, Chater N 1962 The value of hypertonic mannitol solution in decreasing brain mass and lowering cerebrospinal fluid pressure. Journal of Neurosurgery 19:1038

Wise G, Sutter R, Burkholder J 1972 The treatment of brain ischaemia with vasopressor drugs. Stroke 3:135

11

Transient cerebral ischaemia

R. W. Ross Russell

A transient ischaemic attack (TIA) is a focal reduction in cerebral blood supply resulting in a short period of loss of function which recovers rapidly without residual disability. Most attacks last from five to twenty minutes but some do not recover for some hours. The duration allowed within the definition is arbitrary but most authors accept a maximum period of 24 hours.

A sharp distinction is traditionally made on clinical grounds between TIA, in which it is assumed that no structural brain damage has occurred, and minor stroke where a small but permanent ischaemic lesion exists inspite of a good clinical recovery. The distinction has been made on the duration of the deficit and on the presence or absence of residual signs. With modern CT scanning it has become clear that it is impossible to exclude cerebral infarction on clinical signs alone. Furthermore, there is no difference on grounds of aetiology, prognosis or treatment between a true TIA, a prolonged reversible ischaemic neurological deficit (PRIND) and a minor stroke. It has been found neither practical nor helpful to separate these three conditions and they are now considered as a single entity.

Transient cerebral ischaemia is a common symptom though *prevalence* rates are subject to large ethnic and socio-economic variation; its prevalence for instance is 50 per 1000 in white women aged 65–74 living in the Northern United States but 89 per 1000 in black women. *Incidence* rates on the other hand are much more constant, the overall figure for North America being 0.3 per 1000 per year. At ages 55–64 the figure is 0.7 per 1000 per year and at 65–74 it is 2.2. Men with TIA outnumber women except in the over 80 age groups (Heyman et al, 1974).

NATURAL HISTORY OF TIA

TIAs often recur but the number of attacks suffered by individual patients is variable (Table 11.1). One third of patients suffer only a single attack but most have two to ten attacks and only 12 per cent have a total of more than ten (Freidman et al, 1969). There may also be differences between

Table 11.1 Clinical characteristics of transient ischaemic attacks. (Freidman et al, 1969).[a]

	Number of patients	Per cent
Number of attacks		
1	22	37
2	7	12
3	7	12
5	2	3
10	1	2
uncertain < 10	14	23
uncertain > 10	6	10
unknown	1	2
Duration of typical attack		
< 10 min	9	15
10 min–1 hour	21	35
1–24 hours	24	40
Unknown	6	10
Vascular territory involved		
Carotid	47	78
Vertebrobasilar	11	18
Unknown, probably both	2	3
Previous cardiovascular disease		
Hypertension	29	48
Coronary artery disease	27	45
Abnormal ECG	29	48
Enlarged heart on X-ray	9	15
Cardiac failure	9	15
Atrial fibrillation	5	8

[a]Freidman et al studied the occurrence of TIA in a retirement community. Eighteen per cent developed a stroke during 29 months of observation. The following features were correlated with stroke: female sex, age over 70, carotid location, brief TIA. Number of TIAs, blood pressure, and cardiac status showed no correlation.

the two main types of TIA. Vertebrobasilar ischaemic attacks (VBI) are said to be more than twice as frequent as carotid and tend to recur over a longer period (Ziegler & Hassanein, 1973) but diagnostic criteria are not uniform and this opinion has been challenged.

About 30 per cent of patients with stroke give a retrospective history of TIA and the chief importance of transient cerebral ischaemia is as a precursor of a major stroke, myocardial infarction or death. *Expectation of life* assessed in a community study (Cartlidge et al, 1977) is undoubtedly decreased after TIA; after ten years 40 per cent of patients are still alive compared with 60 per cent of age-matched controls. Myocardial infarction is the commonest cause of death. The site of TIA (carotid or VBI) does not affect survival.

As might be expected the *incidence of stroke* is greatly increased after a TIA. In the same study strokes occurred in 17 per cent of patients in the first year after TIA (compared with an expected one per cent). Here again there was no carotid-vertebral difference. The risk of stroke is particularly high in the first month after the first TIA, one quarter of all strokes occurring during this time and one third within six months. After one year the incidence of stroke declines but continues indefinitely at about five per cent per year. approximately five times the incidence for a normal population.

Recent work has also identified other prognostic features; males are more likely to develop *myocardial infarction* after TIA than are females but there is no sex difference in the incidence of cerebral infarction (Heyman et al, 1980). The incidence of stroke is unrelated to duration of individual TIAs and to the number of TIAs but the presence of hypertension or diabetes significantly increases the risk both of myocardial and of cerebral infarction. A past history of myocardial infarction appears to have no effect on the incidence of cerebral infarction but a past history of stroke in a patient suffering TIA signifies an increased risk of both myocardial and cerebral infarction.

The risk of stroke is also influenced by disease in the carotid artery. The presence of an obstructive or ulcerative carotid lesion increases the risk of subsequent development of cerebral infarction, myocardial infarction and sudden death. In TIA patients without a carotid lesion the cumulative risk of cerebral infarction over five years is only 6.4 per cent compared with a figure of 18.2 per cent for the whole group (Heyman et al, 1980).

These studies indicate that a transient cerebral ischaemic attack can be regarded as a symptom of atherosclerosis and as an index of disease in both the coronary and the cerebral circulation.

DIAGNOSIS OF TIA

Carotid ischaemic attacks

The symptomatology of carotid TIA is very variable; although in an individual patient the attacks tend to conform to a single type, there may be differences in severity, duration and distribution. The onset is abrupt and unexpected and affects the patient in the course of everyday activities; the time of day most favoured for attacks is within two hours of rising. In individual patients attacks may be provoked by sudden standing, exertion, coughing, laughing, smoking or anger; most attacks are unprovoked and unpredictable. The disability reaches a maximum within 20 to 30 minutes, occasionally up to 24 hours. Recovery is usually rapid over a few minutes.

The commonest variety affects the territory of a middle cerebral artery and consists of weakness, numbness and heaviness of the contralateral arm and leg. The patient may exhibit slowness and clumsiness of movement out of proportion to weakness or sensory loss. In the usual type of attack facial paresis also occurs but may pass unnoticed by the patient. Other types of attacks affect the arm alone, the leg alone, the face and arm, and arm and leg in that order of frequency (Fisher, 1962). Positive sensory features such as paraesthesiae frequently affect the distal parts of the limb, one side of the face and mouth, and half of the tongue. The march of symptoms characteristic of focal epileptic seizures is not a feature of ischaemic attacks. Visual scintillations in the homonymous half fields do not occur in carotid attacks. A true convulsive seizure is most unusual although the patient may experience a regular jerking or trembling of the affected side.

Examination of the patient during an attack may reveal flaccid weakness of the arm and leg affecting especially abduction of the shoulder, intrinsic muscles of the hand, flexors of the hip and dorsiflexors of the ankle. Sensation may be quite normal, or there may be sensory loss of a cortical type. The reflexes may be somewhat brisker on the affected side, the plantar response extensor in the presence of good power in the leg. Speech disturbance of a dysphasic type may accompany ischaemia of the dominant hemisphere and may be the only symptom. A true dysarthria with preservation of full comprehension and verbal content should raise the suspicion of a brain stem or subcortical lesion. In patients seen some hours after an attack there may be no deficit, but asymmetry of the reflexes or an extensor plantar response may persist. Amaurosis fugax or transient visual uniocular loss in the eye contralateral to the hemiparesis has been calculated to occur in 40 per cent of patients with carotid TIA (Fisher, 1962). Only very exceptionally does it occur at the same time as the hemiparesis. It is a reliable index of carotid disease and is discussed more fully on page 218.

Transient vertebrobasilar ischaemia

Transient vertebrobasilar ischaemia or vertebrobasilar insufficiency (VBI) produce symptoms of disturbed function in the brain stem or the posterior part of the hemisphere either separately or in groups. In a single patient the attacks tend to conform to one type although the intensity may vary. Vertebrobasilar ischaemia is difficult to diagnose because its features may resemble those of syncope or vertigo. There is a tendency to over-diagnosis which probably accounts for the supposed difference in prognosis and natural history between carotid and vertebrobasilar attacks.

The commonest symptom, *vertigo*, occurs in two thirds of patients and is the most difficult to interpret as it cannot easily be distinguished from that originating in disordered labyrinthine function. It is a good general rule that VBI cannot be diagnosed with certainty when recurrent vertigo is the only symptom. Vertigo may be severe, sometimes with vomiting, often related to change in posture or to rotation or extension of the neck. Only very rarely is it accompanied by fluctuating bilateral deafness, or by tinnitus. *Ataxia* on walking is often found in association with vertigo, and there

may be subjective movement of the field of vision. Sometimes there is distortion and apparent tilting of the visual field or oscillopsia. Brief attacks of *diplopia* or rarely polyopia may accompany vertigo and are an important point of distinction from purely labyrinthine disorder. The diplopia may be horizontal or vertical. It usually lasts for five to ten minutes, occasionally for as long as half an hour (Hoyt, 1970). Slurring *dysarthria* may also be experienced with vertigo and the patients may notice *paraesthesiae* and numbness around the mouth and tongue on one or both sides.

Visual disturbances are second in importance only to vertigo and occur in 50 per cent of patients. They consist of abrupt attacks of dimness or loss of focus, often with positive scotomas such as black and white lines or patterns with shimmering scotomas. These may be bilateral, confined to one homonymous half field or to both upper fields. On other occasions vision may be retained but distorted as though looking through water or a moving veil. Complex visual hallucinations, often elaborate and pleasing, are a feature of some attacks (Williams & Wilson, 1962). Total loss of vision or the coloured scotomas of migraine are rare in transient vertebrobasilar attacks. *Headache* is present during an attack to some degree in the majority of patients. It is usually occipital, has a throbbing, bursting quality, and may be intense (Denny-Brown, 1951).

The syndrome of *transient global amnesia* in which the patient loses orientation of time and place and the memory for past events over a period of some hours yet retains personal orientation and remains capable of speech and with no physical defects is usually an isolated event occurring in elderly male patients. Similar attacks however may be encountered in patients with vertebrobasilar insufficiency when the amnesia may be combined with a homonymous hemianopia. Recurrent attacks may leave a permanent amnesic defect (Benson et al, 1973).

Disturbance of consciousness affects only a small minority of patients with vertebrobasilar insufficiency, and a true epileptic seizure rarely if ever occurs. More common are short periods of confusion or loss of awareness without loss of consciousness (Mathew & Meyer, 1974). At other times there may be decorticate posturing, periodic stupor, or akinetic mutism. These symptoms may last some hours and may be followed by complete and rapid recovery. *Leg weakness*, sudden unexpected falling without loss of consciousness or headache (drop attack), is a symptom of vertebrobasilar insufficiency in about 15 per cent of patients. The symptom is commoner in women, usually occurs unexpectedly while walking or standing, and may be provoked by movements of the head or neck (Kremer, 1958). This particular symptom has a number of other causes and vertebrobasilar ischaemia should not be diagnosed when drop attacks are the only feature. Attacks of *weakness or sensory disturbance* localised to one side of the body happen in about 10 per cent of patients. In this type of attack it may be impossible to differentiate carotid from vertebrobasilar TIA. *Alternating attacks* involving the right and left side on different occasions, or marked dysarthria with left sided attacks are suggestive of brain stem localisation. Simultaneous involvement of all four limbs does not occur, although a common feature of basilar occlusion. There is some evidence that patients who experience alternating hemiparesis as a symptom of vertebrobasilar insufficiency are more likely to develop a permanent stroke than those with other symptoms (Marshall, 1964). Abnormal *visceral sensations* such as distortion of taste, feelings of fear or unreality may in rare instances be experienced at the same time as other symptoms of vertebrobasilar insufficiency. They probably relate to ischaemia in the temporal lobes (Williams & Wilson, 1962).

Differential diagnosis

Focal epilepsy may cause attacks of localised limb weakness or positive sensory symptoms, but there is usually additional evidence of an irritative motor lesion shown by repeated jerking or involuntary movements which tend to begin distally and spread up the limb and may on occasion culminate in a generalised seizure. Electroencephalography may indicate an epileptogenic focus whereas the e.e.g. is almost always normal after a TIA.

Focal cerebral symptoms, possibly due to ischaemia, are a feature of many attacks of *migraine*. These are easy to differentiate from TIA when they conform to a classical type with a visual prodrome, followed by unilateral headache and vomiting. The spread of the visual aura in classical migraine to include sensory symptoms in the limbs, face and tongue, sometimes dysphasia but not a severe motor paralysis, is characteristic of migraine but not seen in other forms of vascular disease. Many migrainous patients suffer incomplete attacks where the prodromal symptoms occur without headache. These may be difficult to distinguish from TIA in the posterior cerebral territory. In these cases the diagnosis must rely on the age and sex of the patient and past history of attacks affecting one or other side of the body and on the family history. Vertebrobasilar migraine is commonly found in young women.

In diabetic patients who may be receiving *hypoglycaemic treatment* and some of whom may have latent cerebrovascular disease focal symptoms exactly similar to those of transient cerebral ischaemia may occur during the period of hypoglycaemia (Meyer & Portnoy, 1958; Silas et al, 1981). This cause should be kept in mind particularly when attacks of hemiparesis occur during the night. General hypoglycaemic symptoms may be inconspicuous.

Vertebrobasilar insufficiency may be confused with *labyrinthine disease* such as Menière's syndrome and benign positional vertigo. Deafness, tinnitus and a past history of aural discharge all point to a peripheral labyrinthine disorder.

Acute hypertension by causing local regions of cerebral oedema may present with symptoms resembling a transient ischaemic attack (Kendall & Marshall, 1963). There are usually other symptoms of a more generalised kind such as severe headache, seizures, clouding of consciousness and the onset is seldom as rapid as in TIA.

It is important and sometimes difficult to differentiate focal transient ischaemia from attacks of more *generalised cerebral ischaemia* (syncope) such as that which results from a sudden reduction in cardiac output. Most types of syncope occur only when the patient is upright and the onset may be preceded by feelings of light-headedness, nausea, sweating, pallor, palpitations and heaviness in the limbs. Visual symptoms are also constantly present in syncope and consist of concentric contraction or altitudinal defects of the field of vision, loss of colour vision, spots before the eyes and sometimes complete blindness. Loss of consciousness in the vasovagal type of syncope is rapid and accompanied by bradycardia. The symptoms are rapidly relieved by lying flat.

In summary, the diagnosis of VBI rests on the history of a group of symptoms, the commonest of which are vertigo, visual blurring, ataxia and diplopia occurring in a patient with negative clinical findings and in a setting of arterial degenerative disease. Vascular disease can seldom be diagnosed with confidence on the basis of a single symptom.

PATHOGENESIS OF TRANSIENT ISCHAEMIC ATTACKS

Much of the past disagreement over the aetiology of TIA has been due to the attempt to identify a single factor accounting for all attacks, whereas there are probably many causes. Furthermore the aetiology of a single attack of transient ischaemia may be distinct from the aetiology of multiple repetitive attacks. If the patient recovers completely from an attack it is assumed that no structural damage has been sustained but this assumption is not always justified. Pathological study of the brain of a patient who suffered a single episode of transient ischaemia in life may reveal an unexpected small infarction or even a haemorrhage (Van der Drift & Kok, 1973) and minor alterations in regional blood flow or in oxygen metabolism may be detected for some months after TIA in certain cases (Rees et al, 1970). It must be accepted that if purely clinical criteria are used the definition of TIA will include a number of patients who have sustained a minor infarction or even haemorrhage. As many as 34 per cent have been found to show an abnormality on CT scan (Petrone et al, 1979). When there are repetitive attacks then a TIA without infarction becomes much more likely.

In considering the various causes of transient ischaemia the first major category which can be identified is that due to a temporary defect in the homeostatic mechanisms regulating cerebral blood flow (haemodynamic crisis). This term, introduced by Denny-Brown, was derived from experimental work showing the importance of systemic blood pressure in maintaining blood flow via collateral vessels to a focal region of brain after occlusion of one of the main cerebral arteries (Meyer & Denny-Brown, 1957). Cerebral arteries have an autoregulatory range over which blood flow is maintained irrespective of perfusion pressure. Below a critical point however autoregulation cannot operate and flow becomes passive.

In practice, systemic hypotension appears to be a relatively rare cause of focal TIA; if blood pressure is measured during attacks it is usually normal. Attempts to reproduce focal attacks by artificially reducing blood pressure usually are unsuccessful but if the reduction is excessive loss of consciousness occurs due to generalised cerebral ischaemia (Kendall & Marshall, 1963). This result is not unexpected since the range of blood pressure capable of reducing blood flow to one region of the brain while maintaining adequate flow to other regions is a narrow one. Nevertheless, well-authenticated cases are recorded where systemic hypotension, usually due to sudden cardiac dysrhythmia, blood loss or alteration in posture, has resulted in a focal cerebral deficit (Shanbrom & Levy, 1957). An associated carotid artery lesion may be present (Ruff et al, 1981). When systemic blood pressure is restored the attack comes to an end. Attacks of this type more often affect the vertebrobasilar circulation and this may account for the less serious prognosis of TIA in this territory. In clinical diagnosis, haemodynamic crisis should be suspected when the attacks are related to the upright posture, are accompanied by features of generalised cerebral ischaemia, or by other evidence of reduced cerebral blood flow such as pallor, palpitations or bradycardia or by anginal pain. The onset of attacks is usually less abrupt than in the case of embolism. It must be stressed again that focal symptoms are exceptional. In a large series of patients with ischaemia due to cardiac dysrhythmia only 1.5 per cent had focal rather than general symptoms (Reed et al, 1973).

Stealing and redistribution of blood

An unusual type of haemodynamic crisis may affect the vertebrobasilar circulation when there is a localised proximal occlusion or severe stenosis of one subclavian artery, usually on the left side. The normal pressure gradient in the vertebral artery is reversed, the pressure becoming lower in the neck than in the head. Blood passes up the right vertebral artery, down the left and into the arm. It was originally proposed that vasodilatation in the arm during exercise might increase the amount of diverted blood and lead to temporary cerebral ischaemia (Reivich et al, 1961). In practice such cases are rare; Held et al, (1973) however showed that brachial blood flow on the side of a subclavian occlusion is usually normal but the expected increase in flow during exercise of the arm may be impaired. The reactive hyperaemia test applied to the arm may sometimes provide a brainstem ischaemic attack (Sharon et al, 1981).

Complex patterns of collateral blood flow with reversal of flow in some arteries are a feature of arterial occlusive disease in many sites and do not always imply 'stealing' of blood. In carotid occlusion for instance reversal of blood flow in the ophthalmic artery is a frequent finding and contributes to the cerebral blood supply. The term 'steal' should be reserved for a situation in which increase in flow to one part of a vascular territory is accompanied by features of ischaemia in another. Any change in cerebrovascular resistance in one vascular territory should not have any effect on the blood flow through other territories provided that the blood pressure remains unaltered. However, if one vascular bed is already maximally dilated and a further fall in pressure occurs then the effective blood pressure for the tissue is reduced with a consequent fall in flow in that region. In the case of subclavian steal, hind-brain ischaemia presumably occurs because of the large vasodilatory potential of the arm muscles and the impaired vasodilatation of atherosclerotic cerebral arteries.

The symptomatology of patients with subclavian steal syndrome is little different from other forms of vertebrobasilar insufficiency and consists of recurring occipital headache, dysarthria, vertigo, visual blurring and limb weakness. Tinnitus and loss of consciousness may also occur and the only distinctive symptom is weakness or pain in the arm on the side of the occluded artery which may be provoked by exercise (Toole, 1964).

Other examples of reversed flow and steal may be seen in the extracranial circulation. Blood may flow from the circle of Willis down the right carotid and into the right subclavian artery in patients with occlusion of the brachiocephalic trunk;

extensive anastomoses may develop between the two carotid arteries via thyroid branches, or between the external carotid artery and the vertebral artery via occipital branches. In all these situations the possibility of reduction of cerebral blood flow is present should the effective cerebral blood pressure be reduced by diversion of a large quantity of blood to extra-cerebral tissues.

A similar haemodynamic situation may obtain in arteriovenous fistula or malformation involving the carotid artery. Shunting may occur between carotid branches and one of the venous sinuses or between the vertebral artery and vein. When this happens large volumes of arterial blood may be diverted into a low pressure venous pool, and in some circumstances intermittent focal ischaemia may occur in the territory of the affected vessel (Russell & Green, 1971).

The concept of 'stealing' has also been extended to the intracerebral circulation. An unstable situation in which different areas of brain receive a variable blood supply depending on fluctuations in blood pressure, gas tensions, and intracranial pressure, undoubtedly occurs (Symon, 1969) after acute vascular occlusion (intracerebral steal) and is relevant to the management of cerebral infarction. It has been claimed that this mechanism may cause repeated transient ischaemic attacks by diversion of blood from one hemisphere to the other (Hachinski et al, 1977). The evidence for this is unconvincing except in the presence of a tumour or angioma (Kosary et al, 1973).

Temporary failure of homeostasis may also occur as a result of variations in the cerebral vascular resistance. In polycythaemia, leukaemia, or dysproteinaemia alteration in the relative amounts of plasma and cells or in the physical characteristics of plasma may lead to changes in blood viscosity. The resultant increase in peripheral resistance may be offset to some extent by vasodilatation but the regulatory efficiency of the cerebral circulation may be impaired. Such attacks are usually nonfocal but occasionally resemble vertebrobasilar insufficiency.

Occlusive attacks

The second major cause of transient ischaemia is arterial blockage or narrowing during the period of an attack. This may be caused by embolism or by external compression of an artery. The lumen of an extracranial artery, especially the vertebral (Toole & Tucker, 1960) and to a lesser extent the carotid arteries (Boldrey et al, 1956) may be reduced during movements of the neck and the resistance to blood flow may be increased. This is more likely to occur in the presence of arterial disease, cervical spondylosis or congenital abnormality (Janeway et al, 1966). Because the resistance of the neck arteries is only a part of the total cerebral vascular resistance and because there are alternative routes of blood supply, notably the other extracranial arteries and the circle of Willis, neck movements are seldom the cause of transient cerebral ischaemia except in the presence of extensive extracranial occlusive disease, e.g., in bilateral carotid occlusion. Indentation of the vertebral arteries is produced by lateral protrusion of intervertebral discs and osteophytes and is usually present at a number of levels (Payne & Spillane, 1957). Occasionally obstruction is at a single level and the removal of the lateral disc protrusion has led to cessation of attacks (Gortvai, 1964).

Embolism

Embolism has now become accepted as an important cause of transient ischaemia, especially in the carotid circulation. The clinical and pathological evidence may be summarised as follows: firstly, many attacks develop abruptly and are unrelated to changes in posture, cardiac irregularity or symptoms of systemic hypotension; this sequence of events is consistent with a sudden arterial occlusion in a previously normal vascular bed.

Secondly, separate attacks may affect different parts of the same territory; in the case of the carotid artery patients experience hemisphere ischaemia in some attacks and retinal ischaemia in others. If all were due to a reduction in blood flow through the carotid artery the attacks would be more stereotyped and would consistently tend to affect the same region.

Thirdly, evidence is frequently found of a source of embolism in the heart or major extracranial artery (Symonds, 1927; Gunning et al, 1964). Furthermore, in a patient with carotid stenosis

transient attacks cease when the artery becomes completely blocked (Fisher, 1962).

Fourthly, emboli may be visible in retinal arteries sometimes passing rapidly through the circulation in the course of an attack (Fisher, 1959).

The main objection to embolism as a cause of transient ischaemia is the difficulty of explaining repeated attacks. Research on the composition and behaviour of emboli in the circulation has shown that freshly-formed thrombus composed of platelets and fibrin may break up after causing temporary arrest in the circulation and may pass into smaller arteries. Finally these may disappear completely as a result of lysis or fragmentation. Subsequent emboli tend to take a similar path and may then cause repetitive symptoms.

Carotid TIA: emboli or haemodynamic crisis?

Since the pioneer observations of Fisher (1954) transient ischaemic attacks in the middle cerebral territory and in the retina have come to be associated with disease of the internal carotid artery. How the attacks are produced is still a matter for debate.

Thrombosis of the internal carotid artery has been recognised for many years as a cause of cerebral infarction (Hunt, 1914) but was commonly thought to be less important than thrombosis of intracranial vessels. There were good reasons for this since it was known that surgical ligation of the internal carotid artery in the neck was not usually followed by brain damage, a fact used by Willis to deduce the function of the circular anastomosis at the base of the brain. Even in patients with atherosclerosis, complete carotid occlusion may be asymptomatic and occur as an incidental finding — approximately one to two per cent of patients undergoing angiography for brain tumour show carotid occlusion. On the other hand, in patients with clinical cerebrovascular disease angiography has shown occlusion to be much more prevalent than in patients without vascular disease. A prevalence rate of 17.5 per cent (Bull et al, 1960) agrees closely with that found by Schwartz & Mitchell (1961) in an unselected autopsy series of patients with stroke.

There is thus good reason to incriminate carotid *occlusion* as a factor in cerebral infarction. It may be deduced that in those patients who escape infarction a collateral blood supply is established via the circle of Willis from the contralateral internal carotid and from the basilar system as well as by way of external-internal carotid anastomoses such as the ophthalmic artery.

A link between cerebral infarction and carotid *stenosis* is less clear. Fisher (1954) showed the presence of unsuspected lesions of the carotid artery in 10 per cent of routine autopsies (including patients with cerebral infarction). Hutchinson & Yates (1957), who examined at autopsy the entire extracranial vasculature of 83 patients who had cerebral vascular symptoms during life, found occlusive changes in 40 per cent although they did not separate complete occlusion from severe stenosis. On the other hand, Schwartz & Mitchell (1961) looking at an unselected autopsy population also found 40 per cent to have severe stenosis of one or more extracranial arteries. Less than half of these patients had a history of cerebral symptoms in life.

Since caroticovertebral stenosis seems to be no more frequent at autopsy in cases of stroke than in random population it has been questioned whether a stenosis plays much part in the causation of infarction. Further doubts arise from measurements of pressure in the carotid artery and pial vessels, which show that the major part of the cerebrovascular resistance is in the smaller pial arteries and intracerebral arterioles and that a comparatively small proportion is due to the neck vessels. The calibre of the neck vessels can thus be substantially reduced before having a controlling influence on cerebrovascular resistance. Russell & Cranston (1961) showed that in patients with mild or moderate stenosis of the internal carotid artery the ophthalmic artery pressure was normal and only when stenosis was almost complete was there a reduction in pressure. Similar conclusions were reached by Brice et al (1964), who measured flow in the carotid artery during progressive clamping of the vessel. From these observations it may be deduced that mild or moderate narrowing of a single carotid artery is haemodynamically insignificant and unlikely to cause transient cerebral ischaemia by interference with blood flow. Even

after surgical ligation of the carotid artery (as in the treatment of aneurysm) transient attacks occur very rarely (Fisher, 1962), demonstrating the functional reserves of the collateral circulation. If multiple lesions are present in extracranial arteries, however, haemodynamic factors such as blood pressure may become more critical.

In spite of these reservations there is a strong clinical and angiographic body of evidence linking cerebral ischaemic attacks with all grades of stenosis of the carotid artery and even with atheromatous ulceration of the artery without narrowing (Fisher, 1954). For instance, in patients with unilateral carotid stenosis the symptoms are significantly more frequent on the side of the stenosis than on the contralateral side (Drake & Drake, 1968). In a recent Italian study atherosclerotic lesions were found in patients with TIA in 54 per cent on the side appropriate to the symptom and in 11 per cent on the contralateral side (Fieschi et al, 1981).

It seems that the likeliest mechanism of transient ischaemia in patients with mild stenosis or ulceration of the carotid artery is not a haemodynamic effect but the formation of mural thrombus and embolism to the brain of fragments of thrombus (Fig. 11.1 A–B). Examination of resected specimens of carotid artery from patients with TIAs has confirmed the frequent presence of mural thrombus on the surface of the atheromatous lesion, especially in those patients experiencing recent attacks (Harrison & Marshall, 1976). It is known that some atherosclerotic lesions are enlarged progressively by the accumulation of thrombus over months and years while others remain stationary (Gurdjian et al, 1969). The final effect of successive layering of mural thrombus is to occlude the lumen of the vessel.

ANGIOGRAPHY IN TRANSIENT ISCHAEMIC ATTACKS

The commonest sites of atheromatous narrowing and of occlusion found in patients with all types of transient cerebral ischaemia by four vessel angiography are shown in Figure 11.2 taken from the Cooperative Study (Hass et al, 1968). The frequency of stenotic lesions at the origins of the internal carotid (33.8 per cent) and the vertebral

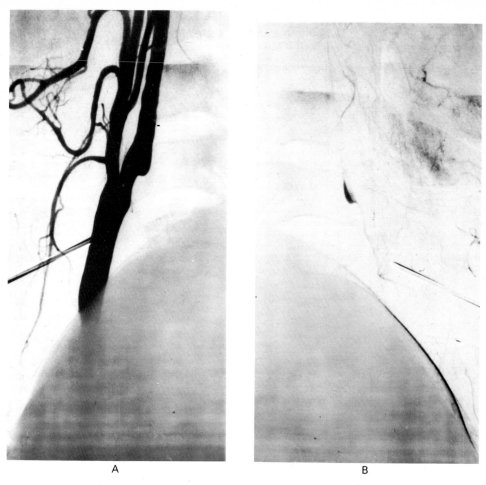

A   B

Fig. 11.1A Carotid angiogram from a patient with transient cerebral ischaemia showing a large atheromatous plaque. There is minimal arterial stenosis.
Fig. 11.1B Later view showing stasis of contrast in an ulcer cavity

artery (20 per cent) is notable. No occlusion was found in 19.4 per cent of patients and in 6.1 per cent changes were present in intracranial vessels only. In carotid occlusion propagation of thrombus takes place throughout the length of the artery so that it is not possible to determine the original site of occlusion. The high proportion of multiple lesions (67.3 per cent) is important and has a bearing both on pathogenesis and treatment.

These findings have been amplified in a more recent study (Swanson et al, 1977) of 100 patients with TIA having angiography of all four main vessels. Atheromatous lesions were graded as either occlusion, severe stenosis (greater than 50 per cent), mild stenosis (less than 50 per cent), or normal. In the group as a whole 60 per cent showed lesions in one or more arteries, although only 32 per cent had single lesions in the artery appropriate to the symptoms. Of those showing angiographic change, there was a wide variety in the degree of narrowing. The commonest finding (47 per cent) was severe stenosis, 33 per cent showed mild stenosis and 26 per cent complete occlusion. Of those patients with one-sided TIA of carotid type 52 per cent has lesions. In 21 per cent this was on the side appropriate to the symptoms, in 22 per cent it was present in both carotids and in 9 per cent in one of the other vessels. All patients having bilateral symptoms showed lesions although not all were on both sides. Of those with vertebrobasilar

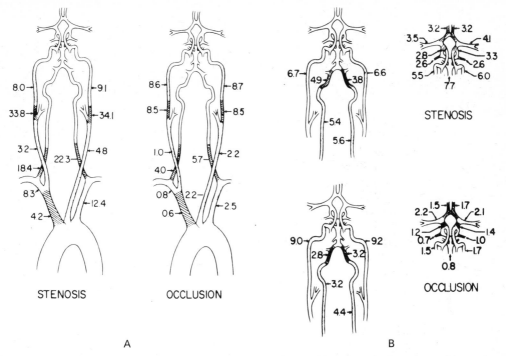

Figs. 11.2A and 11.2B Frequency of stenosis and occlusion found at four vessel angiography on patients with transient cerebral ischaemic attacks. (Reproduced from the joint study of extracranial arterial occlusion by courtesy of Dr W. K. Hass and the editor of the *Journal of the American Medical Association*).

ischaemia 59 per cent showed lesions of one or both vertebral arteries; bilateral lesions were commoner and the left side was more affected than the right. Basilar artery lesions occurred in 16 per cent.

The morbidity and mortality of angiography is decreasing year by year but is still a significant factor in management, especially in the elderly or hypertensive patient or in those with residual signs following a minor stroke. In a recent large multi-centre trial in America including 400 patients having four vessel angiography, transient neurological complications occurred in 5.4 per cent, a permanent deficit in 0.6 per cent and death in 0.25 per cent.

The cause of these complications varies with the technique used. Direct arterial puncture may cause intimal stripping or partial dissection or may dislodge portions of atheromatous plaques. The risk of dissection is particularly high in patients with mesenchymal defects such as the Marfan syndrome. Although indirect techniques are safer the end of the catheter may traumatise the arterial wall, and attempts to pass the catheter through a narrowed vessel may dislodge portions of atheroma causing cerebral embolism. An intramural haematoma or direct pressure from extravasated blood around the artery may cause a delayed occlusion.

Contrast material itself, especially in high concentrations, may have a direct harmful effect on small intracerebral or intraspinal blood vessels. This is most likely when cerebral blood flow is reduced as in cerebral infarction, subarachnoid haemorrhage, polycythaemia, hypertensive cardiac failure or when the patient is anaesthetised.

Non-invasive ultrasound techniques have made recent advances and are now capable of showing moderate or severe grades of stenosis as well as estimating the direction and volume of blood flow. Although these are valuable as screening tests it is not yet possible to distinguish confidently between sub-total and total occlusion; minor grades of stenosis or mural ulceration may also be overlooked. New techniques in *computerised image intensification* may allow arteries to be seen after intravenous injection of contrast with a clarity which approaches that of an arterial injection. These techniques may well replace other methods in the future (Christenson et al, 1980).

In making a clinical decision on whether to do an angiogram it is helpful to keep in mind the likely yield of positive information. An estimate of this can be gained from simple clinical examination. Harrison & Marshall (1975) have shown that the prevalence of carotid lesions is greatest in those patients having ischaemic attacks in both retina and hemisphere and in those with a carotid bruit. Carotid stenosis of a type suitable for surgery was found in 33 per cent and 61 per cent respectively. This compares with the figure of 13 per cent in those patients having hemisphere attacks without a carotid bruit. Wilson & Russell (1977) who studied patients with amaurosis fugax showed that age over 50, hypertension, transient cerebral ischaemia or intermittent claudication as well as the presence of a carotid bruit were all features which correlated with the finding of surgically correctable lesions in the carotid artery. If none of these features was present the angiogram was always negative. These clinical guidelines are useful in the selection of patients for angiography. A localised carotid bruit is the most informative clinical sign but it can indicate stenosis of the external rather than the internal carotid and it can be present without any abnormality, especially when there is increased flow through the vessel as in occlusion on the contralateral side. The bruit also tends to become softer and may even disappear as the arterial lumen becomes very narrow. As many as 20 per cent of those with severe stenosis had no detectable bruit in one series (Swanson et al, 1977). A non-localised carotid bruit heard over the whole length of the common carotid artery in the neck is much less informative and frequently arises in the aorta or the aortic valve. A localised murmur heard over the head of the clavicle on the right side is a common finding of doubtful significance and is associated with lengthening or kinking of the innominate artery.

Although hypertension causes an increase in severity of atheroma in large arteries it also tends to cause intracranial arterial disease in small vessels. This latter change is evidently a more significant cause of stroke. Prineas & Marshall (1966) examining patients with completed stroke showed that extracranial arterial lesions were more frequent in patients with normal blood pressure whereas hypertensive patients had fewer large vessel extracranial occlusions but more intracranial small vessel disease.

SURGICAL TREATMENT

The first successful carotid endarterectomy for transient cerebral ischaemia was published by Eastcott et al in 1954 and the subsequent 25 years have seen reports of many thousands of patients treated by a variety of surgical techniques. Carotid endarterectomy is now said to be the commonest vascular operation in the United States. Unfortunately there has been only one controlled clinical trial to assess its effectiveness and this did not show overall benefit in the surgical group (Fields et al, 1970). However, since it may never be repeated it is worth considering in some detail.

There was a total of 316 patients randomly allocated to surgical and non-surgical categories. All patients had a history of transient cerebral ischaemia in any vascular territory but no fixed neurological deficit; some of the non-surgical group received anticoagulants.

In patients with *unilateral carotid stenosis* with no lesion on the opposite side followed for an average period of three and a half years, 43 per cent of the surgical group continued to experience transient attacks compared with 44 per cent of the control group. However the majority of attacks were vertebrobasilar in type and when carotid attacks were considered separately it was found that only four to five per cent of the surgical group had continuing attacks in this territory compared with 8.3 per cent in the non-surgical group. Of the operated cases 36.3 per cent were asymptomatic compared with 37.5 per cent in the non-surgical group. Completed strokes, fatal and non-fatal, occurred in two surgical patients and five non-surgical patients. There was thus no significant difference between the two groups.

In patients with *bilateral carotid stenosis* the surgical group underwent single or multiple endarterectomy and 45.5 per cent were asymptomatic on follow up compared with 25.4 per cent of the non-surgical group, this difference being significant. Three strokes occurred in the surgical group.

In patients with *carotid stenosis and a contralateral occlusion*, most underwent endarterectomy on the stenosed carotid, and 85 per cent of the surgical patients became asymptomatic; in the non-surgical group 48 per cent were asymptomatic. One permanent stroke occurred in the follow-up period in the surgical group and four in the non-surgical group.

In the whole group over the period of the trial the percentage of asymptomatic surviving patients was significantly greater in the surgical group although in the sub-group with unilateral carotid stenosis no significant difference emerged. TIAs continued in 36 per cent of cases in the surgically treated group as against 47 per cent in the non-surgical group, the difference being not significant. However in all three sub-groups the difference was in favour of surgically treated cases. When TIAs recurred in the surgical group they were usually referred to the territory of a cerebral artery other than the one operated on.

The most important findings were in relation to new strokes. (Table 11.2). When the operative phase was included there were 20 new strokes in 169 surgical patients (12 per cent) compared with 19 in 147 medical patients (13 per cent). Only if the operative complications were disregarded did a significant difference emerge between late strokes in the surgical group (4 per cent in 42 months) compared with the medical group (12 per cent in 42 months).

A number of criticisms can be made of the Cooperative Study, the most serious of which is that the mortality and morbidity of surgical procedure was insufficiently stressed when presenting the results. Furthermore, during the follow-up period strokes arising in the territory of the operated artery were not considered separately from those in other territories. A smaller point is that both groups had a variety of medical treatments so that the trial in fact compared 'medical treatment' with 'medical treatment plus surgery'. It was a condition of the trial that all patients underwent angiography before inclusion; this leads to some confusion since angiography is a necessary preliminary to surgical but not to medical treatment.

The results of this painstaking trial have been largely ignored chiefly because of the assumption that surgical mortality and morbidity have improved since it was carried out. This is probably true and even during the period of the trial a reduction in surgical mortality was evident from 5 to 1.5 per cent. Although no other controlled studies have been carried out the recurrence rate of new strokes after successful surgery has been consistently found to be approximately three per cent per annum (Stanford et al, 1978), about one-half of the expected incidence without surgery.

Many other reports have appeared; most consist of series of patients treated surgically usually from specialist centres. None of these has included a control group but in general they support the claims of surgical efficacy. Wylie & Ehrenfeld (1970) operated on 91 patients with unilateral carotid stenosis who had suffered transient symptoms and showed that 85 were symptom-free during an average follow-up period of 4 years. 3

Table 11.2 The results of the Joint Study of patients with TIAs divided into categories on the basis of the angiographic appearances (Fields et al, 1970)

| | | Number of patients Unilateral carotid stenosis | | Bilateral carotid stenosis | | Unilateral carotid stenosis and contralateral occlusion | | Total | |
	End points	Surgical	Medical	Surgical	Medical	Surgical	Medical	Surgical	Medical
In hospital	Stroke	1 (2%)	1 (2%)	10 (11%)	0	3 (10%)	0	14 (8%)	1 (1%)
	Death	1 (2%)	0	5 (5%)	1 (1%)	0	0	6 (4%)	1 (1%)
Follow-up after hospital	Stroke	2 (5%)	5 (10%)	3 (4%)	9 (12%)	1 (4%)	4 (16%)	6 (4%)	18 (12%)
	Death	7 (16%)	7 (15%)	11 (14%)	14 (19%)	5 (19%)	6 (24%)	23 (15%)	27 (19%)
Total follow-up	Stroke	3 (7%)	6 (12%)	13 (14%)	9 (12%)	4 (13%)	4 (16%)	20 (12%)	19 (13%)
	Death	8 (18%)	7 (14%)	16 (17%)	15 (21%)	5 (17%)	6 (24%)	29 (17%)	28 (19%)
Total number of patients		45	49	94	73	30	25	169	147

patients were unchanged. Operative mortality in patients with transient symptoms improved from 1.7 per cent to 0.5 per cent over the 10 years of this study. In bilateral carotid stenosis in 135 patients 95 per cent were rendered symptom-free after operation on both arteries. In carotid stenosis and contralateral occlusion there were 21 patients of whom 15 had no symptoms on follow-up. On the other hand carotid endarterectomy outside the major centres carries a very different operative complication rate and in one recent report serious complications or death occurred in as many as 21 per cent (Easton & Sherman, 1977).

The great majority of surgical reports refer to stenotic lesions of the internal carotid artery (De Weese et al, 1971). Reconstructive procedures have been used for other lesions such as stenosis of the vertebral artery at its origin or in the bony canal, occlusion or stenosis of the brachiocephalic trunk and of the subclavian arteries. The operative technique used is most commonly endarterectomy and the arterial lumen may be widened by insertion of a homograft or patch graft. If disease extends into the ostia of the great vessels or involves the aorta it may be preferable to employ bypassing procedures from other healthy arteries (De Bakey et al, 1965). Complete occlusion of the internal carotid artery is not operable except in its very early stages since propagation of thrombus occurs throughout the vessel and no back flow can be obtained. It can however be treated by extracranial/intracranial artery bypass (see Ch. 21).

When advising treatment for patients with carotid stenosis and transient cerebral ischaemia the standard of available vascular surgery is thus of the first importance. It has been calculated that to show an overall improvement on the natural history of the condition a surgical series must have a stroke and mortality rate of less than three to four per cent and an operative mortality of less than one per cent (Harrison, 1980). Evidence summarised above and in chapter 21 shows that either medical or surgical treatment slightly improves the prognosis of patients with TIA but neither is clearly superior. If expert surgery is available this is often preferred since it offers a rapid, simple and relatively safe treatment and avoids the risks and inconvenience associated with long term anticoagulant or antiplatelet therapy.

When deciding on treatment for an individual patient the following points may be kept in mind. In favour of *surgical treatment* are: 1. availability of an experienced department of vascular surgery; 2. a young patient without symptoms of generalised peripheral vascular disease; 3. the absence of a history of cardiac ischaemia, severe hypertension and diabetes. If these are present in combination the operative mortality for carotid endarterectomy may be as high as seven per cent; 4. a localised lesion of the internal carotid artery with a moderate degree of stenosis and no extensive intracranial disease in a patient with carotid TIA or amaurosis fugax on the appropriate side; 5. the absence of intravascular thrombus in the carotid artery on angiography.

Conversely *medical treatment* is favoured in those patients who have VBI, have symptoms in a part of the brain not supplied by the stenotic artery, have a higher operative risk for reasons of age, intercurrent illness, cardiac ischaemia, hypertension or diabetes. Many operative stroke deaths occur in patients who have recently suffered cerebral infarction and this factor should be given particular weight. It may happen that a patient known to have carotid stenosis develops a stroke while on medical treatment or while awaiting surgery in hospital. When this occurs there is a strong presumption that the carotid artery has thrombosed and a previously audible bruit may disappear. If such patients are subjected to emergency carotid surgery with or without angiography it is often possible to remove fresh thrombus from the carotid artery. However the results of this are often disappointing. The operation carries a high mortality and rethrombosis of the artery frequently occurs. With the possible exception of postoperative thrombosis when a dissection or periarterial haematoma may be found the early treatment of carotid thrombosis is by medical rather than by surgical means.

MANAGEMENT OF TRANSIENT CEREBRAL ISCHAEMIA DUE TO ATHEROSCLEROSIS

After exclusion of patients with arteritis or haematological disorders and those with a cardiac source for embolism, the remainder (constituting over 90 per cent of those with transient ischaemia) are presumed to have atherosclerotic cerebrovascular disease. Guidelines for the management of this group can be laid down in the light of the natural history and the results of available trials of medical and surgical treatment. The following scheme is orientated towards the detection of extracranial vascular disease on the assumption that expert vascular surgery is available and is the most satisfactory treatment for those patients with accessible lesions of the internal carotid artery. Management of patients can be divided into three main parts — C.T. scanning, clinical examination and angiography (see Table 11.3).

C.T. scanning

Many of the previous uncertainties and dangers of early treatment were due to the inadvertent inclusion in the treated group of patients with other lesions. With C.T. scanning it is now possible to be sure that a brief reversible focal disturbance is not due to a minor haemorrhage or to a cerebral tumour. In ideal circumstances all patients should have a C.T. scan with contrast enhancement as soon as possible after the attack.

Clinical examination

If the scan shows no evidence of haemorrhage a further reappraisal of the patient's vascular state and general health is now necessary. Particular attention is paid to age, blood pressure, cardiac status, diabetes, e.c.g. and arterial pulses. The object is to decide whether the patient is fit for angiography and arterial surgery. If fit, the patient is assigned to the *good risk group*.

Angiography

Good risk patients with carotid TIA proceed to angiography of both carotid arteries and are referred for vascular surgery if a lesion suitable for carotid endarterectomy is found in the appropriate carotid artery. It is important to visualise not only the origin but the intracranial portions of the carotid artery because a proportion of stenotic lesions are found in the distal segment. In those patients found suitable for surgery there is nothing to be gained by delaying operation and this should be carried out as soon as possible.

MEDICAL TREATMENT

The remainder of patients are treated medically but the type of treatment varies according to the time which has elapsed since the last attack. The objective of medical treatment is to prevent further thromboembolism and since the risks of this are greatest in the first few weeks after a TIA medical treatment should begin at once.

General measures

Patients with hypertension or diabetes require optimal control and all patients are strongly advised

Table 11.3 Initial clinical screening of patients with transient cerebral ischaemia

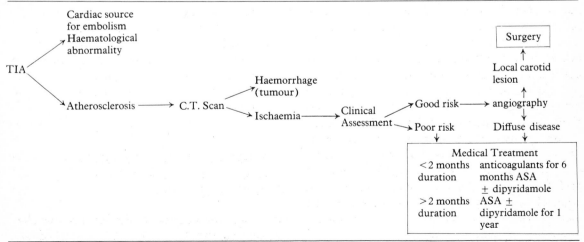

to stop smoking cigarettes. They should remain off work for from two to four weeks after a TIA but should be encouraged to remain ambulant, to take moderate exercise and have a minimum of seven hours sleep at night. Obese patients are advised to lose weight.

Antithrombotic treatment

The choice of antithrombotic treatment is a matter for individual preference depending on the availability and quality of laboratory services, the reliability of the patient and relatives, and the patient's tolerance of a particular drug.

Patients seen soon after an attack (less than two months). Some authorities use anticoagulants (Warfarin) for three months for all patients seen within two months of the event (Sandok et al, 1978). If the condition is stabilized after three months on treatment the anticoagulants are slowly discontinued and replaced by aspirin (300 mg a day), or by dipyridamole for female patients. These are continued for one year.

Other centres have a similar policy to the above except that TIA patients with moderate or severe hypertension are not given anticoagulants. Hypertension is controlled and they are then assigned to aspirin or dipyridamole.

Patients seen more than two months after the attack. The risk of stroke has been substantially reduced by this time and aspirin alone or dipyridamole in female patients is given as above. Hypertension is treated if appropriate.

Patients seen more than one year after the attack. No clinical treatment is advised except general measures and the control of blood pressure.

Vertebrobasilar ischaemic attacks

Management for patients with vertebrobasilar ischaemia is similar except that they are not subjected to angiography unless there is clinical evidence of arterial stenosis or occlusion in the carotid or subclavian arteries. If these features are absent they are treated medically as above.

A difficult question is posed by those patients who have vertebrobasilar symptoms but are found to have carotid stenosis on one or both sides. In my view such patients should be referred for carotid endarterectomy if the degree of stenosis is severe and may be limiting overall cerebral blood flow. Those with minor degrees of stenosis or ulceration are treated medically.

A discussion on the indication for transcranial bypass surgery in TIA is found in Chapter 21.

OCULAR ISCHAEMIA

Since the ophthalmic, middle cerebral and anterior cerebral arteries all originate from the internal carotid artery, ischaemic attacks in the brain and eye have many features in common. The retina derives blood from two sources, the outer layers being nourished by the short ciliary arteries, two or more in number, which also supply the optic disc and the major part of the optic nerve. The inner retina including nerve fibre layer and ganglion cells receive blood from the central retinal artery. Both the central retinal artery and the ciliary arteries arise from the ophthalmic artery.

Temporary reduction in ocular blood supply in either the retinal or choroidal system may produce transient uniocular loss of vision (amaurosis fugax). This symptom should be distinguished from transient loss of the homonymous half field due to ischaemia in one posterior cerebral territory.

As in the brain, there are a number of possible mechanisms which may sometimes be separated by attention to the circumstances of onset of the attack and the type of visual field loss. The number of attacks varies considerably; some patients suffer only a single attack while in others the symptoms may occur many times a day.

Retinal embolism

Embolism is probably the commonest single cause of amaurosis fugax. Emboli which are visible by ophthalmoscopy and which are of the size capable of occluding retinal arteries (50 to 150 microns) may be composed of platelets, cholesterol fragments, mixed thrombus or particles of calcified cardiac valve. The degree and duration of retinal ischaemia depends on the number and composition of the emboli.

Fibrin platelet emboli appear as small, white, friable, non-refractile bodies which have been observed to pass slowly through the retinal circulation breaking up as they do so. They have been shown to be composed of platelet fibrin aggregates (McBrien et al, 1963). The source is commonly mural thrombus in the internal carotid artery formed on the surface of an atheromatous plaque or ulcer. The artery is usually, but not necessarily, narrowed at the point of thrombus formation. Fibrin platelet emboli are thought to be responsible for the majority of attacks of amaurosis fugax, the duration of attacks corresponding to the passage of an embolus through the retinal circulation. The symptoms consist of abrupt painless uniocular visual loss, usually without positive phenomena such as flashing lights or patterns. A horizontal curtain effect is often described and the loss of vision can be limited to the upper or lower half field. The duration is commonly half to five minutes, recovery is rapid and sometimes succeeded by violaceous discolouration of vision for a few minutes. The number of attacks varies widely up to 20 or more per day. Very similar symptoms probably occur with embolic obstruction of ciliary arteries but field loss is not complete and there may be a vertical type of hemianopia. Because they originate in the internal carotid artery fibrin-platelet emboli also pass into the cerebral circulation, usually the middle cerebral branch. These attacks do not occur at the same time as amaurosis fugax and are seldom as frequent.

The natural history of amaurosis fugax of this type probably differs from that of transient cerebral ischaemia, the incidence of stroke being lower than 10 per cent (Marshall & Meadows, 1968). The two conditions should not be equated in therapeutic trials.

Cholesterol emboli

Retinal emboli composed of cholesterol-containing atheromatous debris were described by Hollenhorst (1962) and shown to be derived from the internal carotid artery by David et al (1963). The origin is usually a plaque situated near the origin or in the syphon. In chronic hypertension, where atheroma is more extensive, emboli may be derived from smaller vessels such as the ophthalmic artery. The behaviour of cholesterol emboli differs from that of platelet emboli; the majority impact for a time at the lamina cribrosa before fragmenting into smaller flakes which lodge in retinal arterioles usually in the region of the macula. The amount of visual loss is unpredictable; small numbers of cholesterol emboli may be an incidental finding in hypertensive or diabetic subjects without visual loss. This is probably because the flat cholesterol crystals impact across the vessel without causing significant obstruction of flow. Cholesterol emboli can however cause branch occlusion and permanent visual loss. Finally, cholesterol emboli may be found in patients shortly after an attack of amaurosis fugax when a brief obstruction is presumably followed by fragmentation and restoration of flow. Cholesterol emboli have a characteristic yellow refractile appearance and are usually found at points of branching of the retinal arteries. They usually disappear from retinal vessels within a few weeks leaving behind a short segment of arterial sheathing.

Other types of emboli

Emboli composed of uninfected *mixed thrombus* may originate in the left atrium, in patients with mitral valve disease. They have also been described in atrial septal defect, systemic lupus erythematosis, and endomyocardial fibrosis. They usually cause complete obstruction of retinal branch arteries producing permanent visual loss of sectorial or fibre bundle type. Infected retinal emboli are smaller; they usually cause small, multiple petechial haemorrhages (Roth's spots). These are a feature of subacute bacterial endocarditis.

Calcific emboli form a distinctive sub-group and have frequently been described in the retina. They are derived from degenerate cardiac valve usually calcific aortic stenosis. The mitral valve may also be responsible. The embolus appears as a chalky white single obstruction usually resulting in partial visual loss of fibre bundle type. The visual loss is permanent but recurrence is rare. Patients developing calcific emboli of this type should be referred for cardiac evaluation since the occurrence of embolism may be an early sign that the diseased valve is breaking up and surgical replacement may be indicated. On rare occasions fat, air or tumour emboli from atrial myxoma may be encountered in retinal arteries.

Retinal insufficiency

Though the majority of attacks of amaurosis fugax are due to emboli there are a number of other conditions which may temporarily diminish retinal blood flow and lead to transient uniocular visual impairment. In general the onset is less abrupt, the visual loss less severe. The visual field tends to contract from the periphery and the 'curtain effect' is not described.

Raised intraocular tension must not be overlooked since this also raises venous pressure and reduces trans-capillary pressure gradient. The disc is usually but not always cupped, the veins are dilated and attacks tend to occur in poor light when the pupil is dilated. Features of venous occlusion may co-exist. The intraocular tension should always be checked.

Intracranial *arteriovenous fistula* may also cause similar symptoms since there is a rise in venous and intraocular tension as well as a reduction in arterial blood pressure.

Patients with *severely reduced arterial pressure* due to extensive arterial occlusion affecting both external and internal carotids may suffer from periodic impairment of vision. In these cases uniocular visual loss may be provoked by systemic hypotension, cardiac dysrhythmia, postural change or perhaps by a steal effect to the external carotid territory. Some patients describe a dazzling effect like a photographic negative without much loss of central acuity. (Furlan et al, 1979). Ophthalmoscopic signs of venous stasis retinopathy are often present on careful inspection of the retinal periphery; arterial closure, multiple blocked haemorrhages and microaneurysms may be seen. In more advanced cases extensive arterial closure occurs with peripapillary shunt vessels and permanent visual defect (Takayasu disease).

Amaurosis fugax may also be a symptom in patients with *high retinal resistance* either due to narrowed arteries as in malignant hypertension or arteritis, or to increased blood viscosity as in macroglobulinaemia, sickle cell disease, thrombocythaemia or polycythaemia vera. Retinal *arterial spasm* is another possible mechanism which may affect patients with Raynaud's disease or in migraine. Unilateral *papilloedema* may also present with transient visual loss due in this case to venous obstruction and usually related to posture. Finally amaurosis fugax may occur in the absence of any detectable haematological or vascular abnormality. This type mainly affects young patients and appears to have a benign prognosis. The cause is unknown.

Management

Management of amaurosis fugax should begin with an evaluation of the cause and an enquiry into the circumstances of onset, the occurrence of cerebral TIA, a history of cardiac symptoms or past history of heart disease or intermittent claudication.

Examination will include a careful search for retinal emboli (preferably during an attack), carotid artery murmurs, absent or delayed pulses, and a general vascular survey for hypertension or cardiac valvular abnormality. Preliminary investigations comprise full blood count, estimation of intra-ocular tension, Doppler ultrasound and examination of the carotid artery. When blood disease and local ocular disease have been excluded the great majority of patients with amaurosis fugax will be found to have widespread atherosclerosis. There is a predominance of men and a high prevalence of hypertension, diabetes, heart disease and intermittent claudication. About one-third of patients show clinical evidence of carotid stenosis with a localised bruit over the bifurcation of the artery or a history of transient cerebral ischaemic attacks. A decision to proceed to carotid angiography is often a difficult one. Prevalence of carotid artery disease has been estimated at 78 per cent (Morax et al, 1970) and 50 per cent (Marshall & Meadows, 1968). The abnormality may be complete occlusion, stenosis or atheromatous ulceration. The object of arteriography is to detect those patients suitable for surgical treatment. The proportion of such patients is considerably increased if one or more of the following criteria are present: age over 50, hypertension, carotid bruit, transient cerebral ischaemic attacks (Wilson & Russell, 1979). If the patient is less than 50 and has none of the above features the yield of angiography is so low as to make the investigation superfluous.

Treatment

Patients with amaurosis fugax having localised carotid atheroma at the carotid origin are best treated by carotid endarterectomy if age and general health permit. Other patients are treated by antiplatelet agents such as aspirin in the low dosage (300 mg per day) for six months. Since this has been shown to be effective only in men, dipyridamole is sometimes added to or substituted for aspirin in female patients. In spite of earlier favourable reports there is at present no indication that sulphinpyrazone has any effect on the prognosis of amaurosis fugax. The patients with cholesterol emboli may be suitable for carotid endarterectomy but if not, it seems very unlikely that any medical treatment will influence the release of atheromatous material from the primary lesion. The lesion may heal by endothelial growth over the exposed portion of vessel and in many cases the attacks subside after a few weeks.

REFERENCES

Benson D F, Marsden C D, Meadows J C 1973 The amnesic stroke. Neurology (Minneapolis) 23:400

Boldrey E, Maas L, Miller E R 1956 The role of atlantoid compression in the aetiology of internal carotid thrombosis. Journal of Neurosurgery 13:127

Brice J G, Dowsett D J, Lowe R D 1964 The effect of constriction on carotid blood flow and pressure gradient. Lancet i:84

Bull J W D, Marshall J, Shaw D A 1960 Cerebral angiography in the diagnosis of the acute stroke. Lancet i:562

Cartlidge N E F, Whisnant J P, Elveback L R 1977 Carotid and vertebrobasilar transient cerebral ischaemic attacks. Mayo Clinic Proceedings 52:117

Christenson P C, Ovitt T W, Fisher H D et al 1980 Intravenous angiography using video subtraction. American Journal of Neuroradiology 1:379

David N J, Klintworth G K, Friedberg S J, Dillon M 1963 Fatal atheromatous cerebral embolism associated with bright plaques in the retinal arterioles. Report of a case. Neurology (Minneapolis) 13:708

De Bakey M E, Crawford E S, Cooley D A, Morris G C, Garrett H E, Fields W S 1965 Cerebral arterial insufficiency: one to 11-year results following arterial reconstruction. Annals of Surgery 161:921

Denny-Brown D E 1951 The treatment of recurrent cerebrovascular symptoms and the question of vasospasm. Medical Clinics of North America 35:1457

Desai B, Toole J F 1975 Kinks, coils and carotids: a review. Stroke 6:649

De Weese J A, Rob C G, Satran R, Marsh D D, Joynt R J, Lipchik E O, Zehe D N 1971 Endarterectomy for atherosclerotic lesions of the carotid artery. Journal of Cardiovascular Surgery 112:299

Drake W E, Drake M L 1968 Clinical and angiographic correlates of cerebrovascular insufficiency. American Journal of Medicine 45:253

Eastcott H H G, Pickering G W, Rob C G 1954 Reconstruction of internal carotid artery in a patient with intermittent attacks of hemiplegia. Lancet ii:994

Easton J D, Sherman D G 1977 Stroke and mortality rate in carotid endarterectomy. Stroke 8:565

Faer M J, Mead J H, Lynch R D 1977 Cerebral granulomatous angiitis. American Journal of Roentgenology 129:413

Farlan A J, Whisnant J P, Kearns T P 1979 Unilateral visual loss in bright light. Archives of Neurology 36:675

Fields W S, Maslenikov V, Meyer J S, Hass W K, Remington R D, Macdonald M 1970 Joint study of extracranial arterial occlusion. Progress report of prognosis following surgery or non surgical treatment for transient cerebral ischaemic attacks and cerebral carotid artery lesions. Journal of American Medical Association 211:1993

Fieschi, C, Argentino C, Rasura M 1981 Italian study of reversible ischaemic attacks. Stroke 12:293

Fisher C M 1954 Occlusion of the carotid arteries. Archives of Neurology and Psychiatry 72:187

Fisher C M 1959 Observations of the fundus oculi in transient monocular blindness. Neurology (Minneapolis) 9:333

Fisher C M 1962 Concerning recurrent transient cerebral ischaemic attacks. The Canadian Medical Association Journal 86:1091

Freidman G D, Wilson W S, Mosier J M, Calandrea M A, Nichaman M S 1969 Transient ischaemic attacks in a community. Journal of American Medical Association 210:1428

Gortvai P 1964 Insufficiency of the vertebral artery treated by decompression of the cervical part. British Medical Journal ii:233

Gunning A J, Pickering G W, Robb-Smith A H T, Ross Russell R 1964 Mural thrombosis of the internal carotid artery and subsequent embolism. Quarterly Journal of Medicine 33:155

Gurdjian E S, Darmody W R, Thomas L M 1969 Recurrent stroke due to occlusive disease of extracranial vessels. Archives of Neurology (Chicago) 21:447

Hachinski V, Norris J W, Cooper P, Marshall J 1977 Symptomatic intracranial steal. Archives of Neurology 34:149

Harrison M J G 1980 Vascular surgery for ischaemic stroke. British Journal of Hospital Medicine 24:108

Harrison M J G, Marshall J 1975 Indications for angiography and surgery in carotid artery disease. British Medical Journal i:616

Harrison M J G, Marshall J 1976 Angiographic appearance of carotid bifurcation in patients with completed stroke, TIA and cerebral tumour. British Medical Journal i:205

Hass W K, Fields W S, North R R, Kricheff I I, Chase N E, Bauer R B 1968 Joint study of extracranial arterial occlusion II. Arteriography, techniques, sites and complications. Journal of American Medical Association 203:961

Held K, Jipp P Schreier A 1973 Natural history and muscle blood flow of patients with occlusion in the subclavian arteries and aortic arch syndrome. In: Meyer J S, Lechner H, Reivich M, Eichhorn O (eds.) Cerebrovascular disease 6th international conference, Salzburg, 1972. Thieme, Stuttgart

Heyman A, Leviton A, Millikan C et al 1974 Transient focal cerebral ischaemia: epidemiological and clinical aspects. Stroke 5:277

Heyman A, Wilkinson W E, Heydon S et al 1980 Risk of stroke in asymptomatic patients with cervical arterial bruits. New England Journal of Medicine 302:838

Hollenhorst R W 1962 Carotid and vertebrobasilar arterial stenosis and occlusion: Neuro-ophthalmologic considerations. Transactions of American Academy of Ophthalmology and Otolaryngology 66:166

Hoyt W F 1970 In: Extracranial occlusive cerebrovascular disease diagnosis and management. Eds: Wylie E J & Ehrenfeld W K Philadelphia: Saunders

Hunt J R 1914 The role of the carotid arteries in the causation of vascular lesions of the brain with remarks on certain special features of the symptomatology. American Journal of Medical Science 147:704

Hutchinson E C, Yates P O 1957 Carotico-vertebral stenosis. Lancet i:2

Janeway R, Toole J F, Leinbach L B, Miller H S 1966 Vertebral artery obstruction with basilar impression. Archives of Neurology 15:211

Jick H, Porter J, Rothman K J 1978 Oral contraceptives and nonfatal stroke in healthy young women. Annals of internal medicine 89:58

Kendall R E, Marshall J 1963 Role of hypotension in the genesis of transient focal cerebral ischaemic attacks. British Medical Journal ii:344

Kosary I Z, Triester A, Tadmor R 1973 Transient monocular amaurosis due to a contralateral cerebral vascular malformation. Neurochirurgia 16:127

Kremer M 1958 Sitting, standing and walking. British Medical Journal ii:63

Lieberman A N, Bloom W, Kishore P S, Lin J P 1974 Carotid artery occlusion following ingestion of LSD. Stroke 5:213

Marshall J 1964 The natural history of transient ischaemic cerebrovascular attacks. Quarterly Journal of Medicine 33:309

Marshall J, Meadows S P 1968 The natural history of amaurosis fugax. Brain 91:419

Mathew N T, Meyer J S 1974 Pathogenesis and natural history of transient global amnesia. Stroke 5:303

McBrien D J, Bradley R D, Ashton N 1963 The nature of retinal emboli in stenosis of the internal carotid artery. Lancet i:697

Meyer J S, Denny-Brown D 1957 The cerebral collateral circulation. 1. Factors influencing collateral blood flow. Neurology (Minneapolis) 7:447

Meyer J S, Portnoy H S 1958 Localised cerebral hypoglycaemia simulating stroke. Neurology (Minneapolis) 8:601

Morax P V, Aron-Rosa D, Gautier J C 1970 Symptomes et signes ophthalmologiques des stenoses et occlusions carotidiennes. Bulletin de Societe Ophthalmologique Francais, Suppl. 1:169

North R R, Fields W S, De Bamey M E, Crawford E S 1962 Brachial basilar insufficiency syndrome. Neurology (Minneapolis) 12:810

Payne E E, Spillane J D 1957 The cervical spine: an anatomico-pathological study of 70 specimens with particular reference to the problems of cervical spondylosis. Brain 80:571

Petrone P et al 1979 CT evaluation of patients with transient ischaemic attacks. European Neurology 18:217

Prineas J, Marshall J 1966 Hypertension and cerebral infarction. British Medical Journal i:14

Ramos M, Mandybar T I 1975 Cerebral vasculitis in rheumatoid arthritis. Archives of Neurology 32:271

Reed R L, Siekert R G, Merideth J 1973 Rarity of transient focal cerebral insufficiency in cardiac dysrhythmia. Journal of American Medical Association 223:893

Rees J E, Du Boulay G H, Bull J W D, Marshall J, Ross Russell R W, Symon L 1970 Regional cerebral blood flow in transient ischaemic attacks. Lancet ii:1210

Reivich M, Holling H E, Roberts B, Toole J F 1961 Reversal of blood flow through the vertebral artery and its effect on cerebral circulation. New England Journal of Medicine 265:878

Ruff R L, Talman W T, Petito F 1981 Transient ischaemic attacks associated with hypotension in hypertensive patients with carotid artery stenosis. Stroke 12:303

Russell R W R 1961 Observations on the retinal blood vessels in monocular blindness. Lancet ii:1422

Russell R W R, Cranston W I 1961 Ophthalmodynamometry in carotid artery disease. Journal of Neurology, Neurosurgery and Psychiatry 24:281

Russell R W R, Green M 1971 Mechanisms of transient cerebral ischaemia. British Medical Journal i:646

Sandok B A, Furlan A J, Whisnant J P, Sundt T M 1978 Guidelines for the management of transient ischaemic attacks. Mayo Clinic Proceedings 53:665

Schwartz C J, Mitchell J R A 1961 Atheroma of the carotid and vertebral arterial systems. British Medical Journal ii:1057

Shanbrom E, Levy L 1957 The role of systemic blood pressure in cerebral circulation in carotid and basilar artery thromboses. Clinical implications and therapeutic implications of vasopressor agents. American Journal of Medicine 23:197

Sharon M A, Sunger R W, Hodges M 1981 Reactive hyperaemia for the clinical diagnosis of subclavian steal syndrome. Stroke 12:369

Silas J H, Grant D S, Maddocks J L 1981 Transient hemiparetic attacks due to unrecognised nocturnal hypoglycaemia. British Medical Journal 282:132

Slack J 1969 Risk of ischaemic heart disease in familial hyperlipoproteinaemic states. Lancet ii:1380

Solomon G E, Hilal S U, Gold A P, Carter S 1970 Natural history of acute hemiplegia of childhood. Brain 93:107

Stanford J R, Lubow M, Vasko J S 1978 Prevention of stroke by carotid endarterectomy. Surgery 83:259

Swanson P D, Calanchini P R, Dyken M L et al 1977 Cooperative study of hospital frequency and character of transient ischaemic attacks II Angiography. Journal of American Medical Association 237:2202

Symonds C P 1927 Two cases of thrombosing subclavian artery with contralateral hemiplegia of sudden onset probably embolic. Brain 50:259

Symon L 1969 The concept of intracerebral steal. In: McDowall G (ed.) International anaesthesiology clinics cerebral circulation. Little, Brown and Co. Boston

Thomas J E, Agyar D R 1972 Systemic fat embolism. Archives of Neurology 26:517

Toole J F 1964 Reversed vertebral artery flow: subclavian steal syndrome. Lancet i:872

Toole J F, Tucker S H 1960 Influence of head position upon cerebral circulation. Archives of Neurology 2:616

Van der Drift J H A, Kok N K D 1973 Clinical pathological correlations in transient cerebral ischaemic attacks. In: Meyer J S, Lechner H, Reivich M, Eichhorn O (eds.) Cerebrovascular disease 6th international conference, Salzburg 1972. Thieme. Stuttgart

Williams D, Wilson T G 1962 The diagnosis of the major and minor syndromes of basilar insufficiency. Brain 85:741

Wilson L A, Russell R W R 1977 Amaurosis fugax and carotid artery disease: indications for angiography. British Medical Journal ii:435

Wylie E J, Ehrenfeld W K 1970 Extracranial occlusive cerebrovascular disease: diagnosis and management. W B Saunders. Philadelphia

Ziegler D K, Hassanein R S 1973 Prognosis in patients with transient ischaemic attacks. Stroke 4:666

12

Cerebral ischaemia in hypertension

J. C. Gautier

The adverse effects of high blood pressure on life expectancy are well established (Leishman, 1959; Hodge et al, 1961) and cerebral arterial accidents rank in second place among the causes of death in hypertensives (Breckenridge et al, 1970). Furthermore beneficial results of treating hypertension have been repeatedly reported (Hamilton et al, 1964; Veterans Administration Cooperative Study Group on Antihypertensive Agents, 1967; Breckenridge et al, 1970). The improved prognosis resulting from antihypertensive treatment also holds true after a cerebral arterial accident (Marshall & Kaeser, 1961; Marshall, 1964; Cambier & Gautier, 1965).

Large and small cerebral haemorrhages are almost entirely confined to hypertensives (Cole & Yates, 1968) and it is likely that the merits of reducing hypertension result largely from a decrease in haemorrhagic accidents (Breckenridge et al, 1970; Beevers et al, 1973). However there is also a strong case for hypertension as a significant aetiological factor in cerebral infarction. A prospective study has proved that hypertension is the most common and potent precursor of atherothrombotic brain infarction (Kannel et al, 1970; Kannel, 1971). The fact that hypertension is a major risk factor in brain infarction has been confirmed in other surveys (Whisnant, 1974; Shekelle et al, 1974). In a postmortem controlled series Low-Beer & Phear (1961) showed that patients who die from cerebral infarction have on average a higher blood pressure than the normal population. This is hardly surprising when it is known that arterial hypertension aggravates atherosclerosis (see below). In addition, hypertension appears to be linked to the development of microinfarcts or lacunes which outnumber all other cerebrovascular lesions combined (Fisher, 1969).

Macro- and microinfarction are the main topics of the present chapter. However a brief account will be given of the much rarer diseases Binswanger's encephalopathy and arteriopathic Parkinsonism. Although hypertensive encephalopathy is not strictly an ischaemic disorder and might more correctly be called a hyperaemic disorder (see below), it is convenient to deal with it here.

A short account of the cerebral blood flow disorders and pathological lesions in hypertension is relevant at this stage. An attempt is made to review cerebral arterial lesions in hypertension on the premise that although lesions of large and small arteries are morphologically quite different, there are basic physiopathological and pathological similarities between them.

HYPERTENSION AND THE CEREBRAL CIRCULATION

In acute and chronic hypertension the arteries are subjected to a physical stress which is responsible for a variety of lesions in vessels from the size of the aorta to the smallest intracerebral arteries. However, since the bulk of cerebrovascular resistance depends upon the small (pial and intracerebral) arteries (Figs. 12.1 and 12.2) lesions most specific to arterial hypertension are to be expected and are indeed mainly present on these vessels. It is relevant that pressure in the intracranial internal carotid artery and its main branches is usually only fractionally lower than that recorded in the artery in the neck (Bakay & Sweet, 1952, 1953). More distally the intra-arterial pressure falls gradually and in arteries of 0.4 mm diameter, on the supero-

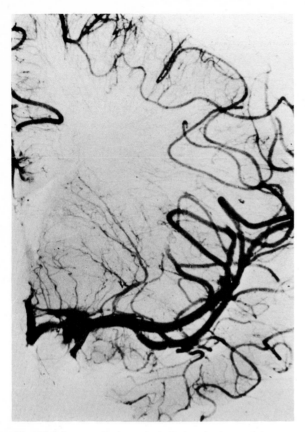

Fig. 12.1 Intracerebral arteries in human brain coronal section. Arteries injected with lead carbonate. Author's specimen.

lateral aspect of the hemisphere, it still ranges from 65 to 92 per cent (mean 83 per cent) of the pressure in the cervical part of the artery (Ibid). For

anatomical features of pial and intracerebral arteries, see Vander Eecken (1959), Baker & Iannone (1959a, b), and Russell (1963). Due to their size and distribution to nervous tissue there are fundamental similarities in behaviour between retinal and the small intracerebral arteries. Therefore much has been gained and is to be gained from the study of the retinal circulation in hypertension. Since there is no anatomic way to distinguish between arteries and arterioles (Kernohan et al, 1929; Cook & Yates, 1972) the word arteriole will not be used here.

Intra-arterial pressure is one of the main stimuli responsible for the tone of arteries by stretching the muscular coat or media of the vessel wall. A rise in intra-arterial pressure causes arterial constriction while a decrease in pressure causes dilatation (Bayliss, 1902). It is not within the scope of this paper to discuss whether arterial vasoconstriction is a primary or secondary event in essential hypertension. Suffice it to say that the basic concomitant arterial reaction in hypertension is arterial constriction. This can be witnessed in retinal arteries in man (Harnish & Pearce, 1973) in rat mesenteric and retinal arteries (Byrom, 1954) and in cerebral arteries of various species (Byrom, 1954, 1969; Meyer et al, 1960a).

For the sake of clarity the circulatory and structural consequences of hypertension will be considered under three categories, keeping in mind that there may be some overlapping and oversimplification.

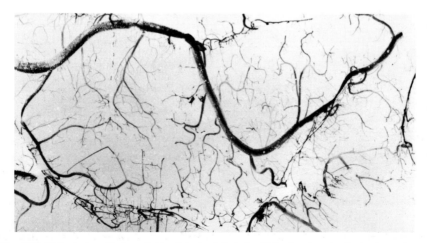

Fig. 12.2 Pial arteries of human brain. Arteries injected with lead carbonate. Author's specimen.

Mild and moderate hypertension

In mild and moderately severe hypertension of some duration diffuse narrowing of the arteries is present. Besides degenerative changes involving hyperplasia of connective tissue and damage to the elastica, the characteristic structural feature is hypertrophy of the muscle cells of the media (Russell, 1963; Cook & Yates, 1972) with an increase in the size of their nuclei. Such muscular hypertrophy may be likened to left ventricular hypertrophy. Histological criteria which are proposed for this 'hypertonus' are distortion of smooth muscle cells and their nuclei, progressive deformation of the internal elastic lamina, crowding of endothelial cells (Van Citters et al, 1962), crowding and spiral twisting of the nuclei of the muscular cells (Rodda & Denny-Brown, 1966a).

In patients with mild or moderately severe chronic hypertension without cerebral complications the cerebral blood flow remains normal. Chronic arterial constriction is the basis of autoregulation of the cerebral blood flow. A similar autoregulation, i.e. myogenic, is likely to be present in the human retinal arterial circulation (Russell, 1973). There is, however, another level of cerebral arterial pressure below which the cerebral autoregulation becomes inadequate and blood flow decreases. In normotensives this lower limit of autoregulation is 60 to 70 mmHg (Lassen, 1959). An increase in oxygen extraction compensates for this decrease in blood flow but only down to a second limit, corresponding to a pressure of 35 to 40 mmHg, below which symptoms of cerebral hypoxia appear. It is of interest for the clinician to keep in mind that in patients with untreated hypertension the lower limit of the autoregulatory range is higher than in normotensives (Finnerty et al, 1954; Lassen, 1959). In one study the average value for this lower limit of autoregulation in severe hypertensives was 120 mmHg and the limit for brain hypoxia was on average 68 mmHg (Strandgaard et al, 1973). Such a shift to a higher level of autoregulation in hypertensives may be explained by the hypertrophy of the small artery walls (Folkow, 1971). It suggests that therapeutic lowering of arterial hypertension should be gradual and cautious (Strandgaard et al, 1973), a fact in keeping with clinical experience. Blindness prob-

ably due to optic nerve damage after rapid reduction of malignant hypertension has been recently reported (Cove et al, 1979).

Acute hypertension

In acute severe hypertension extreme arterial constriction is to be expected. This indeed occurs but it is important to realise that, at least after some time, it appears as a *segmental* constriction (Figs 12.3 and 12.4). This has been the source of terms such as vasospasm and probably of much confusion in understanding the disorders of the

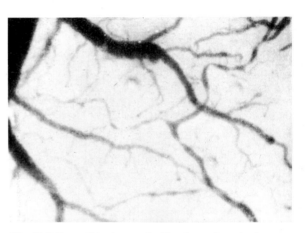

Fig. 12.3 Reversible change of calibre in small cerebral arteries of rat in severe uncomplicated hypertension (× 26). Light ether anesthesia (B.P. 240 mm). Gross irregularity in calibre of small arteries, veins normal.

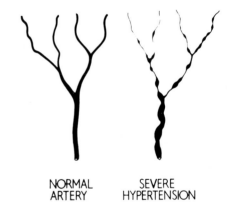

NORMAL ARTERY   SEVERE HYPERTENSION

Fig. 12.4 The typical picture of dilatation, tortuosity, irregularity of largest vessels, tight uniform constriction of smallest vessels, and alternating constriction and dilatation of intermediate vessels. (Figures 12.3 and 12.4 are from F. B. Byrom (1969) *The Hypertensive Vascular Crisis*, London: Heinemann. Reproduced by courtesy of the author.)

cerebral circulation in such circumstances. Since the first observations in retinal and pial arteries in man and animals the segmental arterial constriction has been held responsible by many authorities for ischaemia resulting in damage to the vessel wall and consequently to the tissues supplied by the damaged arteries (Fog, 1939; Byrom, 1954; Meyer et al, 1960b; Rodda & Denny-Brown, 1966b; Dinsdale et al, 1974). However, in the first reports of these carefully designed experiments it had also been mentioned that there existed *dilated* arterial segments as well as constricted ones (Byrom, 1954). By injecting *intravitam* trypan blue Byrom (1954) found conspicuous rounded blue areas on the surface of the brain (Fig 12.5), a finding which implied a break in the blood brain barrier (BBB). The blue areas of cerebral tissue were found to contain a considerably higher content of water than control tissue, i.e., they were oedematous. This seemed to account for the cerebral oedema in

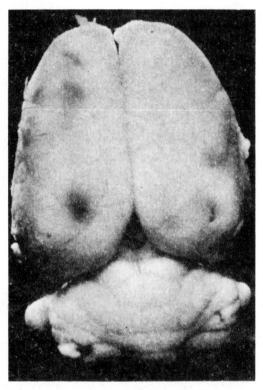

Fig. 12.5 Brain of a rat with encephalopathy, killed soon after an intravenous injection of trypan blue, showing rounded areas of staining on the surface of the cerebral cortex. (From F. B. Byrom (1969) *The Hypertensive Vascular Crisis.* London: Heinemann. Reproduced by courtesy of the author.)

human hypertensive encephalopathy (see below). However it now appears that the leakage of fluid through the arterial wall may not take place in the constricted but in the *dilated* arterial segment. This was elegantly demonstrated by Giese (1966) in a series of experiments with serum labelled by a fluorescent dye and carbon-labelled plasma. This crucial evidence was subsequently confirmed by using Evans blue albumin as an index of breakdown of the BBB and ^{125}I-antipyrine and ^{3}H-ethanol as indicators of blood flow (Johansson, 1974). In short during acute very high hypertension there is a forced arterial dilatation resulting in a 'breakthrough' of autoregulation (Lassen & Agnoli, 1972) and in a pronounced increase in blood flow. This pressure-forced arterial dilatation leads to BBB damage with focal leakage of fluid through the walls of the overstretched arteries (Johansson et al, 1970) and formation of cerebral oedema (Johansson, 1974; Johansson et al, 1974). The characteristic arterial lesion (Figs. 12.6 and 12.7) is necrosis of medial muscle fibres with the presence of erythrocytes and of a substance staining pink with eosin, bright red with PAS, and purple with PTAH. This has been termed hyaline or fibrinoid necrosis (Byrom, 1969; Wilson, 1969). Both hyaline and fibrinoid changes are due to the presence within the vessel wall of material which has the histochemical immunological and ultramicroscopic features of fibrin (Adams, 1967).

In hypertensive monkeys ultrastructural studies of retinal arteries showed seeping of plasma and fibrin deposits into the vessel wall ('insudation of plasmatic vasculosis'). Eventually the muscle cell cavities in the basement membrane contained only plasma, fibrin, muscle cells debris, and lipid, and in some cases large numbers of platelets and occasional red cells. The pathway of the plasma leakage through the endothelium could, however, not be demonstrated (Garner & Ashton, 1970).

With regard to moderately severe hypertension in which hypertrophy of the media is the characteristic lesion (see above) it is of interest to note that the arterial disorders of acute severe hypertension, namely focal leakage of plasma, occur in experimental animals (i.e., in previously normotensive animals) and are almost restricted to clinical conditions in which there is an abrupt onset of severe hypertension in a previously normotensive

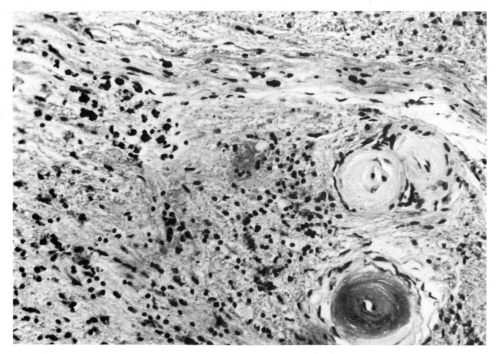

Fig. 12.6 Arterial hyalinosis, at bottom. Two hyalinised occluded arteries, above. On the left, haemosiderin-laden macrophages. H. E. × 120. Female, aged 60 (B.P. 250/150).

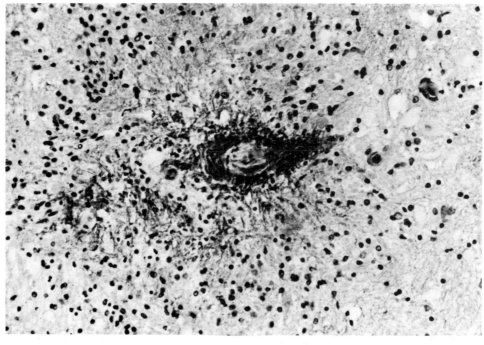

Fig. 12.7 Fibrinoid necrosis of intracerebral artery. H.E. × 120. Same case as Figure 12.6.

patient (e.g., in acute glomerular nephritis or toxaemia of pregnancy). Hypertensive encephalopathy is rarely encountered in other hypertensive conditions; for instance, there was only one case of hypertensive encephalopathy in 190 cases of established malignant hypertension (Clarke & Murphy, 1956), and experimentally hypertensive encephalopathy is rare when blood pressure is increased in a step-wise fashion (Häggendahl and Johansson, 1972). This may be due to the hypertrophy of the muscular coat with an increased resistance to overstretching.

Chronic hypertension

In chronic severe hypertension there exist two distinct though related cerebral arterial changes, namely aggravation of atherosclerosis and the development of specific lesions on the small intracerebral arteries.

Aggravation of atherosclerosis by hypertension

Experimental, clinical, and pathological studies indicate that hypertension accelerates the onset and accentuates the progress of atherosclerosis (see Baker, Resch, and Loewenson, 1969). Fisher et al (1965a) found that stenosis of the cervical and cerebral arteries (i.e., Circle of Willis and stems of the main intracranial arteries) was more frequent and more severe in hypertensives than in normotensives. Increased calcification of the carotid syphon was clearly associated with hypertension (Fisher et al, 1965b). Russell (1963) and Baker et al (1969) found that the severity of atherosclerosis of the Circle of Willis was more pronounced where hypertension had been present. Multiple stenoses of arterial branches on angiography and yellow specks on the leptomeningeal arteries at autopsy are almost a hallmark of severe long-standing hypertension. Fisher (1961a) reported that in his material it had been extremely easy to find hypertensive atherosclerotic cases while it had taken several months to find an adequate sample of normotensive cases with severe cerebral atherosclerosis or hypertensive cases without atherosclerosis. In some hypertensive patients, a particular type of atherosclerosis of cerebral arteries is present, characterised by ladder-like, yellow or orange bars (Arab, 1957) (Fig. 12.8).

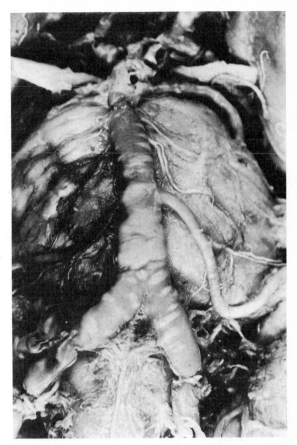

Fig. 12.8 Ladder-like atherosclerosis of vertebral and basilar arteries. Arteries injected with lead carbonate. Author's specimen.

However, besides aggravating atherosclerosis, hypertension exerts a second and most important effect, the production of lesions on smaller arteries. In normotensives atherosclerosis implicates arteries 0.2 or more millimetres in diameter, namely, from vessels of the size of those which penetrate the basal ganglia and pons to the common carotid arteries in the neck (Adams, 1955). Hypertension extends the atheromatous process, seeming to force the fatty deposits upon vessels of lesser size. For instance the penetrating arteries of the internal capsules, basal ganglia, and pons tend to be involved only in patients subject to hypertension, the diabetic being a possible exception (Adams and Fisher, 1961b). Examples of this may be found in intracerebral and retinal arteries. In a study of the arterial lesions underlying 50 lacunes Fisher (1969) reported three cases in which a focal plaque consisting of fatty macrophages had encroached upon or occluded the lumen of the feeding artery. The lesion was typical of microscopic atherosclerosis in small cerebral arteries. It is of interest to note that the involved arteries were larger than in any of the other lacunes, namely 500, 400, and 300 μm, respectively. Atherosclerosis is lacking on retinal arteries since, except for the central retinal artery, all are less than 100 μm in diameter (Adams, 1955). However in hypertensives atherosclerotic lesions of the retinal arteries have been demonstrated (Harnish & Pearce, 1973; patients E and G). Moreover it should be noted that in Harnish & Pearce's patient E an atherosclerotic lesion was present post-mortem where a soft exudate had been observed during life.

Specific hypertensive lesions in intracerebral arteries

In chronic severe hypertension, arterial lesions specific to hypertension are present which to some extent are restricted to cerebral arteries. Unlike arteries of other organs which divide regularly into smaller branches, penetrating or nutrient cerebral arteries enter the brain from main stems or large pericerebral branches (Duret, 1874) (Fig. 12.2). Most of the hypertensive lesions lie in the territories of the basal perforating arteries, and it has been suggested that this could be due to the proximity of large arteries where a high pressure or marked fluctuations in pressure would be more likely to be transmitted to smaller vessels (Russell, 1963). It may be that at the base of the brain the small nutrient arteries are subjected to especially high pressure by virtue of their origin at right angles from the major arterial trunks and that a gradual reduction of pressure is lacking (Fisher, 1961b). Whatever the truth in these considerations, it must be recognised that with regard to atherosclerotic thrombosis the behaviour of penetrating arteries at the base of the brain is different from that of pial arteries on the convexity (Fisher, 1961b), a fact which suggests significant differences in the regime of blood flow.

Intracerebral arterial lesions found chiefly in hypertensives are of two main kinds: (1) lipohyalinosis and (2) miliary aneurysms. Both have in common, it should be noted at once, to be present on small arteries in the range of 40 to 300 μm diameter.

Lipohyalinosis is a word coined by Fisher (1972) to refer to cerebral arterial lesions correlating chiefly with hypertension and which had been described under various names: fibrinoid necrosis, hyaline arterionecrosis, atherosclerosis of small arteries, hyaline fatty changes, plasmatic vascular destruction, hyalinosis, angionecrosis, fibrinoid arteritis (see Fisher, 1972), segmental arterial disorganisation (Fisher, 1969). The essential pathological process may be summarised as follows (Fig. 12.9): mural destruction, focal expansion of the vessel, fatty macrophages or foam cells frequently present in the disorganised wall, thrombotic occlusion, haemorrhagic extravasation and fibrinoid deposit (Fisher, 1969, 1972). The term lipohyalinosis stresses the fact that such lesions stain readily for fat, and it should be reminded that Charcot & Bouchard (1868) had commented on the presence of fatty granulations in some of the lesions. By some features, e.g., fibrinoid deposit, focal enlargements (Fisher (1972) went as far as to use the term 'miliary aneurysms in lipohyalinosis'), lipohyalinosis is reminiscent on one hand of lesions resulting from arterial overstretching under high blood pressure. On the other hand the presence of a lipid-staining material as a prominent constituent of arterial segmental disorganisation strongly suggested to Fisher (1969) that there exists a relation with the fatty plaque of atherosclerosis, a view with which the author agrees. Fisher's (1969, 1972) evidence for this is worth quoting here: (1) severe atherosclerosis of the cerebral arteries accompanies lacunar infarcts (of which lipohyalinosis is the commonest cause); (2) in hypertension the smaller surface cerebral and cerebral arteries are affected by atherosclerosis, hence atherosclerosis of the very small intracerebral twigs might also be expected; (3) it may be significant that vessels larger than 200 μm display atherosclerosis rather than lipohyalinosis and the reverse is also true; (4) the presence of fat combined with macrophages hints that the lesion may be related to atherosclerosis; (5) in hypertension atherosclerotic nodules may be found with concomitant evidence of leakage of red blood cells; (6) in cases showing disorganisation of the smaller twigs plaques filled with typical fatty macrophages were often found in the immediate

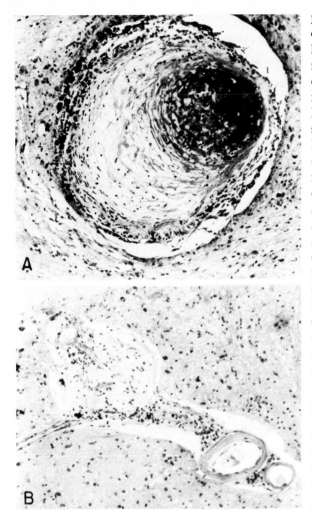

Fig. 12.9A Segmental disorganisation (angionecrosis) with local enlargement of the artery to three times the normal diameter of 130 μm. The dark material is fibrinoid staining (H.E.).
   B. Old segmental enlargement of an 80 μm artery consisting of a nodule of collagenous connective tissue. The edge of the lacune is seen above. (Courtesy of Dr C. Miller Fisher, 1969.)

larger parent branches. On the other hand the presence of fat in the arterial wall could also be explained by insudation of plasma (Russell, 1975).

Miliary aneurysms were described by Charcot and Bouchard (1868) (Fig. 12.10) then more or less discarded or misinterpreted for almost a century. By micropaque injections and pathological observations Russell (1963) put them back into the limelight for neurology. Cole and Yates (1967a) showed that they are hypertension and age-de-

pendent. Fisher (1972) gave a detailed study based on serial sections. Apart from their significance in hypertensive arterial lesions, miliary aneurysms must be considered here for they are likely to be a cause, admittedly an infrequent one, of small infarcts in hypertensive patients (Charcot and Bouchard, 1868; Russell, 1963; Fisher, 1972). The significance of miliary aneurysms with regard to lipohyalinosis must now be considered. Fisher (1972) described saccular and fusiform asymmetric miliary aneurysms but thought that both kinds are closely related and have much in common. He apparently considered lipohyalinosis as a variety of aneurysm and commented that all three types of aneurysms are tied to hypertension, involve arteries of the same size and location and small extravasations of red blood cells occur around each, clearly suggesting a relationship. Although he did not find intermediary forms, he obviously felt that there exists a strong possibility that they all have a common origin and that the three types of aneurysms might really be variations of the same process. If this were true it could be assumed that in hypertensive cerebral arterial disease there is a change in the morphology of lesions where arteries become less than about 300 μm in diameter, i.e. frank atherosclerosis disappear while lipohyalinosis and miliary aneurysms appear. However, this change is probably more apparent than real for atherosclerosis is likely to be closely related to lipohyalinosis while miliary aneurysms may well be closely related to lipohyalinosis. Moreover

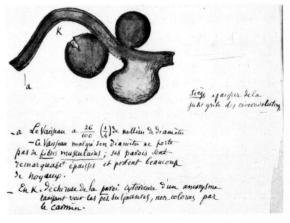

Fig. 12.10 Original drawing and notes by Charcot of miliary aneurysms (Musée de la Salpêtrière).

cerebral arterial lesions in moderately severe or very severe hypertension display mixed features of both aggravated atherosclerosis and overstretching of the vessel wall with resultant enlargement and leakage of plasma. For the student of hypertensive arterial cerebral lesions it is likely that there is a continuum of lesions from the large to the smallest arteries with variations presumably due to differences in pressure and structure of the vessel wall.

HYPERTENSIVE ENCEPHALOPHATHY

Acute cerebral disorders in Bright's disease, mainly convulsions and blindness, were at first ascribed to uraemia ('convulsive uraemia'). However, at the turn of the century it became apparent that they could result from vascular disturbances due to a rise in systolic pressure (Pal, 1905). Oppenheimer & Fishberg (1928) coined the term hypertensive encephalopathy to account for the recurrent fits in a case of acute nephritis with raised blood pressure. They discarded the current views on pathogenesis, namely renal insufficiency or chloride retention, to conclude that hypertension was responsible for the nervous disorders, most likely through 'a widespread and perhaps universal peripheral vasoconstriction'. In the late 1930s and 1940s the nervous lesions were emphasised in French literature under the term of acute meningocerebral oedema (oedéme aigu cérébro-méningé) (Alajouanine & Hornet, 1939; Milliez, 1943). Eventually hypertensive encephalopathy superseded other appellations but came to be used in a restricted sense, i.e., to refer to largely reversible cerebral disorders associated with raised blood pressure in the absence of evidence of cerebral thrombosis or haemorrhage (Jellinek et al, 1964). 'Hypertensive encephalopathy' however is still occasionally encountered referring to vascular ('fibrinoid necrosis of arterioles'; 'thrombosis of arterioles and capillaries') and nervous ('microinfarcts'; 'petechial haemorrhages') lesions found after many years of severe ('malignant') hypertension (Chester et al, 1978). To keep some degree of clarity the restricted appelation of 'hypertensive encephalopathy' is to be preferred.

Cases of hypertensive encephalopathy have been most frequently associated with acute nephritis and toxaemia of pregnancy. In a series of 225 patients with nephritis admitted to the London Hospital in the years before the Second World War hypertensive encephalopathy occurred in 11, an incidence of 6.4 per cent (Wilson, 1963). A few cases have been reported in association with phaeochromocytoma (Milliez, 1943; Graham, 1951) and lead poisoning. As already mentioned the condition appears to be infrequent in the course of malignant hypertension (see above). A case of Jellinek et al (1964) was due to renal arterial occlusion. Meyer (1961) mentioned porphyria as a rare cause. There seems to be few doubts that the condition was formerly overdiagnosed (Ziegler et al, 1965). Nowadays although Finnerty recently claimed (1972) to have treated 'over 400 patients with various types of hypertensive encephalopathy with diazoxide' the condition appears to be very uncommon since conditions which lead to it are either naturally rare or have become rare with the advent of efficient treatments of hypertension. However, a few cases continue to be reported (Strandgaard et al, 1973; Jewett, 1973) and in some parts of the world hypertensive encephalopathy is still frequent.

Disorders of cerebral blood flow with a breakthrough in autoregulation, overstretching of arteries and focal damage to BBB have been mentioned earlier. Cerebral lesions of oedema have been reported by Blackfan (1926) who demonstrated the presence of a medullary pressure cone and consequently concluded that lumbar puncture, which was formerly advocated by some authors as a therapeutic procedure, 'should be used guardedly'. Alajouanine & Hornet (1939) stressed that there was at post-mortem a great quantity of c.s.f. around the brain and that the latter was swollen with flattened gyri and a conspicuous superficial vasodilatation. Arteries, capillaries, and veins appeared to be distended and Virchow-Robin spaces were greatly distended with the presence of an amorphous material which had the features of an albumin-fibrin coagulum. There was in addition a characteristic shredded appearance (état effiloché) of the nervous tissue with acute swelling of the oligodendroglia, sometimes clasmatodendrosis, and ischaemic changes of neurones. The lesions were most marked in cortex and basal ganglia.

The full crisis of hypertensive encephalopathy

is often heralded by weakness, apathy, headache, drowsiness, and vomiting concomitant with a severe rise in blood pressure. Convulsions are common, either generalised or focal. In the absence of treatment they are usually recurrent. Loss of vision is a second main feature. Papilloedema and hypertensive changes in the fundi are frequently lacking (Milliez, 1943; Jellinek et al, 1964), a fact that again sets hypertensive encephalopathy apart from malignant hypertension and obviously suggests occipital blindness. This is supported by cases in which homonymous hemianopia has been recorded. Drowsiness may lead to coma. Various focal cerebral disturbances may occur, e.g., transient paralysis and aphasia. Stiffness of the neck is frequent (Milliez, 1943). The cerebrospinal fluid pressure is usually raised, although this is inconstant. A rise in the c.s.f. protein content is also usual but may also be absent. The cell count is normal.

The electroencephalogram in Jellinek et al's (1964) cases showed in the acute stage bilaterally synchronous often rhythmic occipital sharp and slow activity. The alpha rhythm was lost or impaired during the period of blindness. Some records showed in addition focal abnormalities elsewhere. C.T. scanning may show low density regions affecting the white matter of occipital and parietal lobes (Rail & Perkin, 1980). (Fig. 12.11A & B).

Hypertensive encephalopathy is, as already mentioned, generally concomitant with a severe rise in blood pressure but it must be stressed that this is not always true. The condition may occur with rather moderate hypertension.

The clinical disorder may lead to deep coma and death, or rapidly regress. Sequelae have been recorded, e.g., intellectual impairment and epilepsy (Jellinek et al, 1964). More often emergency therapy (see below) brings dramatic relief by lowering blood pressure. The cerebral disorders may disappear very quickly in a matter of hours or even minutes.

Hypertensive encephalopathy must be differentiated from: (1) infarction due to occlusive arterial disease and haemorrhage; (2) subarachnoid haemorrhage; (3) cerebral abscess or tumour which by raising intracranial pressure could determine hypertension. Finnerty (1972) stated that

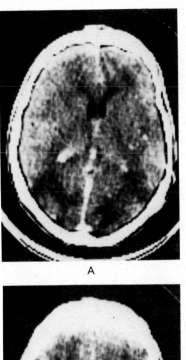

A

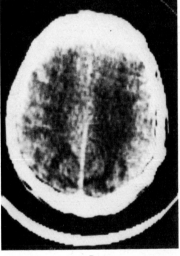

B

Fig. 12.11 A & B C.T. scan appearance of hypertensive encephalopathy showing areas of low density in white matter (courtesy of Dr G. D. Perkin).

acute anxiety states with labile hypertension and acute pulmonary oedema due to hypertensive heart disease may require differentiation from hypertensive encephalopathy.

The treatment is essentially based on a prompt lowering of hypertension. It has been reviewed by Finnerty (1972). From this and present knowledge (e.g., Hypertensive encephalopathy, 1979), it would appear that the main drugs available are: diazoxide, trimetaphan camphor sulfonate, furosemide and sodium nitroprusside. If such drugs are not available in an emergency it should be remembered that venesection was formerly used with success. For reasons stated above, vasodilator drugs such as papaverine and hypercapnia should be avoided. There is a risk of blindness if blood pressure is reduced excessively (Cove et al, 1979).

LACUNES (*ÉTAT LACUNAIRE*)

The term 'lacunes' (Latin, *lacuna, -ae*: a hole or small cavity) was first used by Durand-Fardel (1843, case 78) in the macroscopic description of the striate bodies of a 77-year-old man whose brain showed a wide variety of ischaemic and haemorrhagic lesions. The term '*état lacunaire*' was introduced by Pierre Marie (1901) to refer to the chronic condition of patients affected by lacunes. Marie reported clinical and pathological observations from 50 patients and Ferrand added 38 cases in his monograph which appeared the following year (Ferrand, 1902). For review of what could be called the 'first historical period' of lacunes see Ferrand (1902) and Fisher (1965a). Between the First and Second World Wars a number of clinico-pathological cases were reported, although according to the fashion of the time, nervous lesions and their clinical counterparts and not arterial lesions were the chief interest of the authors. After Foix & Hillemand's (1925) description of the patterns of arterial anatomy in the brain stem, studies took into account the localisation of the lesions in the newly defined territories, but again arterial lesions were too often missed or mentioned without precise qualifications. During the 1940s and 1950s the advent of angiography strongly focused interest upon extracranial arteries and for a time lacunes were the poor relation of cerebral arterial disease. This is no longer the case and for this a special tribute must be paid to Fisher's pathological (1961a, 1965a, 1969, 1972) and clinico-pathological studies.

Lacunes (Figs. 12.12 & 12.13) are small infarcts, mostly found in the chronic or healed stage when they appear as irregular trabeculated usually pale cavities. When of recent origin they show liquefaction necrosis. In the acute stage the area of temporary ischaemia is considerably larger than

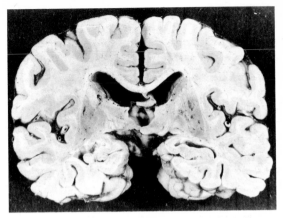

Fig. 12.12 Lacunes in basal ganglia and internal capsule. Moderate ventricular enlargement. The left mamillary body is atrophied.

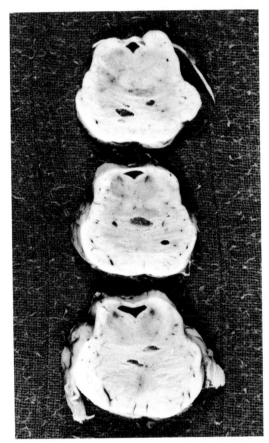

Fig. 12.13 Lacunes in basis pontis. Same case as Figure 12.12. Male, aged 53 (B.P.: 230/125).

the scar, possibly two or three times (Fisher, 1961a) a fact that may account for the partial recovery in clinical episodes resulting from lacunes.

The dimensions of lacunes range on average from 0.5 to 15 mm in diameter but it would be unwarranted to draw a firm line between lacunes and infarcts. To emphasise the unusual size of the larger lacunes Fisher (1965a) suggested to qualify those 10 mm or more in diameter as 'giant' and suggested that preferably the nature and site of the lesion rather than its size should be the chief criterion. However, such qualifications leave the student of cerebral lesions undecided on many of the cases reported in the literature. The author of the present paper believes that the term 'lacune' should be restricted to lesions which can be ascribed to permanent or transient occlusion of *intracerebral* arteries. Admittedly, however, a small number of lacunes may be due to transient occlusion of the mouth or extracerebral part of the penetrating

arteries by transient occlusion of the large parent vessel, e.g., in cardiac embolism.

In a series of 1042 consecutive post-mortems in a general hospital, 114 brains (11 per cent) had one or more lacunes. Seventy-one were male, 43 female (Fisher, 1965a).

The primary or immediate causes of lacunes are likely to be reflected in Fisher's (1969, 1979) series of the arterial lesions underlying lacunes: in the first study 40 were due to occlusive segmental arterial disorganisation or lipohyalinosis (see above) (Figs. 12.14 & 12.15), two resulted from thrombosis in an asymmetric fusiform micro-aneurysm, three from typical microscopic athero-sclerosis in small cerebral arteries, in four the nature of the lesion was questionable, albeit in three there was some disorganisation of the wall.

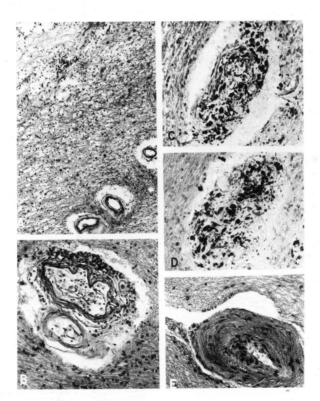

Fig. 12.14 Diseased artery running to 5 × 5 mm lacune in pontine base. Five different levels.

A. Section No. 38 showing three small arteries adjacent to lacunes.

B. Section No. 300. Arteries joining are occluded by fine connective tissues.

C. Section No. 357. Artery disorganised and enlarged, lumen obliterated. Many hemosiderin-filled macrophages. Artery is normally 160 μm.

D. Section No. 381. Chief segment of disorganisation.

E. Section No. 677. Artery entering subarachnoid space acquires lumen. Sections are approximately 10 μm thick. The vascular arrangement is pictured diagrammatically in Figure 12.15.

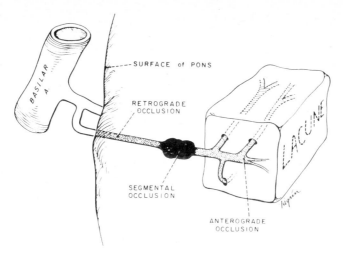

Fig. 12.15 Diagram of pons showing relation of lacune to vascular lesion described in Figure 12.14. (From C. M. Fisher (1969) The arterial lesions underlying lacunes. *Acta Neuropathologica.* (Berlin), 12:1. Reproduced by courtesy of the author.)

Finally, in the fiftieth lacune the nutrient artery was patent and possible embolism with transient occlusion had to be considered. In the second study of 11 lacunes of large size ('Capsular infarcts'), two were due to an atheromatous plaque with superimposed thrombus, in four there was a severe atherosclerotic stenosis, in one lipohyalinosis was present, in one the nature of the obstruction remained uncertain, in one the ostium of the penetrating artery was obstructed by atheroma of a main branch of the middle cerebral artery. In two cases the vessels were patent suggesting embolism.

In the series of 114 patients with lacunes (Fisher, 1965a) correlations were sought for various pathological conditions. It was concluded that lacunes were not related to carotid disease or cerebral embolism (although there may be exceptions to this) or diabetes. On the other hand a strong correlation was found with cerebral, i.e., intracranial atherosclerosis, and in approximately 50 per cent of patients with lacunes atherosclerotic lesions extended up to the small pial cerebral and cerebellar arteries. This, as already mentioned, closely parallels hypertension and indeed the strongest correlation for lacunes was found to be hypertension which was documented in 111 out of 114 patients (in two BP was unknown, one was normotensive and had been treated for neurosyphilis, possibly meningovascular syphilis).

In all studies the first preferential site for lacunes has been found to be the lenticular nucleus, particularly the putamen (Fig. 12.12) followed by pons (Fig. 12.13), thalamus, and caudate nucleus. However it must be stressed that lacunes are by no means rare in the white matter of the brain. Among 100 lacunes in Ferrand's (1902) series, 13 were in the white matter of the brain, and among 376 lacunes of Fisher's (1965a) series 89 (23 per cent) were either in the internal capsule or corona radiata or corpus callosum or white matter of cerebral lobes. Regarding the lacunes of the internal capsule Ferrand (1902) aptly remarked that lacunes usually do not occur in the internal capsule but rather in adjacent lenticular nucleus, thalamus, or caudate nucleus whence they encroach upon the internal capsule (Fig. 12.12), and moreover that it is infrequent that all capsular fibers are interrupted, a fact that may obviously have some clinical implications. Conversely lacunes appear to be absent from cortex, rare in cerebellum, and absent from medulla oblongata and spinal cord. The predominant sites of lacunes are closely similar to those of lipohyalinosis but also to those of microaneurysms. This may be taken as additional evidence that, as suggested above, both arterial lesions are the result of one basic pathological process (Russell, 1979).

It is a common belief that lacunes are very numerous in any one patient but this is far from being always the case. In Farrand's (1902) 88 patients a single lacune was present 14 times (15.9 per cent) and in Fisher's (1965a) 114 patients 29

(25.4 per cent) had also a single lesion. Among the 114 patients 54 had one or two lacunes, i.e., nearly half the total number of patients. Sixty patients had more than two lacunes; among these 2 had 14 and 2 had 15 lesions. Thus more often than is commonly believed lacunes allow a precise clinico-anatomical correlation, a point which will be commended on further. Unfortunately lacunes are often associated with haemorrhages as well as infarcts. In Marie's (1901) series of 50 brains there were haemorrhages in 16 and infarctions in seven. In Fisher's (1965a) series of 114 brains, haemorrhages were associated with lacunes in 35 per cent and infarction in 26 per cent. Also Marie (1901) mentioned that in four brains there existed in the cortex of the frontal or temporal poles, on one or both sides, 'état vermoulu', i.e., worm-eaten condition, consisting of a circumscribed destruction of the cortex with presence of small pits. Although Marie's description does not suggest the usual site of granular atrophy it would seem that this is a likely diagnosis for 'état vermoulu'.

The clinical picture of lacunes and état lacunaire according to Marie (1901) and Ferrand (1902) was mainly that of an hemiplegia of sudden onset, most often without loss of consciousness. After a few hours or days paralysis improved to a great extent but recovery remained usually incomplete. Useful clinical tests for minimal motor skill deficit were to ask the patient to button and unbutton his coat with either hand and for minimal facial paresis to ask the patient to wink either eye. It was frequently noted that one eye could easily be closed alone while this was impossible on the side of the facial paresis. In addition, it was noted that hemianesthesia was rare, and hemianopia was not observed. Dysarthria was common but aphasia was not encountered. No contracture of the limbs occurred. Walking was very characteristic, consisting of marche à petits pas de Dejerine. Psychic functions were impaired, pseudobulbar palsy was common.

It is usual in medicine that the earliest descriptions give an account of a disease in its fully developed form. Since Marie's and Ferrand's descriptions of état lacunaire, numerous attempts have been made to isolate clinical disorders that could be related to specifically located lesions. Many of the infrequent classical eponymic syndromes of the brain stem listed in the textbooks of neurology were the result of small infarcts or lacunes. In the present chapter a short account will be given only of the most frequent of them.

Fisher & Curry (1965) reported 50 clinical cases of pure motor hemiplegia, meaning that there were no clinical signs other than a complete or incomplete paralysis of face, arm, and leg at any time in the illness. All patients except four were hypertensive, hypertension being defined as blood pressure above 150/90 mmHg. One patient (case 10) had atrial fibrillation. In nine cases a post-mortem examination of the brain was performed. In five cases there was an infarct of the internal capsule (as well as of the adjacent basal ganglia), in three there was a lacunar infarct on one side of the basis pontis, not crossing the mid-line nor reaching into the middle cerebellar peduncles. Capsular cases appear to be similar to those reported by Foix & Lévy (1927) under the term 'ramollissements sylviens profonds partiels', i.e., incomplete deep basal infarcts (in the basal territory of the middle cerebral artery, see Fig. 12.1). Pontine cases resemble those previously reported by Lhermitte & Trelles (1934) under the term of 'hemiplégie protubérantielle', i.e., pontine hemiplegia. The same authors reported cases of 'paraplégie protubérantielle', i.e. pontine paraplegia resulting from bilateral small infarcts in basis pontis.

In the capsular as well as in the pontine cases of Fisher & Curry there was hemiparesis or hemiplegia. The extraocular movements may help to distinguish capsular from pontine lesions. In capsular cases, even in the presence of a severe hemiplegia, there usually was no paralysis of gaze; conjugate lateral gaze away from the hemiplegic side was sometimes easier than in the opposite direction. By contrast in one case of pontine lesions conjugate eye movements were easier towards the hemiplegic side. This sign, however, had disappeared within 24 hours.

The prognosis for recovery of the neurological deficit and surviving the illness appeared to be good. Usually recovery began within two weeks and advanced more quickly in the leg than in the arm. There was, however, a tendency to bilateral occurrence. Fisher & Curry concluded that in such cases angiography is not indicated and anticoagulant therapy probably not efficacious. It should be added—and this will hold true for other lacunar syndromes — that since nearly all patients are chronic hypertensives anticoagulant therapy should be considered dangerous for the reason that miliary aneurysms are very likely to be present.

Fisher (1965b) reported 26 patients with a symptomatology limited to a persistent or transient numbness and mild sensory loss over one entire side of the body, including the face, arm and leg. There was no motor deficit and other symptoms and signs were absent. All patients except one had hypertension defined as blood pressure above 150/90 mmHg. A post mortem study of the brain was obtained in one patient showing a single lacune 7 mm in diameter situated in the postero-ventral (sensory) nucleus of the thalamus and it was postulated that in most of the other cases of pure sensory stroke the responsible lesion also lay in the thalamus. Pure hemisensory strokes were nearly always benign and in none of the typical cases were they a harbinger of hemiplegia or other severe accident. It was inferred that the thalamic lesion resulted from thrombotic occlusion of a penetrating artery on the basis of hypertension and atherosclerosis. Therefore it was advised that anticoagulants be withheld and angiography not undertaken.

Pure sensory stroke is reminiscent of the thalamic syndrome, although in the three cases reported by Dejerine & Roussy (1906) there was mild hemiplegia and choreic-athetotic movements in addition to sensory disorders, and the infarcts were a little more extensive, involving the adjacent internal capsule and lenticular nucleus. On the other hand Garcin & Lapresle (1954, 1960) reported two patients in whom the sensory deficit affected only the lips and hand or part of the hand. In both cases the causal lesion was a lacunar infarct partially involving the ventral posterior lateral nucleus of the thalamus.

Fisher & Cole (1965) reported 14 patients in whom arm and leg on one side showed a combination of severe cerebellar-like ataxia and pyramidal signs. The leg was weak more distally than proximally and in some cases only the toes and ankle were involved. The arm showed little or no weakness. The face was spared and usually there was no dysarthria. A Babinski sign was always present and the deep reflexes were exaggerated.

Walking was impossible or almost so without support. Sensation was intact in all but one case. Two patients had nystagmus. Twelve of the 14 patients were hypertensive. The only available post-mortem brain examination was indecisive for there were at least 11 old lesions in the brain, most of them taking the form of lacunes. A clinical case closely resembling this had been reported by Nicolesco et al (1932). Fisher & Cole (1965) were inclined to believe that a supratentorial lesion of the crural pyramidal fibres was responsible for the clinical picture and that it possibly lay in the posterior-superior part of the internal capsule or in the adjacent corona radiata. In 12 of the 14 patients recovery was almost complete, and it was concluded that angiography and any therapy carrying a significant risk (anticoagulants had been used) is to be avoided.

Fisher (1967) reported some 20 patients with mild stroke consisting chiefly of dysarthria and clumsiness of one hand. The cardinal features of the syndrome included in addition: central weakness of one side of the face, deviation of the tongue on protrusion, a trace of dysphagia, a wavering ataxia on the finger-nose test not clearly cerebellar in type, mild imbalance on walking, possibly enhanced tendon reflexes on the affected side, a Babinski sign and reduced arm swing. Hypertension was almost always present. One patient with right hand clumsiness came to post-mortem examination due to a pancreatic carcinoma. The lesion held responsible for the nervous disorders was a lacune on the left side of the base of the pons in its top-most 5 mm. It was situated deeply, almost reaching the medial lemniscus. The cavity lay close to the mid-line and its broadest part may have crossed slightly to the other side. The cause of the lacune was likely to be thrombosis but the possibility of an embolus could not be excluded. The prognosis of this syndrome for virtually complete recovery appeared to be good. Angiography was deemed unnecessary and anticoagulants were not warranted.

Pseudobulbar palsy refers to a clinical condition in which there is paralysis or paresis of those muscles that control movements of the lips, tongue, pharynx, larynx, i.e., muscles that subserve mainly talking and swallowing. According to Broadbent's hypothesis (later demonstrated), 'the more muscles are bilateral in their action the more equally are the muscles of both sides represented in each side' (quoted by Jackson 1874–1876). Therefore muscles innervated from the medulla receive impulses from both hemispheres. This implies that pseudobulbar palsy results from lesions on both corticobulbar tracts, and the word pseudobulbar implies that the lesions are situated above the medulla. For reviews of early cases and of the concept of pseudobulbar paralysis see Comte (1900) and Thurel (1929).

Pseudobulbar palsy of arterial origin is usually due to successive lacunar infarcts resulting in *état lacunaire*. Although the levels of blood pressure are not mentioned in many of the early cases it may be reasonably assumed that patients did not differ from others with lacunes, i.e., they were hypertensives. Present experience supports this view. It is generally admitted that multiple lacunar infarcts involve both internal capsules and/or basis pontis, two elective sites for lacunes (see above).

The clinical picture (Fig. 12.16) includes poor

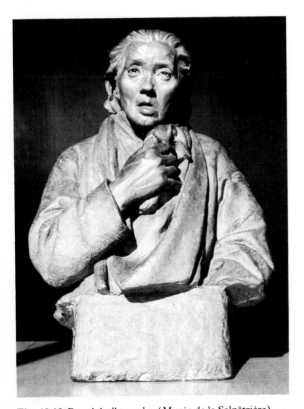

Fig. 12.16 Pseudobulbar palsy (Musée de la Salpêtrière).

mimicry at rest, often facial asymmetry due to uneven facial paresis (since the nuclei of the facial nerve are also often deprived of their normal innervation), drooling of saliva. Most characteristic is a dysarthria with paralytic and dystonic components. Speech is slurred, consonants especially labials and dentals being affected; palilalia may occur (Thurel, 1929; Brain, 1961). Loss of emotional control is common with outbursts of so-called spasmodic laughing or more often weeping. Disorders of swallowing may appear less severe although death may be due to choking as mentioned by Hughes et al (1954) and supported by the author's experience. Impairment of memory and dementia may be present but not necessarily even in severe cases (Hughes et al, 1954).

The limbs are generally clumsy and mildly paretic with bilateral extensor plantar responses, but contracture is usually slight with *marche à petits pas*. Double severe hemiplegia is exceptionally rare; urgency of micturition is common.

There is no doubt that pseudobulbar palsy deserves further studies of the kind that Fisher performed for other lacunar states. In the present state of knowledge the term refers to a galaxy of symptoms and signs which could most probably be broken down into more specific syndromes. Two well-identified syndromes must be mentioned: (1) pseudobulbar palsy resulting from lesions of both rolandic opercula and adjacent part of the third frontal gyrus (Foix et al, 1926; from the short extraneurological notes of this paper it is likely that both infarcts were of cardiac embolic nature) and (2) pseudobulbar palsy due to pontine infarcts with additional cerebellar disorders (L'hermitte & Trelles, 1934; Thurel, 1928).

Another quite different cerebral disorder has been recently tentatively ascribed to lacunes; Earnest et al (1974) reported two hypertensive patients with symptoms and signs suggesting normal pressure hydrocephalus. Pneumoencephalograms showed enlarged lateral and third ventricles in both cases. A right ventriculo-peritoneal shunt in the first patient and a right ventriculojugular shunt in the second one were performed. The first patient improved and did not die until three years later, after the onset of cerebral symptoms from myocardial infarction with cardiac failure plus evidence of new cerebral lesions. The second patient did not improve and died four weeks after the neurosurgical procedure. Post-mortem studies showed numerous lacunes in both cases. Earnest et al suggested that many infarcts in the periventricular matter and basal ganglia could reduce tissue bulk and tensile strength allowing the ventricles to enlarge under the stress of increased intraventricular cerebrospinal fluid pulse pressure of hypertensive vascular disease. The enlarged ventricles could then be subject to an increased total intraventricular force setting up a progressive ventricular enlargement. With en-largement of the ventricles ballooning of the hemispheres could compromise the convexity subarachnoid space by compression against the calvarium, so reducing cerebrospinal fluid drainage and causing a communicating hydrocephalus with convexity or incisural block and abnormal isotope cisternogram (Earnest et al, 1974). Enlargement of the ventricles (Fig. 12.12) is no new fact in *état lacunaire*. Marie (1901) reported that a common feature of lacunar brains was a dilatation of the cerebral ventricles, ... which may be fairly pro-nounced. It has been mentioned by authors in the first half of the nineteenth century under the name of 'senile hydrocephalus'. Ferrand (1902) stated that ventricular dilatation may reach such propor-tions as 'to reduce to almost nothing' the white matter of centrum ovale. Granted that ventricular dilatation is likely to be common in *état lacunaire* it must be recognised that its mechanisms and consequences are poorly understood and that it deserves further study.

Undoubtedly the last word has not been said about lacunes. Studies of recent years have shown that there certainly is much more to be discovered about these disorders by painstaking clinical and pathological correlations. To be sure the results may be disappointing when lacunes are too nu-merous to allow any correlation. On the other hand asymptomatic lacunes or at least lacunes which go by without recognised clinical disorders do exist. Fisher (1968) reported the case of a fit man, aged 71, who attended the neurological clinic because of a brief dizzy spell. A detailed neurologic examina-tion showed no defect. Five days later the patient died unexpectedly as the result of a myocardial infarction and neuropathological examination showed the presence of 44 lacunes in the cerebral hemispheres and brain stem. It is reasonable to hope that detailed study of such cases may one day yield further information.

Binswanger encephalopathy

Binswanger (1894) described a particular chronic progressive subcortical encephalopathy in hyper-tensive patients. Although he reported eight cases this is a very rare disease. Garcin, Lapresle, and Lyon (1960) reported three patients and found 20 reported cases. Mikol (1966) reported two addi-tional patients. Clinical symptoms and signs appear generally between the ages of 50 and 60 and result in progressive pseudobulbar palsy and dementia in three to five years. Some cases, however, have a more protracted course. At neuropathological examination the brunt of the process falls on the white matter. Some of the regions of myelin destruction are sharply demarcated, some have less distinct contours. One or several convolutions may be affected. In most cases myelin lesions predomi-nate in the occipital and temporal lobes. In severe cases nearly all the white matter of the brain is involved. The cortex and subarcuate fibres are spared. Intracerebral arteries show extensive hya-line changes. Figures 12.17A, B, and C (unpub-lished case) are from a man who developed at age 66 disorders of memory and in the following years pseudobulbar palsy and dementia. At first exami-nation blood pressure was recorded at 160/110 and on subsequent examination was often in the range of 200/100. At post-mortem, six years later, there was remarkably little atherosclerosis on the basal arteries.

The mechanisms of lesions in Binswanger's leucoencephalopathy are a riddle. Arterial lesions together with the sparing of the cortex have suggested a particular variety of distal ischaemic necrosis, somewhat similar to watershed infarc-tion, but there is not much more than theoretical reasoning to support this view. Oedema of venous origin has been suspected by Stochdroph & Meesen (1958). Feigin & Popoff (1963) thought that in hypertensive individuals the changes in the white matter indicate that there is a tendency for cerebral oedema to develop around focal lesions or even in the absence of such detectable lesions, a view which is supported by present evidence. Feigin & Popoff

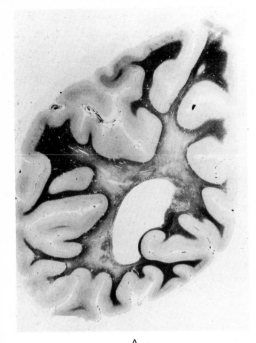
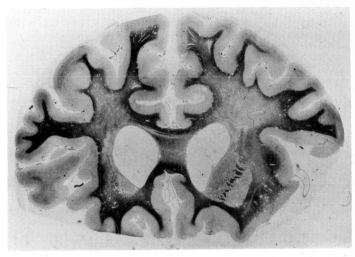

A

B

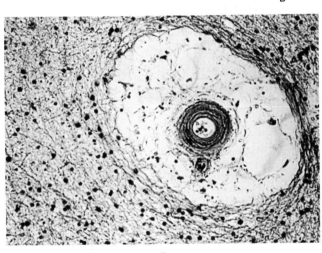

C

Fig. 12.17 Binswanger's encephalopathy.
  A. Coronal section of left hemisphere just behind splenium of corpus callosum.
  B. Coronal section of frontal lobes. Extensive demyelination. Celloidin. Loyez Stain.
  C. Artery in white matter. Hyalinosis. H.E. × 120.

(1963), however, go further and state that 'the basic change [i.e., arterial hyalinosis] is a late effect of cerebral oedema initiated by some aspects of hypertensive disease and that the vascular change is a secondary effect, secondary to the hypertensive disease itself, to the cerebral oedema and most likely to both'. There may obviously be some truth in these views but the role of each component of this rather elaborate hypothesis has yet to be determined.

Arteriopathic Parkinsonism
The term Parkinson's disease should be reserved for true paralysis agitans. According to all available

evidence arterial disease is not an aetiological factor in this disease (Escourolle et al, 1971). Parkinsonism is a syndrome and several aetiological factors may cause the same clinical picture. Among the causes of Parkinsonism, arterial disease is a classical one; in a review of arteriosclerotic Parkinsonism, Critchley (1936) stressed the clinical differences between it and paralysis agitans, in particular he aptly remarked that tremor is usually absent and that blood pressure is often high. He noted that in many cases of arteriosclerotic Parkinsonism there are 'bulbar' signs, emotional incontinence and a variable dementia. Undoubtedly most of the cases which were in the scope of Critchley's paper could as well be classified as pseudobulbar palsy or *état lacunaire*. Their pathological basis may be assumed to be similar (i.e., occlusion of perforating arteries) and their preventive therapy should be treatment of arterial hypertension.

Acknowledgement

Figures 12.3, 12.4, 12.5, 12.9, 12.14, and 12.15 have been reproduced through the courtesy of Drs F. B. Byrom and C. Miller Fisher and with the kind permission of Heinemann Medical Books Ltd., London and Springer Verlag, Berlin.

REFERENCES

Adams C W M 1967 Vascular Histochemistry. Lloyd-Luke, London

Adams R D 1955 Pathology of cerebral vascular disease. In: Millikan C H (ed.) Princeton conferences on cerebrovascular disease. Second conference. Grune & Stratton, New York

Adams R D, Fisher C M 1961 Pathology of cerebral arterial occlusion. In: Fields W S (ed.) Pathogenesis and treatment of cerebrovascular disease. Charles C Thomas, Springfield, Illinois

Alajouanine T, Hornet T 1939 L'oedème cérébral généralisé. Etude anatomique. Annals d'Anatomie Pathologique 16: 133

Arab A 1957 L'artériosclérose cérébrale scalariforme hypertensive. Psychiatrie und Neurologie (Basel) 134: 175

Bakay L, Sweet W H 1952 Cervical and intracranial intra-arterial pressures with and without vascular occlusion. Surgery, Gynecology and Obstetrics 95: 67

Bakay L, Sweet W H 1953 Intra-arterial pressure in the neck and brain. Late changes after carotid closure, acute measurements after vertebral closure. Journal of Neurosurgery 10: 353

Baker A B, Iannone A 1969a Cerebrovascular disease. II. The smaller intracerebral arteries. Neurology (Minneapolis), 9: 391

Baker A B, Iannone A 1959b Cerebrovascular disease. III. The intracerebral arterioles. Neurology (Minneapolis), 9: 441

Baker A B, Resch J A, Loewenson R B 1969 Hypertension and Cerebral Atherosclerosis. Circulation 39: 701

Bayliss W N 1902 On the local reaction of the arterial wall to changes of internal pressure. Journal of Physiology 28: 220

Beevers D G, Hamilton M, Fairman J E, Harpur J E 1973 Antihypertensive treatment and the course of established cerebral vascular disease. Lancet i: 1407

Binswanger O 1894 Die Begrenzung der allgemeinen progressiven Paralysie. Berliner Klinische Wochenschrift 31: 1137

Blackfan K D 1926 Acute nephritis in children with special reference to the treatment of uremia. Bulletin of the Johns Hopkins Hospital 39: 69

Brain, Lord 1961 Speech Disorders, Aphasia, Apraxia and Agnosia. London: Butterworths

Breckenridge A, Dollery C T, Parry E H O 1970 Prognosis of treated hypertension. Quarterly Journal of Medicine 39: 411

Byrom F B 1954 The pathogenesis of hypertensive encephalopathy and its relation to the malignant phase of hypertension: experimental evidence from the hypertensive rat. Lancet ii: 201

Byrom F B 1969 The Hypertensive Vascular Crisis. London: Heinemann

Cambier J, Gautier J C 1965 Pronostic des accidents vasculaires cérébraux de nature ischémique. Achter Internationaler Kongress für Lebensversicherungsmedizin. Schwaba and Co. Verlag, Basel, and Stuttgart

Charcot J M, Bouchard C 1868 Nouvelles recherches sur la pathogénie de l'hémorragie cérébrale. Archives de Physiologie Normale et Pathologique 1: 110, 643, 735

Chester E M, Agamanolis D P, Banker B P, Victor M 1978 Hypertensive encephalopathy: A Clinicopathological Study of 20 cases. Neurology 28: 928

Clarke E, Murphy E A 1956 Neurological manifestations of malignant hypertension. British Medical Journal 2: 1319

Cole F M, Yates P O 1967a The occurrence and significance of intracerebral micro-aneurysms. Journal of Pathology and Bacteriology 93: 393

Cole F M, Yates P O 1967b Intracerebral micro-aneurysms and small cerebrovascular lesions. Brain 90: 759

Cole F M, Yates P O 1968 Comparative incidence of cerebrovascular lesion in normotensive and hypertensive patients. Neurology (Minneapolis) 18: 225

Comte A 1900 Des Paralysies Pseudo-Bulbaire. G. Steinheil, Paris

Cook T A, Yates P O 1972 A histometric study of cerebral and renal arteries in normotensives and chronic hypertensives. Journal of Pathology 108: 129

Cove D H, Seddon M, Fletcher R F, Dukes D C 1979 Blindness after treatment for malignant hypertension, British Medical Journal ii: 245

Critchley M 1936 Arteriosclerotic Parkinsonism. Brain 52: 23

Dejerine J, Roussy G 1906 Le syndrome thalamique. Revue Neurologique 12: 521

Dinsdale H B, Robertson D M, Haas R A 1974 Cerebral blood flow in acute hypertension. Archives of Neurology 31 : 80

Durant-Fardel M 1843 Traité du ramollissement du cerveau. Baillière, Paris and London

Duret H 1874 Recherches anatomiques sur la circulation de l'encéphale. Archives de Physiologie 1 : 60, 316

Earnest M P, Fahn S, Karp J, Rowland L P 1974 Normal pressure hydrocephalus and hypertensive cerebrovascular disease. Archives of Neurology 31 : 262

Escourolle R, de Recondo J, Gray F 1971 Etude anatomopathologique des syndromes parkinsonens. In : Monoamines, Noyaux Gris Centraux et Syndrome de Parkinson. Georg and Cie, Geneva ; Masson et Cie, Paris. p 173

Evans H 1933 Hypertensive encephalopathy in nephritis. Lancet ii : 583

Feigin I, Popoff N 1963 Neuropathological changes late in cerebral edema. The relationship to trauma, hypertensive disease and Binswanger encephalopathy. Journal of Neuropathology and Experimental Neurology 22 : 500

Ferrand J 1902 Essai sur l'Hémiplégie des Vieillards. Les Lacunes de Désintégration Cérébrale. Paris : J Rousset

Finnerty F A, Witkin L, Fazekas J F 1954 Cerebral hemodynamics during ischaemia induced by acute hypotension. Journal of Clinical Investigations 33 : 1227

Finnerty F A 1972 Hypertensive encephalopathy. American Journal of Medicine 52 : 672

Fisher C M 1961a Clinical syndromes in cerebral arterial occlusion. In : Fields W S (ed.) Pathogenesis and treatment of cerebrovascular disease. Charles C Thomas, Springfield, Illinois

Fisher C M 1961b The pathology and pathogenesis of intracerebral hemorrhage. In : Fields W S (ed.) Pathogenesis and treatment of cerebrovascular disease. Charles C Thomas, Springfield, Illinois

Fisher C M 1965a Lacunes : small, deep cerebral infarcts. Neurology (Minneapolis) 15 : 774

Fisher C M 1965b Pure sensory stroke involving face arm and leg. Neurology (Minneapolis) 15 : 76

Fisher C M 1967 Lacunar stroke. The dysarthria–clumsy hand syndrome. Neurology (Minneapolis) 17 : 614

Fisher C M 1969 The arterial lesions underlying lacunes. Acta Neuropathologica (Berlin) 12 : 1

Fisher C M 1972 Cerebral miliary aneurysms in hypertension. American Journal of Pathology 66 : 313

Fisher C M 1979 Capsular Infarcts. The underlying vascular lesions. Archives of Neurology 36 : 65

Fisher C M, Cole M 1965 Homolateral ataxia and crural paresis : a vascular syndrome. Journal of Neurology, Neurosugery and Psychiatry 28 : 48

Fisher C M, Curry H B 1965 Pure motor hemiplegia of vascular origin. Archives of Neurology 13 : 30

Fisher C M, Gore I, Okabe N, White P D 1965a Atherosclerosis of the carotid and vertebral arteries. Extracranial and intracranial. Journal of Neuropathology and Experimental Neurology 24 : 455

Fisher C M, Gore I, Okabe N, White P D 1965b Calcification of the carotid syphon. Circulation 32 : 538

Fog M 1939 Cerebral circulation. II. Reaction of pial arteries to increase in blood pressure. Archives of Neurology and Psychiatry 41 : 260

Foix C, Hillemand P 1925 Les artères de l'axe encéphalique jusqu'au diencéphale inclusivement. Revue Neurologique 2 : 705

Foix C, Chavany A, Marie J 1926 Diplégie facio-linguomasticatrice d'origine cortico sous corticale sans paralysie des membres. Revue Neurologique 1 : 214

Foix C, Lévy M 1927 Les ramollissements sylviens. Syndromes des lésions en foyer du territoire de l'artère sylvienne et de ses branches. Revue Neurologique 2 : 1

Folkow B 1971 The haemodynamic consequences of adaptive structural changes of the resistance vessels. Clinical Science 41 : 1

Garcin R, Lapresle J 1954 Syndrome sensitif de type thalamique et à topographie cheiro-orale par lésion localisée du thalamus. Revue Neurologique 90 : 124

Garcin R, Lapresle J 1960 Deuxième observation personnelle de syndrome sensitif de type thalamique et à topographie cheiro-orale par lésion localisée du thalamus. Revue Neurologique 103 : 474

Garcin R, Lapresle J, Lyon G 1960 Encéphalopathie sous-corticale chronique de Binswanger. Etude anatomoclinique de trois observations. Revue Neurologique 102 : 423

Garner A, Ashton N 1970 Ultrastructure of hypertensive retinopathy. Excerpta Medica International Congress Series No. 222 Ophthalmology

Gautier J C 1970 Histoire naturelle des accidents cérébraux dus à l'athérosclérose, Encéphale 3 : 197

Giese J 1966 The Pathogenesis of Hypertensive Vascular Disease. Copenhagen : Munskgaard

Graham J B 1951 Pheochromocytoma and hypertension. An analysis of 207 cases. International Abstracts of Surgery (Surgery Gynecology Obstetrics. Suppl.) 92 : 105

Häggendahl E, Johansson B 1972 On the pathophysiology of the increased cerebrovascular permeability in acute arterial hypertension in cats. Acta Neurologica Scandinavica 48 : 265

Hamilton M, Thompson E N, Wisniewski T K M 1964 The role of blood pressure control in preventing complications of hypertension. Lancet i : 235

Harnish A, Pearce M L 1973 Evolution of hypertensive retinal vascular disease. Correlations between clinical and post-mortem observations. Medicine 52 : 483

Hodge J V, McQueen E G, Smirk H 1961 Results of hypotensive therapy in arterial hypertension. British Medical Journal i : 1

Hughes W H, Dodgson M C H, MacLennan D C 1954 Chronic cerebral hypertensive disease. Lancet ii : 770

Hypertensive encephalopathy 1979 Editorial British Medical Journal ii : 1387

Jackson J H 1874–1976 ; reprinted 1958 Selected writings. vol. 1. Staples Press, London. p 265

Jellinek E H, Painter M, Prineas J, Ross Russell R 1964 Hypertensive encephalopathy with cortical disorders of vision. Quarterly Journal of Medicine 33 : 239

Jewett J F 1973 Fatal intracranial edema from eclampsia. New England Journal of Medicine 289 : 976

Johansson B 1974 Blood-Brain Barrier Dysfunction in Acute Arterial Hypertension. Göteborg

Johansson B, Li C L, Olsonn Y, Klatzo I 1970 The effect of acute arterial hypertension on the blood brain barrier to protein tracers. Acta Neuropathologica (Berlin) 16 : 117

Johansson B, Strandgaard S, Lassen N A 1974 On the pathogenesis of hypertensive encephalopathy. Circulation Research 34 : 167

Kannel W B 1971 Current status of the epidemiology of brain infarction associated with occlusive arterial disease. Stroke 2 : 295

Kannel W B, Wolf P A, Verter J, McNamara P 1970 Epidemiologic assessment of the role of blood pressure in stroke. The Framingham Study. Journal of the American Medical Association 214: 301

Kernohan J W, Anderson E W, Keith N M 1929 Arterioles in cases of hypertension. Archives of Internal Medicine 44: 395

Lassen N A 1959 Cerebral blood flow and oxygen consumption in man. Physiological Reviews 39: 183

Lassen N A, Agnoli A 1972 The upper limit of autoregulation of cerebral blood flow. On the pathogenesis of hypertensive encephalopathy. Scandinavian Journal of Clinical and Laboratory Investigation 30: 113

Leishman A W D 1959 Hypertension treated and untreated. A study of 400 cases. British Medical Journal i: 1361

Lhermitte J, Trelles J O 1934 L'artériosclérose du tronc basilaire et ses conséquences anatomo-cliniques. Jarhbücher für Psychiatrie und Neurologie 51: 91

Lhermitte F, Gautier J C, Derouesné C 1970 Nature of occlusions of the middle cerebral artery. Neurology (Minneapolis) 20: 82

Lhermitte F, Gautier J C 1975 Sites of cerebral arterial occlusions. In: Modern Trends in Neurology, 6. London: Butterworth

Low-Beer T, Phear D 1961 Cerebral infarction and hypertension. Lancet i: 1303

Marie P 1901 Des foyers lacunaires de désintégration et de différents autres états cavitaires du cerveau. Revue de Médecine 31: 281

Marshall J 1964 A trial of long-term hypotensive therapy in cerebrovascular disease. Lancet i: 10

Marshall J, Kaeser A C 1961 Survival after non-haemorrhagic cerebrovascular accidents. A prospective study. British Medical Journal ii: 73

Medina J L, Rubino F A, Ross E 1974 Agitated delirium caused by infarctions of the hippocampal formation and fusiform and lingual gyri. Neurology (Minneapolis) 24: 1181

Meyer J S 1961 The value of electroencephalography in diagnosis of cerebrovascular disease. In: Fields W S (ed.) Pathogenesis and treatment of cerebrovascular disease. Charles C Thomas, Springfield, Illinois

Meyer J S, Waltz A G, Gotoh F 1960a Pathogenesis of cerebral vasospasm in hypertensive encephalopathy. I. Effects of acute pressure in intraluminal blood pressure on pial blood flow. Neurology (Minneapolis) 10: 735

Meyer J S, Waltz A G, Gotoh F 1960b Pathogenesis of cerebral vasospasm in hypertensive encephalopathy. II. The nature of increased irritability of smooth muscle of pial arterioles in renal hypertension. Neurology (Minneapolis) 10: 859

Mikol J 1966 Contribution à l'Etude des Leucoencéphalopathies Artérioscléreuses: Maladie de Binswanger et Formes Apparentées. Paris

Milliez P 1943 Accidents Cérébraux des Hypertendus et Oedème Méningo-Encéphalique. Thèse Faculté Médecine. J Peyronnet et Cie: Paris

Nicolesco J, Cretu V, Demetresco L 1932 Syndrome de l'artère cérébrale antérieure. Monoplégie crurale droite avec symptomatologie cérébelleuse prédominante. Revue Neurologique 1: 563

Oppenheimer B S, Fishberg A M 1928 Hypertensive encephalopathy. Archives of Internal Medicine 41: 264

Pal J 1905 Die Gefässkrisen. Hirzel, Leipzig

Rail D L, Perkin G D 1980 Computerized tomographic appearance of hypertensive encephalopathy. Archives of Neurology 37: 310–11

Rodda R, Denny-Brown D 1966a The cerebral arteries in experimental hypertension. I. The nature of arteriolar constriction and its effects on the collateral circulation. American Journal of Pathology 49: 53

Rodda R, Denny-Brown D 1966b The cerebral arterioles in experimental hypertension. II. The development of arteriolonecrosis. American Journal of Pathology 49: 365

Russell R W R 1963 Observations on intracerebral aneurysms. Brain 86: 425

Russell R W R 1969 Cerebral embolism: pathogenesis and clinical features. In: Gillespie J A (ed.) Extracranial cerebrovascular disease and its management. Butterworth: London

Russell R W R 1973 Evidence for autoregulation in human retinal circulation. Lancet ii: 1048

Russell R W R 1975 How does blood pressure cause stroke? Lancet ii: 1283

Shekelle R B, Ostfeld A M, Klawans Jr H L 1974 Hypertension and risk of stroke in an elderly population. Stroke 5: 71

Stochdorpf O, Meesen H 1958 Article in Handbuch der Speziellen Pathologischen Anatomie und Histologie. J Springer, Berlin

Strandgaard S, Olesen J, Skinhøj E, Lassen N A 1973 Autoregulation of brain circulation in severe arterial hypertension. British Medical Journal i: 507

Thurel R 1929 Les Pseudo-Bulbaires. Etude Clinique et Anatomo-Pathologique. Paris: G. Doin

Tissot R 1966 Neuropsychopathologie de l'Aphasie. Paris: Masson et Cie

Van Citters R L, Wagner B M, Rushmer R F 1962 Architecture of small arteries during vasoconstriction. Circulation Research 10: 668

Vander Eecken H M 1959 The anastomoses between the leptomeningeal arteries of the brain. Charles C Thomas, Springfield, Illinois

Veterans Administration Cooperative Study Group on Antihypertensive Agents 1967 Effects of treatment on morbidity in hypertension. Journal of the American Medical Association 202: 1028

Whisnant J P 1974 Epidemiology of stroke: emphasis on transient cerebral ischemic attacks and hypertension. Stroke 5: 68

Wilson C 1963 Personal communication to Jellinek et al 1964

Wilson C 1969 Hypertension. In: Schettler F G, Boyd G S (eds.) Atherosclerosis, pathology, physiology, aetiology, diagnosis and clinical management. Elsevier, Amsterdam, London, New York

Ziegler D K, Zosa A, Zileli T 1965 Hypertensive encephalopathy. Archives of Neurology 12: 472

13

Spontaneous intracerebral haemorrhage

Alan Richardson

CEREBRAL HEMISPHERES

Haemorrhage into the substance of the cerebral hemispheres may occur from a variety of causes, but the type for discussion here is that associated with hypertensive disease or atherosclerosis, affecting the cerebral vessels. This group is commonly characterised by haemorrhage into the brain parenchyma in patients with known vascular disease who, at angiography, operation or post-mortem, show no evidence of an associated vascular anomaly such as aneurysm, angioma or tumour. The occurrence of minute angiomas or thrombosed aneurysms in similar cases has of course been described but these are outside the present context.

Pathology

Brief reference to the possible pathological sequence is necessary to understand the clinical and therapeutic problems. Most large clinical or post-mortem series indicate prevalence of hypertension of at least 50 per cent (Locksley et al, 1966; Richardson & Einhorn, 1963), with a peak age incidence between 50 and 59 years (McKissock et al, 1959). Though at first sight it may seem not unreasonable to expect haemorrhage from diseased vessels in hypertensive patients, the definition of the precise pathological substrate has excited much attention starting with Charcot & Bouchard in 1872 who postulated miliary aneurysms as the cause. This has been validated by Ross Russell (1963) who elegantly demonstrated microaneurysms on perforating vessels of 100 to 300 μm diameter, occurring almost exclusively in hypertensive patients. The fact that these were common on vessels at the usual sites of primary haemorrhage

was of great importance. It is naturally difficult to prove that such lesions are always the cause of such haemorrhage, and Fisher (1971) has suggested that the haemorrhage may arise from sequential involvement of a number of small vessels. The microaneurysm hypothesis nevertheless seems the most attractive except that these lesions are relatively rare in normotensive patients under the age of 65 years (Cole & Yates, 1967) whereas primary brain haemorrhage in such patients is not. Such haemorrhage most commonly starts in the putamenocapsular region or the thalamus and then may either arrest as a circumscribed haematoma or may spread. It may suffuse to occupy predominantly the region of the external capsule or proceed further and by splitting along the planes of white matter form a substantial space occupying clot in the frontal, temporal, or parietal lobes. Occasionally it arises from the posterior capsular region and tracks into the occipital lobe. As an alternative, the haemorrhage may remain confined to the ganglionic masses or rupture into the ventricular system. Such rupture may be massive and rapidly fatal or be a secondary event resulting in a communication between the haematoma cavity and the trigone of the lateral ventricle or less commonly between the haematoma and the frontal or temporal horns. Whether the haemorrhage is a single event or is followed by further episodes of bleeding (Fisher, 1971) remains a matter for debate, but it is a surgical fact that clot of varying ages from within the cavity can only occasionally be confirmed.

This brief pathological concept serves to highlight the three important clinical groups: firstly, the destructive massive ganglionic haemorrhages which are rapidly fatal; secondly, more circumscribed lesions in the same area causing maximal neurological deficit but with survival; thirdly, those cases in which the lobar component predominates and therefore present as a space-occupying mass. Additionally one must consider the response of the brain to these sudden insults, and of paramount importance is the disruption of the normal vascular autoregulation in the region of the lesion to which is added the space-occupying character of the lesion, resulting in rapid and often dramatic changes in intracranial pressure. It is well known that spontaneous intracranial bleeding may provoke rises in intracranial pressure approaching arterial systolic levels the persistence of which may cause arrest of the cerebral circulation. Lesser degrees of pressure change may account for brief periods of unconsciousness at the moment of ictus, and slower but more persistent changes associated with brain oedema and loss of autoregulatory capacity are responsible for the brain herniations and secondary brain stem haemorrhages so commonly seen in fatal cases. The origin of the haemorrhage, the vascular tonus at the time and the sequential pathological changes in the brain set the stage for the varied clinical presentation and courses and help to define the therapeutic aims as well as setting limits on their effectiveness.

Clinical features

Consideration of cerebral haemorrhage conjures the picture of sudden onset of severe headache with vomiting and the rapid evolution of a neurological deficit with depression of consciousness. This was the accepted classical description, and less severe clinical events were regarded as thrombotic in aetiology. However, in a series of 244 cases of proven intracerebral haemorrhage (McKissock et al, 1959) it was possible to identify four major presenting groups:

1. Sudden onset without loss of consciousness (89 cases).
2. Sudden onset with loss of consciousness (117 cases).
3. Gradual onset without loss of consciousness (23 cases).
4. Gradual onset with later loss of consciousness (3 cases).

The exact mode of onset in the remaining 12 cases was unknown. Thus about half the patients did not lose consciousness at or within 24 hours of ictus. If we follow the clinical course a little further it is noted that about one-third of those in the first group subsequently showed a depression of conscious level usually within two to five days, and a similar number of those in the second group regained consciousness in the same period of time. It therefore follows that consciousness will be preserved or regained in about half the cases of cerebral haemorrhage. The accurate assessment of neurological signs depends on the state of awareness of the patient. In this series of 244 patients, 86 were either in deep coma or simply capable of reflex protective responses. In the remainder, hemiplegia or hemiparesis was the commonest sign with evidence of hemisensory disturbance in the more deeply placed lesions. Less than 10 per cent of the group were without an identifiable severe deficit, this most commonly amounting to severe confusion, disorientation and often marked behaviour disturbance.

The more definitive clinical features have been described by Fisher (1961), and only brief reference needs to be made to them here. Severe headache was only a feature in 50 per cent of cases whereas vomiting was almost universal. Nuchal rigidity was not invariable and was usually mild in degree and slow of evolution.

Putamenocapsular haemorrhage

This produces the classical abrupt hemiplegic onset with an all-modality sensory disturbance, hemianopic defects and speech deficit in the dominant hemisphere. Loss of conjugate lateral gaze may be a prominent feature. Usually the motor deficit is more severe and persistent than the sensory, but even then may have a non-uniform distribution. Where the haemorrhage is more confined to the region of the caudate head the deficits may be less severe, transient, and associated with more obvious confusion. Alertness is commonly maintained. Rupture into the ventricular system is almost invariable.

Thalamic haemorrhage

Vessel rupture in this region may produce a localised haematoma or a destructive haemorrhage involving the peduncle and/or midbrain. The clinical features may vary from rapidly advancing coma with decerebrate posturing and autonomic failure, to less dramatic forms with global motor and sensory deficits often associated with gross ocular signs. Loss of upward gaze with downward deviation of the eyes may occur, and skew deviation is an even more sinister sign. Pupillary inequality is usual. Lateral gaze palsies were also noted in Fisher's cases (1961). He suggested that these were more likely in the deeply-placed haemorrhage but unfortunately they are also seen in pontine haemorrhage, cerebellar lesions, acute aneurysmal rupture and acute subdural haematomas. Haemorrhage in the region of the thalamus and internal capsule account for about 30 per cent of all cases in most series.

Lobar haematomas

These most commonly originate in the external capsule and split white matter to involve one of the lobes. Confusion and disorientation with more severe headache are common, the neurological signs being referable to the lobe involved, though the severity often seems to bear little relationship to the size of the haematoma unless it is truly massive. Epilepsy as an acute phenomenon is seen in these lesions, often generalised at the onset with a tendency to be focal later. Kaplan (1961) gives a incidence of 30 per cent for epilepsy in acute haemorrhage whereas our own experience would suggest a much lower figure.

DIAGNOSIS

The diagnosis of primary intracerebral haemorrhage is based on a combination of clinical characteristics, such as the nature of onset, and the evolution of events, together with more definitive investigatory procedures designed directly or indirectly to demonstrate the haematoma and to exclude the presence of an associated lesion. An abrupt onset with little preceding history, the absence of trauma and with the other clinical features noted above is still the commonest starting point in the diagnostic procedure. In view of the known tendency for blood to enter the ventricular

system, examination of the c.s.f. was usually the first step. In cases showing depression of consciousness, brain scanning takes precedence.

Lumbar puncture

In the series of 244 cases (McKissock et al, 1959) this investigation had been performed in 201 patients. Evidence of recent haemorrhage was obvious in 161 of them but was absent in the remaining 40 cases. Forty-three patients did not have the lumbar c.s.f. examined; of these the ventricular fluid was blood-stained and xanthochromic in 18 and in nine it was clear. In the remainder the time interval from the ictus was too long for valid conclusion. This study did not allow of any firm conclusion but suggested that in an appreciable proportion of cases the fluid showed no evidence of recent haemorrhage, therefore leaving some initial doubt between the diagnosis of haemorrhage and infarction. It was of further interest that in five cases the cerebrospinal fluid showed a marked pleocytosis such as to suggest the possibility of meningitis. This point had been earlier noted by Bedford (1958). The absence of blood from the c.s.f. in a conscious patient may suggest cerebral infarction rather than haemorrhage, whereas its presence simply indicates the entry of blood into the subarachnoid space and therefore does not exclude the possibility of an underlying causal lesion. Further complicating the problem is the fact that diagnostic lumbar puncture may not be free from hazard. Certainly in a patient showing signs of mesencephalic embarrassment with depression of consciousness, hemiplegia and increasing pupillary inequality the hazards of lumbar puncture in accelerating a progressive haematoma will outweigh the advantage of the information so gained. In the unconscious patient following a deteriorating course the investigation should be employed only if a treatable alternative diagnosis presents itself.

Ultrasound

Leksell (1956) first used transmitted ultrasound to define displacements of the midline cerebral structure. Achar et al (1966) made the case for its use in differentiating haemorrhage from infarction on the basis of the degree of midline displacement. The advent of tomographic brain scanning has largely displaced this atraumatic bedside investigation.

Radioactive brain scanning

Rectilinear brain scanning in neurological diagnosis using various radioisotopes is a well established procedure in many acute brain lesions, particularly brain tumours. Its usefulness in the diagnosis of primary intracerebral haematomas has been less well validated though some authors have suggested that it will demonstrate the lesion in nearly three-quarters of patients (Ojemann, 1973). Extensive experience in our own department does not really substantiate this claim throughout the varied range of such cases. In the general context of acute cerebral lesions it may be useful in excluding other lesions such as massive infarction, tumour, abscess or the occasional acute spontaneous subdural haematoma (Tallala & McKissock, 1971). Computerised scanning now gives a definitive diagnosis.

C.T. scanning

In 1961 Oldendorf devised a system for displaying anatomical structures as a complex demonstration of their radiodensity. This idea was brought to fruition by Hounsfield in 1969, who evolved the radiological system and computer programme to represent the skull and its contents in serial axial slices in relation to their X-ray density. The technique has been fully described (Hounsfield et al, 1973) and needs no amplification except to stress that it is a non-invasive method of investigation uniquely relevant to the accurate diagnosis of intracerebral haematomas. Clotted blood, partly due to its calcium has an X-ray density in striking contrast to that of the surrounding brain and much greater than that of the fluid-filled ventricular system. It therefore allows of accurate assessment of the size, situation and configuration of the haematoma (high density — represented as white), as well as indicating the degree of displacement or distortion of the ventricular system and the presence of any associated oedema in the brain parenchyma (diminished density — represented by black or dark grey areas).

A series of 66 intracerebral haematomas all verified by operation or autopsy were investigated in this way and reported by Paxton & Ambrose (1974). In each case the haematoma was accurately diagnosed and its precise configuration, extent and relationship to the cerebral structures and the ventricular system demonstrated. The overwhelming majority of the lesions were seen as high density areas, with some increase in density noted in those patients subjected to serial examination. This was thought to be due to subsequent clot retraction, loss of fluid and therefore relative increase in calcium ion content. Figure 13.1 shows a typical high density clot in the region of the external capsule with a medial margin of oedema (black), and clearly shows the compression and displacement of the body and part of the frontal horn of the lateral ventricle. A much larger haematoma with more marked ventricular displacement is shown in Figure 13.2, with the lesion dissecting towards a more superficial position in the temporal lobe but also extending far posteriorly. In contrast Figure 13.3 shows a small subependymal haematoma as a small white area in the region of the caudate head on the left side at the junction of the frontal horn and the body of the ventricle. A haemorrhage into

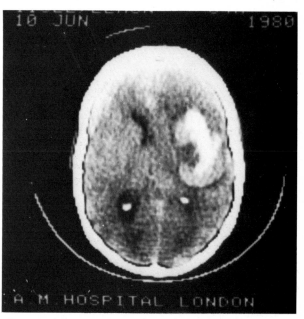

Fig. 13.1 Typical haematoma in external capsule of right hemisphere. Frontal horn displaced. Some oedema around lesion. Clot density diminishing.

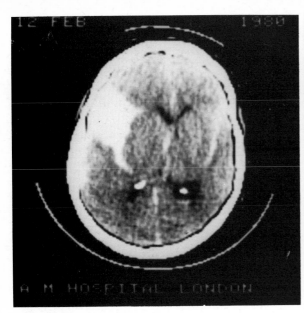

Fig. 13.2 More extensive dissection by haematoma to a superficial position in left temporal lobe with displacement of frontal horn.

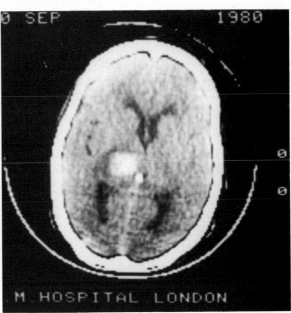

Fig. 13.4 Typical left thalamic haemorrhage with distortion of the third ventricle.

the left thalamus in a restless patient is shown in Figure 13.4. This clearly demonstrates the dilatation of the ventricular system and the distortion of the third ventricle which is almost obliterated. Finally Figure 13.5 shows a large haemorrhage dissecting towards the fronto-temporal operculum, arising from the region of the internal capsule and showing clear evidence of marked ventricular distortion with actual rupture into the ventricular system. In the collected series of Paxton & Ambrose (1974) further examples are shown including primary massive intraventricular rupture.

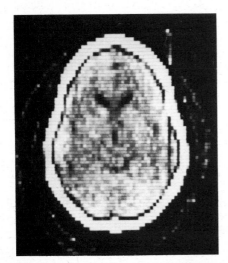

Fig. 13.3 Small, spherical haematoma (white) at point of junction of anterior horn and body of lateral ventricle. Subependymal in position. Virtually no ventricular distortion and certainly no displacement.

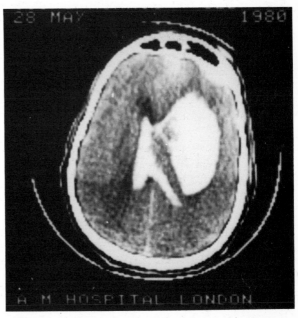

Fig. 13.5 Extensive dissection of a haematoma with rupture into the ventricular system.

There is no doubt that this form of scanning has revolutionised not only the ease of diagnosis of intracerebral haemorrhage but has also provided vital information in relation to associated pathology necessary to the formulation of a logical treatment policy.

Angiography

The widespread use of tomographic brain scanning has influenced the use of angiography in intracranial haemorrhage. As a primary investigation it will give accurate location and configuration of a haematoma in the brain substance and indicate the involvement of the subarachnoid space or ventricular system as well as demonstrating the presence of oedema, displacement or complicating hydrocephalus. The demonstration of a cerebral clot without subarachnoid space involvement then requires the distinction of hypertensive haemorrhage from that due to a demonstrable causal lesion. Analysis of 100 cases of such haematomas by Hayward & O'Reilly (1976) showed an accuracy rate of 90 per cent in predicting the underlying pathology. Three cases of primary haemorrhage were thought to have vascular pathology, but only one case considered as a primary event was found to harbour an aneurysm. Haemorrhage in the internal and external capsules, thalamus and caudate head were rarely other than primary. Whilst accepting that angiomas can be atypical in young people and that tumours may produce haemorrhage anywhere, the typical site and configuration of a hypertensive haemorrhage will certainly justify a pause before performing angiography. In many instances angiography can be omitted entirely especially if the scan can be repeated at a later date. Angiography, perhaps limited to the appropriate territory, is still necessary in young patients and in those other instances in which the haematoma is atypical or in patients in whom tumour pathology is likely. In such cases a delayed scan with enhancement may indicate associated pathology.

Pneumoencephalography

Visualisation of the ventricular system by the direct injection of air via a burrhole or indirectly by air encephalography is rarely indicated in the diagnostic evaluation of cerebral haemorrhage. That it is dangerous in the acute phase is not questioned for it not only causes an acute upset in intracranial pressure dynamics but it may increase brain shifts or cause rupture of the haematomas into the ventricular system with its attendant complications of aseptic ependymitis or mechanical ventricular obstruction by clot. The use of air as a contrast study should be reserved for chronic cases in which there is diagnostic doubt or in cases wherein a late complication of haemorrhage, such as hydrocephalus, is suspected. Such complications are more readily and safely diagnosed by brain scanning.

Initial management

Authors are agreed that of all the factors affecting prognosis, the level of consciousness is the most significant and that any factor influencing this will affect the outcome. Whilst it is true that initial and unremitting coma carries a mortality risk approaching 100 per cent and preservation of consciousness may reduce this to 20 per cent (McKissock et al, 1959), the conscious state may vary for differing reasons and it is therefore logical initially to take all possible medical measures to improve the patient's state optimally before embarking on invasive investigation or contemplating surgical evacuation. Sudden depression of consciousness associated with a space-taking mass and consequent elevation of intracranial pressure has a number of abnormal pathological concomitants. Foremost is depression or alteration of the respiratory cycle with diminution of the cough reflex and the usual pattern of intermittent sighing which aerates the lungs and is characteristic of the normal state. Reduction of coughing leads to retention of normal pulmonary secretion, and this is made worse if there is pulmonary oedema engendered by high intracranial pressure or by a markedly elevated systemic arterial pressure. Cardiac failure may prove rapidly fatal in these circumstances. Total pulmonary care is required utilising expert physiotherapy and skilled suction with meticulous maintenance of the airway. Intubation with an endotracheal tube may be necessary as a temporary expedient with adequate humidification and optimal oxygen concentration. Tracheostomy is best avoided as it may simply prolong a chronic vegetative state in the severely obtunded. Hypertension is a common causally related problem and demands careful treatment in its own right; Meyer et al (1960) showed that brain swelling usually increased at pressures above 180 mmHg systolic when the filtration pressure may well exceed the colloid osmotic pressure. The studies of Strandgaard et al (1973) have shown that autoregulation in hypertensive patients may be more complex with a shift of the whole autoregulatory range to a higher level. Above this range the resistance vessels react passively and below the range they fail to respond to a falling inflow pressure. The balance must therefore be achieved with caution to effect a steady and stable blood pressure within the physiological limits appropriate to the patient's previous vascular status. Without the benefit of cerebral blood flow studies this usually means gradual reduction of blood pressure to levels consistent with the patient's age or known previous levels, modified always by the clinical response. Marked hypertension or a labile state should be treated within 24–48 hours if the patient is conscious and accessible. Thiazides, methyl dopa or beta blocking drugs are used, the choice resting on previous response to treatment or the personal experience of the treating physician. Reduction of blood pressure in an unconscious patient should be deferred until improvement occurs. The acute hypertensive response ascribed to cerebral haemorrhage is rare in previously normotensive patients and if it occurs is relatively transient and therefore requires no treatment.

The biochemical changes following spontaneous subarachnoid haemorrhage have also been studied (Buckell et al, 1966) and highlight the importance of rapid fluid depletion and occasional electrolyte disturbance as a result of inappropriate ADH secretion or pathological sodium redistribution. Where clouding of consciousness dulls thirst or reduces the ability to satisfy it, dehydration rapidly ensues. If this is complicated by hyperventilation or excessive sweating, significant fluid loss can occur in 24–48 hours leading to hypovolaemia and impaired cerebral perfusion. This state may not be obvious clinically but is usually suggested by plasma electrolyte and urea levels and confirmed by estimating simultaneously the osmolality of blood and urine. Correction of dehydration must be accurate but unhurried as sudden transfusion of fluid in a previously hyperosmolar situation may aggravate brain swelling.

These concepts are also important in using osmotherapy, as the objective of such treatment is to withdraw fluid from the brain and not to dehydrate the whole patient. Intravenous mannitol as a 20 per cent solution in a quantity of 250 to 500 ml is occasionally advocated as a short term measure to induce reduction of intracranial pressure. The small risk of provoking further haemorrhage by such a manoeuvre must be accepted. It is certainly a minor hazard particularly if the treatment is reserved for those cases showing early deterioration in whom it is desired to produce a temporary amelioration prior to some more elective form of management.

There has been no conclusive study on the effectiveness of large doses of mineralocorticoids, either to diminish the oedema associated with such lesions or to improve the efficiency of small vessel perfusion. Dramatic improvements may follow their use in patients obtunded by brain tumours but their effects in cerebral haemorrhage seem less predictable. Personal clinical studies (Richardson, 1969) have not shown any convincing beneficial effects, though it is the increasing impression of many surgeons that such treatment is helpful.

SURGICAL MANAGEMENT

The presence of a potentially removable space-occupying lesion in a possibly fatal condition has naturally attracted much surgical interest. Over the years operative enthusiasm has waxed and waned and controversy still exists in relation to the benefits and particularly the timing of surgery. Our own early studies were reported fully in relation to a controlled trial of treatment (McKissock et al, 1961). This compared active medical treatment with global application of surgery performed immediately after diagnosis, when surgery was employed within two hours of the ictus. No superiority for surgery thus randomly applied early was forthcoming but suggested that delayed operation might have some benefit. Some important points emerged from the study and deserve brief comment.

Conscious level

An assessment of conscious level and neurological deficit at 24 hours from the ictus was a good prognostic guide. There was a mortality of 30 per cent for medical treatment in the non-comatose as judged at a six month follow-up; acute surgical results were similar. Patients in coma however suffered a 75 per cent death rate, mostly in the first week.

Sex

The incidence of haemorrhage in men and women was similar but females sustained the lesion with a lower death rate when treated medically. In general they fared less well than men when subjected to early surgery.

Arterial tension

Hypertension seemed to improve the natural history as compared with the small number of normotensive patients, but surgery had the reverse effect having a higher death rate in hypertensive cases and a lower mortality in normotensive patients.

Angiographic findings

For simplicity these were divided into two groups — those with mid-line displacement suggesting a significant space taking mass and those without, indicating a smaller lesion. Absence of mid-line disturbance carried a better natural prognosis (49 per cent survived) as opposed to a natural death rate of 58 per cent where significant displacement was seen. Surgery increased the death rate in the group with no displacement, largely from the complications of attempting to remove deeply placed lesions. An attempt was made to correlate these various factors in hypertensive patients. This showed no striking difference in the cross-section of conscious levels in the two angiographic groups, but again confirmed the relatively good prognosis in untreated females with little angiographic displacement. In the remaining subgroups early surgery appeared to offer little advantage over energetic medical treatment. This study, which has been subject to some valid criticism, did however establish some prognostic criteria for the medically treated group with a global six month mortality of 51 per cent, a figure much lower than that generally accepted at the time. It also demonstrated that the random application of very early surgery produced little overall benefit whilst suggesting that delayed surgery might be more helpful. The diagnostic accuracy has been held in question in the conservative group.

A more recent review by Paillas & Alliez (1973) returns to the contention that the natural death-rate is of the order of 80 per cent, at the same time expressing their belief that many patients who survive after unverified cerebral haemorrhage were in fact afflicted by brain softening. Such an argument is retrograde and will be refuted totally in the future in studies using the EMI scanner as the diagnostic method. For the present our own study must suffice. The trial structure was so designed that the presumptive diagnosis was established and the possibility of surgery confirmed before inclusion in the study and therefore preceding the random allocation to surgery or conservative treatment. One could therefore postulate that the rate of diagnostic error in the surgical group should approximate that of the non-surgically treated. Of the 89 cases allocated to surgery the diagnosis was incorrect in 4 cases, an error rate of 4.5 per cent. There was a subsequently verified error rate of 5.5 per cent in the group of 91 patients allocated to non-surgical treatment. Since the diagnostic criteria were established prior to treatment allocation, and any cases of diagnostic doubt excluded, any gross discrepancy in diagnostic accuracy in the two treatment groups seems unlikely.

Luessenhop et al (1967) in a review of the literature and detailed analysis of 64 cases concluded that patients in a non-comatose condition showing a clear-cut angiographic demonstration of the clot could have their natural mortality reduced to approximately one-third by the use of surgery. They divided their cases into three groups. *Group 1* (seven patients) were fully alert, with minimal or resolving signs clearly destined to make a good recovery. None were subjected to surgery and all survived. *Group 3* (24 patients) were the obverse of group 1 as most were *in extremis* and death seemed almost certain. In these surgery was performed in 13 cases with a total management mortality of 86 per cent. This group probably may be compared with our control group (McKissock et al, 1961) designated as stupor/coma wherein the natural mortality was 76 per cent and the global surgical mortality was 79 per cent. In this group therefore there seems little difference between medical treatment, early surgery or selective surgery.

Their *Group 2* cases are the most interesting. These 33 cases apparently had major neurological deficits and focal signs with conscious levels ranging from drowsiness to deep stupor — the breakdown is unfortunately not further analysed. Craniotomy was performed within 24 hours on 24 patients with two deaths, a mortality of 8 per cent. Operation was not performed in the remaining nine cases of whom one, a man of 90, died. Thus the untreated mortality in this group treated conservatively was only 12 per cent. This suggested the possibility of a rather skew population in this limited study as our own much larger group in a similar category had a natural death rate of 40 per cent.

Their study does confirm earlier views that early surgery in haematomas largely confined to the capsular or immediate paracapsular regions is unrewarding, whilst at the same time suggesting that the mortality for such lesions was of the order of 92 per cent. This is clearly fallacious for they removed from consideration the presumed capsular lesions in Group 2 treated non-surgically with a death rate of only one in nine cases. Confusion of this order is common in published series and highlights the value of the work of Benés et al (1972) who simply differentiated between destructive and limited haemorrhage. They made the important points that destructive haemorrhage much more frequently presents with immediate coma whereas limited haemorrhage, whether capsular or not, is accompanied by less neurological disturbance initially though not precluding subsequent deterioration in some. Thus they differentiate destructive bleeding with massive hemisphere or ganglionic involvement proceeding to rapid brain stem embarrassment or death as opposed to lesions of a more limited character in the basal ganglion or cerebral hemisphere which may be amenable to surgery or may have a good natural history.

A presentation by Paillas & Alliéz (1973) reviews the literature and gives the results in 250 cases of intracerebral haemorrhage treated by surgery but without reference to cases excluded. The number of males was twice that of females in contrast to most other studies and carries a definite augury for more favourable surgical results. The age range was average, diagnosis was by angiography and air studies were not employed in the acute stage. Conscious level is only divided into subnormal and coma without further definition or indication as to the stage at which the conscious level was assessed. A mortality of 24 per cent at one month was achieved in the 'subnormal' group of 58 patients as opposed to a death rate of 63 per cent of 79 patients in 'coma'. Three time groupings for surgery were used, the first being of 61 patients who survived for two to five days and were subjected to clot evacuation. Fifty-four per cent of these died. In the second time scale surgery took place from 5 to 10 days from the ictus with a death rate of 30 per cent of 75 cases. The largest single group of 114 received surgery at an interval of more than 10 days with a mortality of 29 per cent. Though this represents a very mixed series the size of the groups demands attention and suggests that delayed surgery may be optimal even allowing for the inevitable death rate in the interval. They also detail the quality of survival and subsequent death. Of a group of 132 survivors followed for one year it was found that 11 had died and of the remainder about one-third had major deficits, and the remaining third had severe deficits. In the more prolonged follow-up the number of deaths due to further haemorrhage was 11 out of 121 cases. This compares reasonably with our own late death rate in 102 survivors followed for 1 to 10 years in whom five died from a further cerebrovascular accident.

Consideration of our own controlled studies and the reviews and reports of Luessenhop et al (1967) and Paillas & Alliéz (1973), whilst confusing, strongly suggested a selective approach to the surgery of intracerebral haemorrhage both in terms of the patient's clinical status and the timing of surgery, having satisfied the potential necessity of surgery by demonstrating a significant accessible haematoma. A trial of treatment regime reported by Richardson (1969) helped to clarify some of the problems raised by earlier studies and is not refuted by subsequent series. This study concerned the management of 138 cases of intracerebral haemorrhage diagnosed by the usual criteria between 1961 and 1964. Patients who were admitted in coma and remained in that state were excluded as all previous evidence suggested that surgery was of little benefit. By the same token patients in whom the neurological deficit was mild and consciousness was preserved were not considered as surgical intervention was never indicated. These two groups were totally excluded from the study design.

The regime adopted for the trial was that after diagnosis of a potentially removable haematoma a decision relating to immediate therapy was taken. Almost always the primary choice was for active medical management aimed at improving ventilatory function, restoring normal fluid and electrolyte status and managing raised intracranial pressure. Treatment of any complicating medical disease was also immediately commenced. During the next 7 to 10 days careful neurological and general medical assessments were made at the end of which time a decision regarding further treatment was made. In some cases during this interval pre-existing disease such as severe hypertension, renal failure, diabetes became exacerbated and often sufficiently severe to preclude serious consideration of surgery. These together with pulmonary complications were the commonest causes of death in the non-surgical group. Approximately 10 days after the ictus a decision was taken regarding surgery. If at this time the patient had only a mild deficit or was still improving, the decision against surgery was automatic. Where the deficit remained severe but the conscious level was satisfactory, craniotomy evacuation was undertaken within 48

hours. In a small group some deterioration occurred in the waiting period, and these were operated upon as the 'Immediate Operation' group. As will be seen they were small in number and occurred early in the series. Subsequent experience suggested that early deterioration was equally well managed by energetic conservative measures to correct hypoxia, abnormal hydration or raised intracranial pressure.

Table 13.1 shows the overall results as assessed six months following admission. It must be stressed that the treatment groups are not to be compared with each other. The conservative group represents those dying from other causes or recovering to a point where surgery was not thought indicated. Delayed surgery implies a persisting severe deficit at a ten-day interval from the ictus wherein surgical evacuation was designed to reduce the disability. The 'Immediate Operation' group has been explained and though small has a reasonable mortality and acceptable morbidity when compared to the whole series. A global mortality of 20 per cent for this regime may best be compared with the results in the previous controlled study wherein the natural mortality of cases in the combined alert and drowsy categories was 38 per cent and for the same group treated by early surgery was nearly 55 per cent. To draw many conclusions from such a retrospective comparison may be less than valid but sampling of some of the variables is instructive. In the controlled study group the 'alert/drowsy' mortality for patients admitted within three days of the ictus was 20/52 in the untreated group compared with 16/96 in the treatment trial study. This is lower than the total case mortality, the reason being the higher mortality in patients referred more than seven days after the ictus. These patients were often referred because of late but untreated deterioration. Reviewing the conscious status on admission in more detail shows a natural mortality in the controlled

Table 13.1 Quality of survival at six months

	Total	Full recovery	Partial disability	Total disability	Dead
Conservative	60	33	13	1	13 = 21%
Delayed surgery	69	19	31	6	13 = 19%
Immediate operation	9	3	3	1	2 = 22%
	138	55	47	8	28 = 20%

study (1961) of 16 per cent for alert patients and 38 per cent for those drowsy or stuporose, whereas in the treatment trial (1969) of the 37 alert patients only four died (11 per cent) and of the 101 drowsy patients 24 died, a mortality of 24 per cent. A comparison of the timing of operation is excluded by definition as one study was concerned with early surgery and the other with delayed operation.

Many authors have stressed the improved surgical prognosis if the haematoma is predominantly lobar. We were unable to show this in our controlled studies because lobar haematomas were found in many cases to be an extension of a destructive medially-placed haemorrhage. In true lobar haematomas mortality was only 20 per cent, less than that for capsular lesions (McKissock et al, 1961). In the treatment trial study (1969) the non-destructive lobar haematomas had a combined mortality of 12/88 or 14 per cent whereas capsular haematomas had a death rate of 16/50 or 32 per cent, this being increased to 7/14 or 50 per cent if the thalamus was involved. It is interesting that the lobar haematomas were equally distributed between the groups making a good recovery medically and the group subjected to delayed surgery, the latter, however, by definition containing those cases remaining with a severe deficit. Clearly this indicates a fundamentally favourable natural history for this type of haematoma and surgery is only indicated if deterioration occurs or a severe deficit persists after clinical stabilisation. Surgery at this time can confer benefit in about one-third of the cases. Similarly the distribution of ganglionic or paraganglionic haemorrhage was equal in the two major treatment categories, suggesting that if they do not produce coma, though their mortality may be higher, their capacity for recovery may be good (Table 13.2). This conflicts with the view of King (1973), who suggested that quality of survival depends on the site of the haematoma, being good if lobar, but

stating that capsular haematomas always leave severe disabilities. Some of the discrepancy may be due to difference in definition.

The increasing accuracy of information afforded by brain scanning and the evaluation of adverse pathological changes such as oedema, increasing displacement or hydrocephalus has led some surgeons to consider earlier operation. Date et al (1979) compared cases before and during the C.T. scanning era. Early craniotomy was performed in all cases showing progressive brain compression. The summary is brief but indicates that early surgery may benefit younger patients. It is significant that 63 per cent of the cases were less than 50. It is still true to say that patients critically ill from the onset or those harbouring small or very deeply placed haematomas, particularly if associated with ventricular rupture, do not benefit from surgery. Young patients with lobar clots often harbour small angiomas and tolerate surgery well. Surgery is also required in cases stabilising with a marked neurological deficit and in those with accessible haematomas who demonstrate deterioration after preliminary stabilisation. Finally it must be emphasised that non-surgical treatment implies active medical care covering all the aspects of disordered physiology.

CEREBELLUM AND PONS

Non-traumatic spontaneous haemorrhage into the cerebellum represents approximately 10 per cent of all massive brain haemorrhage, this proportion reflecting the relative weights of the cerebellum and cerebral hemispheres. In a post-mortem series of 40 000 cases Courville (1950) described 117 cases of haemorrhage of the cerebellum in a total of 1487 cases of intracerebral bleeding. A similar proportion was found in the clinical series of McKissock et al (1960) wherein 344 cases were analysed in

Table 13.2 Quality of survival by haematoma site

	Total	Dead	Survivors	Full recovery	Partial disability	Total disability
Lobar	88	12	76	40	35	1
Putamenocapsular	36	9	27	13	8	6
Thalamic	14	7	7	2	4	1

which 34 affected the cerebellum. In a more recent study by McCormick & Rosenfield (1973) all cases of massive brain haemorrhage were subject to detailed examination and in the total series of 144 cases no less than 15 involved the cerebellum. This close correspondence of prevalence in clinical and post-mortem series suggests that the mortality of the two conditions is not dissimilar.

Aetiology

Most authors seem in general agreement that hypertension is the commonest causally related process in patients in whom no other pathological entity is identified. Hyland & Levy (1964) made this point but also suggested that blood dyscrasias were more common than generally supposed, finding five such cases in a series of 32 patients. Ransohoff et al (1971), however, suggested that when other aetiological factors are excluded hypertension is present in 90 per cent of cases. In a careful review of the literature and an extensive prospective study of 144 cases, McCormick & Rosenfield (1973) made a strong case for hypertension being a coincidental factor, other lesions being predominantly responsible. Their arguments were more strongly put in relation to lesions of the cerebral hemispheres but in their 15 cases involving the cerebellum a definitive lesion such as aneurysm, angioma or brain tumour were present in 10, with hypertensive vascular disease as a possible cause in four of the remainder. From the practical point of view one need not consider tumour haemorrhage further. Angiomas tend to occur in the age range of 0 to 40 years whereas the hypertensive vasculopathies occur most frequently in the fifth, sixth, and seventh decades. Aneurysms, particularly of the posterior inferior cerebellar arteries, are only rarely associated with massive cerebellar haemorrhage with survival, though the possibility of such a lesion may influence the decisions relating to investigation.

Pathology

The vasculopathy most commonly associated with hypertension is a degenerative process affecting the small perforating brain arteries giving rise to microaneurysms similar in genesis to the more common berry aneurysms of the circle of Willis. Coles & Yates (1967) reported the incidence of these lesions in a series of 200 cases studied in detail. The basis of the study was to exclude cases subject to natural or surgical trauma and only to include those in which the examination could be performed within 24 hours of death. For the purpose of comparison half the studies were in previously hypertensive patients and in the remainder there was no such evidence of pre-existing high blood pressure. Vessel lesions were more common in the pons and brain stem than in the cerebellum, but multiplicity of the lesion in the cerebral and cerebellar hemispheres was common. It was interesting, however, that these small aneurysms were seven times more common in hypertensive patients than they were in normotensive subjects and in this particular series there were no instances of haemorrhage from the lesions in patients with normal blood pressure.

A point of surgical interest is that these lesions were noted most frequently in branches of the superior cerebellar artery in the region of the dentate nucleus, thus explaining the common situation of the more circumscribed haematomas in elderly patients. Lesions were rare in the vermis vessels, whereas, as will be seen, this is a not uncommon situation for angiomas in the younger age groups. Angiomas are usually of arteriovenous type. In a large review article McCormick & Nofzinger (1966) analysed 308 small arteriovenous anomalies of the brain and showed that no less than 44 were situated in the cerebellar hemispheres. The collected series from the literature and their own cases include those that had and had not bled, and so conclusions in relation to responsibility for haemorrhage are tenuous. Nevertheless the relative incidence in the different parts of the brain correlates with the clinical impression of the high proportion of angiomas in clinical cerebellar haemorrhage in the younger age groups. Venous angiomas have also been described by Wolf et al (1967), and were labelled as cryptic due to the difficulty of radiological demonstration. Such terms cannot be regarded as synonymous as it is not uncommon to fail to visualise the more usual arteriovenous lesion, particularly when it was initially small and its rupture has resulted in a large compressing intracerebral haematoma. Many reports describe small angiomas which have been virtually destroyed by the haemorrhage and remnants of angiomas which are found during the course of surgical removal of the consequent haematoma. Again it must be stressed that the majority of such cases occur below the age of 40 years with only an occasional occurrence in the later decades.

Haemorrhage, therefore, most commonly occurs within the white matter or nuclear masses of the cerebellar hemisphere and may be so confined. Some communication with the fourth ventricle is common and accounts for the presence of blood in the subarachnoid space. More massive haemorrhage may involve the fourth ventricle and in severely hypertensive patients may pass in retrograde fashion into the third and lateral ventricles. Direct rupture of the haematoma into the pons or medulla is rare.

Secondary pathological effects may then follow as a result of swelling of the cerebellar white matter causing local compression of the brain stem which may rapidly proceed to obstruction to the ventricular outlet. Obstruction is more likely and more rapid if complicated by solid blood clot in the ventricular system. As the majority of such sequences in older people are on the basis of vasculopathy it is not uncommon to find evidence of previous, or at times co-existent, haemorrhage in the cerebral hemispheres or internal capsule.

Pontine haemorrhage may occur from rupture of microaneurysms in hypertensive patients, particularly in the older age group. Angiomas of similar character to the 'cryptic lesions' of the cerebrum have been discovered in younger people. Tumour is a rare cause but secondary haemorrhage from a separate compressing lesion is common in fatal cases. Pontine haemorrhage may be a devastating and rapidly fatal event but with the use of C.T. scanning more non-fatal lesions are being recognised. These may be small, inaccessible central haematomas, laterally placed elongated lesions within a swollen pons or may rupture to become subependymal in the floor of the fourth ventricle or actually rupture into that cavity. Precise diagnosis of the pathological substrate and location is leading to microsurgical treatment.

Clinical features

In view of these variable basic pathological events the mode of presentation, evolution and outcome are protean, but certain features can be identified which give clues to the probable diagnosis. In a series of 34 cases treated surgically (McKissock et al, 1960) there were three basic patterns. Approximately 20 per cent declared dramatically with rapid and progressive deterioration into coma with death ensuing within 48 hours. A small group presented a very slowly evolving pattern in which the onset was gradual or apparently episodic and in which the course and neurological features were consistent with an expanding cerebellar lesion. In more than half the cases an intermediate onset and course were noted and as these are the most important from the diagnostic and prognostic viewpoint they require more detailed consideration. The original series (McKissock et al, 1960) and a later review by Richardson (1972) stressed the relative infrequency of convincing cerebellar signs in this group, particularly where the conscious level was markedly disturbed. Signs of brain stem embarrassment were, however, common with constricted or asymmetrical pupils and lateral conjugate gaze palsies. Periodic respiration was often detected at some stage in the illness. A true hemiplegia contralateral to the lesion was noted in more than half the more obtunded cases; this should not be confused with the paucity of movement that may typify a cerebellar deficit. Thus in this group presenting as a moderately rapidly or episodically evolving lesion the triad of constricted but reacting pupils with a gaze palsy to the side of the lesion and periodic respiration often raised the diagnostic suspicion.

Fisher et al (1965) presented a detailed review of the literature to which they added their own cases. Their objective was to analyse the clinical course and to differentiate cerebellar lesions from haemorrhage involving the brain stem, cerebral hemispheres and those arising from ruptured saccular aneurysms. Symptom analysis showed vomiting as a consistent early feature with headache as less prominent and true vertigo as infrequent. Consciousness, in their series, was rarely lost early but ataxia often of gross degree was a marked feature. Various permutations of mutism with transient or progressive quadriparesis or paraparesis were noted with evidence of disturbance of ocular movement. It is very relevant that of their 21 personal cases, 13 arrived at the hospital within 2 hours of the ictus and 8 within 8 hours of onset. This very early assessment may explain the rather different clinical features in surgical series as the time interval from ictus to admission to a specialised neurosurgical department may be longer and some of the important initial neurological data may be lost. It is therefore necessary to examine these early cases in some detail.

Of the 21 cases only 14 were sufficiently alert to assist in the examination. Greatest diagnostic importance was placed on the presence of dysarthria; dysphagia was rare. Ocular signs consisted of normal or constricted pupils with disturbance of conjugate gaze to the side of the lesion in 60 per cent, usually a paralysis but in two cases associated with forced deviation of gaze to the opposite side. Forced downward deviation was not seen and vertical eye movements were usually preserved. Nystagmus was only seen in 5 of 12 patients and was virtually confined to the horizontal plane. They suggest that monoplegia or hemiplegia was not seen unless due to an old stroke. Instead cerebellar ataxia is reported initially in four cases and became apparent in a further three patients as the picture evolved, with a marked tendency for truncal ataxia and instability of gait to be more prominent than individual cerebellar signs. With the onset of stupor an ipsilateral facial palsy became apparent in 8 of 13 cases but again hemiparesis was not found. Summarising the situation they stress the relative retention of power and sensation, in contradistinction to pontine or capsular lesions, with small pupils, gaze palsy, cerebellar ataxia and a peripheral facial palsy. Consciousness, they felt, was often preserved initially but supervention of stupor was usually accompanied by marked increase in the neurological deficits.

In a detailed study of 56 cases Ott et al (1974) agreed that hypertension was the commonest cause but mentioned the use of anticoagulants in eight cases. The fifth, sixth, and seventh decades represented the usual age incidence and there was a slight preponderance of males. Good clinical details were available in 44 of the cases and the presenting symptoms in order of frequency are detailed.

Nausea and vomiting, 'dizziness' — i.e., not necessarily true vertigo — ataxia, and headache were most common with vomiting occurring in 42 of the patients. Early loss of consciousness was uncommon but dysarthria or mutism was apparent in one-third of the cases. Of the patients examined within 24 hours, 14 were alert, 22 were drowsy, 5 stuporose, and 15 comatose. In the non-comatose patients ataxia was noted in nearly three-quarters with facial palsy in 60 per cent and an obvious gaze palsy in more than half, with horizontal nystagmus in a similar proportion. They suggested that an abrupt onset with preservation of consciousness with vomiting as a prominent feature and the presence of limb ataxia, gaze palsy and a peripheral facial weakness must arouse strong suspicion of a cerebellar haemorrhage. On these grounds they suggested that the diagnosis was considered in 34 of 53 patients admitted soon after the ictus in a non-comatose state.

Differential diagnosis

The minutiae of clinical differentiation in acute cerebral lesions have had their importance diminished by the diagnostic precision afforded by C.T. scanning. The necessity of and the urgency for the investigation as well as its final evaluation still, however, should have a sound clinical basis. Fisher et al (1965) stressed the predominant motor sign in putamenocapsular haemorrhage together with hemianopia and gaze paresis contralateral to the lesion. Tonic deviation of the eyes to the side of the lesion could be reversed by caloric stimulation. Posterior capsular lesions may accent the sensory disturbance and variably affect the conscious state.

Use of C.T. scanning has shown that pontine haemorrhage is not always the rapidly fatal event ushered in by coma, loss of temperature regulation, pin point pupils and decerebrate posturing frequently described in older text books. Small central lesions can be survived presenting with reduction of consciousness, bilateral gaze palsies or gross abnormalities of vertical control including ocular bobbing, facial weakness and variable motor signs in the limbs. Occasionally these dissect towards the upper portion of the floor of the fourth ventricle and may produce a significant subependymal clot.

At times this may produce obstruction to the lower aqueduct and lead to subsequent hydrocephalus with attendant neurological deterioration. Lateral haemorrhages in the pons, more commonly seen in younger age groups may present with an acute or more slowly evolving lateral medullary syndrome. Facial paralysis with involvement of hearing on the side of the lesion will be combined with loss of lateral gaze to that side together with contralateral hemiparesis. In a review of the literature Doczi & Thomas (1979) indicated the prominence of truncal ataxia as a clinical feature in the more chronic cases and recommended surgery if the neurological deficit was progressive.

The differential diagnostic difficulties associated with ruptured aneurysms particularly those associated with frontal lobe haematomas or subdural collection have largely been resolved by early use of C.T. scanning.

Investigations

In the general context of cerebrovascular accidents or acute neurological disturbance the common first investigation is a diagnostic lumbar puncture. The presence of blood in the subarachnoid space indicates the pathological basis and will determine the urgency of further diagnostic procedures. Blood-stained cerebrospinal fluid is likely to be found in about 80 per cent of cases with cerebellar haemorrhage, due to egress of blood into the fourth ventricle or, rarely, to direct rupture on to the cerebellar surface in cases of angioma or aneurysm. However, in the remainder the clot may be confined within the cerebellar hemisphere, particularly in the more slowly evolving cases presenting a more classical cerebellar syndrome. In these the fluid may be completely clear or contain a slight excess of protein or white cells allowing for confusion with infarction or encephalitis. The dangers of lumbar puncture in a compressing posterior fossa lesion need no emphasis and the possible value of this procedure must be considered in each case. Rapid evolution, and evidence of brain stem embarrassment, may preclude its use and suggest alternative diagnostic measures or in some cases be sufficiently convincing to lead to surgical exploration on clinical grounds alone.

C.T. scanning

In the routine elective radiology pride of place must now be taken by the use of computerised transverse axial tomography (C.T. scan). Numerous publications have described the technique and its application in detail (Ambrose 1973, 1974), and its relevance to the diagnosis of intracranial haematomas (Paxton & Ambrose, 1974).

Preliminary investigation of cerebrovascular accidents of all types has been facilitated by this means (Paxton & Ambrose, 1974) for it not only demonstrates the presence of haematomas or infarcts but will show dilatation, distortion or displacement of the ventricular system. Figure 13.6

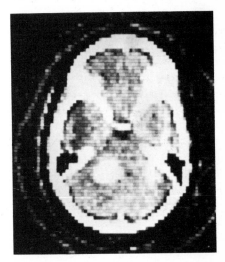

Fig. 13.6 Cerebellar haematoma on left side showing as spherical region of increased density separate from petrous ridge.

shows a basal brain slice. An obvious high density circular area is seen in the position of the left cerebellar hemisphere clearly separate from the petrous ridge. The small low density square on its right side represents the distorted displaced fourth ventricle. Figure 13.7A is the scan of a restless patient, this producing some artefact but not detracting from the diagnosis. A definite haematoma is seen in the region of the right cerebellar hemisphere with the blood-filled fourth ventricle distorted and displaced to the left. Figure 13.7B is a higher level scan showing blood in the lateral and third ventricles and also in the temporal horns.

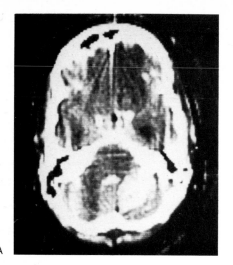
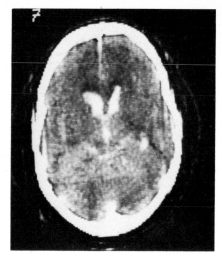

Fig. 13.7 (A) Right cerebellar haematoma with adjacent blood-filled fourth ventricle. **(B)** Haematoma (white) in the lateral ventricles, third ventricle, and the right temporal horn.

The degree of reliability of this benign procedure is so high that further investigative procedures are unnecessary unless the clinical presentation, patient's age, or atypical appearance of the haematoma or surrounding brain suggest the presence of a vascular anomaly of importance to surgical management. Increasing availability of this diagnostic method will diminish the need for any other investigation.

Echoencephalography

In an earlier publication (Richardson, 1972) the use of the simple 'A' mode ultrasonic method was discussed. The investigation requires skill and training but can be performed at the bedside to provide limited but useful information. Ambrose & McKissock (1969) defined the technique for estimating ventricular size and showed that the normal ratio between the width of the lateral ventricle to that of half the brain was one-fifth to one-sixth and that ratios of one-third indicated significant ventricular dilatation. Such enlargement occurs rapidly in most cases of cerebellar haematoma being recorded as early as four to six hours by Dinsdale (1964). This investigation is so limited in terms of accurate information provided that it is rarely used if C.T. scanning facilities are immediately available. In experienced hands, however, it may still be of some value in the assessment of an acute cerebellar lesion particularly if the findings are unequivocal.

Angiography

Selected use of vessel visualisation depends on careful evaluation of the patient's clinical state and the accurate interpretation of the C.T. scan. It is still used in haemorrhage involving the lower brain stem and cerebellum in younger patients to demonstrate or exclude an associated angioma. Only rarely is a pathological circulation demonstrated in significant haemorrhage associated with a tumour, the true causal substrate usually being revealed at surgery or by repeat scanning using enhancing techniques, after a delay, in cases recovering spontaneously. Ruptured aneurysms usually show a subarachnoid haematoma in addition to parenchymal involvement. In classical hypertensive unilateral cerebellar haematomas the C.T. scan usually provides sufficient information for a surgical decision and dispenses with the stress of angiography. If the investigation still requires to be used, the reports of Bull & Kotlowski (1970) suggested the importance of displacement or non-filling of veins, whereas Nornes & Hauge (1972) and Ott et al (1974) placed emphasis on displacement of the posterior inferior cerebellar vessels.

Pneumoencephalography

The experience of most surgeons is strongly against the use of air studies in the acutely evolving haemorrhage causing, as they do, considerable disturbance in intracranial dynamics and necessitating turning the patient into the prone position for radiography. Both lumbar air encephalography and ventriculography often result in significant deterioration of the patient's condition, this being irreversible in a small number. In our earlier studies reliance was placed on this examination (McKissock et al, 1960) but subsequently (Richardson, 1972) it was substantially avoided and much reliance placed on clinical assessment with careful ultrasound investigation and if necessary vertebral angiography or more commonly elective surgical exploration. The advent of C.T. scanning has largely solved this problem but where it is not available a combination of careful clinical assessment with minimal radiological investigation and a willingness for surgical exploration must suffice.

Treatment

Prompt surgical evacuation of the haematoma whilst the patient is still responsive seems to be the accepted method of management. Detailed study of the natural history has been precluded previously by diagnostic failures, complications of investigation and urgent surgery. The series of 67 cases analysed by Richardson (1972) and the 56 patients detailed by Ott et al (1974) show that spontaneous and often unpredictable deterioration in the early stages is very common, this risk only diminishing after complete stabilisation at a high conscious level after 8 to 10 days. Against this must be weighed the unheralded lapses into stupor and coma from a previously alert state and the fact that the major prognostic factor for recovery after surgery is strongly correlated with the conscious state prior to operation. Thus surgical mortality in patients previously responsive is of the order of 20 per cent rising to 75 per cent when stupor or coma supervene.

Analysis of the cause of death most commonly shows tonsillar impaction with brain stem distortion and secondary haemorrhage, but rarely direct implication of brain stem structures by the presenting ictus. More significantly the reaccumulation of clot is recorded in a number of cases, usually in those comatose prior to surgery whose condition remained unchanged and therefore gave no indication of this complication. The absence of primary intrinsic brain stem damage in such patients and the fact that occasionally surgery will enable such previously comatose patients to survive suggests that in some, minor recurrence of haemorrhage may tip the balance. In most of the comatose cases, however, the secondary brain stem vascular lesions have occurred before operation.

The method of surgical evacuation has varied in reported small series but in the larger quoted analyses, formal suboccipital craniectomy and removal of the haematoma with meticulous haemostasis produces the best results. Temporising measures such as ventricular drainage or simple burrhole evacuation of the clot are not to be recommended. If surgery is undertaken promptly and the patient survives, the quality of survival can be gratifying. There were 20 survivors in a total of 32 patients subjected to surgery (Richardson, 1972) observed for periods of 2 to 10 years. Of these 11 have returned to normal life, five have minor cerebellar deficits and the remaining four are partially disabled. Since the advent of C.T. scanning a further 20 cases have been seen, with three further cases being excluded due to associated causal lesions. In 4 cases no surgery was undertaken as the patients were conscious with only mild signs of cerebellar dysfunction. In 3 patients the C.T. scan showed a confined haematoma with normal sized lateral ventricles, whereas in the fourth case modest enlargement of the ventricles had occurred.

Sequential scans showed slow resolution of the clots with no advance in ventricular size. A good recovery was the rule. Sixteen patients were treated surgically due to an unsatisfactory or unstable clinical level associated with evidence of significant displacement of the brainstem or failure to visualise the fourth ventricle. Significant hydrocephalus (ventricular/skull ratio >30 per cent) also prompted surgical intervention. Two patients in coma at the time of surgery died, one failing to improve after clot evacuation and the second suffering a further fatal haemorrhage 12 days after operation with early recovery. A post-mortem was refused. Of the 14 surgical survivors, 9 returned to normal life, 3 had minor cerebellar deficits and 2 were partially disabled. Thus in the total series of 20 cases there were only 2 deaths. Prompt diagnosis with a broad spectrum of information permitted either elective conservative management monitored by scanning or indicated the need for surgical evacuation before brainstem decompensation occurred.

Conclusions

The value of C.T. scanning can only be fully utilised in the diagnosis of cerebellar haemorrhage if the clinical possibility is constantly kept in mind. The immediate use of this diagnostic technique will allow definition of the lesion and more accurate assessment of those factors influencing the correct treatment. Experience is still somewhat limited but a stable and satisfactory clinical state together with a localised haematoma causing minimal brainstem displacement and the absence of ventricular dilatation may commend an expectant policy. If such is elected the patient must be regularly assessed clinically and subjected to sequential scans. At the first hint of neurological deterioration or of adverse scan changes such as increasing displacement or ventricular enlargement immediate surgical evacuation of the haematoma should be considered.

REFERENCES

Archar V S, Coe P K, Marshall J 1966 Echoencephalography in the differential diagnosis of cerebral haemorrhage and infarction. Lancet i: 161

Ambrose J 1973 Computerised transverse axial scanning (tomography). Part 11. Clinical application. British Journal of Radiology, 46: 1023

Ambrose J 1974 Computerised X-ray scanning of the brain. Journal of Neurosurgery 40: 679

Ambrose J, McKissock W 1969 The use of pulsed ultrasound in the detection of space occupying intracranial lesions. In: Measurement and precision in surgery. Blackwell. Oxford

Bedford P D 1958 Intracranial haemorrhage, diagnosis and treatment. Proceedings of the Royal Society of Medicine, 51: 209

Buckell M, Richardson A, Sarner M 1966 Biochemical changes after spontaneous subarachnoid haemorrhage. Journal of Neurology, Neurosurgery and Psychiatry, 29: 291

Bull J, Kotlowski P 1970 The angiographic pattern of the petrosal veins in the normal and pathological. Neuroradiology, 1: 20

Cole F M, Yates P O 1967 The occurrence and significance of intracerebral microaneurysms. Journal of Pathology and Bacteriology, 93: 393

Courville C B 1950 Pathology of the central nervous system. 3rd edn. Pacific Press, Mountain View, California

Date H, Hosoi Y, Watanabe Y 1979 Spontaneous intracerebral haematoma. An analysis of 36 cases in pre-C.T. and C.T. era. Neurological Surgery, 11: 1053

Dinsdale H B 1964 Spontaneous haemorrhage in the posterior fossa. Archives of Neurology (Chicago), 10: 200

Doczi T, Thomas G T 1979 Successful removal of an intrapontine haematoma. Journal of Neurology Neurosurgery and Psychiatry, 42: 1058

Fisher C M 1961 Clinical syndromes in cerebral haemorrhage. In: Fields W S (ed) Pathogenesis and treatment of cerebrovascular disease, Charles C. Thomas, Springfield, Illinois, 13, p. 318

Fisher C M 1971 Radiological observation in hypertensive cerebral haemorrhage. Journal of Neuropathology and Experimental Neurology, 30: 536

Fisher C M, Pickard E H, Polak A, Dalal P, Ojemann R G 1965 Acute hypertensive cerebellar haemorrhage. Diagnosis and surgical treatment. Journal of Nervous and Mental Diseases, 140: 38

Hayward R D, O'Reilly G V A 1976 Intracerebral haemorrhage. Accuracy of computerised scanning in predicting the underlying pathology. Lancet 1: 1

Hounsfield G, Ambrose J, Perry J, Bridger C 1973 Computerised transverse axial scanning. British Journal of Radiology, 46: 1016

Hyland H H, Levy D 1964 Spontaneous cerebellar haemorrhage. Canadian Medical Association Journal, 71: 315

Kaplan H 1961 Clinical syndromes in cerebral haemorrhage. In: Fields W. S. (ed) Pathogenesis and treatment of cerebrovascular disease, Charles C. Thomas, Springfield, Illinois

King T T 1973 Cerebral haemorrhage. British Journal of Hospital Medicine, 10: 250

Leksell L 1956 Detection of intracranial complications following head injury. Acta Chirurgica Scandinavica, 110: 301

Locksley H B, Sahs A L, Sandler R 1966 Report on the co-operative study of intracranial aneurysms and subarachnoid haemorrhage. Journal of Neurosurgery, 24: 1034

Luessenhop A J, Shevlin W A, Ferrero A A, McCullough D C, Barone B 1967 Surgical management of primary intracerebral haemorrhage. Journal of Neurosurgery, 27: 419

McCormick W F, Nofzinger J D 1966 Cryptic vascular malformations of the central nervous system. Journal of Neurosurgery, 24: 892

McCormick W F, Rosenfield D B 1973 Massive brain haemorrhage. A review of 144 cases and an examination of their causes. Stroke, 4: 946

McKissock W, Richardson A, Taylor J 1961 Primary intracerebral haemorrhage. A controlled trial of surgical and medical treatment in 180 unselected cases. Lancet, ii: 221

McKissock W, Richardson A, Walsh L S 1959 Primary intracerebral haemorrhage. Lancet, ii: 683

McKissock W, Richardson A, Walsh L S 1960 Spontaneous cerebellar haemorrhage. A study of 34 consecutive cases treated surgically. Brain, 83: 1

Meyer J, Bauer R 1962 Medical treatment of spontaneous intracranial haemorrhage by the use of hypotensive drugs. Neurology, 12: 36

Nornes H, Hauge T 1972 Spontaneous intracerebellar haemorrhage. Acta Neurologica Scandinavica, Suppl. 51: 253

Odom G L, Tindall G T, Dukes H T 1961 Cerebellar haematoma caused by angiomatous malformation. Journal of Neurosurgery, 18: 777

Ojemann R G 1973 Intracerebral and cerebellar haemorrhage. In: Neurological surgery. Saunders, Philadelphia: vol. 2, ch. 38, p. 844

Oldendorf D 1961 Isolated flying spot detection of radiodensity discontinuities. I. R. E. Transactions on Biomedical Electronics, 8: 68

Ott K H, Kase C S, Ojemann R G, Mohr J P 1974 Cerebellar haemorrhage. Diagnosis and treatment. Archives of Neurology, 31: 160

Paillas J E, Alliez B 1973 Surgical treatment of spontaneous intracerebral haemorrhage. Journal of Neurosurgery, 39: 145

Paxton R, Ambrose J 1974 The E.M.I. Scanner. A brief review of the first 650 patients. British Journal of Radiology, 47: 530

Ransohoff J, Derby B, Kricheff I 1971 Spontaneous intracerebral haemorrhage. Clinical Neurosurgery, 18: 247

Richardson A 1969 Surgical therapy of spontaneous intracerebral haemorrhage. In: Progress in neurological surgery, vol. 3, p. 397. Karger Basle and Year Book, Chicago

Richardson A 1972 Spontaneous cerebellar haemorrhage. In: Handbook of clinical neurology, Venken P J, Bruyn G W (eds) North Holland Publishing Co., Amsterdam

Richardson J C, Einhorn R W 1963 Primary intracerebral haemorrhage. Clinical Neurosurgery, 9: 114

Ross Russell R W 1963 Observations on intracerebral aneurysms. Brain, 86: 425

Strandgaard S, Olesen J, Skinhøj E, Lassen N A 1973 Autoregulation of brain circulation in severe arterial hypertension. British Medical Journal, i: 507

Tallala A, McKissock W 1971 Acute spontaneous subdural haemorrhage. Neurology, 21: 19

Wolf P A, Rosman P N, New P F J 1967 Multiple small cryptic venous angiomas of the brain mimicking cerebral metastases. Neurology (Minneapolis), 17: 491

14

Subarachnoid haemorrhage from intracranial aneurysms and angiomas

Lindsay Symon

In most Western countries, vascular disease of the brain ranks third in the causes of death at the present time. Further analysis reveals that between five and ten per cent of strokes are more properly classified as subarachnoid haemorrhage (SAH), and in this group two of the main causes are potentially surgically treatable. In the extensive cooperative review of SAH undertaken in America some years ago, Locksley (1966) demonstrated that in over 5000 cases of SAH studied with angiography or at autopsy, 51 per cent had as their origin an intracranial aneurysm or aneurysms. Arteriovenous malformations (AVM) with a prevalence of six per cent were much less common. Even in this careful and exhaustive study, just over 20 per cent of cases had no proven aetiology. It is apparent, however, that in general neurosurgical practice, aneurysm is the most frequent cause of SAH, especially in the middle decades of life. In the decade 40 to 49, its frequency is nearly twice that of other causes, and over 25 times that of AVM. In the second decade, however, the frequency of AVM as a cause of SAH equals that of aneurysms; over the age of 70 'other' causes of SAH outweigh both aneurysm and AVM. The high preponderance of aneurysms as the cause of SAH, and the operative and physiopathological problems which still exist in their management, render them of relatively greater importance. AVMs constitute a separate and, in some respects, a simpler problem.

The natural history of subarachnoid haemorrhage from ruptured intracranial aneurysm

Although excellent accounts of SAH have appeared in the standard medical literature since Gull's description in 1859, and occasional descriptions date back to the early eighteenth century, it was not until the development of cerebral angiography by Moniz (1927) and its widespread use in neurological and neurosurgical clinics throughout the world after the Second World War, that a true appreciation of SAH emerged. Thus, it was generally assumed in pre-angiographic days that aneurysmal SAH was predominantly a disease of the young. We now know this to be untrue. It is now certain that while a congenital factor may have a part to play in the origin of intracranial aneurysm (Hassler, 1965), arteriosclerosis and raised blood pressure in later life have an important place in the growth and rupture of aneurysms. Most neurosurgeons have experience of patients with one aneurysm who, in subsequent years, have bled from a second which was either not present or very small at the time of the first study.

While neurosurgery as a whole has operative mortality statistics of acceptably low proportions, in the treatment of intracranial aneurysms the cooperative study from 24 centres suggested that a 30 to 35 per cent overall operative mortality rate might be taken as a guideline. This could in no way be regarded as acceptable. It was already apparent from the publications of McKissock et al (1960) that the prognosis of SAH varied very considerably according to the condition of the patient at the time of admission to hospital, and much study has been devoted to the identification of factors which determine surgical risk. It has emerged that the two most important factors determining surgical mortality are the condition of the patient at the time of surgery and the time which has elapsed from SAH. The earlier operation is undertaken the more dangerous it is, and the sicker the patient at the time of operation, the higher the risks of surgery.

Perhaps not surprisingly, analysis of the mortality rates of cases treated medically shows that these same criteria also apply. Fig. 14.1 which is taken from Locksley's study (1966) shows an attempt to establish graphical analysis of the regression curve

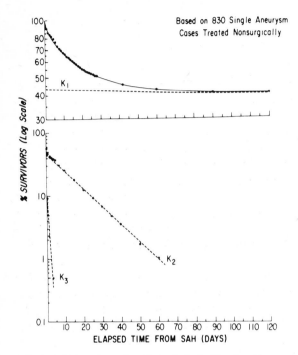

Fig. 14.1 Regression curve of survival of subarachnoid haemorrhage for aneurysm (reproduced by kind permission of Journal of Neurosurgery and of H.B. Locksley from his article (1966) Report of the Co-operative Study of Intracranial aneurysm and subarachnoid haemorrhage Section V, part 1, Natural History of Subarachnoid Haemorrhage, Histology and Aneurysm and Malformation. Journal of Neurosurgery 25:219).

of survival. The determination of such curves is based on the assumption that the number of patients dying during any given period of time is proportional to the number of patients alive at the beginning of this interval. The early portion of this curve, in the first few days following the onset of SAH, has a steep and constantly changing slope, which after six weeks becomes a slow, almost linear, decline. Using the type of exponential stripping familiar to blood flow analysts, the slow tail of the exponential may be stripped from the first portion to reveal three populations at risk. The

slow component describes the behaviour of about 43 per cent of cases of SAH who may be expected to survive beyond the first six weeks. The behaviour of the other 57 per cent can be visualised by subtracting the slow component from the main curve, and this second or slowly decaying curve — K2 in the figure of Locksley — describes the behaviour of about 47 per cent of the initial cases. A third, steeply decaying slope, K3, describes about 9 per cent of patients who die very rapidly within the first few days of SAH. This third group represents patients who are at the moment impossible to treat by any method. It is the second group, about 47 per cent of the total cases, whose numbers decline by about 6.6 per cent per day, who constitute the challenge to neurosurgical treatment. The average survival of this group after the first SAH is about two weeks, and in the absence of treatment designed to improve their survival, few will remain alive at the end of three months.

A careful study by Alvord et al (1972), employing material from the cooperative study and material in an earlier study by Pakarinen (1967) in Finland, has created even more detailed survival probability graphs, taking into account the time of presentation of the patient with SAH to hospital. It will be apparent from Locksley's graph (Fig. 14.1) that if a clinic admits cases only after the rapidly decaying K3 group have died, the expected natural mortality should be very much lower than the grouped mortality of SAH as a whole. Alvord et al from their own and other data constructed the graph shown in Figure 14.2, once again reaching the conclusion that at the end of two months after a SAH only some 40 per cent of cases would be alive, provided the population could include cases studied immediately from the time of the bleeding. If the clinic's admission policy delayed the average time of admission to one day following the haemorrhage, then at the two-month interval nearly 60 per cent of cases would survive. It is therefore apparent that were one to consider the extreme example of a neurosurgical unit operating on all cases presented to it immediately after SAH, a mortality rate of anything better than 60 per cent would constitute an improvement on natural mortality. On the other hand, if the unit admitted only one day after SAH, mortality rate at operation of greater than 40 per cent would be worse than the

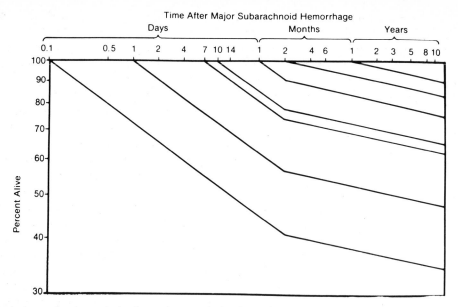

Fig. 14.2 Survival rate of patients admitted to study at particular times after their initial major subarachnoid haemorrhage (reproduced by kind permission of Archives of Neurology, and of Alvord et al (1972) Subarachnoid haemorrhage due to ruptured aneurysm. Archives of Neurology 27:273).

natural survival, and the patient would be better left unoperated. In the same way, a study of Alvord's graph shows that cases presenting one month after SAH will have a natural survival at two months of very nearly 90 per cent, and to operate on aneurysms presenting as late as this, therefore, the surgeon must offer a negligible mortality.

The natural history of arteriovenous malformations

Despite large numbers of neurosurgical publications on the subject of cerebral angiomas, the exact risk which these lesions present is far from clear. There is no doubt that the early re-bleeding rate of angiomas is very much lower than that of aneurysms. Thus, in the cooperative study, only 10 per cent of patients who had survived a single haemorrhage from AVM bled again within six weeks, whereas in survivors from an initial aneurysmal SAH the figure for re-bleeding within six weeks was 30 per cent. The initial mortality rate from haemorrhage from AVM was also appreciably lower. Thus, in the cooperative study, 281 bleeding supratentorial AVMs had a mortality rate from the initial haemorrhage of 10 per cent, whereas of 830

cases of first bleeding single aneurysm patients treated conservatively, 68 per cent had died by the time the study was completed, 93 per cent of them by the end of one year (Graaf, 1971). The cause of death in AVM is almost invariably haemorrhage within the substance of the brain. Indeed, it has been pointed out in more than one series (Perret & Nishioka, 1966; Paterson & McKissock, 1956; Henderson & Gomez, 1967; Morello & Borghi, 1973) that the small angioma is more likely than the large one to be associated with a large haematoma. This has been common surgical experience, perhaps related to the fact that the smaller angiomas tend to lie within the depths of the sulci and therefore to bleed naturally into the white matter rather than on to the surface and into the subarachnoid space. Each centre managing SAH, however, rapidly becomes aware that many patients with AVM re-bleed relatively infrequently, and some survive for many years following several haemorrhages. Kelly et al (1969) followed 33 patients for an average of 15.5 years after an initial haemorrhage from AVM, at which time there had been a mortality rate of 28 per cent, and half the patients had little, if any, disability. In Olivecrona & Ladenheim's (1957) series, 55 per cent of 44 cases which had not been radically operated on, had either complete disability or had died. Pool & Potts (1965), making a retrospective study of cases of angioma, found that 56 per cent of patients conservatively managed either died or were completely incapacitated. Troupp (1965), on the other hand, following 60 patients conservatively managed found that 37 (60 per cent) were in good health and at full work, and 11 were partially disabled, in a follow-up between 17 months and 16 years (mean 5 years) after the diagnosis of angioma had been made.

Where epilepsy alone is the presenting symptom, the management may be somewhat easier, although the enthusiasm of such as Kunc (1965, 1973) indicates that the radical excision of even critically placed AVMs may be attended with success. Where, however, an AVM has presented with haemorrhage, it is likely that further haemorrhage will occur, though probably over a period of years, and the common practice in Britain is to remove the lesion if it is at all surgically accessible, whatever its size. Figures 14.3 and 14.4 indicate two AVMs of considerable size, one supra- and the other infratentorial, successfully excised without increase in neurological deficit. There is no convincing evidence that infratentorial AVMs are associated with a significantly worse prognosis than those placed supratentorially.

The clinical presentation of subarachnoid haemorrhage

The onset of classical SAH presents few diagnostic difficulties. The sudden severe headache, of an intensity such as the patient has never suffered before, sometimes accompanied by the feeling of something giving way inside the head, is a description so clear and so striking that it is not usually overlooked. Retrospective analysis of the history of patients presenting with severe subarachnoid haemorrhage often reveals an incident in the past, sometimes a few weeks before, sometimes in the remote past, in which a similar headache of sudden onset passed off within a few hours. The importance of the early recognition of such warning leaks cannot be over-emphasised. Patients after minor haemorrhage are in excellent condition and their prognosis following surgery is infinitely better than that of a patient precipitated

into coma by severe haemorrhage. On occasion, the initial headache may be overlooked, and the patients come complaining of neckache, a feeling of stiffness in the neck or sometimes even of sciatica. Two patients in the author's experience in fact presented with a second subarachnoid haemorrhage in the post-operative period following the ill-advised excision of a totally blameless lumbo-sacral disc. The 'sciatica' was due to blood in the lumbar canal. Another premonitory sign sometimes seen in subarachnoid haemorrhage is aching pain in the head on the side of the aneurysm. This is perhaps most common in aneurysm in the region of the posterior communicating artery, where aching retro-orbital pain is presumably due to dural stretch or to fifth nerve innervation of the terminal carotid artery itself. This last explanation may presumably serve also for cases of middle cerebral aneurysm presenting with aching pain on the same side of the head.

A number of factors have been thought to predispose to SAH, but the most clearly related of these appears to be the episodic increase in blood pressure related to coitus or straining. Thus in the combined study (Locksley, 1966) SAH occurred during coitus in 3.8 per cent of the patients who bled from intracranial aneurysm, and in 4.1 per cent of the patients who bled from AVM. In a rather nondescript group of 'other SAH', this was the predisposing factor in 2.2 per cent. Lifting or bending was associated with rupture in 12 per cent of aneurysms, and with the onset of haemorrhage in 14 per cent of AVMs. It seems likely that transient severe rises in arterial pressure are responsible for this, although in the case of AVM associated rise in venous pressure may be a factor in rupture of the thin and grossly dilated venous portions of the malformation. The progress after the onset of headache depends a good deal upon the severity of the haemorrhage. Thus, a severe haemorrhage either from aneurysm or AVM will be associated with rapid loss of consciousness, deep coma, and death within a few hours, usually as the result of extensive intracerebral bleeding. More commonly, a transient loss of consciousness succeeds the sudden severe headache, but the onset is normally recalled with great clarity by the patient on recovering from the short period of unconsciousness.

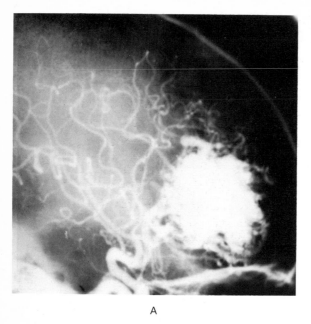

A

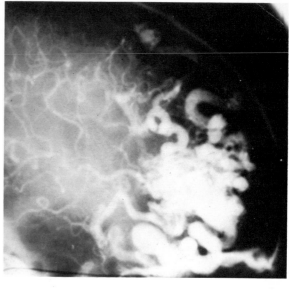

B

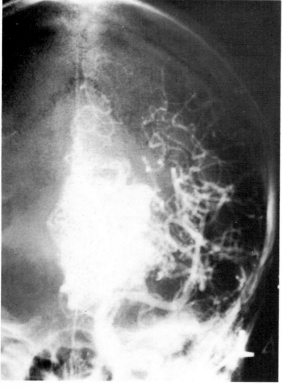

C

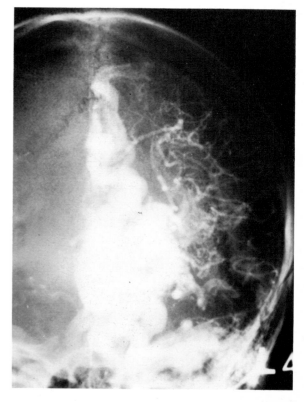

D

Fig. 14.3

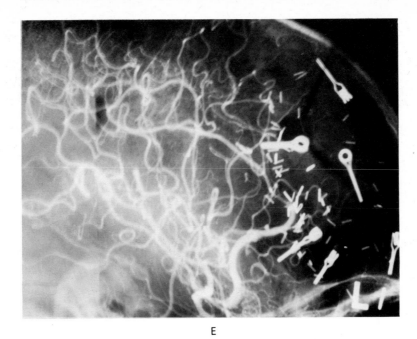

E

Fig. 14.3 Lateral (A & B) and AP (C & D) arterial and venous phases of a large angioma in the left frontal lobe, occasioning troublesome recurrent epilepsy. The malformation was successfully excised. Further view (E) taken soon after surgery shows slight residual swelling of the hemisphere, with complete removal of the malformation. The patient was undisturbed by this procedure. He has remained fit-free on anticonvulsants since that time.

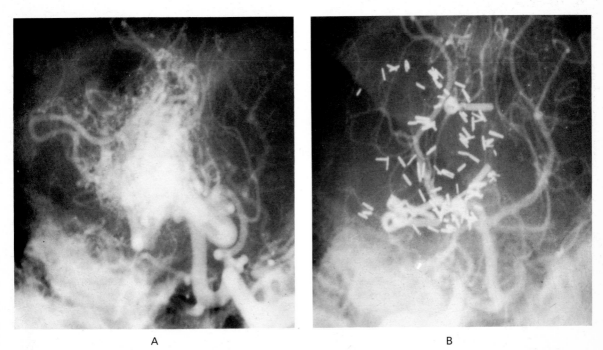

A   B

Fig. 14.4 A large subtentorial, arteriovenous malformation which had presented with four subarachnoid haemorrhages over a period of four-and-a-half years, accompanied by progressive cerebellar deficit. The patient, an 18-year-old boy, showed appreciable neurological improvement postoperatively. Preoperative angiograms are shown in Figure 14.4A. Postoperative angiograms are shown in Figure 14.4B.

Fits as a presenting feature in association with the haemorrhage are not common, although in cases of AVM a preceding history of epilepsy is present in a number of patients (see below). After the onset, the patient may return to full consciousness or may pass through a phase of extreme irritability with or without focal neurological signs, which may give a clue as to the situation of the lesion which has bled. Sometimes immediately or within a few hours, neck stiffness and signs of meningeal irritation, such as a positive Kernig's sign, become apparent even though the patient remains unconscious. Other abnormalities include transient disturbance of vegetative functions manifested by an increase in blood glucose, the development of severe glycosuria, sometimes proteinuria and, not infrequently, abnormalities in the electrocardiogram which may suggest ischaemia and which have been attributed to high concentration of circulating catecholamines as a result of the stress induced by haemorrhage (Cruickshank et al, 1974). The pattern of any focal neurological deficit may give a clue to the site of the offending lesion. Thus, the complaint by the patient that the onset of the headache was associated with a severe feeling of weakness in the legs may be a clue to the haemorrhage having arisen from anterior communicating complex, while the development of a facio-brachial weakness may suggest an origin within the distribution of the middle cerebral artery.

Sudden dense hemiplegia is uncommon in SAH unless the lesion has resulted in bleeding into the deep nuclei in the region of the internal capsule, and this may occur of course either with the deep AVMs or with upward rupture of aneurysms in the region of the posterior communicating artery or in the middle cerebral complex. While a long period of confusion and irrationality may occur in SAH of any origin, it is often seen in lesions involving diencephalic structures, of which anterior communicating aneurysms and aneurysms at the top of the basilar artery are perhaps the most specific. While a focal neurological deficit may be of some clinical value in localisation of the lesion, its value is slight in comparison with angiography. Of even less value is any focally sited headache, with the possible exception of the aching unilateral peri-orbital or frontal headache which, preceding

sudden rupture, may betoken an aneurysm in the region of the terminal carotid artery, near the origin of the posterior communicating branch (Okawara, 1973). These aneurysms more than any other may manifest their presence very clearly by progressive enlargement over some days or weeks prior to subsequent rupture and, if this is so, then the associated third nerve palsy is of absolute diagnostic significance. Less commonly, aneurysms on the proximal portion of the posterior cerebral artery may also involve the third nerve, but the relative infrequency of this last group renders a third nerve palsy almost diagnostic of posterior communicating aneurysm. Impairment of the corneal reflex, while it may occur in aneurysms of the terminal carotid or upper basilar arteries which subsequently bleed into the subarachnoid space, is more often associated with aneurysms of the internal carotid within the cavernous sinus and, as a rule, these do not produce SAH.

Particular features of the presentation of arteriovenous malformations

AVMs differ from intracranial aneurysms in that a substantial proportion present not with SAH, but with epilepsy. SAH may appear at any later stage in development, although there is a tendency for each AVM to run true to type, that is, more patients who develop epilepsy continue with epilepsy as their only symptom than subsequently develop haemorrhage. This may be, as pointed out by Morello & Borghi (1973), because epilepsy occurs in its major form particularly with very large lesions, and there is a slight but definite tendency for subarachnoid or intracerebral haemorrhage to occur with rather smaller lesions. However, a clear history of epilepsy followed by the development of SAH is a valuable diagnostic point, and since the prognosis for SAH following rupture of AVMs and of aneurysms is very different — the latter having a much more serious outlook — the differentiation is worthwhile from the point of view of management of relatives, even at an early stage before angiography has confirmed the nature of the lesion.

The particular presenting features of intracranial AVM in six recent large series (Paterson &

McKissock, 1956; Olivecrona & Riives, 1948; Mackenzie, 1953; Kelly et al, 1969, Perret & Nishioka, 1966; Morello & Borghi, 1973) are shown in Table 14.1. There is general agreement that between 30 and 60 per cent of these lesions present with haemorrhage as the first sign, and that between 25 and 40 per cent present with epileptic seizures. Rather less frequently, progressive neurological deficit is the mode of presentation, while curious neurological signs such as those of the cerebello-pontine angle, may betoken AVMs in unusual sites.

Later features associated with subarachnoid haemorrhage

One of the most interesting complicating features of massive SAH, either from intracranial aneurysm or angioma, results from the extensive blockage of the absorption of cerebrospinal fluid or from direct adhesions induced in the subarachnoid space by the breakdown products of the haemorrhage (Gallera & Greitz, 1970; Shulman et al, 1963). Thus, in a series presented by Yasargil et al (1973) 10 per cent of the 280 cases with intracranial aneurysm developed communicating hydrocephalus. This complication usually follows within one to three weeks after haemorrhage, and it may occur either when the patient is managed conservatively or by craniotomy. Although it has been recorded following AVM, it is relatively infrequent. The usual picture is for the patient apparently recovering from severe SAH to become increasingly obtunded. Gradual confusion, disorientation, memory impairment and a decrease in mental and physical activity are early symptoms, and the condition, although progressing no further, may yet thereby mar an otherwise reasonable recovery.

Bilateral pyramidal and extrapyramidal signs may then appear, there is quite commonly increasing neck stiffness, increasing papilloedema and a gradual descent, at the worst, to akinetic mutism. Where SAH has been severe, the coma associated with the original haemorrhage — perhaps with focal hypothalamic damage as in the case of an anterior communicating artery aneurysm, in its own turn producing akinesia and mutism — may merge imperceptibly into the prolonged unconsciousness and severely raised intracranial pressure of communicating hydrocephalus (Fig. 14.5). In these cases, the development of severe and persistent papilloedema may be the only sign giving the clue to the nature of the progressive and continuing pathology. This form of communicating hydrocephalus responds particularly well to ventriculoatrial shunt procedures and the diagnosis should, therefore, be considered in all cases of SAH where the level of consciousness shows an unexpected decline some weeks after haemorrhage, or where prolonged unconsciousness is associated with papilloedema.

Less commonly, the communicating hydrocephalus may prove of the 'normal pressure' or, more properly, infrequently raised pressure type, when its recognition may prove less easy, demanding careful continuous pressure measurement over some days to detect the abnormal pressure wave phenomena (Symon et al, 1972; Symon & Dorsch, 1975). Treatment by bypass shunt operation is no less necessary in such cases, and is often equally rewarding.

Grading of patients with subarachnoid haemorrhage from aneurysm

The accumulated experience over almost 40 years from the Second World War has produced general

Table 14.1 Initial symptoms of intracranial arteriovenous malformations

Symptoms	Paterson & McKissock 110 cases (1956)	Mackenzie 50 cases (1953)	Olivecrona 43 cases (1948)	Kelly et al 70 cases (1969)	Perret & Nishioka 453 cases (1966)	Morello & Borghi 154 cases (1973)
Haemorrhage	46 (42%)	15 (30%)	17 (40%)	36 (51%)	307 (68%)	86 (56%)
Epilepsy	29 (26%)	16 (32%)	17 (40%)	26 (37%)	119 (28%)	31 (20%)
Progressive hemianopia	16 (15%)	12 (24%)	—	2 (3%)	Uncertain	
Migraine or other headache, and other neurological symptoms	8 (7%)	6 (12%)	—	6 (9%)	44 (10%)	14 (9%)

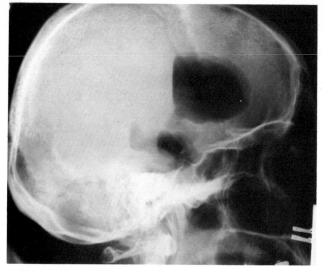

A

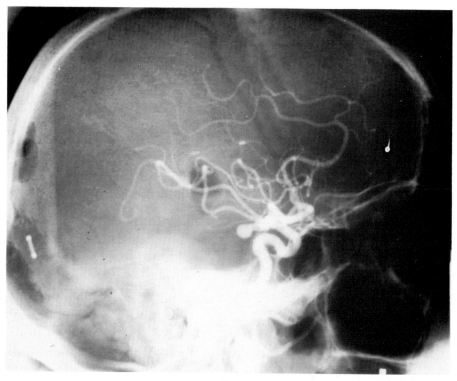

Fig. 14.5

B

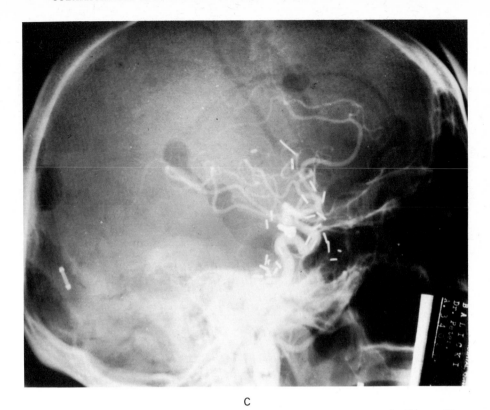

C

Fig. 14.5 A 60-year-old general practitioner who became akinetic and mute after a severe subarachnoid haemorrhage. Figure 14.5A shows the evident communicating hydrocephalus on air encephalogram. Figure 14.5B, the reduction in size of the ventricles following shunt surgery and the continued presence of the posterior communicating aneurysm which became active again about five weeks following the first haemorrhage when a complete third nerve palsy developed. The aneurysm was then satisfactorily occluded, as shown in Figure 14.5C.

agreement among neurosurgeons that the risks of operation on patients with SAH from intracranial aneurysm are closely related to the condition of the patient at the time of surgery. The first serious attempt to codify the condition of patients suffering from SAH was made by Botterell et al (1956), and it is a modification of this original classification developed by Hunt & Hess (1968) which has been adopted in most neurosurgical units to describe a patient's condition either on admission or at surgery. The adoption of this simple classification has been one of the most useful aspects of aneurysm study in recent years, since it has enabled the comparison of data from one clinic to another and, if stated in association with the time of operation from the time of SAH, enables the calculation of surgical contribution to survival in comparison with natural mortality, as Alvord et al (1972) have made clear.

The classification which in most features approximates to that used by Nishioka (1966) in the combined study is expressed in Table 14.2 from Hunt & Hess's original work. Their suggestion that 'serious systemic disease such as hypertension,

Table 14.2 The grading of patients with subarachnoid haemorrhage

Grade 1	Asymptomatic, or minimal headache, and slight neck stiffness.
Grade 2	Moderate to severe headache, neck stiffness, no neurological deficit other than cranial nerve palsy.
Grade 3	Drowsiness, confusion, or mild focal deficit.
Grade 4	Stupor, moderate to severe hemiparesis, possible early decerebrate rigidity and vegetative disturbances.
Grade 5	Deep coma, decerebrate rigidity, moribund appearance.

(After Hunt and Hess (1968) Surgical risk as related to time of intervention in the repair of intracranial aneurysms. Journal of Neurosurgery, 28 : 14. By kind permission of the authors and publishers.)

diabetes, severe arteriosclerosis, chronic pulmonary disease and severe vasospasm seen in arteriography, results in placement of the patient in the next less favourable category' is less uniformly applied, and if this amendment to the grading of patients is employed it is advisable that it be stated in the breakdown of patient data. Analysing 275 cases of their own, Hunt & Hess showed that the overall mortality from the time of admission varied from 11 per cent in Grade 1 patients to 100 per cent in Grade 5 patients, giving a total mortality rate of 35 per cent. Separating off those patients whom they were able to submit to surgery, the mortality figures of a group of 156 cases subjected to operation ranged from 1.4 per cent in Grade 1 to 43 per cent in Grade 4. They operated on no patients in Grade 5, and their total operative mortality was 16 per cent.

The objection is often raised, however, that in the usual surgical series a number of cases have died in the interval between admission and surgery. These being abstracted from the surgical mortality inevitably favour the surgical results in relation to natural mortality. This frequent criticism of surgically analysed series led Alvord et al (1972) to create a matrix of probability in relation to clinical grade, in which they combined the time after the last SAH with the clinical grade (Table 14.3). Their analysis had previously indicated that there was little difference in the natural decay curves for aneurysm cases, whether one constructed the tables in relation to either the first or the last SAH. This related to two factors: firstly, each SAH rendered the prognosis worse; secondly, recurrence of bleeding took place in only about 25 to 30 per cent of patients. This impressive work has enabled us to relate surgical results corrected for time following haemorrhage and grade at operation to Alvord et al's predictions of natural mortality, and has enabled for example the analysis of 300 personal cases treated by intracranial operation following SAH, shown in Table 14.4.

It appears from this table that the surgical mortality has improved on natural mortality significantly in Grades 1, 2, and 3, most particularly in Grade 3. Evidence of improvement in relation to surgery is less impressive in Grade 4, and operation is less frequently undertaken on such patients. A recent remarkable series from Krayenbuhl et al (1972) reported an overall mortality rate in 250 operations for intracranial aneurysm of 5 per cent. The mortality rate for operations on Grades 1, 2, and 3 patients was 1.6 per cent, and there were no deaths in 112 patients operated on in Grades 1 and 2. Twenty four per cent of the cases were operated on within one week of haemorrhage and 52 per cent within two weeks. Although it is impossible to place this series in relation to Alvord et al's criteria without further details, the remarkably low mortality rate in good-risk patients is clearly superior to natural mortality.

Assessment of the comparative morbidity of conservative and surgical treatment is less easy, largely because of inadequate information concerning the natural morbidity. It is however, regrettably true that a proportion of surgical survivors are intellectually or physically handicapped (Logue et al, 1968), but once again the general surgical experience has been that unsatisfactory results are, like deaths, commoner in bad-risk cases.

Table 14.3 Matrix of probability in relation to clinical grade. (Reproduced by kind permission of the Archives of Neurology and of Alvord et al, from Subarachnoid haemorrhage due to ruptured aneurysms. Archives of Neurology, 27:283 1972.)

| Clinical grade | Probabilities Days after subarachnoid haemorrhage | | | | | | |
	0 to 1	1 to 3	3 to 7	7 to 21	21 to 60	60+	All intervals
1	65	80	90	95	95	95	90
2	55	70	75	90	95	95	75
3	45	55	65	75	85	95	65
4	30	40	45	50	60	70	45
5	5	5	5	5	5	5	5
All grades	45	55	65	75	85	95	65

Table 14.4 Predicted (Alvord) and surgical survival in 300 supratentorial aneurysms with subarachnoid haemorrhage

Clinical grade	Days post haemorrhage 0–1	2–3	4–7	8–21	22–60	Total
1	70 0	85 0	95 100	100	100	95 100
	0	0	(10)	(9)	(13)	(32)
2	60 0	75 100	80 93	90 93	95 100	80 93.7
	0	(5)	(42)	(42)	(6)	(95)
3	50 0	60 100	70 96	80 100	90 100	70 98.3
	0	(15)	(47)	(44)	(8)	(114)
4	40 75	45 62.5	50 87.5	55 65.5	60 100	50 73
	(4)	(8)	(16)	(29)	(2)	(59)

A comparison of predicted mortality in terms of grade and time following haemorrhage, with the actual mortality of surgery under the same conditions. The Matrix is prepared by Alvord's criteria, using 300 personal intracranial aneurysm operations of the author. The two figures in the top line in each column are two months survival rates from Alvord's prediction on the left, and in the surgical series on the right. The figure in brackets below represents the number of surgical cases.

Timing of investigation and operation in cases of aneurysmal subarachnoid haemorrhage

The advent of C.T. scan has added a new dimension to the analysis of subarachnoid haemorrhage. In most clinics, C.T. scan would be performed at once when the patient is admitted. Immediate information as to the presence of haematoma is thereby obtained. In addition, the amount and distribution of blood in the subarachnoid space may be assessed, together with a presence of low density lesions, suggesting ischaemia such as may appear within a few days of subarachnoid haemorrhage. From the distribution of the blood, the approximate site of the aneurysm may be defined, and there is some evidence (Fisher, 1980; Bell et al, 1980) that the amount of blood in the subarachnoid space correlates well with the development of possible episodes of reduced perfusion, often described by the term vasospasm.

From the careful analytical work of the Cooperative Study and other authors, it is clear that operation on intracranial aneurysms following SAH cannot be undertaken in all cases immediately the patient presents in the clinic. It follows, therefore, that if immediate operation is not to be undertaken, one must first make a decision about the propriety and extent of angiographic investigation. Complete angiographic investigation in our hands, particularly in the unconscious or restless patient, almost invariably requires general anaesthesia. Provided that the patient is in a condition to sustain a general anaesthetic lasting perhaps two to three hours, immediate angiography is recommended. Only in this way will the information as to the site and accessibility of the aneurysm be available, the presence or absence of intracranial haematomas be defined, and detailed planning of any surgical intervention put on a rational basis.

Much has been written about delayed angiography with the caveat that immediate angiography soon after SAH increases the risk, but this has not been the author's experience. Careful angiography performed by skilled radiologists early after SAH has not contributed significantly to morbidity or mortality. The question of extent of angiography must also be considered. Here, the C.T. scan data are of considerable value. Where the distribution of blood clearly indicates a supratentorial lesion, then bilateral carotid arteriography alone is probably all that is required for management, although it is the author's practice still to arrange a four vessel arteriography in patients under the age of 60, so that a full delineation of other possible aneurysm sites may be undertaken. In the elderly, however, vertebral angiography should be omitted if C.T. scan, clinical evidence and angiography together point to supratentorial origin. It is usually wise, however, to undertake bilateral carotid arteriography to define any possible anomalies in the circulation which might alter surgical management.

Having established the site and accessibility of the aneurysm responsible for the SAH, the question of timing of operation arises. It is apparent from numerous studies that there is nothing to be said for intervention in cases of Grade 4 or Grade 5 early after haemorrhage, unless an intracranial haematoma appears to threaten life. In that event a judicious burrhole with evacuation of the clot may enable the patient's condition to be sufficiently improved to warrant further surgery at a later date. A word of caution is necessary here, however. The mere presence of an intracranial haematoma does not demand immediate evacuation. The work of Löfgren & Zwetnow (1972) and Nornes (1973) has indicated that changes in intracranial pressure may provoke further rupture from aneurysms, so that if the patient's life is not threatened by the intracranial haematoma and the condition appears to be improving, then the haematoma is best left. The presence of a haematoma of moderate size may well enhance the accessibility of an aneurysm at the time of definitive surgery and make the whole procedure very much easier. Thus patients of Grade 5 should not be subjected to surgery at all unless a life-threatening haematoma is present, and operation after the first week should be undertaken only advisedly in such cases as, for example, in younger patients with a reasonable prospect of a worthwhile long-term neurological recovery. Patients in this grade over the age of 60, are probably best left unoperated.

The decision for or against surgery reaches its maximum difficulty in patients of Grade 3. Here the rewards for success are high, and conversely the sharp post-operative deterioration of a patient apparently improving in Grade 3 is a burden which every neurosurgeon carries. The author's view is that the patients who are stable over a period of 48 hours in Grade 2 or who show signs of improvement from Grade 3 merit surgery as soon as may be. Circumstances which may alter this decision are the presence of marked hypertension or extreme neck stiffness in association with drowsiness or hemispheral signs, since there is a strong clinical impression, not backed by any significant statistical analyses, that these patients are more likely than others to develop extensive vasospasm following surgery. Operation is delayed, therefore, on Grade 3 cases associated with very marked neck stiffness and very heavy blood staining in the c.s.f.

In patients of Grades 1 or 2, there can be little justification for delay. The probability is only that such patients will get worse if bleeding should recur, and there is little doubt that in skilled hands at this time the mortality of surgery in these grades is appreciably lower than the risk which these patients run of recurrent haemorrhage. The careful work of Drake (1968a) some years ago, which proposed that surgery even in good-risk patients be deferred to the end of the first week, has been so at variance with the author's and other colleagues' practice that early surgery in good-risk patients has continued. The mortality rate may be somewhat higher but this is off-set by the absence of re-bleeding during the week of delay.

Some recent advances in general techniques of management

Technical surgical changes

There have been two principal changes in surgical technique in recent years. The first of these has been the development of the torsion bar clip, in which the clip is applied to the neck of the aneurysm, not with the surgeon's musculature under active contraction, but with a relaxing grip. The likelihood of the neck of the aneurysm being torn by the vibration of muscular tremor, is markedly reduced by this development. Figure 14.6 shows the e.m.g. recorded from the author's adductor pollicis applying a straightforward MacKenzie clip in one instance and releasing a Scoville clip in the other. The comparison in muscular effort is quite striking and justifies the complete abandonment of clips which are not applied in this way.

The second great technical advance has been the increased use of the operating microscope. To this, neurosurgeons owe a great debt to Professor Yasargil of Zurich, who developed the neurosurgical aspects of Jacobson's original work in Burlington, Vermont, taken up locally by Dr. Peardon Donaghy. Yasargil created a full range of neurosurgical instruments suitable for use under the microscope and developed operating microscopes for neurosurgical use. Yasargil's own views of the advantages of the microscopic technique are: firstly, the production of excellent illumination; secondly, the early recognition of field detail and accurate delineation of blood vessels; thirdly,

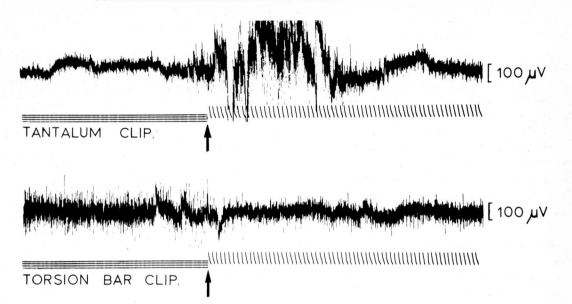

Fig. 14.6 The electromyogram of the author's adductor pollicis during the application of a tantalum clip (top panel) and a torsion bar clip (bottom panel) (under test conditions).

increased safety in clip placement because of clear vision and dissecting ease; and, fourthly, minimal retraction necessary for satisfactory completion of the operation.

Personal experience has fully borne out these contentions. The decreased retraction associated with aneurysmal surgery under the microscope is one of the main advantages of the method. Self-retaining retractors with constant and gentle pressure enable dissection even of such difficult sites as the anterior communicating complex under direct vision, with minimal distortion of neuraxial structures, and there is no doubt that the magnification and intensity of illumination enable the recognition of blood vessel detail behind covering arachnoid, so that accurate dissection through the arachnoid results, rather than the previous tentative opening hoping to avoid important underlying vessels. No young surgeon who proposes taking up aneurysmal surgery can today omit the development of microscopic techniques.

Recent pathophysiological developments concerned with subarachnoid haemorrhage

The past three decades have seen a vast increase in the knowledge and understanding of the cerebral circulation and its reactions. A series of interna-tional meeting since the first meetings in Lund and Copenhagen in 1965 have resulted in a wealth of physiological detail culled from both the experimental laboratory and the clinic, associated with the development of increasingly accurate techniques for regional and quantitative measurement of cerebral blood flow. Recent work in clinics both in North America and in Europe has indicated the generalised depression in hemispheral blood flow associated with recent SAH and the focal reduction in blood flow in areas supplied by spastic arteries (Heilbrun et al, 1972; Symon et al, 1972). The realisation that these problems are open to physiological analysis has encouraged others to take up analytical techniques. As a result of greater understanding of the cerebral circulation and its reactivity, assisted ventilation in anaesthesia has become the norm in surgery of intracranial aneurysms, and hypotensive anaesthesia has become safer with the understanding of the diminished autoregulatory capacity of areas of the circulation already exposed to stress such as vasospasm or swelling. There has been a gradually increasing use of monitoring techniques before, after and even during surgery for intracranial aneurysms, which have charted neurological function, either assessed by direct cortical stimulation (Eisenberg et al, 1979) or by the analysis of central conduction time (Symon et al, 1979; Symon et al, work in preparation) or have assessed the capacity of the circulation to withstand hypotensive stress of varying degree (Pickard et al, 1980).

Also in the past decade, the increased use of steroids such as dexamethasone, which protect the blood brain barrier and diminish the tendency for oedema to follow transient vascular occlusion encouraged by vasospasm, has resulted in a decreased incidence of the swollen brain with which many were familiar in the past.

The use of anti-fibrinolytic and hypotensive agents in conservative management, or as an adjunct to surgery

In recent years, a number of authors have reported on drugs designed to prevent clot lysis, which it is presumed is responsible for re-bleeding from aneurysms. The bleeding tendency is known to rise to a maximum around the end of the first week, and thereafter to fall to a relatively low level after the third week, although the exact timing varies from one particular aneurysm to another. There is thus evidence that aneurysms of the internal carotid artery, for example, show a tendency to remain active longer than other intracranial aneurysms, but on the whole the incidence of re-bleeding after three months has fallen to very low levels. The rationale of antifibrinolytic drugs is to protect the aneurysm from re-bleeding during the early period when other circulatory disturbances are at their maximum, and when experience has shown that operation carries a higher mortality than later.

In 1967, Norlen & Thulin reported experiences with epsilon aminocaproic acid (EACA) in neurosurgery. This drug acts principally by competitive inhibition of the activator substances converting plasminogen into the proteolytic enzyme plasmin, and also to a lesser extent by direct plasmin inhibition. Since the initial report, therapeutic trials have been published by Mullan & Dawley (1968), with the encouraging suggestion that a re-bleed rate of 2 out of 35 patients constitutes an improvement on natural re-bleeding rate, although the design of their trial was not a standard one and the duration of the treatment varied from periods of several days to six weeks. A further trial, reported by Ransohoff et al (1972), combined

antifibrinolytic drugs (again EACA) with hypotension for two weeks following the period of haemorrhage, and concluded that both ancillary methods were probably of value, since in 50 cases in which the two techniques were used together there were only six re-bleeding incidents, the latest occurring on the twenty-fifth day of treatment in one case. A more recent brief report of the use of tranexamic acid (AMCA) in 182 patients with SAH (Uttley & Richardson, 1974), indicated that the re-bleeding rate in the first 14 days from the original ictus was 12.1 per cent. A cooperative multicentre study of the use of antifibrinolytic agents in 502 patients was reported by Nibbelink et al in 1975. They concluded that this treatment reduced the frequency of re-bleeding by approximately 50 per cent. Even more impressive results were claimed by Sengupta et al in a clinical trial of 142 patients, where none of the 66 patients treated with EACA suffered recurrent haemorrhage (Sengupta et al, 1976).

There have been isolated reports of toxic reactions (Charytan & Purtilo, 1969; Naeye, 1962). These have included peripheral gangrene, vascular thrombosis and pulmonary embolism, although not in neurosurgical patients, and angiographic appearances suggesting arteritis or thrombosis in association with a deteriorating clinical course in patients treated with the drug following SAH (Sonntag & Stein, 1974). In Norlen & Thulin's initial report of 14 cases, one death occurred due to bilateral thrombosis of the anterior cerebral arteries 10 days after surgery. It is of course not certain that this could be attributed to the use of the drug, but it is certainly a most unusual post-operative complication. The standard regime for the use of EACA is an oral dose of 4 g four-hourly. The closely related drug tranexamic acid (AMCA), which appears to act in the same way although in a much lower concentration, is usually given in divided doses to a total of 12 g in 24 hours.

The use of hypotensive agents in the management of subarachnoid cases early after the ictus was suggested by Slosberg (1973), but there is as yet no firm statistical evidence of a significant protective effect. In 109 cases of aneurysmal bleeding treated with hypotension alone in the cooperative aneurysm study (Sahs, 1966), there was a 48 per cent mortality rate and no clear evidence of protective effect of the treatment. In addition, the maintenance of a steady level of blood pressure in the course of treatment with antihypertensive drugs may prove difficult. In more recent years, attempts to modulate blood pressure, in particular to avoid the surges of hypertension occasionally seen in aneurysm patients in poor condition, have been reported using beta-blocking agents such as propranolol. Thus Walter & Neil-Dwyer have used a regime of propranolol and phentolamine for several weeks following subarachnoid haemorrhage in a double-blind study, and have reported 'a strong trend' in favour of the treated group. It is likely that further information, particularly on beta-blockade preoperatively, will emerge within the next few years. (Walter & Neil-Dwyer, 1980).

As a rule, the conservative management of SAH cases in most centres is restricted to supportive treatment of the chest and respiration in comatose cases and the maintenance of strict bed rest for a period of four to six weeks following the ictus. Many would take the view that bed rest should not exclude the patient arising for toilet purposes.

The specific technical approach to aneurysms in various situations

The great majority of intracranial aneurysms — 95 per cent in the combined series — are in the anterior part of the circle of Willis, affecting either the region of the anterior communicating complex, the middle cerebral artery, or the terminal carotid artery in the region of the origin of the posterior communicating artery. The distribution of aneurysms in the combined study and in a personal series is shown in Table 14.5.

It is generally agreed now that the approach to anterior circle aneurysms is best made by a small

Table 14.5 Per cent probability of survival after SAH

	Combined series (%)	Personal series (%)
Anterior communicating complex	39.1	28.0
Distal anterior cerebral artery	1.6	2.6
Middle cerebral artery	18.3	20.0
Posterior communicating artery	32.5	25.0
Terminal carotid artery	5.0	9.0
Posterior circulation	3.3	3.5

fronto-temporal craniotomy, with excision of the outer part of the sphenoidal wing. This approach, used by many surgeons and most specifically advocated in recent years by Yasargil, has the considerable merit that the surgeon, who may deal with a relatively small number of these cases in the course of a year, makes what is essentially the same initial approach to the common aneurysms. Dissection, under the operating microscope assisted by appropriate self-retaining retractors, is pursued down to the terminal carotid artery, and the branches of the internal carotid followed to the aneurysm-bearing area.

Anterior communicating artery aneurysms

While the usual approach now, following the initial stages common to all aneurysms, is to excise a portion of the gyrus rectus just above and in front of the optic nerve and to dissect into the anterior communicating complex through the gyrus rectus, some surgeons still find merit in the interhemispheric approach, with excision of the medial portion of the frontal pole, popular a number of years ago. The use of this approach is particularly favoured by some in aneurysms lying above and behind the plane of the anterior communicating artery. The gyrus rectus approach, however, although it is certainly more difficult in such cases, is still satisfactory and has the great advantage of familiarity of approach, which the interhemispheric approach does not possess. An example of an aneurysm attacked by the subfrontal approach is shown in Figure 14.7, while Figure 14.8 shows a large aneurysm above the level of the complex attacked by the interhemispheric route. Both are satisfactory, but the simplicity of surgery in the former route along the sphenoidal wing renders it the most suitable at the present time, in the author's experience.

Posterior communicating artery aneurysms and aneurysms of the terminal carotid artery

Here there is little debate. The direct access along the wing brings the terminal carotid artery closer than any other approach, and the exact siting of the flap may be varied a little according to whether one wishes to approach the aneurysm more from

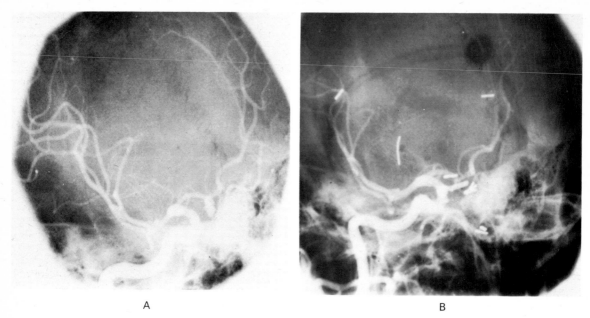

A   B

Fig. 14.7A & B Pre- and postoperative views of an anterior communicating artery aneurysm clipped by an approach along the sphenoidal wing.

anteriorly or from laterally. It is the author's current practice to divide the polar temporal veins to enable self-retaining retraction of the tip of the temporal lobe in aneurysms of the posterior communicating complex which are directed downwards and backwards so that the fundus of the aneurysm lies entirely behind the tentorium. By

this method, excellent visualisation of the origin of the neck, of the anterior choroidal artery, and of the posterior communicating artery, may be assured. The anterior choroidal artery, if it is clearly visualised on angiography and is demonstrably some distance from the origin of the aneurysm, need not be visualised at surgery; the

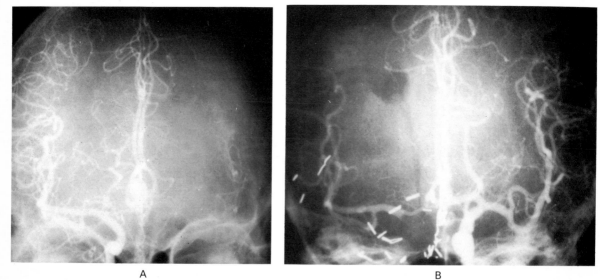

A   B

Fig. 14.8A & B Pre- and postoperative views of an anterior communicating artery aneurysm clipped by the inter-hemispheric route.

minimum of dissection in the region of aneurysms necessary to ensure satisfactory clipping is the ideal. The posterior communicating artery need not necessarily be preserved, the artery itself usually being a 'no-flow' vessel, but if careful angiography has demonstrated that the artery is in fact a fetal posterior cerebral artery with the ipsilateral posterior cerebral filling preferentially or entirely from the carotid, great care must be taken to preserve the posterior communicating artery itself. Extreme care is necessary also in those instances where, either from the size or multiplicity of aneurysms, the exact relationship of the neck to the anterior choroidal artery is in doubt (Drake et al, 1968).

Terminal carotid aneurysms present problems in proportion to their association with the perforating branches of the proximal middle cerebral artery. The terminal carotid itself and the region of the first centimetre of its main branches are, as pointed out by Shellshear (1920) many years ago, commonly entirely devoid of branches, but the situation of the fundus of an aneurysm arising from the terminal carotid in relation to the

perforating vessels determines not only the degree of deficit which the SAH may produce, but also the operative difficulty of exposure of the aneurysm. If, however, the neck can be shown angiographically to be free from perforating vessels, then dissection of the parent artery and the neck alone may prevent disturbance and distortion of the perforating vessels in attempted dissection of the fundus. The greatest degree of difficulty arises where the neck itself is in close relation to perforating vessels, and here the great advantages of illumination and magnification afforded by the operating microscope have their greatest reward.

Middle cerebral artery aneurysms

Aneurysms of the middle cerebral artery commonly have their origin at the first bifurcation of the vessel. They are there in close relationship with the major insular branches, frequently being embraced by them as Figure 14.9 shows; and even now, with the advantages of the operating microscope and its illumination, the surgeon may feel it unwise to dissect these vessels with sharp dissection from the

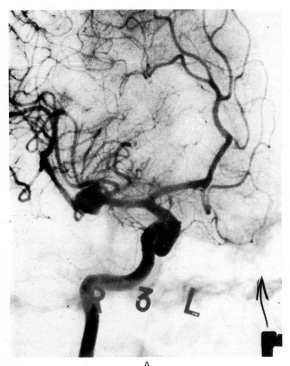

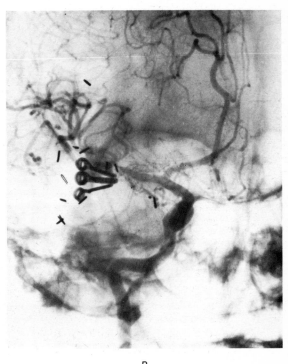

A   B

Fig. 14.9A & B Pre- and postoperative views of a typical middle cerebral trifurcation aneurysm clipped by an approach through the superior temporal gyrus.

fundus of the aneurysm to enable a clippable neck to be created. In this aneurysm there is still a place for gauze reinforced with acrylic applied as an investment to the whole complex. There is no doubt, however, that the proportion of aneurysms invested, in the author's own experience, has declined since microscopic techniques have been employed, but the ease and safety of the investment technique should not be entirely abandoned. More proximal aneurysms in the middle cerebral artery are certainly most easily approached by following the main vessel out along the sphenoidal wing from the terminal carotid artery. Peripheral aneurysms, as for example in a very lateral trifurcation of the vessel, may be approached by dissection through the superior temporal gyrus. This is particularly so if a temporal haematoma is present; dissection through the haematoma will often bring the surgeon directly on to the aneurysm without the necessity of disturbing the perforating-bearing area of the middle cerebral complex. It does, of course, carry the disadvantage of approaching the

fundus of the aneurysm first, and each individual approach and aneurysm must be considered on its own merits in this sometimes most difficult technical dissection.

Less common anterior circle aneurysms lie distally on the branches of the carotid. Of these, perhaps the commonest is the distal anterior cerebral artery aneurysm, which is often associated with congenital anomalies of the anterior communicating complex such as a single anterior cerebral artery bifurcating at the level of the genu of the corpus callosum (Fig. 14.10). This aneurysm has a sinister reputation, so that although the approach to it is straightforward and easy, clipping of the aneurysm is not infrequently followed by intense spasm of the distal pericallosal vessels and considerable damage to the medial aspect of both motor strips. Indeed, some experienced surgeons regard this aneurysm with such misgiving that they invariably wrap the region with gauze or gauze and acrylic rather than attempt to clip it. Yasargil & Carter (1974) recently reported on a

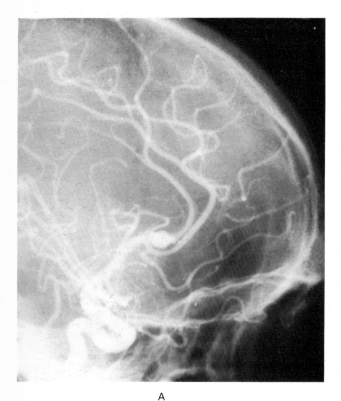
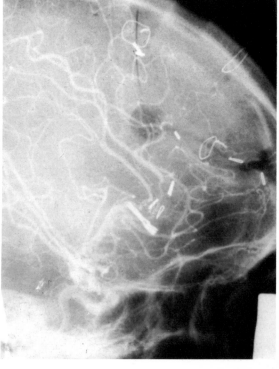

A   B

Fig. 14.10A & B Pre- and postoperative views of a pericallosal artery aneurysm clipped by the interhemispheric approach.

group of distal communicating aneurysms clipped with excellent results, and no doubt this will encourage the majority of surgeons to attempt the standard obliteration techniques even with this less common and widely feared lesion.

Aneurysms of the vertebro-basilar system

These aneurysms have a sinister surgical reputation since the majority of surgeons have limited experience of their management. Aneurysms of the vertebro-basilar trunk were very commonly regarded as inoperable until the work of Drake (1961, 1965, 1968b) in which he showed that while the results were far from satisfactory, it was possible to approach these lesions with careful technique, and in a number of instances, to occlude them. His vast experience, which now extends to over 600 vertebro-basilar aneurysms, has encouraged him and others in this belief. Surgeons throughout the world are now less inclined to treat these aneurysms by conservative methods. Successful reports from

Japan by Sugita and his colleagues (1979), from the United States (Wilson & U, 1976) and from Europe (Yasargil et al, 1976) have reported acceptable results in significant numbers of aneurysms of the posterior circulation. Lesions in the distribution of the basilar artery however continue to be formidable technical dissections, and few would consider it feasible to attack them in the conditions of patient grade at which surgery would now be thought feasible for anterior circle aneurysms. Few would consider for example, operation on upper basilar aneurysms in Grade 3. A detailed analysis by grade and time following subarachnoid haemorrhage, similar to that applied in relation to anterior circle aneurysms, is still awaited in relation to aneurysms of the posterior circulation. It seems likely however, that surgery is now offering more than conservative management, remembering that the rate of late re-bleeding in untreated vertebro-basilar aneurysms has been suspected to be greater than that of the more common sites.

Figures 14.11 and 14.12 show that even the

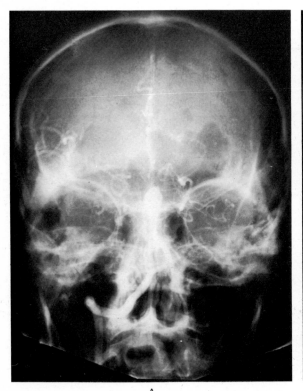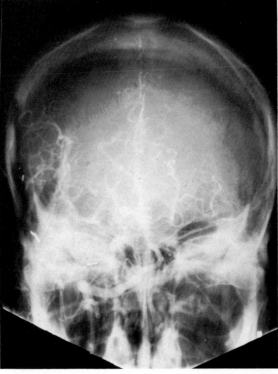

A   B

Fig. 14.11A & B Pre- and postoperative views of a terminal basilar artery aneurysm approached along the petrous ridge by the mid-temporal approach of Drake.

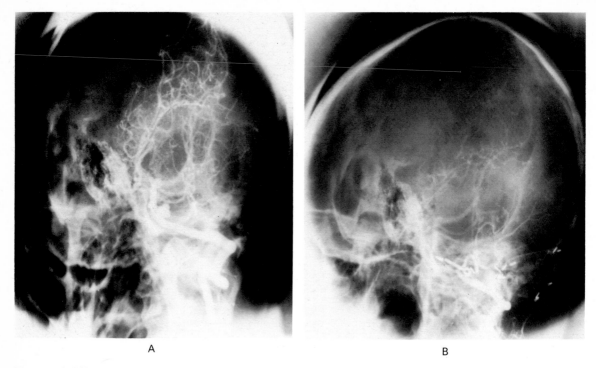

A   B

Fig. 14.12A & B Pre- and postoperative views of an aneurysm at the junction of vertebral and basilar arteries in the pre-pontine cistern. This aneurysm was clipped by a lateral posterior fossa approach.

'occasional vertebro-basilar surgeon' will have success from time to time, but against this must be set the disasters which vertebro-basilar surgery, even in careful and experienced hands, will continue to present.

The problem of the giant aneurysm

Giant aneurysms may present either in association with SAH or as space occupying lesions in their own right. In the second group, of course, they fall outside the scope of the present article, but the technical problems are no less severe when they present with SAH. Indeed, the question of the patient's condition is superimposed on the technical difficulty of the separation of a large sac from its parent vessel. Possibly the main hazard is that the angiographic visualisation of the sac may fall far short of its true mass. Distortion of the surrounding vessels apparently round a circular and non-opacified region should arouse suspicion; as Figure 14.13 shows, the true size of the sac may well exceed the central area opacified by dye. Since

these lesions commonly take many years to reach the presenting size, dissection of vessels from their close attachment to a thickly fibrous sac presents enormous problems and is really technically feasible only with magnification and excellent lighting. In the author's experience with direct approach to some 20 giant aneurysms, the essential feature is the capacity to occlude temporarily the aneurysm-bearing artery proximal to the neck of the aneurysm.

It is perhaps surprising that even the more proximal middle cerebral artery may be occluded for some appreciable time — in one of the author's own cases a period of 45 minutes — without infarction of the peripheral distribution of the vessel, the reason being given by the angiographic appearances. For example, in the case shown in Figure 14.14, the distal distribution of the middle cerebral branches and partly backward reflux from peripheral anastomoses. The territory had therefore been accustomed to hyperfusion from its main trunk for some little time and had established some degree of leptomeningeal collateral circulation elsewhere. Figure 14.14 shows that occlusion of the

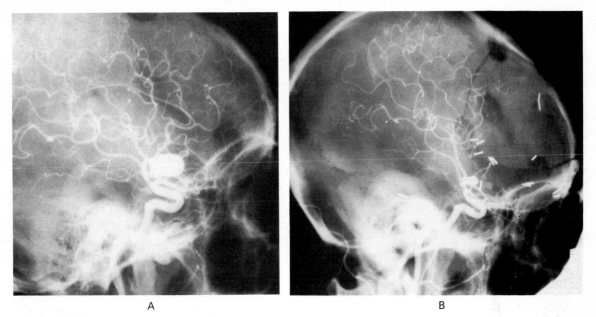

Fig. 14.13 Pre-and postoperative views of a giant anterior communicating artery aneurysm. The upward displacement of the proximal anterior cerebral artery (Fig. 14.13A) is a clue to the fact that only a portion of the sac is opacified, the sac itself extending into close contact with the planum sphenoidale. The displacement of the proximal portion of the artery has disappeared following excision of the sac (Fig. 14.13B).

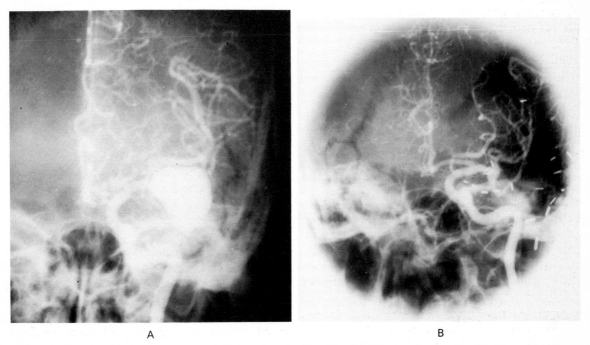

Fig. 14.14 A giant middle cerebral aneurysm which presented with subarachnoid haemorrhage as shown in Figure 14.14A, with postoperative view (Fig. 14.14B) following successful ligation and excision of the sac.

parent vessel for some 20 minutes may be followed by successful ligation of the aneurysm, facilitated by direct opening of the aneurysm and the clearance of contained clot. The application of a circumferential ligature is often difficult in the presence of contained clot, but much easier when the aneurysmal sac has been collapsed. While this is technically feasible in middle cerebral aneurysms and no doubt in aneurysms of the anterior cerebral complex, the difficulties and dangers of such techniques in the vertebro-basilar situation makes the giant vertebrobasilar aneurysm still usually an inoperable lesion.

A number of reports have indicated the usefulness of this technique in the handling of various giant aneurysms. Thus, Spetzler and his associates (1980) have used elective extracranial-intracranial arterial bypass in treatment of inoperable giant aneurysms of the internal carotid artery, while Sundt & Piepgras have reported the utility of bypass grafts in the management of giant middle cerebral aneurysms (1979). Hosobuchi (1979) has summarised his experience in 40 cases as yielding respectable results, provided the technique best suited to the particular aneurysm is carefully selected. In his view, neck occlusion, trapping and aneurysmorrhaphy are best for giant aneurysms of the anterior circulation, and intramural thrombosis best for those of the posterior circulation.

Multiple aneurysms

In the cooperative study on aneurysms, Perret & Nishioka (1966) reported an autopsy study of 888 cases in which single aneurysms had been found in 78 per cent, a second aneurysm in 17 per cent and three or more aneurysms in the remaining 5 per cent of cases. The data from a very much larger angiographic series of over 3000 cases showed a very similar distribution, suggesting that unless full angiography is carried out a second aneurysm may occasionally be missed. The problem of management of cases with multiple aneurysms, therefore, is a very real one. Sometimes there is no doubt from the clinical features as to the origin of the haemorrhage. On occasions, although the clinical features are non-specific, the angiographic appearances may give a strong indication. Thus,

irregularity in the shape of one aneurysm, the presence of focal associated vascular spasm near one of the aneurysms, or the presence of small vascular displacements suggesting the presence of a perivascular haematoma may provide an adequate guide. Where there is neither angiographic nor clinical clue, the difficulties of management are maximal.

Other special investigations may assist in the decision as to which aneurysm has bled. Some days after SAH focal disturbances in the e.e.g may assist at least in lateralising the hemisphere most affected by the bleeding, while the C.T. scan by showing small intrasylvian haematomata scarcely detectable by angiography, or changes in brain density suggestive of the presence of focal oedema, may assist in the attribution of haemorrhage to one particular aneurysm.

The author's practice is to operate only on the aneurysm which has bled, but if several aneurysms may be reached comfortably in one craniotomy, then all may be clipped at the same time. It is probably bad practice, however, to prolong aneurysm surgery where the management of the bleeding aneurysms has proved technically difficult. In a recent series (Heiskanen & Martila, 1970), a six-year follow-up of 76 patients with a known unoperated second aneurysm showed that over this period of time there was a five per cent mortality. This, of course, represents a similar mortality to that of the majority of centres in the management of aneurysmal SAH in Grades 1 and 2 cases, and it is clear that serious consideration should now be given to operations on aneurysms which are demonstrated either incidentally at angiography or are known to be present in patients who have had SAH from another aneurysm. Studies recently reported demonstrating an appreciable late mortality in unoperated single aneurysms (Winn et al, 1973) tend to support this decision, although there is as yet no clear evidence that the behaviour of an aneurysm which is known to have bled on one occasion is necessarily the same as that of an aneurysm present which has never occasioned SAH. The decision will clearly remain a highly personal one and will probably continue to be influenced mainly by the accessibility of the second aneurysm and the age and clinical state of the patient.

Other possible surgical manoeuvres in the treatment of intracranial aneurysms

In past years, the procedure of carotid ligation was widely practised, particularly for treatment of aneurysms of the terminal carotid artery, and the series presented by McKissock et al (1960) demonstrated beyond question, in a randomised clinical trial, that ligation reduced mortality in single bleeding aneurysms as compared with the expected natural survival. Most surgeons, however, have experience of re-bleeding in subsequent years from aneurysms in the region of the posterior communicating artery, which had remained patent and re-bled through collateral supply either from the vertebro-basilar system or from the opposite carotid. Figure 14.15 shows such a case. The increasing experience with intracranial surgery, particularly the very low mortality rate reported by Paterson (1968) in a series of posterior communicating aneurysms directly attacked, has encouraged the majority of centres to pusue direct attack on these aneurysms and to reserve carotid ligation solely for aneurysms in the region of the terminal carotid artery closely involved with perforating vessels, where the technical difficulties of surgery are likely to be great and the risks of surgical morbidity appreciable. The technique of proximal ligation of the anterior cerebral artery for aneurysms of the anterior communicating complex, which was originally described by Logue (1956), was practised by the author and his colleagues for a number of years, but with the introduction of microscopic techniques it is now little used.

Other techniques which have been used are piloinjection — the injection of bristles by a special apparatus (Gallagher, 1964) — particularly used

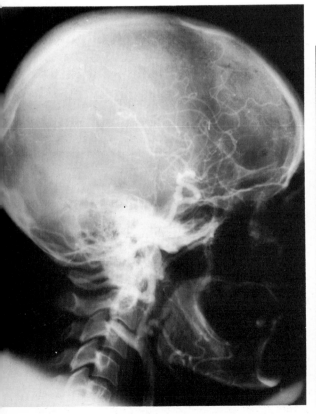
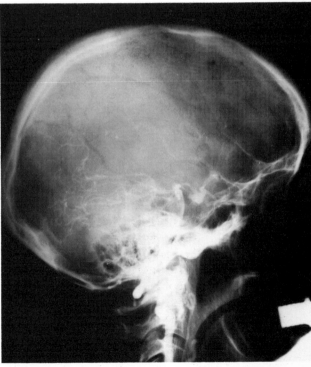

A   B

Fig. 14.15 A posterior communicating aneurysm (Fig. 14.15A) was treated by carotid ligation. Seven years later (Fig. 14.15B) recurrent subarachnoid haemorrhage from the same aneurysm occurred, and filling from the vertebrobasilar circulation with enlargement of the posterior communicating artery is shown.

in the treatment of very large aneurysms, and endo-aneurysmorrhaphy by fine copper needles (Mullan et al, 1965), or the obliteration of the aneurysm by the injection of iron filings, whose position is maintained by a magnet. This technique (Alksne, 1971) can be performed either by direct puncture of the aneurysm or by injection of the filings through a catheter introduced into a proximal artery. Perhaps not surprisingly, none of these methods has obtained widespread favour, and Drake's experience (1968b) would suggest that permanent occlusion of giant aneurysms by the piloinjection method cannot be relied upon.

Continuing problems in the management of aneurysmal subarachnoid haemorrhage

It will be apparent from this review that technical advances have now made the surgery of anterior circle aneurysms relatively routine. The results in good-risk cases are excellent, and although the technical complexities of operations on the posterior circle mean that surgical results here will continue to lag behind until more surgeons have had experience of these dangerous lesions, there is no reason to suppose that technical problems in the posterior circle lesions will prove any more insurmountable than in the more common lesions in the anterior part. The unsatisfactory results in patients in poor clinical grades however leave the surgeon in no doubt that the major problem still to be solved in the surgery of SAH is the effect of the haemorrhage on the cerebral circulation, with the attendant problems of brain swelling and infarction.

The reason for the unsatisfactory state of the brain in patients after recent SAH is still not certain. The concept of intracranial vasospasm has been brought forward to explain reduction in peripheral perfusion in the territory of an aneurysm-bearing artery, and neurosurgeons in general are familiar with the angiographic appearances of marked vascular narrowing in the immediate area of intracranial aneurysms at some time following SAH (Symon, 1971). The association of vasospasm with the severity of the patient's illness has varied, however; Allcock & Drake (1963), in the analysis of post-operative vasospasm, noted that 27 per cent of patients with satisfactory recovery showed

evidence of vasospasm, but that vasospasm was present post-operatively in 71 per cent of patients with unsatisfactory results. In a series analysed by the author (Symon, 1966) it has appeared that vasospasm is commoner in patients who are severely ill. Of 33 patients who died, 14 showed significant vasospasm; of 53 patients who survived, only 17 showed vasospasm. In individual cases, however, the frequent failure to establish correlation between the severity of vasospasm and the severity of the patient's illness has made it clear that factors other than the apparent luminal reduction must be playing a part. Some patients with quite severe vasospasm are clinically alert and without neurological deficit; others with severe neurological deficit have little or no vasospasm. In recent years however, there has been a considerable amount of work to show that vasospasm has an influence upon the state of perfusion of the brain distal to the vasospastic vessels. Thus, Symon et al (1972) showed in an analysis of post-operative angiograms and blood flow good correlation between angiographic demonstration of vasospasm and focal reduction in blood flow in brain supplied by the spastic segments. Similar conclusions were reported by Heilbrun et al (1972) and have also been confirmed by Overgaard (1973). Studies of regional perfusion by Kelly & Grossman (1977) and Pitts et al (1980) have made it clear that there is a better relationship between the state of hemispheral perfusion and the clinical signs than there is with the appearances at angiography. Hemispheral blood flow has correlated more clearly with the level of consciousness, for example, than with the presence or absence of vasospasm, although Du Boulay has pointed out (1980) that the appearance of middle cerebral arterial spasm has a high correlation with the appearance of a hemispheric deficit. Possible complicating factors here are the presence or absence of an adequate collateral circulation, since the perfusion pressure distal to a vasospastic segment may remain almost unchanged if the vasospasm, though focally intense, has no effect on adequate collateral circulation. If, however, the collateral vessels are also involved, a much lesser degree of vasospasm may induce considerable fall in hemispheral perfusion, with the production of clinical symptoms.

Once perfusion has fallen, there may be prompt

damage to the blood-brain barrier, with the development of vasogenic oedema and locally raised tissue pressure. If the area involved is sufficiently large, secondary gradual rises in intracranial pressure will result, maximal first in the supratentorial compartment in the initial swelling. This will further reduce the available perfusion pressure and lead to sequential changes in blood brain barrier, the consequence of the fall of perfusion to critical vasodilatation (vasoparalysis) and global loss of autoregulation (Lassen, 1966). The way becomes open to the development of 'intracerebral steals', and the full pattern of circulatory abnormality demonstrated in experimental infarction. Heilbrun et al (1972) demonstrated such global loss of autoregulation in patients who had deteriorated following SAH, suggesting that while angiographic and CBF correlations are best on a focal level, the general effects of tissue acidosis and diminution of perfusion are much more widespread.

Increased understanding of the role of reduced perfusion in the production of ischaemia following subarachnoid haemorrhage has led to one of the principal advances in the management of such events following surgery. Kosnik & Hunt (1976) and the author (1978) have shown that the elevation of systemic perfusion pressure may reverse focal ischaemic deficits occurring following operations for intracranial aneurysms. There is abundant experimental evidence (Symon et al, 1978: Branston et al, 1977; Strong et al, 1977) that the effects of ischaemia on electrical function and ionic shifts in the ischaemic brain can be reversed by the induction of hypertension experimentally without removal of the initial cause of the ischaemia. A common regime used clinically therefore (which of course is applicable only to situations where the aneurysm has already been clipped) is to increase the circulating blood volume by a fluid load of 500–1000 mls of a low molecular weight dextran, and to increase the systemic blood pressure by sympathomimetic drugs. The author's preference is meteraminol intravenously, the drip rate being adjusted to elevate the systemic blood pressure by 30 or 40 mms Hg. Before employing this method of induced hypertension, it is important that a C.T. scan be performed to exclude the presence of a space-occupying low density region

with shift. This might suggest the transudation of fluid into the infarct had already occurred, and induced hypertension thereafter could be expected to be dangerous. Where, as is commonly the case soon after such transient ischaemic episodes, no shift is demonstrable, then the induction of hypertension may safely be performed and has resulted in a dramatic resolution of hemiparesis in a number of the author's and other reported cases. Parallel measures of cerebral blood flow (Symon et al, 1979) and of central conduction time (Symon et al, 1980) have shown the expected flow increase and improvement in electrophysiological function.

Current investigations of the aetiology of vasospasm

Experimental production of vasospasm, either by trauma to cerebral arteries (Echlin, 1965; Symon, 1967; Simeone et al 1968), or by the infusion of blood into the subarachnoid space (Ogata et al, 1973; Crompton, 1964), have led analyses of vasospasm to concentrate either on direct vascular damage or upon the effects of vaso-active material released into the c.s.f. from effused blood. Damage to vessels in the area of SAH has been well documented (Crompton, 1964; Conway & McDonald, 1972). Direct damage to basal cerebral vessels in the experimental animal induced marked vasoconstriction indistinguishable angiographically from the appearances of clinical vasospasm, although it is a much more transient phenomenon lasting, in an intense form, as a rule less than half-a-hour.

A possible biphasic type of spasm (Brawley et al, 1968), suggested that later secondary phenomena may superimpose upon the initial vasospasm induced by trauma to the blood vessel. The appearances of experimental vasospasm strongly suggest the local release of vaso-active material, possibly from the wall of the damaged artery, possibly from effused blood, and the potential nature of this material has been subjected to a great deal of investigation (Arutiunov et al, 1970; Kapp et al, 1968a, b; Wilkins et al, 1967; Landau & Ransohoff, 1968; Weir et al, 1970). Serotonin (Raynor et al, 1961) or some serotonin-like factor (Wilkins et al, 1966) was at first a common suggestion but, more recently, the potential role of prostaglandins (Yamamoto et al, 1972) has been advanced, since these substances have been found to be present in effused blood and to reduce the calibre of epicerebral vessels. Recent work in North America (Rice-Edwards, 1973) has suggested that the role of platelet aggregation on vessel walls deserves further investigation. Degeneration of the catecholamine plexus has been put forward as the basis (Nielsen & Owman, 1971), and elaborated in the form of a hypothesis by Symon (1971) and Du Boulay et al (1972), with the suggestion that the initial SAH produced degeneration of catechol-amine-containing nerve endings, which subsequently became sensitive to normal levels of adrenergic amine in the familiar delayed denervation hypersensitivity.

What seems clear, however, is that vasospasm is more likely to occur where the SAH has been massive, and re-analysis of the role of blood constituents on cerebral vasoconstriction is under way in several centres in Europe and the United States at the present time. This is particularly welcome in view of the disappointing results obtained by alpha blockade. C.T. scan studies, by Fisher in Boston (1980) and by Symon et al in Queen Square (1980), have indicated a clear correlation between the presence of blood in appreciable quantity in the basal cisterns, and a poor clinical outcome. In Fisher's view, blood in C.T. scans of 1.5 mm or more in extent on straightforward measurement of a plain scan was invariably associated with vasospasm and with appropriate deficit which in the middle cerebral field would be manifest as hemiparesis. A further potential link between tissue damage and muscular contraction has been the work of Peterson et al (1973), who have demonstrated that certain aden-osine compounds dilate vessels in states of vaso-spasm induced by effused blood. They suggested that disorder of the endogenous myogenic meta-bolism of the spastic vessel had been induced by ischaemia, and that re-supply of exogenous aden-osine compounds resulted in the resolution of this abnormality. Work in Japan from Sano's depart-ment (1980) has suggested that reduction of oxyhaemoglobin to methaemoglobin may initiate free radical lipid peroxidation of polyunsaturated fatty acids. An increase in malonaldehyde, a good indicator of lipid peroxidation of polyunsaturated

fatty acids, was found by this group in the c.s.f. patients with cerebral vasospasm. A possible link with the prostaglandin chain is the inhibition of prostacylcine synthesis by such polyunsaturated fatty acids. The presence of this powerful natural vasodilator might encourage the development of pathological constriction.

A final further facet of the aetiology of vasospasm has been raised by the suggestion (Kassel et al, 1980) that vasospasm may be a proliferative vascular angiopathy. He demonstrated that in patients with cerebral vasospasm who died within eight days of subarachnoid haemorrhage, cerebral basal vessels showed loss of smooth endothelial surface, whereas those who died between 9 and 60 days afterwards, showed smooth muscle prolifer-ation. They suggested that this might be a progressive change due to a mitogenic factor, similar to that proposed by Ross (1974) in atherosclerotic lesions.

Most neurosurgeons concerned with the treat-ment of SAH agree that the problems of the technical approach to aneurysms have now largely been solved. Clear guidelines to the preservation of the cerebral circulation by pharmacological tech-niques, particularly during anaesthesia, have emerged in the past 10 years, and it would not be too optimistic to say that the clear recognition of the salient remaining problem — the unspecified origin of impaired cerebral perfusion consequent upon SAH — has focused the attention of both pharmacologists and neurosurgeons on this major continuing problem. Within the next 10 years or so, we have good ground to expect further encouraging improvements in the prognosis of this most serious disease.

The treatment of subarachnoid haemorrhage from arteriovenous malformation

Although at this time there can be no conclusive proof that the surgical management of haemor-rhage from arteriovenous malformation is associ-ated with a lesser mortality than the death rate by natural re-bleeding, the experience of several large series (Olivecrona & Ladenheim, 1957; Morello & Borghi, 1973; Pool & Potts, 1965) would suggest that this is so. Indeed, it would now appear that complete excision of the AVM is the most satisfactory treatment following the presentation of such a lesion with subarachnoid or intracerebral haemorrhage. It is clear, however, that this conclusion cannot be applied in all cases, since the location of the lesion involving brain stem or inaccessible in deep structures may make surgical treatment impossible. Figure 14.16 shows such a lesion which, although it had not in fact presented with SAH, clearly would have been technically inoperable however it had presented. Careful angiography however, may demonstrate that even in infratentorial lesions which at first sight appear to involve important arteries supplying the brain stem, the AVM may be entirely extracerebral and removable by meticulous dissection under the microscope. Figure 14.4 shows such a case, which had been deemed technically inoperable after angiography some five years before the final presentation, during which time the young man had suffered four recurrent haemorrhages and developed a progressive cerebellar deficit. Angiography indicated that although the lesion was fed by branches of the anterior inferior cerebellar artery, the brain stem distribution of this vessel was uninvolved, and the lesion was successfully and totally removed. A group of such cases of posterior fossa AVM

demonstrably extracerebral on careful angiography has been reported by Drake (1973).

Even where AVMs are in close relation to major vessels so that extensive feeding arteries pass straight into the malformation from major portions, for example, of the middle cerebral artery, careful dissection under the operating microscope in association with hypotensive anaesthesia will result in these lesions being accessible to dissection in an increasing proportion of cases, with an acceptable mortality. Thus, Moody & Poppen (1970) radically removed 51 angiomas, with a mortality rate of 12 per cent; Muller et al (1970) operated on 88 mixed supra- and infratentorial AVMs, with a mortality rate of 20.5 per cent; Maspes & Marini (1970) excised 60 cases, with an 8 per cent mortality; Krayenbuhl's mortality (Wegmann, 1970) for the resection of 69 angiomas was 8.7 per cent; Morello & Borghi (1973) completely excised 88 angiomas in their series of 150, with an operative mortality of 9 per cent. Comparing their mortality rate with those of conservatively treated cases, it was approximately half the death rate from recurrent haemorrhage in 44 conservatively managed cases.

While of course this appears impressive and convincing, surgical series on the whole tend to divide themselves into those cases which are

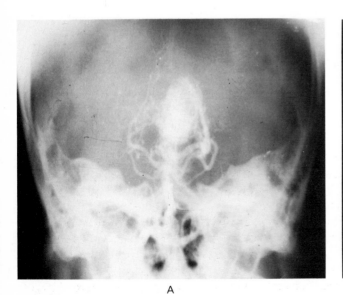

A

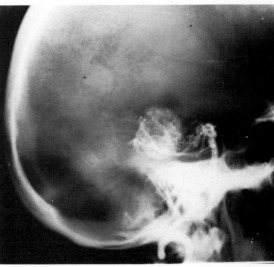

B

Fig. 14.16A & B An arteriovenous malformation of the upper brain stem which presented as aqueduct stenosis. The location of such an AVM renders surgery impossible.

considered operable by the surgeon and those which are not, and it is scarcely fair to compare the two groups in order to indicate a superior mortality for surgery when such selection has already been applied. As Moody & Poppen (1970) commented, however, it is in general good judgment to avoid surgery for the asymptomatic malformation, or where the symptoms are those of the occasional seizure which may be adequately controlled by anticonvulsants. Otherwise, in the case of haemorrhage as a presenting feature, surgery should certainly be considered, provided adequate anaesthesia and meticulous technique is used.

There is general agreement in the management of AVMs that, with the rare exception of occasional deep lesions feeding from single vessels, ligation of the feeding vessels has nothing to offer (Poole, 1968). This is almost invariably followed within a short time by the refilling of the angioma from feeding vessels which were not visualised at the time of the original angiography; similar restrictions apply to the previously used practice of carotid ligation.

More recently, embolisation of portions of AVMs (Luessenhop et al, 1965; Kusske & Kelly, 1974), thermocoagulation by stereotactic techniques, or operative excision after partial obliteration of the lesion by cryosurgical means have been recommended. More refined techniques (Mullen et al 1979) have allowed the introduction of small emboli deep in arteriovenous malformations, both supratentorial and infratentorial, or even the endovascular catheterisation of the feeding vessels of such lesions, and their obliteration by rapidly setting cyanoacrylate or silastic compounds. These techniques must be regarded as under trial, and have so far yielded acceptable results only in a few hands.

REFERENCES

Alksne J F 1971 Stereotactic thrombosis of intracranial aneurysms. New England Journal of Medicine 284:171

Allcock J M, Drake C G 1963 Post-operative angiography in cases of ruptured intracranial aneurysms. Journal of Neurosurgery 20:752

Alvord E C, Loeser J D, Bailey W L Compass M K 1972 Subarachnoid haemorrhage due to ruptured aneurysms. Archives of Neurology 27:273

Arutiunov A J, Baron M A, Majarova N A 1970 Experimental and clinical study of the development of spasm of the cerebral arteries related to subarachnoid haemorrhage. Journal of Neurosurgery 32:617

Asano T, Tanishima T, Sesaki T, Sano K 1980 Possible participation of free radical reactions initiated by clot lysis in the pathogenesis of vasospasm after subarachnoid haemorrhage. In: Wilkins R H (ed) Cerebral arterial vasospasm. Proceedings of the 2nd international workshop 1979. Williams & Wilkins, Baltimore, p 409–411

Bell B A, Kendall B E, Symon L 1979 Computerized tomography in aneurysmal subarachnoid haemorrhage. Journal of Neurology, Neurosurgery & Psychiatry 43:522–524

Botterell E H, Lougheed W M, Scott J W, Vandewater S L 1956 Hypothermia, and interruption of carotid or carotid and vertebral circulation, in the surgical management of intracranial aneurysms. Journal of Neurosurgery 13:1

Branston N M, Strong A J, Symon L 1977 Extracellular potassium activity, evoked potential and tissue blood flow: Relationship during progressive ischaemia in baboon cerebral cortex. Journal of Neurological Sciences 32:305–321

Brawley B W, Strandness D E, Kelly W A 1968 The biphasic response of cerebral vasospasm in experimental subarachnoid haemorrhage. Journal of Neurosurgery 28:1

Charytan C, Purtilo D 1969 Glomerular capillary thrombosis and acute renal failure after Epsilon-aminocaproic acid. New England Journal of Medicine 280:1102

Conway L W, McDonald L W 1972 Structural changes of the intradural arteries following subarachnoid hemorrhage. Journal of Neurosurgery 37:715

Crompton M R 1964 The pathogenesis of cerebral infarction following the rupture of cerebral berry aneurysms. Brain 87:491

Cruickshank K M, Neil-Dwyer G, Brice J 1974 Electrocardio-graphic changes and their prognostic significances in subarachnoid haemorrhage. Journal of Neurology, Neurosurgery & Psychiatry 37:755–759

Drake C G, 1961 Bleeding aneurysms of the basilar artery: Direct surgical management in four cases. Journal of Neurosurgery 18:230

Drake C G 1965 Surgical treatment of ruptured aneurysms of the basilar artery. Journal of Neurosurgery 29:372

Drake C G 1968a Discussion of the paper by Hunt and Hess. Journal of Neurosurgery 28:19

Drake C G 1968b Further experience with surgical treatment of aneurysms of the basilar artery: Experience with 14 cases. Journal of Surgery 29:372

Drake C G 1973 Cerebello-pontine angle arteriovenous malformations. In: Shurmann K, Broch M, Reulen H-J & Voth D (eds) Advances in Neurosurgery. Springer-Verlag, Berlin

Drake C G, Vanderlinden R G, Amacher A L 1968 Carotid-choroidal aneurysms. Journal of Neurosurgery 29:32

Du Boulay G, Symon L, Shah S, Dorsch N, Ackerman A L 1972 Cerebral arterial reactivity and spasm after subarachnoid haemorrhage. Proceedings of the Royal Society of Medicine 65:80

Du Boulay G, Marshall J, Merory J, Symon L 1980 The location of spasm and its relation to symptoms In: Wilkins R H (Ed) Cerebral Arterial Spasm. Proceedings of the 2nd International Workshop 1979. Williams & Wilkins, Baltimore, p 394–396

Echlin F A 1965 Spasm of basilar and vertebral arteries caused by experimental subarachnoid hemorrhage. Journal of Neurosurgery 23:1

Eisenberg H M, Turner J W, Teasdale G, Rowan J, Feinstein R, Grossman R G 1979 Monitoring of cortical exitability during induced hypotension in aneurysm operation. Journal of Neurosurgery 50:595–602

Fisher C M, Kistler J B, Davis J M 1980 Relation of cerebral vasospasm to subarachnoid haemorrhage, visualised by computerised tomographic scanning. Neurosurgery 6:1–9

Gallagher J P 1964 Piloinjection for intracranial aneurysms. Report of progress. Journal of Neurosurgery 21:129

Gallera R G, Greitz T 1970 Hydrocephalus in the adult secondary to the rupture of intracranial arterial aneurysms. Journal of Neurosurgery 32:634

Graaf C J 1971 Prognosis for patients with non-surgically treated aneurysms. Analysis of the co-operative study of aneurysms and subarachnoid haemorrhage. Journal of Neurosurgery 35:438

Gull W 1859 Cases of aneurysm of the cerebral vessels. Guy's Hospital Report (S3) 5:281

Hassler O 1965 On the etiology of intracranial aneurysms. In: Fields W S, Sahs A L (eds) Intracranial aneurysms and subarachnoid hemorrhage. Charles C Thomas, Springfield, Illinois

Heilbrun M P, Olesen J, Lassen N A 1972 Regional cerebral blood flow studies in subarachnoid hemorrhage. Journal of Neurosurgery 27:36

Heiskanen O, Martila I 1970 Risk of rupture of a second aneurysm in patients with multiple aneurysms. Journal of Neurosurgery. 32:295

Henderson W R, Gomez R L 1967 Natural history of cerebral angiomas. British Medical Journal iv:571

Hosobuchi Y 1980 Direct surgical treatment of giant intracranial aneurysms. Journal of Neurosurgery 51:743–756

Hunt W E, Hess R M 1968 Surgical risk as related to time of intervention in the repair of intracranial aneurysms. Journal of Neurosurgery 28:14

Kapp J, Mahaley M S Jr, Odom G L 1968a Cerebral arterial spasm. Part 2: Experimental evaluation of mechanical and humoral factors in pathogenesis. Journal of Neurosurgery 29:339

Kapp J, Mahaley M S Jr, Odom G L 1968b Cerebral arterial spasm Part 3: Partial purification and characterization of a spasmogenic substance in feline platelets. Journal of Neurosurgery 29:350

Kassel N F, Peerless S J, Drake C H 1980 Cerebral vasospasm; acute proliferated vasculopathy? 1: hypothesis. In: Wilkins R H (ed) Cerebral arterial spasm. Proceedings of the 2nd international workshop 1979. Williams & Wilkins, Baltimore, p 85–87

Kelly D L, Alexander E, Davis C H, Maynard D C 1969 Intracranial arteriovenous malformations. Clinical review and evaluation of brain scans. Journal of Neurosurgery 31:422

Kelly P J, Gorten R J, Grossman R G, Isenberg H M 1977 Cerebral perfusion, vascular spasm and outcome in patients with ruptured intracranial aneurysms. Journal of Neurosurgery 47:44–49

Kosnik E J, Hunt W E 1976 Post-operative hypertension in the management of patients with intracranial aneurysms. Journal of Neurosurgery 45:148–149

Krayenbuhl H A, Yasargil M G, Flamm E S, Trew J M 1972 Microsurgical treatment of intracranial saccular aneurysms. Journal of Neurosurgery 37:678

Kunc Z 1965 The possibility of surgical treatment of arteriovenous malformations in anatomically important cortical regions of the brain. Acta Neurochirurgica 13:361

Kunc Z 1973 Surgery of arteriovenous malformations in the speech and motor sensory regions. Journal of Neurosurgery 40:293

Kusske J A, Kelly W A 1974 Embolism and reduction of the steal syndrome in cerebral arteriovenous malformations. Journal of Neurosurgery 40:313

Landau B, Ransohoff J 1968 Prolonged cerebral vasospasm in experimental subarachnoid hemorrhage. Neurology (Minneapolis) 18:1056

Lassen N A 1966 The luxury perfusion syndrome and its possible relation to acute metabolic acidosis localised within the brain. Lancet ii:1113

Locksley H B 1966 Report on the co-operative study of intracranial aneurysms and subarachnoid hemorrhage. Section V. Part 1: Natural history of subarachnoid hemorrhage, intracranial aneurysms and ateriovenous malformations. Journal of Neurosurgery 25:219

Lofgren J, Zwetnow N N 1972 Kinetics of arterial and venous haemorrhage in the skull cavity. In: Brock M, Dietz H (eds) Intracranial pressure, Springer-Verlag, Berlin

Logue V 1956 Surgery in spontaneous subarachnoid haemorrhage. British Medical Journal i:473

Logue V, Durward M, Pratt R T C, Piercy M. Nixon W L B 1968 The quality of survival after rupture of an anterior cerebral aneurysm. British Journal of Psychiatry 114:137

Luessenhop A J, Kochman R Jnr, Shevlin W et al 1965 Clinical evaluation of artificial embolisation in the management of large cerebral arteriovenous malformations. Journal of Neurosurgery 23:400

Luessenhop A J, Spence W T 1960 Artificial embolisation of cerebral arteries. Report of the use in a case of arteriovenous malformation. Journal of Neurosurgery 17:762

Mackenzie I 1953 The clinical presentation of a cerebral angioma. Review of 50 cases. Brain 76:184

McKissock W, Paine K W E, Walsh L S 1960 An analysis of the results of treatment of ruptured intracranial aneurysms. Journal of Neurosurgery 17:762

Maspes P E, Marini G 1970 Results of the surgical treatment of intracranial arteriovenous malformations. Vascular Surgery 4:164

Moniz E 1927 L'encephalographie arterielle son importance dans la localisation des tumeurs cerebrales. Revue Neurologique 2:72

Moody R A, Poppen J L 1970 Arteriovenous malformations. Journal of Neurosurgery 32:503

Morello G, Borhgi G P 1973 Cerebral angiomas. A report of 154 personal cases and a comparison between the results of surgical excision and conservative management. Acta Neurochirurgica 28:135

Mullan S, Dawley J 1968 Antifibrinolytic therapy for intracranial aneurysms. Journal of Neurosurgery 28:21

Muller N L, Koller L, Titgemeyer A 1970 Katamnestische Untersuchungen nach Operation eines intrakraniellen Rankenangiomas. Acta Neurochirurgica 22:53

Naeye R L 1962 Thrombotic state after haemorrhagic diathesis: a possible complication of therapy with Epsilon-aminocaproic acid. Blood 19:694

Nielsen K C, Owman C 1971 Adrenergic innervation of pial arteries related to the Circle of Willis. Brain Research 27:25

Nibbelink D W, Torner J C, Henderson W G 1975 Intracranial aneurysms in subarachnoid haemorrhage. A co-operative study. Antifibrinolytic therapy in recent onset subarachnoid haemorrhage. Stroke 6:622–629

Nishioka H 1966 Evaluation of conservative management of ruptured intracranial aneurysms. Journal of Neurosurgery 25:574

Norlen G, Thulin C A 1967 Experiences with Epsilon-aminocaproic acid in neurosurgery. A preliminary report. Journal of Neurosurgery 39:226

Ogata M, Marshall B M, Lougheed W M 1973 Observations on the effects of intrathecal papaverine in experimental vasospasm. Journal of Neurosurgery 38:20

Okawara S-H 1973 Warning signs prior to rupture of intracranial aneurysm. Journal of Neurosurgery 38:575

Olivecrona H, Riives J 1948 Arteriovenous aneurysms of the brain. Archives of Neurology and Psychiatry 59:567

Overgaard J 1973 Personal communication

Pakarinen S 1967 Incidence, aetiology and prognosis of primary subarachnoid haemorrhage. A study based on 589 cases diagnosed in a defined urban population during a defined period. Acta Neurologica Scandinavica 43:Suppl. 29. 1.

Paterson A 1968 Direct surgery in the treatment of posterior communicating aneurysms. Lancet ii:808

Paterson J H, McKissock W 1956 Intracranial angiomas. A clinical survey of, with special reference to their mode of progression and surgical treatment. A report of 10 cases. Brain 70:233

Perret G, Nishioka H 1966 Arteriovenous malformations. An analysis of 545 cases of craniocerebral arteriovenous malformations and fistulae in the co-operative study. Journal of Neurosurgery 25:467

Peterson E W, Searle R W, Mandy F F, Leblanc R 1973 The reversal of experimental vasospasm by Dibutryl-3′5′ adenosine monophosphate. Journal of Neurosurgery 39:730

Pickard J D, Matheson M, Patterson J, Wyper D 1980 The prediction of late ishaemic complications after cerebral aneurysm surgery by the intra-operative measurement of cerebral blood flow. Journal of Neurosurgery 53:305–308

Pitts L H, McPherson B, Wyper D J, Jennett B, Blair I, Cook M B D 1980 Effects of vasospasm on cerebral blood flow after subarachnoid haemorrhage. In: Wilkins R H (ed) Cerebral arterial spasm. Proceedings of the 2nd international workshop 1979. Williams & Wilkins, Baltimore p 333–337

Pool J L 1968 Excision of cerebral arteriovenous malformations. Journal of Neurosurgery 29:312

Pool J L, Potts D G 1965 Aneurysms and Arteriovenous Anomalies of the Brain: Diagnosis and treatment. New York, Evanston, London: Harper and Row

Ransohoff J, Goodgold A, Vallo Benjamin M 1972 Pre-operative management of patients with ruptured intracranial aneurysms. Journal of Neurosurgery 36:525

Raynor R B, McMurty J G, Pool J L 1961 Cerebrovascular effects of topically applied serotonin in the cat. Neurology (Minneapolis) 11:190

Rice Edwards J M 1973 Personal communication

Ross R, Glosmet J, Kariya B, Harker L 1974 A platelet dependent serum factor that stimulates the proliferation of arterial smooth muscle cells in vitro. Proceedings of National Academy of Science. U.S.A. 71:1207–1210

Sahs A L 1966 Report on the cooperative study of intracranial aneurysms and subarachnoid haemorrhage. Section VII. Part 2: Hypotension and hypothermia in the treatment of intracranial aneurysms. Journal of Neurosurgery 25:593

Sengupta R P, So S C, Villarejo-Ortega F J 1976 Use of epsilonaminocaproic acid (EACA) in the pre-operative management of ruptured cranial aneurysms. Journal of Neurosurgery 44:479–484

Shellshear J L 1920 The basal arteries of the forebrain and their functional significance. Journal of Anatomy (London) 55:27

Shulman K, Martin B F, Popoff N, Ransohoff J 1963 Recognition and treatment of hydrocephalus. Journal of Neurosurgery 40:480

Simeone R A, Ryan K G, Kotter J A 1968 Prolonged experimental cerebral vasospasm. Journal of Neurosurgery 29:357

Slosberg P 1973 Treatment and prevention of stroke. 1: Subarachnoid hemorrhage due to ruptured intracranial aneurysms. New York State Journal of Medicine. 73:679

Sonntag V K H, Stein B M 1974 Arteriopathic complications during treatment of subarachnoid hemorrhage with Epsilon-aminocaproic acid. Journal of Neurosurgery 40:480

Spetzler R F, Schuster H, Roski R 1980 Arterial bypass in giant carotid aneurysms. Journal of Neurosurgery 53:22–27

Strong A J, Goodhardt M J, Branston N M, Symon L 1977 A comparison of the effects of ischaemia on tissue flow, electrical activity and extracellular potassium ion concentration in cerebral cortex of baboons. Biochemistry Society Transactions. Journal of Biochemistry 5:158–160

Sugita K, Kobayashi S, Shintani A, Mutsuga N 1979 Microneurosurgery for aneurysms of the basilar artery. Journal of Neurosurgery 51:615–620

Sundt T M, Piepgras D G 1979 Surgical approach to giant intracranial aneurysms. Journal of Neurosurgery 53:22–27

Symon L 1966 Vascular spasm in the cerebral circulation. In: Smith R (ed) Background to migraine. First migraine symposium, Nov. 8–9, 1966 Heinemann, London

Symon L 1967 An experimental study of traumatic cerebral vascular spasm. Journal of Neurology, Neurosurgery & Psychiatry 30:497

Symon L 1971 Vasospasm in aneurysm. In: Smith R (ed) Cerebral vascular diseases. Proceedings of the 7th Princeton conference on cerebrovascular diseases. 1970. Heinemann, London

Symon L 1978 Control of intracranial tension. Operative Surgery (Neurosurgery) 3rd edn. Butterworths, London, p 1–12

Symon L, Ackerman R et al 1972 The use of the Xenon clearance method in subarachnoid haemorrhage: post-operative studies with clinical and angiographic correlation. In: Fieschi C (ed) Cerebral blood flow and intracranial pressure: Proceedings of the 5th international symposium, Roma-Siena. 1971. Part II, European Neurology. Karger, Basel

Symon L 1978 Disordered cerebrovascular physiology in aneurysmal subarachnoid haemorrhage. Acta Neurochirurgica (Wein) 41:7–22

Symon L, Dorsch N W C, Stephens R J 1972 Pressure waves in so-called low-pressure hydrocephalus. Lancet ii:1291

Symon L, Dorsch N W C 1975 The use of long-term intracranial pressure measurement in the assessment of hydrocephalic patients prior to shunt preparation. Journal of Neurosurgery 42:258–273

Symon L, Hargadine J, Zawirski M, Branston N M 1979 Central conduction time as an index of ischaemia in subarachnoid haemorrhage. Journal of Neurological Sciences. 44:95–103

Symon L, Bell B A, Kendall B E 1980 Relationship between effused blood and clinical course and prognosis in aneurysmal subarachnoid haemorrhage; a preliminary computerised tomography scan study. In: Wilkins R H (ed) Cerebral Arterial Spasm. Proceedings of the 2nd International Workshop 1979. Williams & Wilkins, Baltimore, p 409–411

Troupp H 1965 Arteriovenous malformations of the brain. Prognosis without operation. Acta Neurologica Scandinavica. 41:39

Uttley D, Richardson A E 1974 E-aminocaproic and subarachnoid haemorrhage. Lancet ii:1080

Walter P H, Neil-Dwyer G Proceedings of the Society of British Neurological Surgeons, 1980. Journal of Neurology, Neurosurgery & Psychiatry. (in press)

Wegmann H D 1970 Dass Shicksal operierter Patienten met arterial venosen Aneurysma des Gehirns. Schweizer Archiv fur Neurologie, Neurochirurgie und Psychiatrie 106:53

Weir B, Erasmo R, Miller J, MacIntyre J, Secord D, Mielke B 1970 Vasospasm in response to repeated subarachnoid hemorrhage in the monkey. Journal of Neurosurgery 33:395

Wilkins R H, Levitt P 1970 Intracranial arterial spasm in the dog. A chronic experimental model. Journal of Neurosurgery 27:490

Wilkins R H, Silver D, Odom G L 1966 The role of circulating substances in intracranial arterial spasm. 1: Serotonin and histamine. Neurology (Minneapolis) 16:482

Wilkins R H, Wilkins G K, Gunnells J C, Odom G L 1967 Experimental studies of intracranial arterial spasm using aortic strip assays. Journal of Neurosurgery 27:490

Wilson C, U. H. 1976 Surgical treatment for aneurysms of the upper basilar artery. Journal of Neurosurgery 44:537–543

Yamamoto Y L, Feindel W, Wolfe L S, Katoh H, Hodge C P 1972 Experimental vasoconstriction of cerebral arteries by prostaglandins. Journal of Neurosurgery 37:385

Yasargil M G, Yonekawea Y, Zumstein B, Stahl H-J 1973 Hydrocephalus following spontaneous subarachnoid haemorrhage. Clinical features and treatment. Journal of Neurosurgery. 39:474

Yasargil M G, Carter L P 1974 Saccular aneurysms of the distal anterior cerebral artery. Journal of Neurosurgery 40:218

Yasargil M G, Antic J, Lacigar B, Jain K K, Hodosh R M, Smith R D 1976 Microsurgical pterional approach to aneurysms of the basilar bifurcation. Surgical Neurology 6:83–91

15

Angiomas and fistulae involving the nervous system

Michael J. Aminoff

Angiomas are congenital vascular malformations due to a localized maldevelopment of part of the primitive vascular plexus. Several different types of these anomalies can be recognized. *Capillary telangiectasias* are reddish-brown unencapsulated lesions that are characterized by pathologically enlarged capillaries and are usually found within the substance of the brain or brainstem, often in the pons or basal ganglia. They are generally of little clinical significance, tending to be an incidental finding at postmortem examination, but occasionally lead to repeated hemorrhages. In most instances they are solitary, but multiple lesions may occur, sometimes on a familial basis. *Cavernous angiomas* are well defined, compact, lobulated masses containing a tangled web of vascular spaces, without intervening neural parenchyma. They are regarded by some as a form of telangiectasia and by others as arteriovenous malformations. *Venous angiomas* are described as an abnormal mass of sinuous, engorged veins, but most probably represent arteriovenous malformations in which the arterial component is relatively inconspicuous. Except in rare instances (Wendling et al, 1976), it is generally not possible to distinguish venous from arteriovenous angiomas either angiographically or pathologically. The most common and important types of angioma relating to the nervous system are the so-called *arteriovenous malformations*, and it is to these that attention will be directed primarily. They consist of an abnormal arteriovenous communication, without intervening capillaries. They may be small lesions that are not clearly visualized angiographically and are sometimes difficult to identify in the brain ('cryptic malformations'), or massive lesions fed by multiple vessels and lying on or within a large part of the brain and spinal cord, with abnormal gliotic parenchyma interposed between the component vessels. At operation, cerebral malformations are seen to consist commonly of a wedge-shaped mass of tortuous, engorged pulsating vessels located on the lateral aspect of the hemisphere, with the apex of the wedge directed toward the ventricles. Besides the major arterial feeders that are visualized at angiography, there may be numerous other small arterial branches supplying the mass of vessels. Venous drainage may be toward the ventricles and toward the surface, and venous structures may be seen pulsating and engorged with red arterial blood.

Both cerebral and spinal arteriovenous malformations may be associated with arterial aneurysms. The association of arterial aneurysms with cerebral arteriovenous malformations occurs in approximately 10 per cent of cases (Stein, 1979), while 1.4 per cent of patients with intracranial aneurysms have been found to have coexistent angiomas (Perret & Nishioka, 1966).

In the present chapter, attention is confined to intracranial (cerebral and dural) and spinal (intradural and epidural) angiomas, and to carotid-cavernous fistulae. Vascular malformations located primarily in the scalp or calvarium are not considered.

CEREBRAL ANGIOMAS

The development of cerebral angiography led to considerable interest in cerebral angiomas, and thus to a greater awareness of the neurological disturbances that they may cause. Angiography markedly facilitated the preoperative diagnosis of these lesions, and it soon came to be realized that they are not as rare as was once believed. Despite this, however, their management has often seemed to depend more on the ready availability of a skilled neurosurgeon than on a critical evaluation of therapeutic alternatives.

Some of the clinical features of angiomas may relate to maldevelopment of part of the brain occurring in association with the anomaly of blood vessels. However, angiomas can themselves lead to neurological disturbances in several different ways. First, hemorrhage may occur into the brain or subarachnoid space from one of the vessels involved in the malformation, or from a coexisting arterial aneurysm. Second, cerebral ischemia may result from diversion of blood from the normal cerebral circulation to the anomalous arteriovenous shunt ('steal'), or from venous stagnation secondary to the increased venous pressure that occurs as a sequel to the shunt. Thirdly, enlarged anomalous vessels may compress or distort adjacent cerebral tissue, or interfere with the normal circulation of cerebrospinal fluid, thereby causing an obstructive hydrocephalus, whereas a communicating hydrocephalus may occur as a sequel to previous hemorrhage. Finally, mechanical and ischemic factors may lead to progressive gliosis of surrounding brain tissue.

Clinical features of supratentorial angiomas

Cerebral angiomas may present at any age, in patients of either sex and show no preferential lateralization. They are located supratentorially in at least 70 per cent of cases, and usually then lie in the territory of the middle cerebral artery, most commonly in the Rolandic area. Patients may present with subarachnoid or intracerebral hemorrhage, or with seizures, headache, or a focal neurological deficit. The initial symptoms recorded in several different series are shown in Table 15.1. Some of the apparent differences between series may relate to patterns of patient referral, for example a higher incidence of hemorrhage is more likely among patients referred to a neurosurgical unit than elsewhere.

Hemorrhage

Intracranial or subarachnoid hemorrhage is a common presentation, and approximately 50–70 per cent of angiomas bleed at some time in their natural history. In general there does not appear to be any correlation between the tendency of angiomas to bleed and their site, or the age and sex of the patient. Similarly, these factors do not influence the prognosis following hemorrhage.

Some authors have reported that small angiomas are more likely to bleed than large ones (e.g., Henderson & Gomez, 1967; Waltimo, 1973; Luessenhop, 1976), although this has not been the experience of all (Troupp, 1965; Forster et al, 1972). The peak age for hemorrhage is between 15 and 20 years, and by the age of 40 about three-quarters of all angiomas (supratentorial and infratentorial) that will bleed have done so (Perret & Nishioka, 1966). The hemorrhage is typically into the subarachnoid space, but is commonly partly intracerebral as well. Patients characteristically present with intense headache, neck stiffness, photophobia, and — in about 50 per cent of cases — a focal neurological deficit, and consciousness may initially be lost. The mortality rate from the

Table 15.1 Initial symptoms of patients with cerebral angiomas (expressed as percentages)

	Olivecrona & Riives (1948)	Mackenzie (1953)	Paterson & McKissock (1956)	Troupp (1965)	Kelly et al (1969)
Epilepsy	40	32	26	20	37
Hemorrhage	40	30	42	57	51
Headache	—	24	21	8	—
Miscellaneous (including focal deficits)	—	14	10	13	12
Incidental	—	—	—	2	—
Source of patients	surgical	mixed medical and surgical	surgical	surgical	surgical

initial hemorrhage is approximately 10 per cent which is less than that from an aneurysm. The recurrence rate of recurrent hemorrhage from supratentorial lesions was 23 per cent in the study of Perret & Nishioka (1966), and there is general agreement that the chances of hemorrhage are greater in those patients with an angioma that has already bled than in other patients with angioma.

Seizures

Most patients presenting with hemorrhage do not give a history of epilepsy (Perret & Nishioka, 1966), but fits may certainly accompany or follow the bleed. In many patients, however, seizures are the initial symptom of the malformation (Table 15.1). In all, the prevalence of epilepsy in patients with supratentorial malformations is between 28 per cent (Perret & Nishioka, 1966) and 50 per cent (Houdart & Le Besnerais, 1963) in different series. Seizures are especially likely to occur if the malformation is frontal or parietal in location, and they may be either focal or generalized; when focal, they are usually Jacksonian in type. The seizures themselves are usually readily controlled by anticonvulsant drugs, but may occasionally be intractable. In patients presenting with seizures alone, Perret & Nishioka (1966) found that the prevalence of subsequent hemorrhage was 18 per cent, while Forster et al (1972) reported that the chance of a hemorrhage occurring in the next 15 years was approximately 25 per cent.

Headache

Headache unrelated to hemorrhage is a conspicuous feature in the history of many patients with cerebral angiomas, and indeed may be the sole complaint, especially when the external carotid arteries are involved in the malformation. In some instances, the headache has migrainous features, but visual or other prodromata are likely to be lateralized consistently to one side, and auras may accompany or follow the headache, rather than preceding it as in classical migraine. The headache itself may also be unilateral, and then generally occurs on the side of the underlying vascular malformation. More commonly, headaches are non-specific in character, with nothing to suggest that there may be an underlying structural lesion to account for them; evaluation is then difficult since headache is such a common, general complaint.

Other presenting symptoms

Non-specific neurological symptoms such as vertigo or disequilibrium, confusion, or focal, sometimes progressive, neurological deficits may occur, and occasionally cause patients to seek medical advice. Bruit or pulsatile tinnitus is rarely a presenting symptom unless the lesion is dural, at least in part.

Intellectual deterioration has sometimes been reported (Olivecrona & Riives, 1948; Mackenzie, 1953; Paterson & McKissock, 1956), but Waltimo & Putkonen (1974) found no psychometric evidence that angiomas had any general influence on the intellectual level of patients, and the full scale IQ did not correlate with the size or clinical manifestations of malformations among their patients. Dementia may, however, result from hydrocephalus secondary to previous subarachnoid hemorrhage.

Physical signs

Neurological signs may help to localize the lesion clinically, and fundoscopic examination may reveal papilloedema, especially following a massive hemorrhage. The presence of a systolic bruit over the eye or head may suggest the possibility of an underlying angioma in patients with a neurological disorder of uncertain etiology, but a bruit may also be found in patients with an aneurysm, meningioma, or acquired arteriovenous fistula, or an orbital, scalp or calvarial vascular anomaly. The prevalence of bruit varies considerably in different series but is usually between 15 and 40 per cent of cases, a lower figure being reported in patients presenting with hemorrhage (Mackenzie, 1953; Paterson & McKissock, 1956). A bruit is especially common if branches of the external carotid arteries are involved in the malformation, and is best heard over the ipsilateral eye or mastoid region. In addition to auscultation for a bruit, it is important to palpate the scalp and neck for large, pulsatile vessels, and to examine the skin and retina for other vascular abnormalities. Angiomas with an arteriovenous shunt of large volume may also be associated with tachycardia, cardiomegaly and even cardiac failure, especially in infants and children, and particularly when the vein of Galen is involved.

Clinical features of infratentorial angiomas

The frequency of infratentorial angiomas varies considerably in different series, but up to about 30 per cent of intracranial vascular malformations may be located in the posterior fossa. Their anatomical classification is discussed by Verbiest (1968). Cerebellar angiomas may be clinically inconspicuous, but hemorrhage can cause signs of meningeal irritation and an acute cerebellar syndrome, sometimes associated with a sixth nerve palsy and minor pyramidal signs (Logue & Monckton, 1954). In other instances they may lead to an obstructive hydrocephalus or to a brainstem syndrome.

Brainstem angiomas, especially telangiectasias, are often clinically silent, being discovered incidentally at autopsy (McCormick et al, 1968). They may, however, lead to subarachnoid or intracerebral hemorrhage, or to an acute obstructive hydrocephalus (Logue & Monckton, 1954). Focal brainstem symptoms and signs may also develop, and follow a progressive or relapsing course. Irrespective of the type of malformation, there may be a combination of cranial nerve (often oculomotor), pyramidal and cerebellar signs, sometimes accompanied by sensory disturbances. Such a deficit is too often attributed to multiple sclerosis, even though the clinical findings can all be accounted for by a lesion at a single site in the nervous system.

Diagnostic investigations

The way in which patients are investigated is governed by their manner of presentation.

Presentation with hemorrhage

The computed tomography (C.T.) scan is a reliable indicator of recent subarachnoid or intracerebral hemorrhage, and may help to localize the source of bleeding. It is usually the first diagnostic study now performed in patients presenting with hemorrhage, and has facilitated the early recognition of angiomatous malformations (Pressman et al, 1975). Non-homogeneous areas of mixed density with irregular — often tubular — calcifications are typical of these malformations, while serpiginous areas of enhancement are seen after infusion of contrast material (Fig. 15.1). Malformations drain-

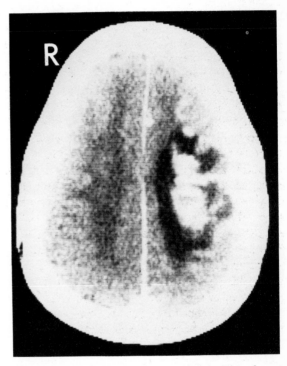

Fig. 15.1 C.T. scan after intravenous administration of contrast medium, showing irregular zone of contrast enhancement in the left parietal region, surrounded by a zone of low density. The patient had an angiographically-verified cerebral arteriovenous malformation.

ing through transparenchymal veins often have a typical wedge shape, the apex of which extends toward the lateral ventricle. There may be associated atrophy on the affected side, while large malformations or an intracerebral hematoma may lead to distortion of normal intracranial anatomy.

Diagnostic changes were present in the C.T. scans of 27 (66 per cent) of 41 patients with intracranial angiomas reported by Kendall & Claveria (1976), and a focal abnormality, often suggestive of the diagnosis, was present in a further

11 patients (27.5 per cent). The presence of such C.T. abnormalities indicates the need for angiography to define the malformation more completely. Even if the C.T. findings are normal, however, angiography should follow if the cerebrospinal fluid is blood-stained or xanthochromic.

Angiography is the definitive investigation (Fig. 15.2) in patients with a suspected angioma, since it permits the nature of the lesion to be established with certainty, and its anatomical features, especially its blood supply and venous drainage, to be characterized. All of the arteries supplying the malformation must be visualized, and in consequence the examination must generally include bilateral opacification of both the internal and external carotid arteries, and the vertebral arteries. This is important since Newton & Cronqvist (1969) found that meningeal arteries, sometimes from the contralateral side, contributed to the blood supply of 15 per cent of cerebral arteriovenous malformations. The typical angiographic appearance is of a tangled vascular mass with distended tortuous afferent and efferent vessels. The circulation time through the lesion is rapid, with arteriovenous shunting. There is usually no displacement of other vessels or structures unless an intracerebral hematoma is present, when an avascular mass is seen in relation to the angioma. It can sometimes be difficult to distinguish a small angioma from a highly vascularized malignant glioma, and the interested reader is referred to the account by Goree and Dukes (1963) of features that may be helpful in this regard. Cerebral cavernous angiomas, which are rare, usually cause arterial displacement, but neovasculature, a stain, and early venous filling have also been described (Jonutis et al, 1971).

Other methods of presentation

In patients presenting with headache or epilepsy, consistently focal or lateralized electroencephalographic abnormalities may first suggest the pres-

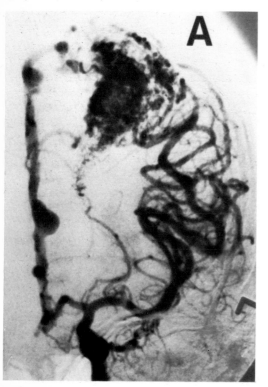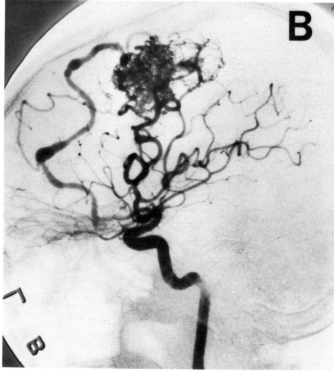

Fig. 15.2 Left internal carotid angiogram, frontal (A) and lateral (B) projections. An arteriovenous malformation supplied by branches of the pericallosal and middle cerebral arteries is shown.

ence of an underlying structural abnormality, but provide no information about its nature.

Radiographs of the skull are often normal, especially in patients with small malformations, unless an intracerebral hematoma is also present. Localized thinning or an increase in thickness of the cranial vault is an occasional non-specific finding. Abnormal calcification is sometimes found, but often resembles that seen occasionally in patients with tumors or aneurysms (Rumbaugh & Potts, 1966). Displacement of a calcified pineal or choroid plexus suggests a space-occupying lesion, and so is especially likely if an intracerebral hematoma is present. Enlargement of vessels feeding or draining the malformation may also be discerned from the plain films, particularly if meningeal vessels supply the anomaly.

C.T. scanning is clearly indicated in patients with clinical or electroencephalographic evidence of a focal neurological lesion. It also has an important role in the investigation of a seizure disorder that is focal, progressive, intractable or of late onset, and in the evaluation of patients with intellectual deterioration. If the C.T. findings suggest the presence of a cerebral arteriovenous malformation (Fig. 15.1), angiography is necessary to delineate the malformation, as discussed earlier. In occasional cases, however, angiography fails to demonstrate an underlying vascular malformation despite suggestive findings on the C.T. scan, usually because of partial or complete thrombotic occlusion of feeding vessels, and the greatest problem is then to distinguish the lesion from a partially calcified, avascular low-grade glioma (Kramer & Wing, 1977).

In patients with signs of a brainstem lesion, C.T. scanning may be helpful in detecting the underlying malformation or any associated hemorrhage. Such patients are often erroneously thought to have multiple sclerosis, but the presence of a cranial bruit, the lack of changes (such as increased IgG levels or the presence of oligoclonal IgG bands) in the cerebrospinal fluid, and a normal visual evoked response should raise the possibility of another pathology (Stahl et al, 1980).

Other investigative procedures
Certain other investigative procedures merit brief comment. Static or dynamic scintigraphy has been used to detect arteriovenous malformations, with varying results depending on technical and anatomical factors (Landman & Ross, 1973; Waltimo et al, 1973; Gates et al, 1978). Such methods have the merit of low cost and no requirement for iodinated contrast agents, but the additional information provided by the C.T. scan concerning hemorrhagic complications and the intracranial architecture clearly make it a superior screening procedure. Regional cerebral blood flow studies in patients with arteriovenous malformations show that blood flow is increased in the involved hemisphere compared to the other, especially when the lesion is superficial (Menon & Weir, 1979). Despite the development of a non-invasive technique, however, the method has more relevance as a means of monitoring the development of ischemic cerebral changes in patients with known malformations than as a diagnostic procedure.

Treatment

The treatment of cerebral angiomas is essentially surgical. The mere presence of a malformation is not an indication for its removal, however, and a wide divergence of opinion exists concerning the precise indications for surgery. This is due in part to lack of detailed knowledge about the natural history of untreated lesions. Moreover, comparison of the results within and between published series of cases is confounded by the bias of case selection; by differences in length of follow-up, technical facilities and surgical expertise, and by continual advances in the investigation and management of cases. In the circumstances, only a few general statements will be made.

Operative treatment to prevent further hemorrhage from lesions that have already bled is justifiable provided that the lesion is surgically accessible, the surgeon is experienced, and the patient otherwise has a reasonable life expectancy. Bearing in mind the likely operative morbidity and that rebleeding may not occur for some years, Forster et al (1972) have stressed that the advantages of surgery only become apparent statistically after a follow-up period approaching 10 years. Operative intervention is clearly justified when intracranial pressure is increased, or when cardiac decompensation occurs in children, and it can sometimes prevent further progression of a focal neurological deficit. Since surgical resection is more likely to cause epilepsy than relieve it, however, patients presenting just with a seizure disorder should generally be managed pharmacologically.

The technical aspects and outcome of surgical treatment are considered in detail elsewhere in this book, but some comment concerning embolization procedures will be made here.

Embolization of the afferent blood supply using an intravascular catheter technique has recently emerged as a simple, relatively safe adjunct to more definitive surgical treatment, its main use being to reduce the size of the malformation before surgical removal is attempted. The feasibility of embolization depends especially upon the characteristics of the blood vessels supplying the malformation. When the main feeders are large compared to vessels supplying adjacent cerebral tissue, successful embolization is facilitated. The angle at which a feeder comes off its parent artery is also important, since a gentle angulation poses no problems but an acute or right angle makes embolization difficult. Finally, emboli are more likely to stray if the malformation is supplied by distal branches of a long tortuous artery rather than from proximal branches of a relatively straight vessel (Wolpert & Stein, 1979). Complications may result if embolic material lodges in a site other than the intended one, but Wolpert & Stein (1979) reported that permanent complications occurred in only 1 patient among a series of 34 patients subjected to 59 embolization procedures.

Embolization is sometimes used as the sole means of treating angiomas deemed inoperable because of their inaccessible location, or because they involve a critical area of the brain. Small feeding vessels are likely to remain patent, however, and will enlarge with time unless the fistulous portion of the malformation is removed. Partial embolic obliteration of an arteriovenous malformation is not a very satisfactory solution, since the incidence of hemorrhage from the anomaly remains high (Luessenhop & Presper, 1975). Nevertheless, headache associated with the malformation may be relieved, and progressive neurological deterioration may stabilize or reverse, provided that the deficit is of relatively short duration and

has not resulted from previous hemorrhage (Kusske & Kelly, 1974; Luessenhop & Presper, 1975).

A somewhat different approach has been employed by Serbinenko (1974) and involves a technique for the temporary or permanent occlusion of major cerebral vessels using balloon catheters. Temporary occlusion of specific vessels can provide prognostic information concerning the consequences of obliterating or embolizing the vessels feeding an angioma, and this may be of particular relevance when the malformation is located in a functionally important area. At the same time, any blood supply to the malformation from neighboring vessels can be studied angiographically. Permanent occlusion of the vessels feeding a malformation is achieved with the help of a detachable balloon that is positioned in the desired site and then inflated with quickly-solidifying contrast material.

Others have developed a microcatheter that can be flow-guided into third- and fourth-order branches of the intracranial arteries, and through which controlled amounts of a vascular occlusive polymer can be deposited in the malformation (Kerber et al, 1979). Evaluation of the technique must await publication of the detailed results in a series of patients with intracranial malformations.

INTRACRANIAL DURAL VASCULAR ANOMALIES

Abnormal intracranial arteriovenous shunts may occur in the dura mater, where they involve meningeal branches of the carotid (internal and external) and/or vertebral arteries, and drain through the dural veins and sinuses. The origin of these shunts is not always clear, but they are often presumed to represent congenital malformations. Angiography sometimes shows the feeding arteries to divide into branches which communicate with a dural sinus at several different points along its length (Aminoff & Kendall, 1973), thereby suggesting that congenital maldevelopment is indeed responsible. In other instances, however, the shunt seems to be acquired in adult life, often in response to trauma, presumably because of the close anatomical relationship of certain meningeal arteries to venous structures (Wilson & Cronic, 1964; Newton & Hoyt, 1970). Similar lesions have also developed following dural sinus thrombosis (Houser et al, 1979), possibly because the resulting alteration in regional hemodynamics influences flow through a coexistent dural shunt, rendering it symptomatic and angiographically evident (Aminoff & Kendall, 1973). Once a dural arteriovenous fistula has been acquired, the angiographic appearance of a congenital vascular malformation may be simulated by progressive dilatation of pre-existing anastomotic channels from arterial sources that are not directly involved in the fistula. Pathological examination of excised specimens in patients with abnormal dural arteriovenous shunts reveals a mass of blood vessels but does not usually permit conclusions to be reached on the nature and cause of the abnormality (Aminoff, 1973), although some dural vascular lesions have the microscopical features of cavernous angiomas (McCormick & Boulter, 1966). Accordingly, these dural lesions will be referred to here simply as vascular abnormalities or anomalies, rather than malformations or angiomas, to avoid any general etiological implications.

The *normal arterial supply to the dura* is complex and merits brief preliminary discussion. The dura receives a major supply by the middle meningeal artery from the external carotid circulation, but small meningeal branches from the ascending pharyngeal and occipital arteries also contribute. In addition, the accessory meningeal artery, a branch of the middle meningeal or maxillary arteries, passes through the foramen ovale to supply adjacent dura. The basal dura is supplied by small branches from the cavernous portion of the internal carotid artery; the meningo-hypophyseal trunk supplies part of the tentorium and dura adjacent to the cavernous sinus and clivus, by tentorial, dorsal meningeal and inferior hypophyseal branches, while the artery to the inferior cavernous sinus (Parkinson, 1964) and the capsular arteries of McConnell (1953) also supply adjacent dura. Additional meningeal vessels arise from the ophthalmic artery and several of its branches; its ethmoidal branches give off vessels to supply the floor of the anterior fossa, and anterior part of the falx and adjacent dura, while its lacrimal branch

may contribute to the supply of the dura of the middle fossa. Small infratentorial meningeal branches from the posterior cerebral artery supply the midline strip of the tentorium, while meningeal branches of the vertebral artery supply the falx cerebelli and adjacent dura. There are normally extensive anastomoses between these meningeal branches, and numerous arteriovenous shunts also exist in the dura, especially parasagittally (Rowbotham & Little, 1965).

The dural venous sinuses can be classified into an anterior-inferior group (cavernous, intercavernous, sphenoparietal, superior and inferior petrosal sinuses, and basilar plexus) and a superiorposterior group (superior and inferior sagittal, straight, transverse, sigmoid and occipital sinuses) which are interconnected. Their anatomy is well known and warrants no further description. The vascular anomalies occurring in the dura are, however, best considered in relation to their venous drainage, as in the following discussion.

The clinical features of abnormal dural arteriovenous shunts may be indistinguishable from those of cerebral angiomas. In general, however, headache and tinnitus are common presenting symptoms, and a bruit is found more often than in patients with cerebral lesions. The presence of a bruit is helpful in suggesting a structural basis for symptoms and in lateralizing the lesion, but is of much lesser value in defining the site of the anomaly with any confidence. Seizures and focal neurological deficits occur less often than in patients with cerebral angiomas, but hemorrhage has a similar incidence (Aminoff, 1973). Radiographs of the skull sometimes reveal prominent vascular markings and/or an enlarged foramen spinosum when the main arterial supply to the anomaly is from the external carotid circulation, but the definitive investigation is arteriography. Selective, bilateral internal and external carotid angiography, and vertebral angiography, are usually necessary, as feeders may originate from many different sources. Furthermore, the malformation can only be localized radiologically to the dura if both its arterial and venous components are durally situated, since, as already emphasized, dural arteries may supply an intracerebral lesion (Newton & Cronqvist, 1969).

Arteriovenous shunts to the anterior-inferior group of dural sinuses

The clinical features of an arteriovenous shunt between meningeal branches of the internal and/or external carotid artery and the cavernous sinus, or a venous structure draining into it, have been described by numerous authors (including Hayes, 1963; Pool & Potts, 1965; Castaigne et al, 1966; Mingrino & Moro, 1967; Clemens & Lodin, 1968a; Rosenbaum & Schechter, 1969) and reviewed in a series of 11 patients by Newton & Hoyt (1970). They occur more commonly in women than in men, usually in middle or later life. Unilateral head pain is commonly the initial symptom, and is localized to the orbit, frontal or temporal region. Diplopia caused by a sixth nerve palsy is also a fairly common early symptom, while other patients may present with a red eye, unilateral tinnitus, or mild protrusion of the eye. On examination (Fig. 15.3), mild proptosis, dilated conjunctival veins, increased intraocular pressure, and sometimes a transient, unilateral sixth nerve palsy are typically found on the involved side. An orbital bruit is present in about 50 per cent of cases. Patients are often misdiagnosed as having a direct carotid-cavernous fistula, but ocular pulsations are absent and marked proptosis, with chemosis and swelling of the eyelid, is uncommon. Spontaneous thrombosis occurs frequently in part of the cavernous sinus and some of its draining veins (Brismar & Brismar, 1976) and may result in closure of the fistulous communication, in some instances shortly after angiography (Newton & Hoyt, 1970). Intolerable symptoms or failing vision may, however, necessitate an attempt to occlude at least some of the feeding arteries, and embolization may be helpful in such circumstances (Aminoff, 1973; Hilal & Michelsen, 1975).

The etiology of these anomalous shunts is unclear. Signs appeared spontaneously in 10 of the 11 patients of Newton and Hoyt, and followed definite head trauma in only one. Congenital anomalies may have been responsible in some of the 10 patients with symptoms that developed spontaneously, but in other instances rupture of the thin-walled dural arteries traversing the cavernous sinus — either spontaneously, following mild trauma, or for other reasons — may have

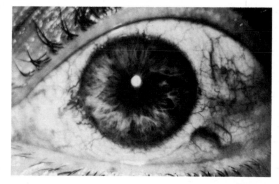
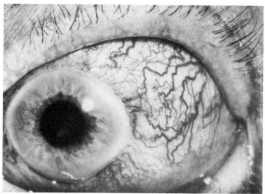
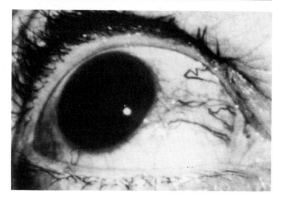

Fig. 15.3 Minimal proptosis and mild conjunctival injection in three separate patients with dural vascular anomalies involving the cavernous sinus. (Courtesy of Dr W. F. Hoyt.)

been responsible. Trauma was directly implicated in all three cases described by Hayes (1963), and in some of the individual cases reported by others. The onset of symptoms sometimes relates to the post-partum period (Newton & Hoyt, 1970; Taniguchi et al, 1971), possibly because of straining during labor or the circulatory changes that occur during pregnancy.

Angiography shows that the dural shunt is

usually of low volume, and that its arterial supply is derived from meningeal branches of the internal and/or external carotid arteries, sometimes from the contralateral side. Very occasionally, there may be a major contribution from the vertebral artery through one of its meningeal branches (Laine et al, 1963; Edwards & Connolly, 1977). The most common sources from the external carotid are terminal meningeal branches of the internal maxillary artery, and from the internal carotid the meningohypophyseal artery. The venous drainage is usually anteriorly into the ophthalmic veins, especially the superior ophthalmic vein. There may be some posterior drainage through the petrosal sinuses or the venous plexus of the clivus, but this is rarely the sole venous drainage.

Newton & Hoyt (1970) subdivided these anomalies into those draining directly into the cavernous sinus, and those involving a more distant dural sinus or a venous structure that communicates with the cavernous sinus. Two of their 11 patients had shunts of the latter type, emptying into a dural vein and thence into the cavernous sinus (Fig. 15.4).

Taniguchi et al (1971) reported a further 11 patients with spontaneous onset of symptoms reminiscent of a carotid-cavernous fistula, in whom angiography revealed abnormal arteriovenous communications about the cavernous sinus. In nearly all cases there was some degree of proptosis and conjunctival injection; chemosis, when present, was minimal and a bruit was found in only five patients. One patient presented solely because of tinnitus, and had no ocular symptoms whatever. The extent to which the patients were investigated angiographically, and the precise sources of feeders to the shunts, are not clear, but venous drainage was primarily through the inferior petrosal sinus, ophthalmic veins and/or the superficial Sylvian veins.

Anomalous dural arteriovenous shunts may also occur between the middle meningeal artery and the superior petrosal or sphenoparietal sinuses, either as a sequel to head injury (Fincher, 1951; Pakarinen, 1965) or without apparent cause (Markham, 1961). The main, often sole, complaint is of tinnitus which may be pulsatile. Examination generally reveals no abnormality other than a bruit that is often restricted to, or maximal in, the region

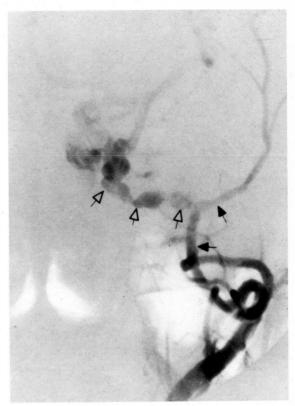

Fig. 15.4 Left external carotid arteriogram, frontal projection. An arteriovenous communication exists between the proximal middle meningeal artery (solid arrows) and a venous structure (open arrows), which drains medially into the cavernous sinus. (Reproduced from Newton T H, Hoyt W F 1970 Neuroradiology 1:71–81.)

about the ear. Simple ligation of the external carotid artery is sometimes effective, but in other instances resection of the fistula is necessary for relief of symptoms. Rare instances of a fistulous communication between meningeal arteries and other venous structures, such as the basilar venous plexus (Houser et al, 1972), have also been described.

Arteriovenous shunts to the superior-posterior group of dural sinuses

Anomalous dural arteriovenous shunts involving the transverse-sigmoid sinus are the most common of these anomalies, and their clinical features, described in individual cases by numerous authors, have been reviewed in detail by Aminoff (1973),

Obrador et al (1975), Kuhner et al (1976), and Houser et al (1979). There is a female predominance among the reported cases and most patients are over 40 years old at the time of presentation. Symptoms and signs can be attributed either to the shunt itself, or to subarachnoid hemorrhage, increased intracranial pressure or cerebral ischemia. Increased intracranial pressure may relate to an elevation of venous pressure in sinuses involved in the anomaly or to associated venous sinus thrombosis (Aminoff & Kendall, 1973); hydrocephalus may also occur as a sequel to subarachnoid hemorrhage or to aneurysmal dilatation of the vein of Galen. Cerebral ischemia results from 'steal' of blood by the anomalous shunt, or perhaps from focal venous stagnation (Houser et al, 1979). Tinnitus is the most common presenting complaint, but headache, progressive visual failure due to increased intracranial pressure, subarachnoid hemorrhage, focal or generalized seizures and various neurological deficits may occur. On examination, a bruit is often, but not always, present and may be the sole finding. It is generally best heard in the mastoid region or behind the ear. Papilledema may be present and other, often focal, neurological signs are found occasionally. In some patients, however, the vascular anomaly is asymptomatic, being an incidental finding at angiography (Aminoff & Kendall, 1973) or postmortem examination (McCormick & Boulter, 1966). Its blood supply is often derived from multiple sources, but contributions from the ipsilateral and/or contralateral occipital artery, middle meningeal artery, tentorial branches of the internal carotid artery and meningeal branches of the vertebral artery are especially common. Other meningeal arteries, including branches of the ophthalmic artery, may also be involved and occasionally there is a contribution from cervical branches of the subclavian artery (Urdanibia et al, 1974). The venous drainage is sometimes to a large dural lake that drains secondarily into the transverse-sigmoid sinus.

Abnormal dural arteriovenous shunts to the superior sagittal sinus have been described in several patients without any history of antecedent trauma (e.g., Ramamurthi & Balasubraminian, 1966; Newton et al, 1968; Kunc & Bret, 1969; Aminoff, 1973), and also following head injury

(Dennery & Ignacio, 1967). Anomalies involving the vein of Galen, the torcular (Fig. 15.5), or the superficial cerebral or cerebellar veins may also occur (Ciminello & Sachs, 1962; Newton et al, 1968; Kunc & Bret, 1969; Aminoff, 1973). Once again, the anomaly may be fed from multiple sources derived from the carotid (external and/or internal) and vertebral circulations. The usual clinical presentation is with papilledema, headache, subarachnoid hemorrhage or tinnitus.

Venous sinus thrombosis sometimes occurs spontaneously in patients with vascular anomalies involving the superior-posterior group of dural sinuses (Handa et al, 1975; Houser et al, 1979) and may lead to resolution of symptoms (Magidson & Weinberg, 1976). In other instances, ligation of individual feeding vessels may produce relief of symptoms, but the outcome of this procedure is often disappointing. Benefit has been reported to follow embolization of feeders (Hilal & Michelsen, 1975; Lamas et al, 1977), but evaluation is difficult because of the limited number of cases treated in this manner, the paucity of reported clinical details, and the relatively short period of follow-up. Surgical extirpation of the vascular anomaly, with occlusion of all its feeding vessels, is the most satisfactory treatment of patients with disabling symptoms or a history of hemorrhage. An alternative approach to the treatment of lesions involving the transverse and sigmoid sinuses has been reported by Hugosson & Bergstrom (1974), who surgically isolated these sinuses from all dural attachments, with apparent benefit (partial or complete relief of pulsatile tinnitus).

INTRADURAL SPINAL ANGIOMAS

Most symptomatic spinal angiomas are of the arteriovenous variety, and their prevalence ranges between 3 and 11 per cent of verified spinal tumours in different series. They have been reported in patients with cerebral, cerebellar or brainstem angiomas, and in patients with intracranial (Brion et al, 1952; Doppman & DiChiro, 1965) or spinal (Herdt et al, 1971; Caroscio et al, 1980) arterial aneurysms. They may also occur in the Rendu-Osler-Weber syndrome and with other vascular or lymphatic anomalies (Aminoff, 1976),

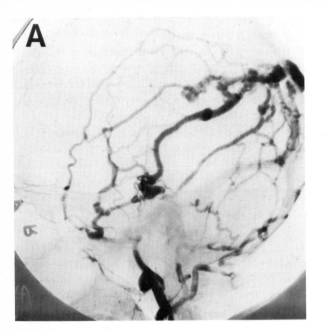
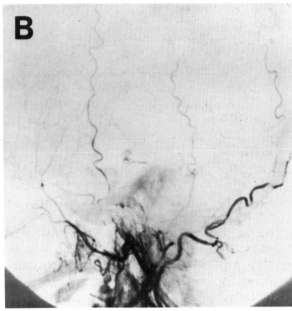

Fig. 15.5 A and B. Right external carotid angiogram, lateral projection. In A, an extensive dural arteriovenous malformation is shown. It is supplied by meningeal and scalp arteries, and drains into the torcular region. Six weeks after embolization of feeding vessels with polyvinyl alcohol sponge particles by Dr T. H. Newton, B shows that the abnormal arteriovenous communication is obliterated, with reduction in the size of visualized scalp and meningeal branches.

and are the responsible lesion in many cases of subacute necrotic myelopathy (Antoni, 1962). In most (80 per cent) cases, the abnormal fistula is mainly or completely extramedullary in location, usually lying behind the cord where it is fed by one or more arteries that do not supply the cord at all, or contribute only to the posterior spinal circulation.

The clinical and radiological features of spinal angiomas depend upon the location of the anomaly. Most (80 per cent) are located below the 2nd or 3rd thoracic segment of the cord, where they occur two or three times more frequently in males than females. Patients may present at any age, but the diagnosis is established most commonly when they are middle-aged. These malformations are usually extramedullary, tending to lie behind the cord where they are usually supplied by no more than one or two feeding vessels which generally do not supply the cord at all. In contrast, cervical malformations have an approximately equal sex incidence and tend to be diagnosed at an earlier age because they are more likely to bleed. They usually lie in front of the cord, are commonly partly

intramedullary, frequently have multiple feeding vessels and generally derive at least part of their blood supply from vessels supplying the cord as well.

Clinical features

Arteriovenous malformations present either with spinal subarachnoid hemorrhage or, more commonly, with a myelopathy or radiculopathy. Numerous case reports have been published, and are reviewed by Wyburn-Mason (1943), Aminoff (1976), and by others.

Spinal subarachnoid hemorrhage

Non-traumatic spinal subarachnoid hemorrhage is relatively rare. Its most common cause is an arteriovenous malformation, but it occurs occasionally in patients with telangiectasias, mycotic or other aneurysms of a spinal artery, coarctation of the aorta, various tumors (including ependymomas, neurofibromas, and meningeal sarcomas), blood dyscrasias, vasculitis (polyarteritis nodosa, systemic lupus erythematosus), and in certain infective states (Aminoff, 1976). Hemorrhage occurs in about 10–15 per cent of patients with spinal angiomas, and is especially liable to occur when the malformation is located in the cervical region (Aminoff, 1976). When an arterial aneurysm is also present, however, it may be a more likely source of bleeding (Herdt et al, 1971; Caroscio et al, 1980).

At the onset of the hemorrhage, sudden severe pain occurs in the region overlying its source. The pain spreads rapidly to the rest of the back and may be accompanied by radicular pain, especially in the legs. Signs of meningeal irritation may be accompanied by headache, a disturbance of consciousness, papilledema, cranial nerve palsies and other more widespread signs if blood passes intracranially, and this can lead to the mistaken assumption that the hemorrhage originated intracranially. Unless a spinal source is indicated by signs of hematomyelia or cord compression from hematoma, diagnosis may be delayed until the later development of a myelopathy or radiculopathy due to the underlying vascular malformation. The presence of a cutaneous angioma, especially on the back, or of a spinal bruit, suggest the possibility of a spinal lesion, however, and should specifically be searched for.

Subarachnoid hemorrhage from spinal arteriovenous malformations has an overall mortality of at least 15 per cent (Aminoff, 1976). Approximately half of the survivors from a first hemorrhage will have a second, and this occurs within a year of the initial bleed in about 40 per cent of patients with recurrent hemorrhage. Half of the subsequent survivors will have further episodes of bleeding unless the underlying malformation is treated.

Myeloradiculopathy

A myeloradiculopathy may develop either gradually (80 per cent of cases) or acutely (20 per cent) in patients with spinal angiomas, and is the usual mode of presentation. The individual symptoms and signs are similar to those caused by cord compression from any cause, but usually indicate extensive involvement along the length of the cord. In one series of 60 patients (Aminoff & Logue, 1974a), the most common initial symptom was

pain, and this occurred either alone or with other symptoms in 42 per cent of patients, being radicular in 23 per cent, localized to the back in 12 per cent, and remote, non-specific pain in 7 per cent. The other initial symptoms consisted of sensory disturbances in 33 per cent, leg weakness in 32 per cent, a disturbance of micturition, defecation or sexual function in 10 per cent, and subarachnoid hemorrhage in 5 per cent. Symptoms usually progress either steadily or episodically after their onset, but this downhill course can sometimes be interrupted by periods of partial remission that can last for several years. By the time of diagnosis, 65 per cent of the patients reported by Aminoff & Logue (1974a) complained of leg weakness, sensory symptoms, pain and a disturbance of micturition.

Certain features of the history may suggest an underlying vascular malformation when patients with a myelopathy or radiculopathy of uncertain etiology are being evaluated. In 19 of the 60 patients reported by Aminoff & Logue (1974a), for example, symptoms, especially pain, were precipitated or enhanced by exercise and relieved by rest. The pain was either localized to the back or legs, or occurred in both sites. Leg pain was usually radicular in distribution, unlike that produced by peripheral vascular disease, and was sometimes accompanied by other symptoms. A few patients developed motor or sensory disturbances without associated pain in response to exercise. The exercise tolerance varied considerably in different patients, but tended to diminish with time. In 14 of the 60 patients, pain or other symptoms were provoked or aggravated by a specific posture, such as sitting or bending forward. Less commonly, symptoms were related to pregnancy, infection, increased body temperature, or trauma. A relationship of symptoms to the menstrual cycle, breath-holding or straining at stool has also been reported (Aminoff, 1976), and recurrent, transient postprandial paresis of the legs has been described (Oliver et al, 1973).

Neurological examination commonly reveals a combined upper and lower motor neuron deficit in the legs, with an accompanying sensory deficit that is often extensive but sometimes confined to a radicular distribution. The motor deficit may consist solely of an upper or lower motor neuron disturbance, however, and there may be no accompanying sensory changes. Certain additional clinical signs may be present and they suggest the possibility of a vascular malformation as the cause of the neurological deficit. The presence of cutaneous angiomas, especially if related segmentally to the level of the spinal lesion, can be especially helpful. These skin lesions can be recognized more easily while patients perform the Valsalva maneuver. Cutaneous lesions were present in only two of the 60 patients reported by Aminoff & Logue (1974a) and were unrelated segmentally to the spinal malformation, but the prevalence of segmentally-related cutaneous angiomas was 12 per cent (Djindjian et al, 1970) and 21 per cent (Doppman et al, 1969) in other recent series of patients. The presence of such a skin lesion may aid in the angiographic work-up of the patient and influence the approach to surgical treatment, as is discussed below.

A bruit is sometimes audible in the region overlying a vascular malformation, as reported originally by Hook & Lidvall (1958), and by Matthews (1959). Accordingly, careful auscultation over the spine should never be omitted when patients with subarachnoid hemorrhage, myelopathy or a radiculopathy of obscure etiology are evaluated. The absence of a bruit does not, however, exclude an underlying angioma.

Substantial disability is likely to result in many untreated patients with symptomatic angiomas. Of the 60 patients evaluated by Aminoff & Logue (1974b), 33 eventually became unable to walk at all or required two sticks or crutches to get about; 10 patients were so disabled within six months, and 28 within three years, of the onset of any leg weakness or disturbance in walking.

Diagnostic investigations

Radiographs of the spine usually show no significant abnormality, but occasionally there is widening of the interpedicular distance or other radiological evidence of an intraspinal space-occupying lesion. Signs of an associated vertebral angioma are also encountered occasionally. A scoliosis or kyphoscoliosis may be present, but is of little diagnostic help.

The cerebrospinal fluid is often abnormal, but the findings are of little diagnostic help except to confirm that subarachnoid hemorrhage has occurred. In patients presenting without a bleed, the protein concentration is frequently increased in the absence of obstruction and there may be an accompanying pleocytosis. In a few patients, however, an increased cell content is the sole abnormality.

The diagnosis is usually suggested by positive contrast myelography, when the length of the cord should be visualized in both prone and supine positions, using a large volume (at least 20 ml) of contrast material. The characteristic finding (Fig. 15.6) is of tortuous filling defects due to vascular impressions in the column of contrast material, without any obstruction in the subarachnoid space. These defects may be localized to a few segments or extend along a considerable length of the cord and into the posterior fossa; in the thoracic region they may only be shown on supine films. The vascular impressions sometimes converge on one point which usually corresponds to the site of the fistula as shown at angiography (Fig. 15.6), and in such instances there may be a smooth projection from the cord shadow caused by the vessels forming the shunt itself (Logue et al, 1974).

Characteristic myelographic findings have been reported in at least 80 per cent of patients with spinal angiomas by several authors (Lombardi & Migliavacca, 1959; Svien & Baker, 1961; Aminoff & Logue, 1974a), but less commonly by others. Thus, Djindjian et al (1970) reported them in only about half of their patients, although less typical changes were found in many of the others.

Myelographic appearances simulating those of an angioma are sometimes encountered in patients with vascular tumors having prominent draining veins. Tortuous, redundant lumbar nerve roots may also have a similar appearance, but any doubt can be resolved by examining the spine in slight flexion to straighten them (Kendall, 1976).

Selective spinal angiography should be undertaken if the myelographic appearance is suggestive of an angioma. Angiography is generally unrewarding when myelography reveals no abnormality in patients with a suspected vascular malformation, but any decision in this regard can only be made on an individual basis. Angiography is undertaken to confirm the presence of a malformation, to determine its level and extent, to define the position of

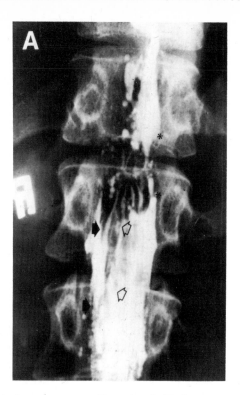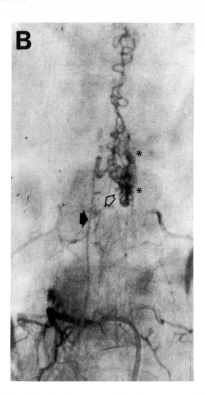

Fig. 15.6 Spinal arteriovenous malformation. A, Myelogram, prone film. The feeding artery (black arrows) and descending vein (hollow arrows) are outlined. These vessels converge towards a constant defect (asterisks) caused by the nidus of vessels in the region of the shunt. The theca above the shunt is incompletely filled, but draining veins are partly outlined in this region also. B, Spinal angiogram, selective injection of right 2nd lumbar artery. The feeding artery (black arrow) ascends along the right side of the theca to T12–L1 vertebral level before crossing the midline to supply the shunt (asterisks). Draining veins mainly ascend, but a fairly large descending vein is indicated (hollow arrow). (Reproduced from Logue et al, 1974 Journal of Neurology, Neurosurgery, and Psychiatry 37:1074–1081.)

the vascular shunt in relation to the spinal cord, and to identify all of its feeding vessels. In addition, the normal blood supply to the spinal cord in the vicinity of the malformation, and especially the regional supply to the anterior spinal artery, must be determined so that damage to it can be avoided at operation. This is achieved by injecting with contrast medium the orifices of the segmental arteries coming off the aorta, so that the segmental vessels entering the spinal canal are opacified. The clinical or myelographic findings will determine which vessels are injected first, but the presence of a cutaneous angioma may suggest the likely level and side of vessels feeding the spinal lesion. The reader is referred to the account by Kendall (1976) for procedural details of the technique.

The site of the fistulous portion of the malformation as determined at angiography does not necessarily coincide with the clinical level of the

lesion, or the site of maximal abnormality at myelography. Three types of angiographic appearance have been described (DiChiro & Wener, 1973). The most common appearance, Type 1, is of an angioma fed by only one or two vessels that do not supply the cord at all. The bulk of the malformation consists of long tortuous vessels on the posterior surface of the cord, and blood flow through the malformation is slow. A more compact coil of vessels characterizes Type 2 ('Glomus') malformations, which are otherwise similar to the preceding variety. Type 3 malformations occur predominantly in children and young adults and have multiple feeders that may also contribute to the spinal cord circulation. The fistulous portion of the malformation may be anterior or posterior to the cord and is often intramedullary, at least in part; transit time through the malformation is generally rapid. The angiographic appearances seem to depend in part upon the location of the lesion (Aminoff, 1976). Angiomas in the cervical region are often of the juvenile (Type 3) variety, while more caudally placed lesions generally appear as Types 1 or 2.

Vascular malformations can also be visualized with contrast-enhanced C.T. scans (DiChiro et al, 1977), and the method shows promise of being useful as a screening procedure for patients with these vascular anomalies. However its place in this regard remains to be defined and at the present time myelography and angiography are the investigative methods of choice.

Pathology and pathophysiology

At autopsy or operation, a collection of abnormal distended intradural vessels are seen to overlie, usually without compressing, part of the posterior surface of the cord, but sometimes only a single coiled vessel is present. The anomalous vessels are sometimes more conspicuous anteriorly, especially if the angioma is located in the cervical region. Vessels may run between these surface vessels and the cord, particularly when the malformation lies anteriorly. Save in exceptional cases (Antoni, 1962), it is usually not possible to define the precise site of shunting between arterial and venous systems except by injection techniques, and it may be hard to determine the individual vessels. The cord may be expanded due to hemorrhage, edema, or an intramedullary component of the malformation, or shrunken due to ischemic necrosis. Leptomeningeal thickening, staining and adhesions are common. Microscopically, the surface vessels are atypical and deformed, with defects in the elastica and media, and hypertrophied walls of irregular thickness; some may be occluded by thrombus. Within the cord, small vessels with thickened hyalinized walls, are prolific, especially posteriorly and laterally. There is variable degeneration of neurons and axons, demyelination of fiber tracks, and glial proliferation. Intravascular thrombosis is sometimes conspicuous but may be completely absent. Cystic infarction of the cord or hematomyelic changes may also be present, as may enlarged abnormal arteries and veins and a mass of sinusoidal vascular channels, if the malformation is intramedullary, at least in part.

The acute onset of neurological symptoms and signs may be due to intramedullary (Odom et al, 1957) or subarachnoid hemorrhage (Henson & Croft, 1956), or to intravascular thrombosis (Wyburn-Mason, 1943). The mechanism by which symptoms develop gradually and progressively is, however, less clear. There is usually little evidence of compression when the cord is examined radiologically, at operation, or at autopsy. Cord ischemia due to diversion of blood through the malformation from the normal intraspinal circulation as a 'steal' phenomenon may sometimes be responsible. However, except in the cervical region arteries supplying the malformation do not commonly arise from a vessel feeding the anterior or posterior spinal arteries, and arteries to angioma and cord are not derived from the same segmental stem; moreover, the circulations through the angioma and the cord are usually distinct (Aminoff et al, 1974). For these reasons, it seems unlikely that 'steal' accounts for the production of symptoms in most cases.

Aminoff et al (1974) suggested that neurological dysfunction related to increased pressure in the coronal veins draining the malformation. These veins, which form an interconnected plexus, drain part of the intramedullary circulation, and as the pressure in them increases the arteriovenous pressure gradient across the spinal cord will be reduced. This, in turn, will reduce intramedullary blood flow, and thus lead to ischemic hypoxia. Such a concept helps to explain the common relationship of symptoms to mechanical factors such as posture. It also accounts for the cord syndrome described by Logue (1979) in a patient with an angioma that was supplied by the left lateral sacral artery and lay in the hollow of the sacrum below the termination of the dural sac; the only vessel entering the theca was a large vein running up in the filum terminals to ascend on the surface of the cord, and division of this vein led to improvement in symptoms.

Treatment

No satisfactory medical treatment is available and surgical treatment should be reserved for malformations that are symptomatic. The prospects for complete recovery after surgery are generally greater in patients with mild symptoms and no incapacity than in those with marked disability. Surgery is indicated in patients with rapidly progressive symptoms or with functional incapacity clearly influencing the pattern of daily life. It is also indicated in patients with a history of subarachnoid hemorrhage because of the risk of further bleeding. When symptoms are mild and there is no significant disability, however, decisions concerning surgical treatment will be influenced by such factors as the age and general condition of the patient, the experience of the surgeon, the availability of such facilities as the operating microscope and the angiographic character of the lesion.

Most (80 per cent) malformations are predominantly extramedullary, lie behind the cord, and are fed by vessels not contributing to the anterior spinal circulation, so their surgical treatment usually poses no particular problem. In contrast, malformations located mainly anterior to, or within, the cord are difficult to treat because of their inaccessibility. Moreover, such malformations are commonly fed by the anterior spinal artery or by one or more of its feeding vessels, occlusion of which may further impair the cord circulation. Most of these inaccessible malformations are located in the cervical region, but occasionally a thoracolumbar malformation supplied either by the anterior spinal artery or the artery of Adamkiewicz is encountered. Occlusion of the artery of Adamkiewicz in such circumstances is sometimes well tolerated (Newton & Adams, 1968; DiChiro & Wener, 1973), but this is not always so. Controlled embolization may well be a useful alternative approach in such circumstances (Djindjian, 1975), the aim being to occlude the feeding branches but preserve the main arterial supply to the cord.

Unless the malformation has an extradural location, surgical treatment is directed to abolishing the blood supply of the malformation by intradural ligation, and is best combined with excision of the fistulous portion of the malformation in an attempt to reduce any possibility of its revascularization. Further details of the surgical technique concerned and of the outcome that can be expected, are given elsewhere (Aminoff, 1976; Logue, 1979). A previously progressive downhill course will generally be arrested by surgery and pain is usually relieved. Undoubted improvement in gait can be expected in at least 60 per cent of cases, and disturbances of sphincter function may also improve, although less frequently. The degree of motor improvement can be very worthwhile; of the seven chairbound patients operated on by Logue (1979), two were subsequently enabled to walk without support, one to get about with a stick, and two to walk with crutches, while only two remained unable to walk at all. Modest improvement in sensory disturbances may also occur, but can be hard to evaluate.

Percutaneous embolization of feeding vessels is a simple, safe technique which was first applied to the treatment of spinal arteriovenous malformations by Doppman et al (1968) and by Newton & Adams (1968). Progressive neurological improvement was subsequently reported by Doppman et al (1971) in three of five patients in whom embolization was successfully achieved under local anesthesia. In the series of patients reported by Djindjian (1976), however, the results of embolization were often disappointing, perhaps reflecting the complexity of the cases that were managed in this way. Thus among his 10 patients with retromedullary angiomas, embolization with gelfoam was definitely ineffective in seven, and probably ineffective in another two patients.

The technique of embolization would seem to have particular appeal when direct operative treatment is especially hazardous or is otherwise not feasible. For example, in the case reported by Doppman and his colleagues (1968), embolization was undertaken because a large overlying cutaneous angioma precluded any approach by laminectomy. In patients with established paraplegia and gross sphincteric dysfunction, embolization is sometimes worthwhile even if a direct surgical approach is deemed unjustifiable, since it may reduce pain and lessen the risk of subarachnoid hemorrhage. There are complications of the procedure, however, and these include occlusion of vessels other than the intended ones. Enlargement of the malformation may also occur if the embolus passes through to block its draining veins, and in such instances hemorrhage may result. In expert hands, selective embolization of certain intramedullary malformations supplied via the anterior spinal circulation is sometimes feasible (Djindjian, 1975), but there is then the very real risk of causing a gross neurological deficit if a block occurs in the main vessels feeding the cord itself.

Another possible therapeutic approach is to inject intra-arterially a material that will form an intravascular cast within the malformation, thereby occluding all of the feeding vessels. At the present time, it is not clear that such a technique has any practical relevance, but the results in one recent preliminary study, using intra-arterial cyanoacrylate, were encouraging (Kerber et al, 1978).

EPIDURAL SPINAL ANGIOMAS

Epidural angiomas are less common than the intrathecal malformations just described. Angiomas that are purely epidural are usually located in the thoracic region (Guthkelch, 1948), but epidural malformations may coexist with cutaneous (Johnston, 1938), vertebral or intradural spinal angiomas (Van Bogaert, 1950; Newquist & Mayfield, 1960; Pia, 1973).

Epidural angiomas may lead to a complete or incomplete cord syndrome and this can develop either gradually or acutely, occasionally in relation to pregnancy (Guthkelch, 1948). Hemorrhage sometimes accounts for the cord disturbance when it has an acute onset, but the c.s.f. findings are usually of no diagnostic help because of the extradural location of the bleed.

The efferent components of epidural angiomas may drain into the coronal venous plexus on the surface of the cord (Kendall & Logue, 1977), and the myelographic appearances are then indistinguishable from those of intradural spinal angiomas. Angiography generally permits the epidural site of the arteriovenous shunt to be recognized, however, and usually indicates also that no more than one or two feeding vessels are involved. The extradural location of these malformations usually makes them readily amenable to surgical excision and the risks of damage to the cord are reduced because the vessels on its surface can be left undisturbed (Logue, 1979).

MISCELLANEOUS SYNDROMES

Wyburn-Mason syndrome

The eponymous designation of Wyburn-Mason syndrome is often used in the English-language literature to refer to the rare association of a mesencephalic arteriovenous malformation with an ipsilateral retinal angioma and facial nevus (Wyburn-Mason, 1943b). Its clinical and radiological features have been reviewed by Theron et al (1974), who reported three new cases and reviewed the findings in 22 previously published ones.

The cerebral lesion is unilateral and deeply placed, frequently implicates the optic pathway, and is supplied from the carotid and/or vertebral circulations. It most often involves the chiasm, hypothalamus, basal ganglia and mid-brain, and sometimes the vermis as well, but the entire optic pathway from retina to occipital cortex (Figs. 15.7 & 15.8) may be affected (Theron et al, 1974). Symptoms include seizures, headaches, bruit, hemorrhage or focal neurological deficits but the lesion is occasionally asymptomatic. Clinical examination frequently reveals homonymous field defects, pyramidal signs, and/or mental retardation, while cerebral or subarachnoid hemorrhage, cerebellar deficits or a Parinaud syndrome are less common manifestations. In rare instances a dural

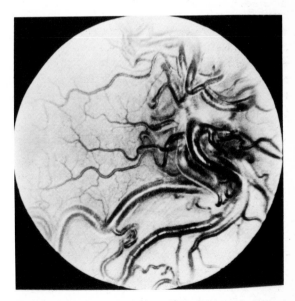

Fig. 15.7 Arteriovenous malformation of right optic disc and retina in a patient with the Wyburn-Mason syndrome. There is gross dilatation of superior and inferior retinal arteries and veins. The optic nerve is completely obscured by the malformation. (Reproduced from Theron et al, 1974 Neuroradiology 7:185–196.)

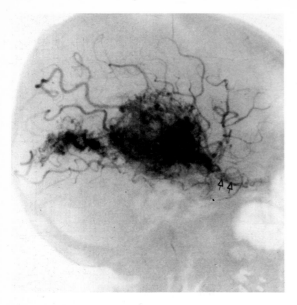

Fig. 15.8 Right internal carotid angiogram, lateral projection, late arterial phase; same patient as in Figure 15.7. An extensive vascular malformation involves the optic nerve (arrow), hypothalamus, basal ganglia and calcarine cortex. (Reproduced from Theron et al, 1974 Neuroradiology 7:185–196.)

angioma may coexist with the cerebral one (Tamaki et al, 1971).

Among the 25 cases reviewed by Theron et al (1974), a cutaneous vascular nevus involving the ipsilateral face or eyelids was present in six patients, but was sometimes very inconspicuous. Facial asymmetry was also evident in some and presumably related to hypoplasia. A vascular malformation involving the jaws, nose or mouth was found in 10 patients and sometimes led to recurrent bleeding from the nose, gums, or tonsils. The associated ipsilateral retinal arteriovenous malformation was of variable appearance, was always unilateral and was easily recognized with an ophthalmoscope. Clusters of peripherally-situated microaneurysms were also sometimes present in the retina. Involvement by the malformation of retrobulbar tissue was frequent; dilated vascular channels were often evident within the optic nerve at angiography, and in one patient the nerve was replaced almost entirely by a tangle of dilated vascular channels. There was often a mild non-pulsatile proptosis, dilatation of conjunctival vessels and a decrease in visual acuity, but acuity was occasionally normal.

It is difficult to establish the incidence of this rare syndrome. The extent of the malformation in the brain and facial tissues cannot be predicted from the clinical symptoms or signs. Most patients present with monocular amblyopia, and ophthalmological examination then reveals the retinal vascular malformation. Unless such patients are investigated further, a coexisting cerebral lesion may be missed if neurological manifestations are clinically inconspicuous. Moreover, two patients with vascular malformations involving the basal ganglia and ipsilateral optic nerve, but sparing the retina, have recently been described (Brown et al, 1973).

Sturge-Weber syndrome

The Sturge-Weber syndrome of encephalofacial angiomatosis is characterized by a congenital, usually unilateral, cutaneous capillary angioma of the upper part of the face, leptomeningeal angiomatosis and, in many patients, a choroidal angioma. The disorder affects both sexes equally and usually occurs sporadically. The cutaneous angioma may have an extensive distribution over the head and neck and is usually very disfiguring except in black patients, especially if there is associated overgrowth of connective tissue. Focal or generalized seizures are generally the presenting feature of neurological involvement and often commence during infancy. Intracranial bleeding is unusual. Examination commonly reveals, in addition to the cutaneous lesion, a contralateral homonymous hemianopia, hemiparesis, hemisensory disturbance and mental subnormality, and the contralateral limbs are often small and poorly developed. There is no cranial bruit. Buphthalmos or glaucoma may be found on the same side as the facial nevus. A number of variants of the classical syndrome have been described, and are reviewed by Alexander (1972).

Skull radiographs usually reveal gyriform ('tramline') intracranial calcification after the first two years of life, especially in the occipital and posterior parietal region, due to mineral deposition in the cortex beneath the intracranial vascular malformation. The distance between the gyriform opacities and the inner table of the skull may be increased due to cerebral atrophy, while the overlying skull vault may be thickened and show an enlarged diploic space (Nellhaus, et al, 1967).

Electroencephalograms generally show depressed normal background activity over the affected hemisphere and irregular slow activity and sharp transients may occur ipsilaterally (Brenner & Sharbrough, 1976).

Although some authorities consider that the lesion is too extensive for neurosurgical intervention, others have recommended occipital lobectomy in the hope of alleviating or preventing the seizure disorder and limiting the intellectual decline (Alexander, 1972). Medical treatment should be directed at controlling seizures and ophthalmological advice should be sought concerning any choroidal angioma and increased intraocular pressure.

Hereditary hemorrhagic telangiectasia (Rendu-Osler-Weber syndrome)

This is a familial disorder with an autosomal dominant mode of inheritance, in which recurrent hemorrhage occurs from multiple cutaneous, mucosal and visceral telangiectasias (Figs. 15.9 & 15.10). The commonest neurological manifestations relate to complications of the pulmonary arteriovenous fistulae that are a feature of the disorder, and include cerebral abscess, hypoxia and embolic phenomena. In addition, however, various types of vascular anomalies, including telangiectasias, cavernous angiomas, arteriovenous malformations and aneurysms, may occur in the brain or spinal cord, and the reader is referred to the paper of Ronan et al (1978) for an extensive recent review of the literature. The telangiectasias are usually asymptomatic, but may lead to hemorrhage that occasionally is devastatingly severe. The disorder may be associated with seizures, progressive hydrocephalus and/or focal neurological deficits that are sometimes a sequel of minor hemorrhage.

Malformations involving the vein of Galen

Arteriovenous malformations involving the vein of Galen are rare. Presentation in the neonatal period is usually with congestive cardiac failure that often has a fatal outcome and other congenital anomalies may also be present (Gold et al, 1964). Infants usually present with hydrocephalus (due to aqueductal compression by the dilated vein of Galen),

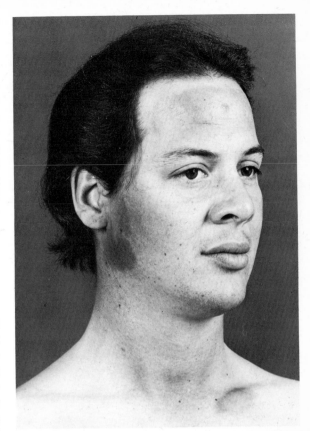

Fig. 15.9 Multiple cutaneous telangiectasias in a patient with Rendu-Osler-Weber syndrome.

convulsions or distended tortuous scalp veins and this may be followed by psychomotor retardation, enlargement of the heart and the development of diffuse pyramidal and other neurological signs. The presence of a cranial bruit is usual but not invariable. In older patients, headaches and/or subarachnoid hemorrhage are common presenting features, but the main complaint is sometimes of a seizure disorder. Focal neurological deficits indicative of brainstem or hemispheric dysfunction subsequently develop and may include a Parinaud syndrome but a cranial bruit is rare. In infants and young children, cardiomegaly is evident on chest radiographs and increased intracranial pressure on skull films, while in older teenagers and adults the wall of the vein of Galen may be outlined by calcification on the skull radiographs (Thomson, 1959). Bilateral carotid and vertebral angiography excludes a tumor, indicates the nature of the lesion,

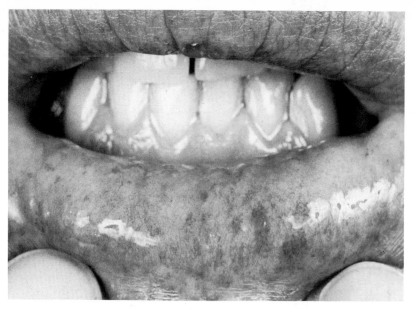

Fig. 15.10 Mucosal telangiectasias in a patient with Rendu-Osler-Weber syndrome.

and is necessary to define all of the vessels involved in the malformation. A midline collection of contrast material is seen, with enlargement of feeders (often one or both posterior cerebral arteries, and frequently other vessels as well), and marked dilatation of draining sinuses. Medical management is directed at maintaining cardiac function and controlling seizures, definitive treatment of the malformation being surgical.

Carotid-cavernous fistulae

A carotid-cavernous arteriovenous fistula results from rupture of the wall of either the intracavernous carotid artery or one of its branches. This occurs most commonly following orbitocranial perforating injuries or after blunt head injury that often involves the ipsilateral frontal region and is usually associated with basal skull fracture. Fistulae may also develop spontaneously, perhaps, in some instances, because of a developmental anomaly, rupture of an intracavernous aneurysm (Obrador et al, 1974; Morley, 1976), or atherosclerotic degeneration of the arterial wall. Spontaneous fistulae have also been reported in patients with Ehlers-Danlos syndrome (Graf, 1965) pseudo-xanthoma elasticum (Rios-Montenegro et al, 1972), or hereditary hemorrhagic telangiectasia

(Von Rad & Tornow, 1975). In many spontaneous cases, however, the fistula is not a direct carotid-cavernous one, but involves meningeal branches of the internal carotid and other major arteries, and such anomalies are considered separately on pp. 303–5. Skull radiographs may show abnormalities relating to causal head trauma, but are otherwise of little diagnostic help. Angiography is the definitive investigation and should involve selective bilateral opacification of both internal and external carotid vessels and the vertebral arteries to establish the nature and extent of the fistula. The characteristic findings (Fig. 15.11) are early dense opacification of the cavernous sinus and of the veins that normally drain it, and poor opacification of the cerebral veins. The cavernous sinus itself may be enlarged or aneurysmally dilated. Its venous drainage is mainly to the superior ophthalmic vein but may also involve the inferior ophthalmic vein, the other cavernous sinus, the pterygoid plexus, the petrosal sinuses or the Sylvian veins (Clemens & Lodin, 1968b; Newton & Troost, 1974).

The fistula diminishes ophthalmic artery pressure and increases venous pressure, causing a reduced retinal arteriovenous pressure gradient and perfusion pressure that lead in turn to capillary shunting and distension, and to venous dilation (Sanders & Hoyt, 1969). Similar hemodynamic

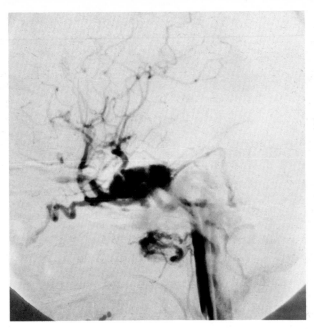

Fig. 15.11 Left internal carotid angiogram, lateral projection. An internal carotid-cavernous sinus fistula is demonstrated, with drainage into the ophthalmic veins, inferior petrosal sinus and Sylvian veins. There is poor opacification of the left middle cerebral artery.

changes also occur in the orbit. Cerebral ischemia does not occur unless attempts are made to correct the fistula by vascular occlusive procedures (Stern et al, 1967), arterial anastomoses presumably compensating for any 'steal' that may occur. Cerebral symptoms in untreated cases usually relate to preceding trauma.

In a review of 224 previously published cases, Martin & Mabon (1943) reported a bruit in 85 per cent, pulsatile proptosis in 80 per cent, chemosis in 70 per cent, diplopia in 34 per cent, headache in 32 per cent and visual disturbances in 30 per cent. The bruit can be so troublesome that it leads to demands for surgical treatment. It is often present over much of the head, but is best heard over the eye on the affected side; it can generally be reduced by ipsilateral carotid compression, except in long-standing cases. Proptosis is usually present ipsilaterally, is sometimes slowly progressive over several weeks and may limit ocular mobility. Contralateral proptosis may also occur, often at the same time or within a few weeks of that developing ipsilaterally, and presumably relates to shunting of arterial blood through the intercavernous sinuses from the involved to the opposite cavernous sinus. Trans-mission of the pulse wave from the carotid or ophthalmic arteries to the ophthalmic vein causes visible or palpable ocular pulsations in most patients, and distension and dilatation of periorbital vessels (Fig. 15.12) may be associated with chronic skin changes. Involvement of the sixth nerve, and/or the third or fourth nerves, may result from the injury causing the fistula, or from compression by a preexisting carotid aneurysm or a dilated, arterialized cavernous sinus. There may also be involvement of the first or second division of the fifth nerve.

Sanders & Hoyt (1969) directed attention particularly at the ocular findings. Examination of 25 patients generally revealed extreme tortuosity of conjunctival vessels with dilatation and thickening of veins and ipsilateral proptosis. In three cases, conjunctival changes and proptosis occurred bilaterally, but were clearly more conspicuous on the side of the fistula. Lid swelling and chemosis occurred in all patients with ocular symptoms of rapid onset. Seven patients had preoperative ischemic changes in the anterior segment of the eye, accompanied in all cases by hypoxic fundal abnormalities. Dilated retinal veins were the most

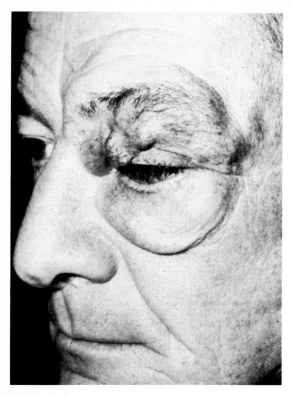

Fig. 15.12 Chronic carotid-cavernous fistula. There is marked dilatation of subcutaneous palpebral veins which have been arterialized by the fistula. (Reproduced from Walsh F B, Hoyt W F 1969 Clinical neuro-ophthalmology. Williams & Wilkins, Baltimore.)

frequent fundoscopic finding, and were present in all patients who complained of a constricted visual field and dimming in the involved eye. Scattered punctate or perivenous hemorrhages were also found in some, and multiple microaneurysms were occasionally conspicuous. Vitreous hemorrhage from microaneurysms was a complicating factor in only one patient, and definite swelling of the optic disc was found only once. These findings suggested that hypoxia was generally the pathophysiological basis of visual failure, except when direct ocular or optic nerve involvement occurred in traumatic cases.

Surgical procedures, such as single or multiple arterial ligations, which lower the local arterial pressure without concomitant reduction in venous or intraocular pressure will aggravate the already-impaired ocular circulation, and may cause further visual deterioration (Stern et al, 1967; Sanders &

Hoyt, 1969), even though proptosis and conjunctival swelling diminish. Accordingly, careful consideration of the aims and risks of treatment must precede surgical intervention. The rare presence of an aneurysm enlarging beyond the cavernous sinus is an indication for operation to prevent fatal rupture. Treatment to maintain or improve visual function is also justified but the presence of hypoxic retinopathy does not necessarily signify imminent blindness (Sanders & Hoyt, 1969). Patients occasionally demand treatment of disfiguring proptosis or a bruit, and rational discussion of the potential hazards may be dissuasive in such circumstances.

Spontaneous closure of the fistula sometimes occurs, and apparently did so in 4 of 11 untreated patients reported by Morley (1976). Only brief comment can be made here concerning surgical approaches to treatment. The various techniques employed include cervical ligation of the internal, external or common carotid arteries, either alone or in various combinations. Various trapping procedures, in which the internal carotid artery is occluded both cervically and intracranially (Hamby, 1964), have also been devised. Intracranial occlusion distal to the fistula is intended to prevent flow into the fistula from above and 'steal' of blood to the fistula from the contralateral hemisphere through the normal intracranial arterial anastomoses, thereby reducing the likelihood of ischemic cerebral complications.

Summarizing the surgical experience at Toronto General Hospital, Morley (1976) reported a high incidence of persistent fistulae and of ocular or ischemic cerebral complications, following proximal arterial occlusion. Ocular, but not cerebral, complications were also common with 'trapping' procedures, due presumably to aggravation of the already-impaired ocular circulation, as discussed earlier.

When 'trapping' procedures were combined with the direct introduction of macerated muscle into the intracavernous carotid artery, to ensure that fistulae were completely and permanently plugged, no ocular or cerebral complications occurred in any of 8 patients reported by Morley (1976). Similarly, local intracarotid injection of acrylic has been successful in a patient previously subjected to multiple arterial ligations (El Gindi & Andrew, 1967). Nevertheless, such procedures carry a definite risk of serious cerebral complications, as the carotid circulation is obliterated.

Several methods have been developed that preserve the carotid circulation. That described by Hosobuchi (1975) involved electrothrombosis of the fistula, and publication of his latest results is awaited with interest. Mullan (1979) reported the occlusion of 33 carotid-cavernous fistulae, without mortality and little morbidity, using a variety of thrombogenic techniques. Visual symptoms were relieved in all patients who were not already blind. A direct surgical approach, with repair of the fistula and preservation of carotid artery flow, has also proved feasible in some instances (Parkinson, 1973).

Treatment by muscle embolization was advocated by Brooks (1930) and Lang & Bucy (1965), but the embolus may enter the cerebral circulation, or pass on in the cavernous sinus to the arterialized veins draining it (Sedzimir & Occleshaw, 1967). Embolization can be combined with a 'trapping' procedure, in which the cerebral circulation is protected by occlusion of the internal carotid artery immediately above the cavernous sinus, and the cervical internal carotid artery is ligated after the embolus has lodged in the fistula, to prevent the embolus from passing on (Jaeger, 1949; Hamby, 1964). The results of this combined approach are not, however, substantially better than with the 'trapping' procedure alone (Morley, 1976).

Others have used a muscle embolus bearing a metal marker and attached to a long thread. The embolus is introduced through the cervical carotid artery and the thread permits its withdrawal if its final position, as determined radiographically, is not adequate; once it is positioned, the carotid artery is ligated in the neck (Arutiunov et al, 1968). This technique was successfully modified by Black et al (1973) who preserved intact the carotid circulation, attaching the thread to cervical fascia to tether the embolus and prevent its passage beyond the target. A somewhat similar technique, but employing emboli of polyurethane foam, was also used with success by Ohta et al (1973).

Perhaps the most promising therapeutic development is the use of balloon catheters, as pioneered by Serbinenko (1974). The method is simple and safe, and the balloon itself can be positioned correctly under radiographic control. In the technique developed by Prolo & Hanbery (1971),

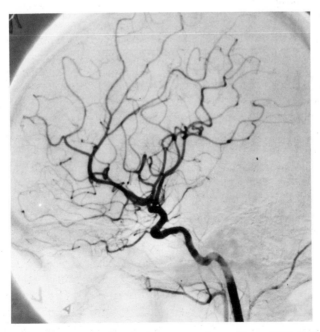

Fig. 15.13 Left internal carotid angiogram, lateral projection; same patient as Figure 15.11. Following placement of a detachable balloon in the left cavernous sinus by Dr T. H. Newton, the previously demonstrated carotid-cavernous fistula is closed, with maintenance of flow in the internal carotid artery and excellent opacification of the intracerebral vessels.

proximal ligation of the carotid artery is included as part of the procedure, but occlusion of the fistula by a balloon placed within the intracavernous carotid artery at a point proximal to the origin of the ophthalmic artery, preserves flow through this artery while lowering venous pressure. When a detachable balloon is used, it is not necessary to ligate the carotid artery (Fig. 15.13). Encouraging results with the use of a balloon catheter technique have been reported (Grunert & Sunder-Plass-

mann, 1971; Markham, 1974; Prolo & Hanbery, 1976; Newton, personal communication), and the method may well become the future treatment of choice for direct fistulae.

Whether selective irradiation by a radiosurgical technique has any useful therapeutic role awaits further study but the method was successful in one recent case involving a fistula between a branch of the intracavernous carotid artery and cavernous sinus (Barcia-Salorio et al, 1979).

REFERENCES

Alexander G L 1972 Sturge-Weber syndrome. In: Vinken P J, Bruyn G W (eds) Handbook of clinical neurology. North-Holland, Amsterdam, vol 14, p 223

Aminoff M J 1973 Vascular anomalies in the intracranial dura mater. Brain 96:601–612

Aminoff M J 1976 Spinal angiomas. Blackwell, Oxford

Aminoff M J, Kendall B E 1973 Asymptomatic dural vascular anomalies. British Journal of Radiology 46:662–667

Aminoff M J, Logue V 1974a Clinical features of spinal vascular malformations. Brain 97:197–210

Aminoff M J, Logue V 1974b The prognosis of patients with spinal vascular malformations. Brain 97:211–218

Aminoff M J, Barnard R O, Logue V 1974 The pathophysiology of spinal vascular malformations. Journal of the Neurological Sciences 23:255–263

Antoni N 1962 Spinal vascular malformations (angiomas) and myelomalacia. Neurology 12:795–804

Arutiunov, A I, Serbinenko F A, Shlykov A A 1968 Surgical treatment of carotid-cavernous fistulas. Progress in Brain Research 30:441–444

Barcia-Salorio J L, Hernandez G, Broseta J, Ballester B, Masbout G 1979 Radiosurgical treatment of a carotid-cavernous fistula. Case report. In: Szikla G (ed) Stereotactic cerebral irradiation, I.N.S.E.R.M. Symposium No. 12. Elsevier, Amsterdam, p 251

Black P, Uematsu S, Perovic M, Walker A E 1973 Carotid-cavernous fistula: a controlled embolus technique for occlusion of fistula with preservation of carotid blood flow. Technical note. Journal of Neurosurgery 38:113–118

Brenner R P, Sharbrough F W 1976 Electroencephalographic evaluation in Sturge-Weber syndrome. Neurology 26:629–632

Brion S, Netsky M G, Zimmerman H M 1952 Vascular malformations of the spinal cord. Archives of Neurology and Psychiatry 68:339–361

Brismar G, Brismar J 1976 Spontaneous carotid-cavernous fistulas. Phlebographic appearance and relation to thrombosis. Acta Radiologica (Diagnosis) 17:180–192

Brooks B 1930 Discussion of paper by Noland L, Taylor A S. Transactions of the Southern Surgical Association 43:176–177

Brown D G, Hilal S K, Tenner M S 1973 Wyburn-Mason syndrome. Report of two cases without retinal involvement. Archives of Neurology 28:67–68

Caroscio J T, Brannan T, Budabin M, Huang Y P, Yahr M D 1980 Subarachnoid hemorrhage secondary to spinal arteriovenous malformation and aneurysm. Archives of Neurology 37:101–103

Castaigne P, Laplane D, Djindjian R, Bories J, Augustin P 1966 Communication arterio-veineuse spontanee entre la carotide externe et le sinus caverneux. Revue Neurologique 114:5–14

Ciminello V J, Sachs E 1962 Arteriovenous malformations of the posterior fossa. Journal of Neurosurgery 19:602–604

Clemens F, Lodin H 1968a Non-traumatic external carotid-cavernous sinus fistula. Clinical Radiology 19:201–203

Clemens F, Lodin H 1968b Some viewpoints on the venous outflow pathways in cavernous sinus fistulas: angiographic study of five traumatic cases. Clinical Radiology 19:196–200

Dennery J M, Ignacio B S 1967 Post-traumatic arteriovenous fistula between the external carotid arteries and the superior longitudinal sinus: report of a case. Canadian Journal of Surgery 10:333–336

Di Chiro G, Wener L 1973 Angiography of the spinal cord. A review of contemporary techniques and applications. Journal of Neurosurgery 39:1–29

Di Chiro G, Doppman J L, Wener L 1977 Computed tomography of spinal cord arteriovenous malformations. Radiology 123:351–354

Djindjian M 1976 Les malformations arterio-veineuses de la moelle epiniere et leur traitement. These pour le doctorat en medicine, Universite de Paris VI

Djindjian R 1975 Embolization of angiomas of the spinal cord. Surgical Neurology 4:411–420

Djindjian R, Hurth M, Houdart R 1970 L'Angiographie de la moelle epiniere. Masson, Paris

Doppman J L, Di Chiro G 1965 Subtraction-angiography of spinal cord vascular malformations. Report of a case. Journal of Neurosurgery 23:440–443

Doppman J L, Di Chiro G, Ommaya A 1968 Obliteration of spinal-cord arteriovenous malformation by percutaneous embolisation. Lancet 1:477

Doppman J L, Di Chiro G, Ommaya G 1971 Percutaneous embolization of spinal cord arteriovenous malformations. Journal of Neurosurgery 34:48–55

Doppman J L, Wirth F P, Di Chiro G, Ommaya A K 1969 Value of cutaneous angiomas in the arteriographic localization of spinal-cord arteriovenous malformations. New England Journal of Medicine 281:1440–1444

Edwards M S, Connolly E S 1977 Cavernous sinus syndrome produced by communication between the external carotid artery and cavernous sinus. Journal of Neurosurgery 46:92–96

El Gindi S, Andrew J 1967 Successful closure of carotid cavernous fistula by the use of acrylic. Case report. Journal of Neurosurgery 27:153–156

Fincher E F 1951 Arteriovenous fistula between the middle meningeal artery and the greater petrosal sinus. Case report. Annals of Surgery 133:886–888

Forster D M C, Steiner L, Hakanson S 1972 Arteriovenous malformations of the brain. A long-term clinical study. Journal of Neurosurgery 37:562–570

Gates G F, Fishman L S, Segall H D 1978 Scintigraphic detection of congenital intracranial vascular malformations. Journal of Nuclear Medicine 19:235–244

Gold A P, Ransohoff J, Carter S 1964 Vein of Galen malformation. Acta Neurologica Scandinavica 40, Suppl. 11:1–31

Goree J A, Dukes H T 1963 The angiographic differential diagnosis between the vascularized malignant glioma and the intracranial arteriovenous malformation. American Journal of Roentgenology, Radium Therapy, and Nuclear Medicine 90:512–521

Graf C J 1965 Spontaneous carotid-cavernous fistula. Ehlers-Danlos syndrome and related conditions. Archives of Neurology 13:662–672

Grunert V, Sunder-Plassmann M 1971 Beitrag zur chirurgischen Therapie der Karotis-Kavernosus-Fisteln. Acta Neurochirurgica 25:109–114

Guthkelch A N 1948 Haemangiomas involving the spinal epidural space. Journal of Neurology, Neurosurgery, and Psychiatry 11:199–210

Hamby W B 1964 Carotid-cavernous fistula. Report of 32 surgically treated cases and suggestions for definitive operation. Journal of Neurosurgery 21:859–866

Handa J, Yoneda S, Handa H 1975 Venous sinus occlusion with a dural arteriovenous malformation of the posterior fossa. Surgical Neurology 4:433–437

Hayes G J 1963 External carotid-cavernous sinus fistulas. Journal of Neurosurgery 20:692–700

Henderson W R, Gomez R de R L 1967 Natural history of cerebral angiomas. British Medical Journal 4:571–574

Henson R A, Croft P B 1956 Spontaneous spinal subarachnoid haemorrhage. Quarterly Journal of Medicine 25:53–66

Herdt J R, Di Chiro G, Doppman J L 1971 Combined arterial and arteriovenous aneurysms of the spinal cord. Radiology 99:589–593

Hilal S K, Michelsen J W 1975 Therapeutic percutaneous embolization for extra-axial vascular lesions of the head, neck, and spine. Journal of Neurosurgery 43:275–287

Hook O, Lidvall H 1958 Arteriovenous aneurysms of the spinal cord. A report of two cases investigated by vertebral angiography. Journal of Neurosurgery 15:84–91

Hosobuchi Y 1975 Electrothrombosis of carotid-cavernous fistula. Journal of Neurosurgery 42:76–85

Houdart R, Le Besnerais Y 1963 Les aneurysmes arterio-veineux des hemispheres cerebraux. Masson, Paris

Houser O W, Baker H L, Rhoton A L, Okazaki H 1972 Intracranial dural arteriovenous malformations. Radiology 105:55–64

Houser O W, Campbell J K, Campbell R J, Sundt T M 1979 Arteriovenous malformation affecting the transverse dural venous sinus — an acquired lesion. Mayo Clinic Proceedings 54:651–661

Hugosson R, Bergstrom K 1974 Surgical treatment of dural arteriovenous malformation in the region of the sigmoid sinus. Journal of Neurology, Neurosurgery, and Psychiatry 37:97–101

Jaeger R 1949 Intracranial aneurysms. Southern Surgeon 15:205–217

Johnston L M 1938 Epidural hemangioma with compression of spinal cord. Journal of the American Medical Association 110:119–122

Jonutis A J, Sondheimer F K, Klein H Z, Wise B L 1971 Intracerebral cavernous hemangioma with angiographically demonstrated pathologic vasculature. Neuroradiology 3:57–63

Kelly D L, Alexander E, Davis C H, Maynard D C 1969 Intracranial arteriovenous malformations: clinical review and evaluation of brain scans. Journal of Neurosurgery 31:422–428

Kendall B E 1976 Radiological investigations. In: Aminoff M J Spinal angiomas. Blackwell, Oxford, p 97

Kendall B E, Claveria L E 1976 The use of computed axial tomography (CAT) for the diagnosis and management of intracranial angiomas. Neuroradiology 12:141–160

Kendall B E, Logue V 1977 Spinal epidural angiomatous malformations draining into intrathecal veins. Neuroradiology 13:181–189

Kerber C W, Bank W O, Cromwell L D 1979 Calibrated leak balloon microcatheter: a device for arterial exploration and occlusive therapy. American Journal of Roentgenology 132:207–212

Kerber C W, Cromwell L D, Sheptak P E 1978 Intraarterial cyanoacrylate: an adjunct in the treatment of spinal/paraspinal arteriovenous malformations. American Journal of Roentgenology 130:99–103

Kramer R A, Wing S D 1977 Computed tomography of angiographically occult cerebral vascular malformations. Radiology 123:649–652

Kuhner A, Krastel A, Stoll W 1976 Arteriovenous malformations of the transverse dural sinus. Journal of Neurosurgery 45:12–19

Kunc Z, Bret J 1969 Congenital arterio-sinusal fistulae. Acta Neurochirurgica 20:85–103

Kusske J A, Kelly W A 1974 Embolization and reduction of the 'steal' syndrome in cerebral arteriovenous malformations. Journal of Neurosurgery 40:313–321

Laine E, Galibert P, Lopez C, Delahousse J, Delandtsheer J M, Christiaens J L 1963 Anevrysmes arterio-veineux intra-duraux (developpes dans l'epaisseur de la dure-mere) de la fosse posterieure. Neuro-Chirurgie (Paris) 9:147–158

Lamas E, Lobato R D, Esparza J, Escudero L 1977 Dural posterior fossa AVM producing raised sagittal sinus pressure. Case report. Journal of Neurosurgery 46:804–810

Landman S, Ross P 1973 Radionuclides in the diagnosis of arteriovenous malformations of the brain. Radiology 108:635–639

Lang E R, Bucy P C 1965 Treatment of carotid-cavernous fistula by muscle embolization alone. The Brooks method. Journal of Neurosurgery 22:387–392

Logue V 1979 Angiomas of the spinal cord: review of the pathogenesis, clinical features, and results of surgery. Journal of Neurology, Neurosurgery, and Psychiatry 42:1–11

Logue V, Monckton G 1954 Posterior fossa angiomas. A clinical presentation of nine cases. Brain 77:252–273

Logue V, Aminoff M J, Kendall B E 1974 Results of surgical treatment for patients with a spinal angioma. Journal of Neurology, Neurosurgery, and Psychiatry 37:1074–1081

Lombardi G, Migliavacca F 1959 Angiomas of the spinal cord. British Journal of Radiology 32:810–814

Luessenhop A J 1976 Operative treatment of arteriovenous malformations of the brain. In: Morley T P (ed) Current controversies in neurosurgery. Saunders, Philadelphia, p 203

Luessenhop A J, Presper J H 1975 Surgical embolization of cerebral arteriovenous malformations through internal carotid and vertebral arteries. Long-term results. Journal of Neurosurgery 42:443–451

Mackenzie I 1953 The clinical prsentation of the cerebral angioma. A review of 50 cases. Brain 78:184–214

Magidson M A, Weinberg P E 1976 Spontaneous closure of a dural arteriovenous malformation. Surgical Neurology 6:107–110

Markham J W 1961 Arteriovenous fistula of the middle meningeal artery and the greater petrosal sinus. Journal of Neurosurgery 18:847–848

Markham J W 1974 Carotid-cavernous sinus fistula treated by intravascular occlusion with a balloon catheter. Report of two cases. Journal of Neurosurgery 40:535–538

Martin J D, Mabon R F 1943 Pulsating exophthalmos. Review of all reported cases. Journal of the American Medical Association 121:330–334

Matthews W B 1959 The spinal bruit. Lancet 2:1117–1118

McConnell E M 1953 The arterial blood supply of the human hypophysis cerebri. Anatomical Record 115:175–203

McCormick W F, Boulter T R 1966 Vascular malformations ('angiomas') of the dura mater. Report of two cases. Journal of Neurosurgery 25:309–311

McCormick W F, Harman J M, Boulter T R 1968 Vascular malformations ('angiomas') of the brain, with special reference to those occurring in the posterior fossa. Journal of Neurosurgery 28:241–251

Menon D, Weir B 1979 Evaluation of cerebral blood flow in arteriovenous malformations by the Xenon 133 inhalation method. Canadian Journal of Neurological Sciences 6:411–416

Mingrino S, Moro F 1967 Fistula between the external carotid artery and cavernous sinus. Case report. Journal of Neurosurgery 27:157–160

Morley T P 1976 Appraisal of various forms of management in 41 cases of carotid-cavernous fistula. In: Morley T P (ed) Current controversies in neurosurgery. Saunders, Philadelphia, p 223

Mullan S 1979 Treatment of carotid-cavernous fistulas by cavernous sinus occlusion. Journal of Neurosurgery 50:131–144

Nellhaus G, Haberland C, Hill B J 1967 Sturge-Weber disease with bilateral intracranial calcifications at birth and unusual pathologic findings. Acta Neurologica Scandinavica 43:314–347

Newquist R E, Mayfield F H 1960 Spinal angioma presenting during pregnancy. Journal of Neurosurgery 17:541–545

Newton T H, Adams J E 1968 Angiographic demonstration and nonsurgical embolization of spinal cord angioma. Radiology 91:873–876

Newton T H, Cronqvist S 1969 Involvement of dural arteries in intracranial arteriovenous malformations. Radiology 93:1071–1078

Newton T H, Hoyt W F 1970 Dural arteriovenous shunts in the region of the cavernous sinus. Neuroradiology 1:71–81

Newton T H, Troost B T 1974 Arteriovenous malformations and fistulae. In: Newton T H, Potts D G (eds) Radiology of the skull and brain: angiography. Mosby, St Louis, vol 2, book 4, p 2490

Newton T H, Weidner W, Greitz T 1968 Dural arteriovenous malformation in the posterior fossa. Radiology 90:27–35

Obrador S, Gomez-Bueno J, Silvela J 1974 Spontaneous carotid-cavernous fistula produced by ruptured aneurysm of the meningohypophyseal branch of the internal carotid artery. Case report. Journal of Neurosurgery 40:539–543

Obrador S, Soto M, Silvela J 1975 Clinical syndromes of arteriovenous malformations of the transverse-sigmoid sinus. Journal of Neurology, Neurosurgery, and Psychiatry 38:436–451

Odom G L, Woodhall B, Margolis G 1957 Spontaneous hematomyelia and angiomas of the spinal cord. Journal of Neurosurgery 14:192–202

Ohta T, Nishimura S, Kikuchi H, Toyama M 1973 Closure of carotid-cavernous fistula with polyurethane foam embolus. Technical note. Journal of Neurosurgery 38:107–112

Olivecrona H, Riives J 1948 Arteriovenous aneurysms of the brain. Their diagnosis and treatment. Archives of Neurology and Psychiatry 59:567–602

Oliver A D, Wilson C B, Boldrey E B 1973 Transient postprandial paresis associated with arteriovenous malformations of the spinal cord. Report of two cases. Journal of Neurosurgery 39:652–655

Pakarinen S 1965 Arteriovenous fistula between the middle meningeal artery and the sphenoparietal sinus. A case report. Journal of Neurosurgery 23:438–439

Parkinson D 1964 Collateral circulation of cavernous carotid artery: anatomy. Canadian Journal of Surgery 7:251–268

Parkinson D 1973 Carotid cavernous fistula: direct repair with preservation of the carotid artery. Technical note. Journal of Neurosurgery 38:99–106

Paterson J H, McKissock W 1956 A clinical survey of intracranial angiomas with special reference to their mode of progression and surgical treatment: a report of 110 cases. Brain 79:233–266

Perret G, Nishioka H 1966 Report on the cooperative study of intracranial aneurysms and subarachnoid hemorrhage. Section VI. Arteriovenous malformations. Journal of Neurosurgery 25:467–490

Pia H W 1973 Diagnosis and treatment of spinal angiomas. Acta Neurochirurgica 28:1–12

Pool J L, Potts D G 1965 Aneurysms and arteriovenous anomalies of the brain. Diagnosis and treatment. Harper & Row, New York

Pressman B D, Kirkwood J R, Davis D O 1975 Computerized transverse tomography of vascular lesions of the brain. Part I: Arteriovenous malformations. American Journal of Roentgenology, Radium Therapy and Nuclear Medicine 124:208–214

Prolo D J, Hanbery J W 1971 Intraluminal occlusion of a carotid-cavernous sinus fistula with a balloon catheter. Technical note. Journal of Neurosurgery 35:237–242

Prolo D J, Hanbery J W 1976 Treatment of carotid-cavernous fistula with catheter and balloon. In: Morley T P (ed) Current controversies in neurosurgery. Saunders, Philadelphia, p 250

Ramamurthi B, Balasubramanian V 1966 Arteriovenous malformations with a purely external carotid contribution. Report of two cases. Journal of Neurosurgery 25:643–647

Rios-Montenegro E N, Behrens M M, Hoyt W F 1972 Pseudoxanthoma elasticum. Association with bilateral carotid rete mirabile and unilateral carotid-cavernous sinus fistula. Archives of Neurology 26:151–155

Roman G, Fisher M, Perl D P, Poser C M 1978 Neurological manifestations of hereditary hemorrhagic telangiectasia (Rendu-Osler-Weber disease): report of 2 cases and review of the literature. Annals of Neurology 4:130–144

Rosenbaum A E, Schechter M M 1969 External carotid-cavernous fistulae. Acta Radiologica (Diagnosis) 9:440–444

Rowbotham G F, Little E 1965 Circulations of the cerebral hemispheres. British Journal of Surgery 52:8–21

Rumbaugh C L, Potts D G 1966 Skull changes associated with intracranial arteriovenous malformations. American Journal of Roentgenology, Radium Therapy, and Nuclear Medicine 98:525–534

Sanders M D, Hoyt W F 1969 Hypoxic ocular sequelae of carotid-cavernous fistulae. Study of the causes of visual failure before and after neurosurgical treatment in a series of 25 cases. British Journal of Ophthalmology 53:82–97

Sedzimir C B, Occleshaw J V 1967 Treatment of carotid-cavernous fistula by muscle embolization and Jaeger's maneuver. Journal of Neurosurgery 27:309–314

Serbinenko F A 1974 Balloon catheterization and occlusion of major cerebral vessels. Journal of Neurosurgery 41:125–145

Stahl S M, Johnson K P, Malamud N 1980 The clinical and pathological spectrum of brain-stem vascular malformations. Archives of Neurology 37:25–29

Stein B 1979 Arteriovenous malformations of the brain and spinal cord. In: Hoff J (ed) Neurosurgery volume in Goldsmith's practice of surgery. Harper & Row, Hagerstown, ch. 17, p 1

Stern W E, Brown W J, Alksne J F 1967 The surgical challenge of carotid-cavernous fistula: the critical role of intracranial circulatory dynamics. Journal of Neurosurgery 22:298–308

Svien H J, Baker H L 1961 Roentgenographic and surgical aspects of vascular anomalies of the spinal cord. Surgery, Gynecology and Obstetrics 112:729–735

Tamaki N, Fujita K, Yamashita H 1971 Multiple arteriovenous malformations involving the scalp, dura, retina, cerebrum, and posterior fossa. Case report. Journal of Neurosurgery 34:95–98

Taniguchi R M, Goree J A, Odom G L 1971 Spontaneous carotid-cavernous shunts presenting diagnostic problems. Journal of Neurosurgery 35:384–391

Theron J, Newton T H, Hoyt W F 1974 Unilateral retinocephalic vascular malformations. Neuroradiology 7:185–196

Thomson J L G 1959 Aneurysm of the vein of Galen. British Journal of Radiology 32:680–684

Troupp H 1965 Arteriovenous malformations of the brain: prognosis without operation. Acta Neurologica Scandinavica 41:39–42

Urdanibia J F, Silvela J, Soto M 1974 Occipital dural arteriovenous malformations. Neuroradiology 7:57–64

Van Bogaert L 1950 Pathologie des angiomatoses. Acta Neurologica et Psychiatrica Belgica 50:525–610

Verbiest H 1968 Arteriovenous aneurysms of the posterior fossa. Progress in Brain Research 30:383–396

Von Rad M, Tornow K 1975 Spontane Carotis-cavernosus-Fistel bei Morbus Osler-Rendu (Teleangiektasia hereditaria). Journal of Neurology 209:237–242

Waltimo O 1973 The relationship of size, density and localization of intracranial arteriovenous malformations to the type of initial symptom. Journal of the Neurological Sciences 19:13–19

Waltimo O, Putkonen A-R 1974 Intellectual performance of patients with intracranial arteriovenous malformations. Brain 97:511–520

Waltimo O, Eistola P, Vuolio M 1973 Brain scanning in detection of intracranial arteriovenous malformations. Acta Neurologica Scandinavica 49:434–442

Wendling L R, Moore J S, Kieffer S A, Goldberg H I, Latchaw R E 1976 Intracerebral venous angioma. Radiology 119:141–147

Wilson C B, Cronic F 1964 Traumatic arteriovenous fistulas involving middle meningeal vessels. Journal of the American Medical Association 188:953–957

Wolpert S M, Stein B M 1979 Factors governing the course of emboli in the therapeutic embolization of cerebral arteriovenous malformations. Radiology 131:125–131

Wyburn-Mason R 1943a The vascular abnormalities and tumours of the spinal cord and its membranes. Kimpton, London

Wyburn-Mason R 1943b Arteriovenous aneurysm of mid-brain and retina, facial naevi and mental changes. Brain 66:163–203

16

Cardiac causes of stroke

David de Bono

Undoubtedly the most important way in which cardiac disease can be a direct cause of stroke is through the formation of cerebral emboli. Emboli from the left side of the heart may reach any part of the systemic arterial tree, but because brain and retina are so sensitive to ischaemia, neurological or visual symptoms are very often an early, or even the only, manifestation. This chapter attempts to assess the embolic risk for a variety of cardiac lesions in the light of available clinical evidence. It will also consider the ways in which cardiac arrhythmias may be associated with stroke or TIA and will outline a suggested scheme for the cardiological assessment of stroke patients.

CARDIAC SOURCES OF THROMBOEMBOLI

Mitral stenosis

It is generally accepted that mitral stenosis is attended by an increased risk of cerebral thromboembolism, which is greater if there is coexisting atrial fibrillation (Wood, 1954). Stagnation of blood in a dilated, poorly contracting left atrium is regarded as the main causative factor, though an increased risk of embolism is still found in the subgroup of patients who have small left atria and remain in sinus rhythm. Blood flow is turbulent across the deformed valve leaflets and in some patients it is possible to show a shortened platelet survival time. This may reflect a 'thrombotic tendency' which is due either to local platelet activation, or to some effect of pulmonary congestion on the production of an endogenous antithrombotic agent such as prostacyclin in the lung. The most extensive data on the risk of embolism in patients with mitral stenosis not treated with anticoagulant drugs come from the retrospective series of Coulshed et al (1970) and Fleming & Bailey (1971).

Coulshed et al studied 737 patients with mitral stenosis. In the group aged 35 years or younger 4.5 per cent of those in sinus rhythm and 27 per cent of those in atrial fibrillation had emboli. In patients aged 36 or over the incidence was 11.2 per cent of those in sinus rhythm and 32 per cent of those in atrial fibrillation. Fleming & Bailey reported on 329 patients with dominant mitral stenosis, and 116 (35 per cent) of this group had suffered systemic emboli. A further 104 patients were seen with dominant mitral incompetence and nine of these had had emboli. In the overall series 35 per cent of the patients in atrial fibrillation and 11 per cent of those in sinus rhythm had emboli. In both series a substantial proportion of the patients who had emboli had mild or trivial symptoms, and there was little correlation between embolism and radiographically-estimated left atrial size. The embolic risk is increased in the first few months after the onset of atrial fibrillation (Szekely, 1964; Coulshed et al, 1970) and most recurrences occur within a year of the first embolic event but some degree of increased embolic risk persists indefinitely. The annual incidence rate of systemic embolism in patients not treated with anticoagulants has been estimated at 4 per cent per annum for patients without a previous history of embolism and 8 per cent per annum for those with previous emboli, but these estimates are based on limited numbers of somewhat selected cases. There is excellent evidence that adequate treatment with anticoagulant drugs reduces the embolic risk in mitral stenosis, but this is considered in detail elsewhere (see Ch. 20).

Mitral incompetence and mitral leaflet prolapse (MLP)

Unlike mitral stenosis, which except for the rare congenital form is invariably attributed to rheumatic heart disease, the pathology of mitral incompetence is extremely diverse. The extent of this diversity has only been fully appreciated since the introduction of echocardiography. The mitral valve abnormalities traditionally associated with chronic rheumatic disease may produce mitral incompetence as well as, or predominating over, mitral stenosis, but the majority of cases of pure mitral regurgitation presenting in the United Kingdom today are probably due either to excessive dilatation of the mitral annulus or to abnormalities of mitral closure, encompassing the various mitral leaflet prolapse syndromes. Recognition of the latter, principally by echocardiography, and the discovery of an association between MLP and TIA or stroke has led to an explosive growth of not always critical literature on this subject. Mitral

prolapse in its more extreme forms resulting from balloon deformity of the mitral valve or from rupture of chordae tendinae has long been familiar to pathologists (Pomerance, 1969), but the belated recognition of its milder variants rests partly on the appreciation of the auscultatory significance of a mid systolic click and late systolic murmur (Fig. 16.1) and partly on the correlation of these observations with echo- and angio-cardiographic findings (Barlow & Pocock, 1975; Jeresaty, 1979). Because of the variability of the physical signs and the extent to which satisfactory echocardiography depends on the skill of the operator, the frequency of MLP in 'normal' populations has been controversial. There is now fairly good evidence, based on objective criteria, that MLP occurs in about five per cent of the young adult North American population (Procacci et al, 1976; Darsee et al, 1979): it is therefore by far the commonest cardiac abnormality in this age group. The underlying pathology is probably diverse. Many patients with MLP are tall and slim but this is not universal. Collagen abnormalities, anomalies in the distribution of coronary arteries and incoordinate left ventricular contraction have all been suggested. In

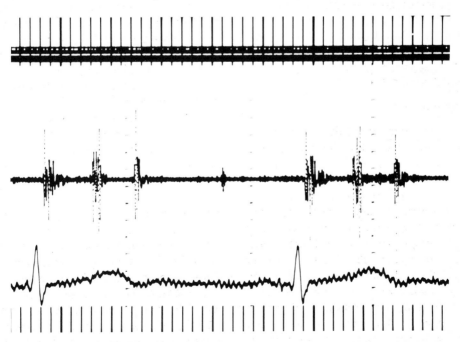

Fig. 16.1 Phonocardiogram showing mid-systolic click and variable late systolic murmur, from a normotensive 42 year old man with a right hemiparesis of sudden onset. Echocardiography confirmed mitral prolapse, blood cultures were negative and carotid angiography showed normal cerebral vessels apart from occlusion of a branch of the left middle cerebral artery.

older patients MLP may result from ischaemic heart disease.

The possibility of an association between mitral incompetence and stroke may be studied either by considering the incidence of stroke in patients already known to have mitral incompetence or, conversely, by looking for mitral valve disease in patients presenting with TIA or stroke. Studies using the former approach tend to concern patients with more severe grades of mitral incompetence and have not attempted to segregate cases according to the underlying pathology. They are in general agreement that the risk of embolism in mitral incompetence associated with sinus rhythm is low, but mitral incompetence with atrial fibrillation has almost as great a propensity for producing emboli as mitral stenosis (Fleming & Bailey 1971). The role of atrial fibrillation will be further considered below. Approaching the problem from the opposite angle, there have been several reports suggesting an excessive incidence of MLP in patients with TIA or stroke (e.g., Kostuk et al, 1977). The most extensive series to date is that of Barnett et al (1980). They studied 141 patients aged 45 or over who had 'transient cerebral ischaemia or partial strokes' and found evidence of MLP in 5.7 per cent; however the incidence of MLP in age-matched control patients was 7.1 per cent. On the other hand, in 60 patients with TIA or stroke aged under 45 MLP was detected in 24 (40 per cent) compared with 6.8 per cent of controls. Even allowing for other possible causes of cerebral ischaemia in 6 of the 24, this is convincing evidence that MLP is a significant cause of stroke in young patients. With regard to older patients, it becomes increasingly difficult to distinguish the effects of MLP from those of other risk factors.

Granted that there is an association between MLP and cerebral emboli, it is clear that the situation is very different from that found in, say, mitral stenosis. Although the latter will be a factor in only a small proportion of strokes, the stroke risk in individual patients with mitral stenosis is very high. In contrast, the overall risk of stroke in individual patients with MLP is very small, and indeed cerebral embolism was not encountered as a complication in either of two long-term follow-up studies (Allen et al, 1974; Mills et al, 1976). Because MLP is so common however it may still

be the cause of a substantial proportion of strokes. It may also be expected to be a frequent finding in patients whose strokes are due to other causes and its discovery does not release the clinician from a search for these alternatives.

Is there any way of predicting which patients with MLP are at special risk from cerebral embolism? Steele et al (1979) found a shortened platelet survival time in a small group of patients with MLP who had had strokes and had normal cerebral arteriograms. The prevalence of a shortened platelet survival time in unselected patients with MLP was considerably less (33 per cent vs. 78 per cent) than in patients with rheumatic heart disease, but even so this test does not seem to be sufficiently predictive to be a guide to therapy. In the series of Barnett et al, 6 of 24 patients with MLP had recurrent emboli, suggesting that an increased embolic risk persists in these patients. A further complicating issue is the association of MLP, in some patients, with recurrent arrhythmias or paroxysmal atrial fibrillation, which may carry an embolic risk of their own. There is at present no justification for the indiscriminate treatment of asymptomatic patients with MLP with either coumarin anticoagulants or platelet anti-aggregant drugs, except possibly in the context of a prospective controlled trial. A logical case could be made for treating patients who have suffered a cerebral ischaemic episode with a platelet anti-aggregant, especially if platelet survival time is shortened or plasma β-thromboglobulin elevated, but formal evidence for the efficacy of such treatment is not yet available.

Aortic valve disease

Less attention has been paid to aortic than to mitral valve disease as a potential source of cerebral emboli. Whereas mitral disease may be associated with stroke in relatively young patients, aortic valve disease (excepting infective endocarditis) can rarely be implicated as a cause of stroke in patients under the age of 45, and in the older age groups the picture is confused by a proliferation of other risk factors. It is also possible that the emboli associated with aortic valve disease are relatively small, and thus more likely to be undetected or to cause transient ischaemia rather than completed stroke. Twenty per cent of patients in one series of cases referred for aortic valve surgery had had symptoms of focal cerebral ischaemia (McDonald et al, 1968). Aortic stenosis was the commonest single cardiac lesion in a recent series of 103 patients with retinal artery occlusion, affecting 11 out of 29 patients with 'structural' cardiac disease (Wilson et al, 1979). In a personal series of 117 patients presenting with amaurosis fugax or TIA haemodynamically significant aortic valve disease occurred in 4, but a further 13 had systolic murmurs which probably originated from the aortic valve although the degree of obstruction to blood flow was thought to be trivial (de Bono & Warlow, 1980). A prospective study of embolic risk in patients with aortic valve disease does not appear to have been undertaken.

Retinal artery emboli associated with aortic valve disease tend to be white and refractile (von Graefe, 1859; Penner & Font 1969), most are probably composed of aggregated platelets, but some may include calcific material extruded from the valve. Studies of surgically-excised stenotic aortic valves at both light microscope (Stein et al, 1977) and electron microscope level (Riddle et al, 1980) emphasise the frequency with which the endothelium is found to be disrupted and the defects covered with platelets and fibrin. It is difficult to conceive of large thrombi being able to form at these sites (although this is known to occur in infective endocarditis). An alternative potential embolic source might be the interstices of a hypertrophied and excessively trabeculated left ventricle, but direct evidence is lacking for this mechanism, which would apply equally in systemic hypertension or hypertrophic cardiomyopathy.

Arrhythmias as a cause of cerebral emboli

Atrial fibrillation increases the risk of systemic embolism in patients with mitral stenosis or incompetence, as already discussed above. Electrical conversion of atrial fibrillation to sinus rhythm (cardioversion) in non-anticoagulated patients with mitral valve disease carries an embolic risk of approximately 6 per cent (Turner & Towers 1965), but the risk of embolism following cardioversion in previously anticoagulated patients is very small (Bjerkelund & Orning 1969). Atrial fibrillation in

the absence of mitral valve disease may be due to a variety of causes, of which thyrotoxicosis, which may be occult (Forfar et al, 1979), is probably more common than previously suspected. It was formerly taught that systemic embolism was rare in thyrotoxic atrial fibrillation, because the hyperdynamic action of the heart would prevent atrial thrombosis but this was disproved by Staffurth et al (1977), who described 17 cases of systemic embolism in 262 patients with thyrotoxicosis. Three of these episodes occurred at the time of cardioversion or of spontaneous reversion to sinus rhythm. Anticoagulation is advisable at least for younger patients with thyrotoxic atrial fibrillation, particularly as the arrhythmia is frequently intermittent and the chances of ultimately restoring regular rhythm are good.

The desirability of anticoagulation prior to cardioversion has to be balanced against the increased chances of success if this is carried out as soon as possible after the onset of fibrillation. My current policy is to advise anticoagulation in all patients with mitral valve disease, or whose arrhythmia has persisted for longer than 48 hours, but this is based on intuition rather than firm evidence. Anticoagulant therapy should be continued for a month after successful cardioversion, as a return to fibrillation is not uncommon.

The assessment of embolic risk in patients with stable 'lone atrial fibrillation' in whom cardioversion is not contemplated is difficult, not least because many of them are elderly and have other risk factors for cerebrovascular disease. Paul Wood (1968) described a 6 per cent risk of 'systemic or pulmonary embolism' in a personal series of 70 patients followed for an average of 8.5 years. My present impression is that the theoretical advantages of anticoagulation in this situation are largely outweighed by the practical disadvantages; however a previous embolism, an enlarged left atrium or a large or dyskinetic left ventricle would alter the balance in favour of anticoagulation.

Sinu-atrial disease and 'sick sinus' syndrome. Fairfax et al (1976), found an increased incidence of focal cerebral ischaemic events in patients with chronic sinu-atrial disorder (tachycardia bradycardia syndrome) considered for pacemaker implantation when they were compared with age-matched controls suffering from stable complete heart block. These events appeared to be independent of syncopal episodes and were attributed to thrombus formation in the left atrium during periods of paroxysmal arrhythmia. Most of their patients were elderly and there is as yet little evidence of an increased embolic risk in young patients with sporadic supraventricular tachycardia (Flensted-Jensen, 1969).

Thromboembolism from the left ventricle

Thrombosis within the cavity of the left ventricle is normally prevented by the combination of a non-thrombogenic endocardium and coordinated left ventricular contraction. Both of these functions may be disturbed acutely after myocardial infarction, and chronically in the presence of a left ventricular aneurysm. 'Transmural' myocardial infarction usually spares a thin layer of myocardium adjacent to the ventricular cavity but the endocardium is nevertheless frequently damaged, perhaps by migrating neutrophils. Hilden et al (1971) found a 58 per cent prevalence of mural thrombosis in patients dying shortly after myocardial infarction, with a lower prevalence in those who had been given anticoagulants. In the multicentre Veterans Administration (1973) trial of anticoagulants in acute myocardial infarction, cerebral embolism accounted for 0.6 per cent of deaths in a series of 500 patients. There was a 3.8 per cent incidence of systemic embolism in control, and a 0.8 per cent incidence in anticoagulated patients. Similar results were obtained in the British Medical Research Council Trial (1969). Most episodes of systemic embolism occur between 5 and 20 days after infarction. There is some evidence that the risk of embolism increases with the size of infarct and is greater with anterior than with inferior infarcts. It is current policy in our unit to administer warfarin to patients admitted with myocardial infarction but to discontinue this therapy prior to discharge from hospital. The efficacy of this policy in preventing systemic embolism has not been fully assessed.

Left ventricular aneurysms, which are usually the consequence of previous myocardial infarction, are almost invariably lined with a layer of thrombus, fragments of which may detach as emboli. The quoted incidence of systemic embolism in post-mortem series of patients with aneurysms is high, but on the other hand none of the 32 patients in the surgical series of Donaldson et al (1976) had had clinical evidence of embolism, though all of them had thrombus in the aneurysm at operation.

Cardiomyopathies, both congestive and hypertrophic, are also associated with an increased risk of systemic embolism. In congestive cardiomyopathy there is frequently left atrial dilatation and a tendency to arrhythmias in addition to poor left ventricular function (Fleming & Wood 1959). Hypertrophic cardiomyopathy is very commonly associated with mitral valve abnormalities, including mitral regurgitation, and at post-mortem examination a characteristic ridge on the aortic surface of the anterior mitral leaflet probably reflects repeated endothelial trauma from contact either with the interventricular septum or the posterior papillary muscle. Thrombosis within the left ventricular cavity appears to be a primary pathogenetic process in certain 'obliterative' cardiomyopathies, but these are rare in the United Kingdom.

Thromboembolism in congenital heart disease (CHD)

Mitral leaflet prolapse and congenital aortic valve disease should strictly come under this heading but have already been discussed. Congenital heart lesions are frequently complex and individual features of a complex which would be associated with increased embolic risk on their own will continue to do so in the context of multiple cardiac lesions. This section is however principally concerned with the risk of cerebral vascular disease in cyanotic CHD. Intracardiac 'right to left' blood shunting will, in addition to conferring cyanosis and a tendency to polycythaemia, make it possible for thrombus originating on the systemic venous side of the circulation to reach the cerebral arteries: so called 'paradoxical embolism'. Persistent right to left shunting is most commonly due to the tetralogy of Fallot but is also found in patients with ventricular septal defect or persistent ductus arteriosus who have pulmonary hypertension. Although lesions such as tetralogy of Fallot are now surgically correctable, advances in care have also meant that more children with complex cyanotic defects are surviving into adulthood. Phornphutkul et al (1973) reviewed the aetiology of cerebrovascular accidents in a series of infants and children with cyanotic CHD. They reported 30 events in 29 patients; 220 other children with similar heart lesions but no cerebrovascular symptoms were seen over the same period. Relative anaemia appeared to be a contributing factor in patients under the age of five years but older patients tended to be severely polycythaemic. By no means all of the ischaemic episodes were due to emboli; necropsy revealed cerebral venous thrombosis in two of the patients who died shortly after the CVA, and arterial thrombosis in another. Patients with cyanotic CHD also have an increased incidence of brain abscess, possibly because bacteria-laden microemboli can reach the brain without passing through the lungs. The incidence of brain abscess was two per cent in the series of Fischbein et al (1974), and this diagnosis should be considered in all patients with cyanotic CHD who develop neurological symptoms.

Patients with atrial septal defects usually have predominant left to right shunts in the absence of pulmonary vascular disease, but a small right to left component, which may be intermittent, can nearly always be demonstrated. In spite of this, and of much speculation to the contrary, paradoxical embolism in patients with atrial septal defect but no pulmonary vascular disease is very rare. Cerebral embolism has however been described following surgical closure of atrial septal defects with patches of prosthetic materials. A totally different situation affects patients with thromboembolic pulmonary hypertension, in whom a raised right atrial pressure may force open a valve-patent foramen ovale. These patients have a high incidence of cerebral embolism, though their comparative rarity makes it hard to quantitate.

Cardiac surgery and valve replacement

Stroke is an important complication of cardiac surgery both in the perioperative and late postoperative periods. The former is outside the scope of this discussion; stroke risk in long surviving patients will depend on the nature of the operation and the technique used.

Mitral valvotomy. Mitral valvotomy does not abolish the risk of thromboembolism. The risk is probably minimal in patients with a good valvotomy, small left atrium and sinus rhythm, but even these need to be kept under observation, as eventual restenosis is not uncommon.

Mitral valve repair. This has been used with great success in some centres for cases of non-rheumatic mitral incompetence. The risk of late thromboembolism is very small, especially if sinus rhythm is maintained.

Mitral valve replacement. This is now accepted as the definitive treatment for most cases of severe mitral valve disease. The first mechanically-satisfactory prosthetic heart valve was the Starr-Edwards ball valve. It soon became apparent that patients with these valves in the mitral position had an unacceptably high rate of thromboembolic complications unless treated with anticoagulants. Technical improvements to the valve and routine anticoagulation have reduced the frequency of thromboembolism to 1.9 events per 100 patient-years (Bonchek & Starr 1975). It has been suggested that combination of warfarin anticoagulation with dipyridamole may reduce the risk still further (Sullivan et al, 1971). Tilting disc prostheses such as the Bjork-Shiley valve may have certain haemodynamic advantages but are still associated with an unacceptable thromboembolism risk in the absence of adequate anticoagulation (Messmer et al, 1972). An alternative approach is to use a 'biological' valve such as a human or pig aortic valve, usually mounted inside a rigid ring or stent for ease of handling. It was originally hoped that long-term anticoagulation would be unnecessary with these valves but it is becoming clear that although the embolic risk is less than with mechanical prostheses it is not negligible, especially if the patient remains in atrial fibrillation. It may well be that any procedure which places a rigid ring in the position of the mitral annulus inevitably interferes with atrial emptying and increases the risk of thrombus formation (Tsakiris et al, 1966; Thiene et al, 1980).

Aortic valve replacement. The risk of thromboembolism following valve replacement is less in the aortic than in the mitral position; nevertheless it is sufficiently high for patients with ball or tilting disc prostheses to require some form of anticoagulant therapy (Roberts et al, 1975). 'Biological' valves in the aortic position carry a very low thromboembolism risk.

Other cardiac surgery. There is no long-term increased risk of thromboembolism after coronary artery bypass grafting or after surgical closure of ventricular or atrial septal defects where no prosthetic material has been used. If such material is required as a 'patch', or if muscular resection leaves a large area denuded of endothelium, many surgeons would recommend anticoagulation for up to six months, by which time these areas are assumed to have been covered by endothelium.

INFECTIVE ENDOCARDITIS

In a recent series (Pruitt et al, 1978) 39 per cent of 218 patients with bacterial endocarditis had neurological complications and in 36 patients the initial presentation was on account of neurological symptoms. The occurrence of neurological complications is of sinister prognostic significance in endocarditis and in this series 58 per cent of the affected patients died. Although *Streptococcus viridans* remains the most common causative organism in bacterial endocarditis, the proportion of patients with cerebral emboli appears to be greater in those with endocarditis due to *Staphylococcus aureus, Streptococcus pneumoniae,* anaerobic streptococci or Enterobacter species, possibly because these infections cause more florid and friable vegetations on the affected heart valves. Another form of endocarditis particularly likely to be the cause of embolism is fungal endocarditis, which usually occurs in immunosuppressed patients or those who have had a prosthetic valve replacement.

The possibility of bacterial endocarditis should be considered in any patient with symptoms of cerebral embolism who has a heart murmur, who has had cardiac surgery or who has a pyrexia of uncertain origin. There is little correlation between the risk of bacterial endocarditis and the haemodynamic effect of the cardiac lesion: haemodynamically mild lesions such as mitral leaflet prolapse or bicuspid aortic valve are the basis for many infections. The single most important step in the diagnosis and effective treatment of bacterial endocarditis is the isolation of a causative organism in blood culture. It is irresponsible to initiate antibiotic therapy in any patient who might have bacterial endocarditis without securing blood cultures. If there is an urgent need to start antibiotics, six cultures may be taken at 20 minute intervals before this is done. If the diagnosis of endocarditis seems likely and the clinical situation permits, at least 12 cultures should be taken. Cultures should be incubated under both aerobic and anaerobic conditions, and blood should also be taken for the measurement of fungal and rickettsial antibodies. In the acutely ill patient antibiotic therapy should be initiated as soon as the cultures have been taken — it may be modified later in the light of the results.

Echocardiography has added a dimension to the investigation of bacterial endocarditis by permitting vegetations on heart valves to be visualised (Fig. 16.2A & B). Using two-dimensional echocardiographic equipment it may be possible to see vegetations as small as 2 mm in diameter on mitral or aortic valves. However such 'optimal' results are dependent on operator skill and appropriate equipment, and may be impossible in obese, emphysematous or very restless patients. Echocardiography is therefore best regarded as complementary to traditional diagnostic methods. Wann et al (1979) have suggested that patients in whom large vegetations are demonstrated echocardiographically on left-sided heart valves are at particular risk from embolism, and consideration should be given to early surgical exploration. On the other hand Stewart et al (1980) have shown that with adequate antibiotic therapy large vegetations may regress or disappear. Appropriate management for individual patients has to be decided in close consultation with both bacteriologists and surgical colleagues. A recently described technique for detecting and estimating the size of vegetations involves the injection of radioactively-labelled platelets, which adhere to the endocarditic vegetations and can be detected using a gamma-camera (Riba et al, 1979). The scope of this technique merits further evaluation.

Discussion of the treatment of infective endocarditis is outside the scope of this chapter but several reviews are available (Pankey, 1979; Oakley, 1980). There is an increasing trend towards early surgical intervention and this is particularly so in the case of prosthetic valve endocarditis,

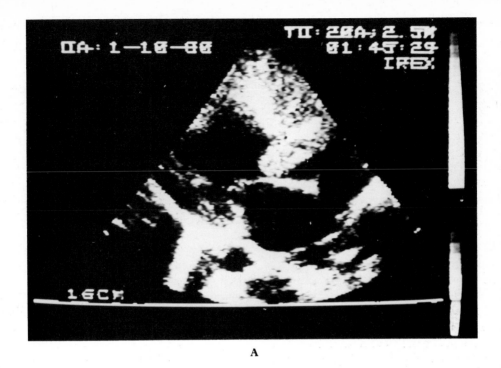

A

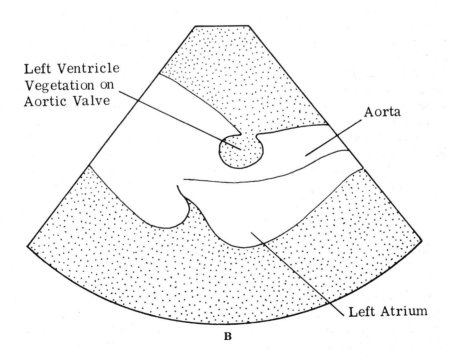

Left Ventricle
Vegetation on
Aortic Valve

Aorta

Left Atrium

B

Fig. 16.2A & B Two-dimensional echocardiogram showing a massive, ball-valve like endocarditic vegetation on the aortic valve. From a 25-year-old woman who had had a minor stroke two weeks before. Shortly after this echocardiogram was recorded, she had an episode of sudden loss of consciousness almost certainly due to left ventricular outflow obstruction. Emergency aortic valve replacement was performed (by courtesy of Drs H C Miller and K Fox).

where good results appear to depend on the removal of infected foreign material (Wilson et al, 1978).

OTHER TYPES OF EMBOLISM

Calcific emboli

Degenerative changes may result in the accumulation of calcified material in the cusps of damaged aortic or mitral valves, or in the mitral annulus. Calcification may also occur within organised thrombi, either in the left atrium or, it has been suggested, in the mitral sulcus. Usually the calcified tissue is rigid and hard (and may cause aortic or mitral obstruction) but sometimes the centre of the calcified mass softens and is partially extruded. This may happen spontaneously or during the course of cardiac surgery. The association of emboli with aortic stenosis was mentioned above; since the stenosed valve is usually calcified it may be hard to decide whether the embolic material consists of platelet aggregates, calcific material or both.

Calcific emboli have frequently been seen in the coronary arteries of patients dying with aortic stenosis, particularly after attempted valve surgery (Holley et al, 1963; Steiner et al, 1976). The reported incidence of calcific emboli in cerebral vessels is low, but this may result from less thorough examination.

Mitral annulus calcification (Fulkerson et al, 1979) is a common degenerative condition principally found in elderly women and sometimes associated with cerebral, retinal or systemic emboli. In our own series (de Bono & Warlow 1979) the retinal emboli seen in patients with mitral annulus calcification were all 'white emboli' suggesting an origin from calcified material in the valve ring rather than from left atrial thrombus. Some patients do however have obstruction to left atrial emptying and are thus also at risk from thromboembolism. Echocardiography is of value in making the diagnosis.

Calcific embolism has been reported as a complication of mitral valvotomy in patients with heavily calcified mitral valves, but mitral replacement is now preferred in these cases.

Tumour emboli

The commonest source for tumour emboli large enough to occlude named cerebral arteries is an intracardiac myxoma. These usually originate from the left atrial wall in the region of the fossa ovalis but may arise from other sites such as the orifice of a pulmonary vein or the mitral valve. The surface of the tumour may be smooth or villous and the latter variety are particularly likely to cause emboli (Fig. 16.3). Physical signs are variable, and depend on the extent to which the tumour is able to cause mitral obstruction. They include variable mid-diastolic murmurs, and a diastolic sound evocatively called a 'tumour plop'. There may be no physical signs with sessile myxomas. Chest radiographs may be normal or show pulmonary congestion. Many, but not all, patients have systemic symptoms, a raised erythrocyte sedimentation rate and abnormal plasma proteins. Echocardiography is useful; the m-mode echocardiogram characteristically showing multiple echoes behind the anterior mitral leaflet. Sessile myxomas on the posterior wall may be missed unless carefully looked for, and two-dimensional echocardiography is likely to be more reliable. Pulmonary arteriography can be used to confirm the diagnosis prior to surgery but may be unnecessary after good echocardiography. Surgical removal of the myxoma is the definitive treatment.

Tumour emboli may also result from other primary tumours arising in the heart, such as angiosarcoma or rhabdomyosarcoma, or from secondary tumour metastasising to or invading the heart, but such causes are rare.

Marantic and paraneoplastic endocarditis

Patients who are in the terminal phases of a severe illness sometimes develop signs of cerebral embolism and at autopsy can be shown to have sterile, but sometimes exuberant, vegetations attached to one or more heart valves (Rosen & Armstrong 1973). Occasionally, cerebral embolism is a presenting or early feature of an illness which subsequently turns out to be due to an occult neoplasm especially a mucus-secreting carcinoma. In both these situations there is increasing evidence for a disseminated abnormality of blood coagulation, which can be detected by appropriate

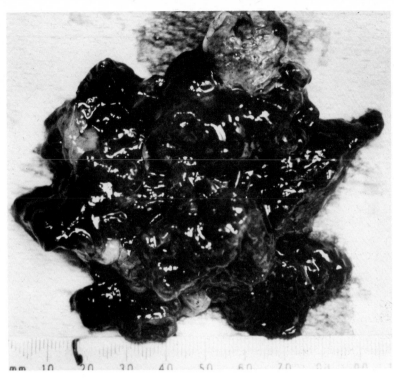

Fig. 16.3 A villous left atrial myxoma (by courtesy of Mr P. R. Walbaum).

haematological tests (Vecht et al, 1978; Zieger, 1979). Treatment with heparin has been recommended but evidence of its efficacy is anecdotal.

Acute rheumatic fever may be associated with small vegetations on the mitral valve, but these are extremely unlikely to cause embolic complications.

Systemic lupus erythematosus may be the cause of damage to heart valves, and particularly the mitral valve, characterised by 'verrucous' vegetations on the valve leaflets. It is conceivable that such vegetations could give rise to emboli and the valve damage may occasionally be severe enough to produce haemodynamically significant mitral stenosis or incompetence. Focal neurological symptoms in this condition are however much more likely to result from local vascular lesions than from embolism.

CARDIAC CAUSES OF NON-EMBOLIC STROKE

Both hypertensive disease and atherosclerosis are important causes of cardiac as well as cerebrovas-cular pathology but they and their associations with thrombotic and haemorrhagic stroke are considered elsewhere in this book. It is conceivable that in circumstances where some cardiac disorder causes prolonged or profound hypotension the perfusion in a localised cerebral region downstream of a critical arterial stenosis might be so reduced as to permit infarction or local vascular thrombosis or failing this, some transient impairment of focal neurological function. In one of the earliest clinical accounts of complete heart block the Edinburgh physician Spens (1793) described the development of a terminal hemiparesis, albeit only after several hours of extreme bradycardia. It has also long been known that elderly patients presenting clinically as cases of stroke frequently have e.c.g. evidence of recent myocardial infarction or ischaemia (Glathe & Achor 1958). It is difficult to be certain that stroke in these cases did not result from embolism and it is possible that the stress engendered by a stroke may even provoke myocardial infarction. The availability of equipment for ambulatory e.c.g. monitoring has revived interest in the possible association of transient brady or tachyarrhythmias with neurological symptoms. Unfortunately an element of confusion has been introduced because some authors have applied the term 'transient ischaemic attack' (TIA) to both focal neurological symptoms and to non-focal black-outs or dizzy spells, whereas others have insisted on the focal nature of TIA. There is no doubt that transient arrhythmias are an important cause of transient non-focal neurological problems and that ambulatory e.c.g. monitoring plays an essential role in their investigation (MacAllen & Marshall, 1973; Jonas et al, 1977). Other possible causes of a sudden fall in cardiac output which need to be considered include severe aortic or pulmonary stenosis, hypertrophic obstructive cardiomyopathy (idiopathic hypertrophic subaortic stenosis) and 'ball valve' obstruction by an endocarditic vegetation (Fig 16.2) or by a myxoma. There is much less evidence that arrhythmias play an important role in causing *focal* neurological symptoms other than via the formation of thromboemboli as mentioned above. Fairfax et al (1976) found only a 1.3 per cent incidence of focal neurological problems in a series of patients receiving pacemakers for symptomatic complete heart block not due to the tachycardia-bradycardia syndrome. Reed et al (1973) found that only 4 out of 290 patients requiring pacemakers had focal symptoms, and in only 2 was there a correlation between the occurrence of a documented arrhythmia and the development of focal symptoms. In a personal series of over 100 patients with transient focal neurological symptoms studied by ambulatory e.c.g. monitoring we were able to show coincidence between the symptoms and an arrhythmia in only one man, who also had a subclavian artery stenosis. Although it is unusual for carotid territory TIA to be due to arrhythmia and it is doubtful if ambulatory e.c.g. monitoring of these patients is worthwhile, caution is needed in respect of 'vertebrobasilar' TIA, which may be much harder to distinguish from the effects of generalised hypoperfusion.

CARDIAC INVESTIGATION OF PATIENTS WITH STROKE OR TIA

There are three principal reasons why a proper cardiac assessment is important in patients presenting with stroke or TIA. Firstly, because treatment of a cardiac lesion may be important in preventing further neurological damage — for example in cases of mitral stenosis, bacterial endocarditis or atrial myxoma. Secondly, because neurological symptoms, though mild in themselves, may be the first indication of serious cardiac disease, such as aortic stenosis. Thirdly, because the detection and documentation of 'minor' cardiac lesions, even where, as in the case of mitral prolapse, there is no consensus yet as to optimal treatment, are important to our understanding of their natural history and prognosis.

The basis of this assessment is a conscientious history with specific enquiry about palpitations and chest pain; physical examination with attention paid to palpation of all the peripheral pulses, to accurate recording of blood pressure and in particular to auscultation of the heart (including auscultation in the left lateral, erect and supine positions, in full inspiration and expiration and with the patient standing); a 12-lead electrocardiogram and chest radiographs in posteroanterior and oblique or lateral projections. Valvular calcification is usually obscured in standard PA chest radiographs. Blood cultures must be taken if there is any suspicion of endocarditis. Echocardiography should be done in those patients who have murmurs and probably in any patient under the age of 45. Since many of the echocardiographic features of particular interest in these patients are subtle, it is important that this test is performed or supervised by a skilled operator who is fully familiar with the clinical picture. Routine ambulatory e.c.g. monitoring is not indicated in patients with focal neurological symptoms unless the occurrence of paroxysmal arrhythmias is suggested by the history. Invasive cardiac investigations such as angiocardiography are very seldom indicated unless urgent surgery is contemplated, since most of the information they provide can be gained more simply by non-invasive means.

Multiple vascular accidents in the territories of different major cerebral vessels within a short period of time are very likely to be due to emboli from the heart (or to a multifocal vasculitis). Isolated events are much more common and much more difficult to ascribe to a cardiac cause even if a potentially causative cardiac abnormality is found. In a personal series (de Bono & Warlow 1980) 15 per cent of patients presenting with TIA had both cardiac and carotid lesions which might have been the source of an embolus. In the face of such uncertainty, considerable weight still has to be allotted to clinical judgement and to an objective assessment of the relative risk associated with particular lesions.

REFERENCES

Allen H, Harris A, Leatham A 1974 Significance and prognosis of an isolated late systolic murmur. British Heart Journal 36:525

Barlow J B, Pocock W A 1975 The problem of non-injection systolic clicks and associated mitral systolic murmurs: emphasis on the billowing mitral leaflet syndrome. American Heart Journal 90:635

Barnett H J M, Baughner D R, Taylor D W, Cooper P E, Kostuk W J, Nichol P M 1980 Further evidence relating mitral valve prolapse to cerebral ischemic events. New England Journal of Medicine 302:139

Bjerkelund C J, Orning O M 1969 The efficacy of anticoagulant therapy in preventing embolism related to DC cardioversion of atrial fibrillation. American Journal of Cardiology 23:208

Bonchek L I, Starr A 1975 Ball valve prostheses — current appraisal of late results. American Journal of Cardiology 35:843

British Medical Research Council — Report of the working party on anticoagulant therapy in coronary thrombosis 1969 Assessment of short term anticoagulant administration after cardiac infarction. British Medical Journal i:335

Coulshed N, Epstein E J, McKendrick C S, Galloway R W, Walker E 1970 Systemic embolism in mitral valve disease. British Heart Journal 32:26

Darsee J R, Mikolich J R, Nicoloff N B, Lesser L E 1979 Prevalence of mitral valve prolapse in presumably healthy young men. Circulation 59:619

de Bono D P, Warlow C P 1979 Mitral annulus calcification and cerebral or retinal ischaemia. Lancet ii:383

de Bono D P, Warlow C P 1981 Potential sources of emboli in transient cerebral and retinal ischaemia. Lancet i:343

Donaldson R M, Honey M, Balcon R, Banim S O, Sturridge M F, Wright J E C 1976 Surgical treatment of postinfarction left ventricular aneurysm in 32 patients. British Heart Journal 38:1223

Fischbein C A, Rosenthal A, Fischer E, Nadas A S, Welch K 1974 Risk factors for brain abscess in patients with congenital heart disease. American Journal of Cardiology 34:97

Fairfax A J, Lambert C D, Leatham A 1976 Systemic embolism in chronic sinu-atrial disorder. New England Journal of Medicine 295:190

Fleming H A, Bailey S M 1971 Mitral valve disease, systemic embolism and anticoagulants. Postgraduate Medical Journal 47:599

Fleming H A, Wood P H 1959 The myocardial factor in mitral valve disease. British Heart Journal 21:117

Flensted-Jensen E 1969 Wolff-Parkinson-White syndrome: a long term follow up of 47 cases. Acta medica Scandinavica 186:65

Forfar J C, Miller H C, Toft A D 1979 Occult thyrotoxicosis: a correctable cause of 'idiopathic' atrial fibrillation. American Journal of Cardiology 44:9

Fulkerson P K, Beaver B M, Ansean J-C, Graber H L 1979 Calcification of the mitral annulus: etiology, clinical associations, complications and therapy. American Journal of Medicine 66:967

Glathe J P, Achor R W P 1958 Frequency of cardiac disease in patients with strokes. Proceedings of the Staff Meetings of the Mayo Clinic 33:417

Graefe A von 1859 Uber Embolie der Arteria centralis retinae als Ursache plötslicher Erblindung. von Graefe's Archiv fur Ophthalmologie 5:136

Hilden T, Raaschou F, Iversen K, Schwartz M 1971 Anticoagulants in acute myocardial infarction. Lancet ii:327

Holley K E, Balm R C, McGoon D C, Mankin H T 1963 Spontaneous calcific embolism associated with calcific aortic stenosis. Circulation 27:197

Jeresaty M 1979 Mitral Valve Prolapse. Raven Press, New York

Jonas S, Klein I, Dimant J 1977 Importance of Holter monitoring in patients with periodic cerebral symptoms. Annals of Neurology 1:470

Kostuk W J, Baughner D R, Barnett H J M, Silver M D 1977 Strokes: a complication of mitral leaflet prolapse? Lancet ii:313

MacAllen P M, Marshall J 1973 Cardiac dysrhythmia and transient cerebral ischaemic attacks. Lancet i:1212

McDonald L, McDonald A, Resnekov L, Robinson R, Ross D 1968 Homograft replacement of the aortic valve. Lancet ii:469

Messmer B J, Okies J E, Holman G I 1972 Early and late thromboembolic complications after mitral valve replacement. Journal of Cardiovascular Surgery 13:281

Mills P, Rose J, Hollingsworth J, Amora J, Craige E 1977 Long term prognosis of mitral valve prolapse. New England Journal of Medicine 297:13

Oakley C M 1980 Infective endocarditis. British Journal of Hospital Medicine 24:232

Pankey G A 1979 The prevention and treatment of bacterial endocarditis. American Heart Journal 98:102

Penner W, Font L 1969 Retinal embolism from calcified vegetations of the aortic valve. Archives of Ophthalmology 81:565

Phornphutkul C, Rosenthal A, Nadas A S, Berenberg W 1973 Cerebrovascular accidents in infants and children with cyanotic congenital heart disease. American Journal of Cardiology 32:329

Pomerance A 1969 Ballooning deformity (mucoid degeneration) of atrioventricular valves. British Heart Journal 31:343

Procacci P M, Savran S V, Schreiter S L, Bryson A L 1976 Prevalence of clinical mitral valve prolapse in 1169 young women. New England Journal of Medicine 294:1086

Pruitt A, Rubin R, Korchmer A, Duncan G W 1978 Neurological complications of bacterial endocarditis. Medicine (Baltimore) 57:329

Reed R L, Siekert R G, Merideth J 1975 The rarity of transient focal cerebral ischemia in cardiac dysrhythmias. Journal of the American Medical Association 223:893

Riba A L, Thakur M L, Gottschalk M D, Andriole V T, Zaret B L 1979 Imaging experimental infective endocarditis with indium 111 labelled blood cellular components. Circulation 59:336

Riddle J M, Magilligan D J, Stein P D 1980 Surface topography of stenotic aortic valves by scanning electron microscopy. Circulation 61:496

Robert W C, Fischbein M C, Golden A 1975 Cardiac pathology after valve replacement by disc prostheses. American Journal of Cardiology 35:749

Rosen P, Armstrong D 1973 Non-bacterial thrombotic endocarditis in patients with malignant neoplastic diseases. American Journal of Medicine 54:23

Spens T 1793 History of a case in which there took place a remarkable slowness of the pulse. Medical Commentaries, Edinburgh, 8:463

Staffurth J S, Gibberd M C, Ng Tang Fui S 1977 Arterial embolism in thyrotoxicosis with atrial fibrillation. British Medical Journal iii:688

Steele P P, Weily H, Rainwater J, Vogel R 1979 Platelet survival time in patients with thromboembolism and mitral valve prolapse. Circulation 60:43

Stein P D, Sabbah H N, Pitha J V 1977 Continuing disease process of calcific aortic stenosis: role of microthrombi and turbulent flow. American Journal of Cardiology 39:159

Steiner I, Hlava A, Procházka J 1976 Calcific coronary embolization associated with cardiac valve replacement. British Heart Journal 38:816

Stewart J A, Silimperi D, Harris P, Wise N K, Froker T D, Kisslo J A 1980 Echocardiographic documentation of vegetative lesions in infective endocarditis: clinical implications. Circulation 61:374

Sullivan J M, Harken D E, Gorlin R 1971 Pharmacologic control of thromboembolic complications of cardiac valve replacement. New England Journal of Medicine 284:1391

Szekeley P 1964 Systemic embolism and anticoagulant prophylaxis in rheumatic heart disease. British Medical Journal i:1209

Thiene G, Bartolotti U, Pannizzon G, Milano A, Gallucci V 1980 Pathological substrates of thrombus formation after heart valve replacement with the Hancock prosthesis. Journal of Thoracic and Cardiovascular Surgery 80:414

Tsakiris A G, Rastelli G C, Bonchero N, Kirklin J W, Wood E H 1966 Haemodynamic effects of implanting a rigid ring in the annulus of the mitral valve. American Journal of Cardiology 17:141

Turner J R B, Towers J R H 1965 Complications of cardioversion. Lancet ii:612

Vecht C J, van Aken W G, Becker A E 1978 The triad 'cerebrovascular occlusion, nonbacterial thrombotic endocarditis and malignant tumours' (in Dutch, English abstract) Nederlandsche Tijdschrift voor Geneeskunde 122:1881

Veterans Administration Cooperative Study 1969 Long term anticoagulant therapy after myocardial infarction. Journal of the American Medical Association 207:2263

Wann L S, Hallam C C, Dillon J C, Weyman A E, Feigenbaum H 1979 Comparison of M mode and cross sectional echocardiography in infective endocarditis. Circulation 60:728

Wilson L A, Warlow C P, Ross Russell R W 1979 Cardiovascular disease in patients with retinal artery occlusion. Lancet i:292

Wilson W R, Danielson G K, Giuliani E R, Washington J A, Joumin P M, Geraci J E 1978 Valve replacement in patients with active infective endocarditis. Circulation 58:585

Wood P H 1954 An appreciation of mitral stenosis. British Medical Journal i:1051

Wood P H 1968 Diseases of the heart and circulation, 3rd edn, Eyre and Spottiswood, London, p 278

Zieger A 1979 On relapsing paraneoplastic cerebral embolism. Case report and survey of literature. Fortschritte Neurologie Psychiatrie 47:377 (in German, English abstract)

17

Haematological aspects of cerebral arterial disease

D. J. Thomas

There are two clinical situations which may bring the haematologist and the neurologist to the bedside of the same patient. The first is that of a patient, known to suffer from a blood disorder, who develops a neurological complication such as a cerebral haemorrhage. In the second a patient presenting with cerebral vascular symptoms is discovered to have a haematological abnormality in the course of routine investigation.

The main diseases which have cerebrovascular aspects will be discussed in turn but an initial cautionary note is in order. It should not be assumed that a neurological event in such a patient is necessarily caused by the blood disorder. The possibility of an unrelated neurological or neuro-surgical condition should always be kept in mind.

THE POLYCYTHAEMIAS

The diagnosis of polycythaemia is usually considered when a high haemoglobin (Hb) and haematocrit (PCV) are found on a routine blood count. However, at the first outpatient visit or on admission to hospital a patient's PCV is often higher than on subsequent measurement because the stress of these occasions may be associated with a contraction of plasma volume. If on a second examination the PCV still exceeds 0.47 in women or 0.50 in men, on a sample taken without venous stasis, then one of the polycythaemias must be considered and further investigation undertaken. Measurements of red cell mass using chromium-labelled red cells and of plasma volume using ml/kg method of expressing these results is unsatisfactory because it gives erroneously normal results for short, fat, polycythaemic individuals. It is prefer-able to consider the patient's lean body mass and to express the results with reference to the expected normal mean red cell mass and plasma volume for his height and weight (Pearson et al, 1978). Definite polycythaemia is present when the measured red cell mass exceeds the predicted value by more than 25 per cent in men and 30 per cent in women. The polycythaemia may be primary, due to a myeloproliferative disorder (polycythaemia rubra vera or primary proliferative polycythaemia PPP), or secondary to excess erythropoietin production, usually from hypoxia or renal disease. If the red cell mass is not significantly increased the patient is said to have apparent polycythaemia. Idiopathic erythrocytosis is the term used to describe patients with a definite polycythaemia with no obvious cause and none of the associated characteristics of PPP when first investigated. A significant proportion of patients with idiopathic erythrocytosis go on to develop PPP (Pearson & Wetherley-Mein, 1979).

Primary proliferative polycythaemia (PPP)

All forms of thrombotic events are increased in PPP. The incidence of stroke is very much greater than in the general population whereas that of myocardial infarction is only marginally increased (Chievitz & Thiede, 1962; Videbaek, 1950; Barabas et al, 1973; Pearson & Wetherley-Mein, 1978). The explanation for this difference may be the different flow characteristics in brain and heart. There is little doubt that treatment favourably influences prognosis (Harman & Ledlie, 1967; Pearson & Wetherley-Mein, 1978).

There are several reasons for this thrombotic

tendency. The platelet count is often high, sometimes dramatically so, and platelet function may be enhanced in the presence of increased numbers of red cells. This effect may be mechanical, large numbers of erythrocytes forcing the smaller platelets to the periphery and thereby increasing platelet-vessel wall contact, or it may be biochemical as a result of more red cell ADP (Harrison & Mitchell, 1966).

Whole blood viscosity is high in untreated polycythaemia because of the increased concentration of circulating particles. Cerebral blood flow (c.b.f.) is reduced not only in those patients with very high PCV but also in those whose PCV is only marginally elevated (Thomas et al, 1977a).

Flow appears to be reduced for two main reasons. Firstly, the higher Hb of polycythaemic blood enables it to carry more oxygen per unit volume. A lower blood flow is therefore adequate to achieve the same oxygen delivery. Secondly, the higher viscosity tends to reduce flow. Cerebral blood flow may be reduced below optimal levels in some individuals and their alertness may be affected (Willison et al, 1980). Reducing PCV and viscosity by venesection produces in some patients an increase in alertness and an increase in c.b.f. Similarly reduction of the oxygen carrying capacity of the blood by venesection is more than compensated for by the improvement in c.b.f. in some individuals (Wade, 1981). Removal of small quantities of blood (250 ml) at a time is usually safe and an equal volume of fluid may be replaced if transient hypotension is judged to be hazardous (Kiraly et al, 1976).

As far as thrombogenesis is concerned, the cause of the low c.b.f. may be immaterial. A sluggish circulation may be less efficient both at removing thrombogenic factors from sites of endothelial damage and at dispersing emboli. Pearson & Wetherley-Mein (1978), have shown that the incidence of occlusive vascular episodes in PPP depends on the PCV. In order to minimise the chance of thrombotic episodes the PCV should be maintained below 0.45. Thomas et al (1977a) have shown that c.b.f. is likely to be restored to normal when the PCV is reduced to this level.

In some cases it is also necessary to reduce the number of platelets in order to reduce the risks of occlusive vascular events. Dawson & Ogston (1970)

found the incidence of thrombosis increased when the platelets exceeded 270×10^9/litre. However, Pearson & Wetherley-Mein (1978) recommend a limit of 400×10^9/litre when venesecting patients. In those with a high platelet count it may be advisable to give an antiplatelet combination, say aspirin and dipyridamole, to minimise the potential dangers of a reactive thrombocytosis.

Apparent polycythaemia (Spurious, stress, relative or pseudo-polycythaemia)

The high PCV in this group is not due to an absolute increase in the red cell mass and there is no associated increase in the white cell or platelet counts. Haematologists have tended not to be very interested in these patients, because they do not have a 'blood disease'. However, there is evidence that they are at risk from vascular occlusion (Burge et al, 1975; Weinreb & Shih, 1975). It is a heterogeneous group and includes the following:

1. Those with high normal red cell mass; some of these patients will go on to develop true polycythaemia, others may be heavy cigarette smokers (Smith & Landaw, 1978) with more than 10 per cent of their haemoglobin in the carboxy form.
2. Those with a reduction in plasma volume — relative polycythaemia. Dehydration is a common cause for this state. In the chronic situation a low plasma volume may be found in 'stressed' individuals, but the reason for this remains obscure. Those in whom the PCV fluctuates considerably are likely to be in this group.
3. Those who do not conform to either of these groups and have been called physiological variants (Pearson et al, 1978).

Weinreb & Shih (1975) indicated that those with a reduced plasma volume were most at risk. These patients are often hypertensive (Lawrence & Berlin, 1952).

Cerebral blood flow has been shown to be low in these patients whatever their subgroup (Humphrey et al, 1979). When PCV was reduced by courses of venesection, c.b.f. increased. Cerebral blood flow also rose when PCV and blood viscosity were reduced by infusions of low molecular weight dextran. Apart from the blood flow findings, clinical improvement has been documented to follow venesection (Burch & De Pasquale, 1963; Cranley et al, 1963).

Clearly no single treatment is appropriate to this heterogeneous group. If the red cell mass is above the patient's predicted value venesection is advisable. It is more difficult to modify the PCV in the low plasma volume group, although surprisingly a proportion of patients do respond to venesection (Thomas, 1977; Humphrey et al, 1980b, c). This form of treatment should not be pursued if the PCV stays high on weekly venesection because of the danger of progressively lowering blood volume. Attempts to increase plasma volume seem more logical. Unfortunately, the use of fludrocortisone is potentially hazardous in those prone to hypertension and has not proved effective in a small series (Humphrey et al, 1980,b,c). In those who are chronically under stress a small dose of an anxiolytic may be of benefit.

Concurrent hypertension should be treated, preferably not with a diuretic in the low plasma volume group. Smoking should be discouraged.

'High normal' haematocrit

This group is of interest because stroke has been reported to be commoner than in those with a 'low normal' PCV (Kannel et al, 1972, Tohgi et al, 1978). The differentiation from those with apparent polycythaemia is somewhat arbitrary. A simple definition might be men with PCV between 0.46 and 0.52 and women with PCV between 0.43 and 0.47. Those with higher values are labelled polycythaemic.

The Framingham study (Kannel et al, 1972) has indicated that men with Hb exceeding 15 g/dl (i.e., PCV of 0.45) and women with Hb over 14 g/dl (i.e., PCV of 0.42) had twice the chance of developing a stroke; those with coincident hypertension were particularly at risk. A large pathological study (Tohgi et al, 1978) has shown that elderly people with high normal PCV before death are more likely to have evidence of cerebral infarction at autopsy. People with high PCV but no cerebral atheroma suffered very few strokes, but those showing both features were particularly vulnerable. It is noteworthy that Pearson & Wetherley-Mein (1978) in patients with true polycythaemia found the same PCV threshold above which occlusive vascular events were more common.

Cerebral blood flow has been found to be lower in people with high normal PCV than in those with low normal PCV (Thomas et al, 1977b). Reducing PCV by venesection in the high normal PCV group improves flow. It could be argued that the lower initial flow is due to blood with high Hb having a higher oxygen carrying capacity and therefore a lower flow required to achieve the same oxygen delivery to the brain (Paulson et al, 1979). However, two observations suggest that in some cases this low flow is sub-optimal. Firstly, patients may have impaired alertness which improves on reducing PCV and secondly they seem predisposed to vascular problems. The Hb/PCV level that is optimal from the viewpoint of oxygen delivery to the brain has yet to be determined. It is possible that a PCV level that is optimal for oxygen delivery may not be optimal for preventing occlusive vascular disease, especially in patients who have other risk factors.

As yet there is little evidence to suggest that reducing and maintaining PCV below 0.46 helps prevent occlusive vascular episodes in this high normal PCV group. It is likely to be beneficial in those with other risk factors, as it is in true polycythaemia, but a prospective trial is necessary.

Patients with high normal PCV are more prone to thrombosis postoperatively (Bouhoutsos et al, 1974). It would therefore seem appropriate to reduce the PCV before elective surgery and to store the blood in case it is needed peri-operatively.

Secondary polycythaemia

Plasma erythropoietin stimulates the marrow to produce red cells. Erythropoietin is produced predominantly from the kidney in response to hypoxia. The causes of secondary polycythaemia therefore include:

1. Renal ischaemia.
2. Pulmonary disease: chronic obstructive airways disease, hypoventilation syndromes.
3. Cyanotic heart disease.
4. High altitude.

5. High oxygen-affinity haemoglobins.
6. Tumours in which there is inappropriate erythropoietin production or activation, notably hypernephroma and haemangioblastoma.

Renal polycythaemia

Almost any type of renal disease in which there is an ischaemic component may produce secondary polycythaemia. The main thrust of treatment must obviously be towards the underlying renal problem. However repeated venesection is usually necessary to reduce the haematocrit until the erythropoietin drive has been corrected. This is particularly important pre-operatively because of the increased risk of thrombotic events following surgery in patients with high normal or raised haematocrit (Bouhoutsos et al, 1974). An elevated PCV may continue to be a problem after renal transplantation. Swales & Evans (1969) reported thrombotic episodes in six out of seven patients whose polycythaemia, following transplantation, had not been corrected.

Pulmonary polycythaemia

This is a common cause of polycythaemia that is usually suspected from the history and physical findings and confirmed by an PaO_2 below 70 mmHg. A moderate increase in PCV is to be expected as a response to hypoxia and probably should be left untreated. However, a minority of patients are found with extremely high PCV. These patients are often slow mentally and very lethargic (Harrison et al, 1973). These symptoms are often attributed to hypercarbia and poor respiratory reserve but the considerable increase in blood viscosity may be partly responsible. Viscosity is increased not only because of the very high PCV but also because of the high fibrinogen levels that accompany frequent chest infections.

Patients with severe pulmonary polycythaemia usually have advanced cardiopulmonary disease and have a short expectation of life. There is no definite evidence of an increased incidence of stroke, possibly because in most cases survival is too short for it to develop (Burrows & Earle, 1969). However, another factor is that c.b.f. is not as low

in this group as in PPP patients with a comparable PCV (Wade, 1981). This may be because of vasodilatation produced by the accompanying hypercarbia and hypoxia.

Obviously attempts to improve ventilatory function, to reduce the frequency of infection and to correct hypoxia with chronic oxygen therapy are indicated, but should PCV be reduced by venesection? Harrison et al, (1973) found an improvement in work capacity and reduction in pulmonary artery pressure after reducing the PCV from a mean of 0.63 to 0.48. Wade (1981) found an improvement in patients' alertness and lethargy and a mean increase in c.b.f. of 21 per cent after venesection.

It is therefore proposed that patients with severe pulmonary polycythaemia and cerebral symptoms might benefit from a gradual reduction in PCV to approximately 0.50. A lower level may not be necessary because of the 'protective' effect of high Pco_2 partially correcting the low c.b.f., but more work needs to be done on this complex group before firm recommendations can be made. Some patients may need a PCV of 0.55 and others only 0.45. Chronic oxygen therapy is advisable in these patients to reduce the hypoxic drive to erythropoiesis.

Cyanotic heart disease

Occlusive vascular events occur in patients with CHD despite their youth (Rich, 1948; Berthrong & Sabiston, 1951; Ferencz, 1960; Cottrill & Kaplan, 1973). Some patients may develop an increase in PCV above the level required to compensate for the hypoxia. The resultant high viscosity may substantially impede flow in certain tissues and trigger excess erythropoietin which in turn raises PCV and viscosity and reduces flow further. Reducing PCV may reduce peripheral resistance and increase flow and oxygen carriage (Rosenthal et al, 1971).

The risks of corrective cardiac surgery in this group are increased if a high PCV is present. These patients are prone to peri-operative bleeding abnormalities which are minimised if they are venesected pre-operatively (Wedemeyer & Lewis, 1973).

It is difficult to suggest an optimal PCV for this

very varied group. Some patients may require higher levels than others. However, in the individual patient any level at which an occlusive event has occured or which is associated with lethargy is probably too high. Measuring c.b.f., blood viscosity and fibrinogen may be of some assistance but a therapeutic trial of repeated isovolaemic haemodilution, of no more than 250 ml at a time, is advised until a PCV level is found at which the patient is relatively free from symptoms of hyperviscosity.

However there are also theoretical problems when the patient becomes iron deficient (Cottril & Kaplan, 1973) and has numerous hypochromic microcytic cells despite a normal Hb. It has been suggested that these cells are more rigid than normal and may impede flow through the capillaries (Card & Weintraub, 1971).

High oxygen affinity haemoglobins

These are an extremely uncommon cause of polycythaemia but illustrate an important point about the regulation of c.b.f. Oxygen is taken up avidly by the abnormal Hb when passing through the lungs but released reluctantly in the tissues. There is thus tissue hypoxia, increased erythropoietin release and marrow stimulation.

An abnormal haemoglobin is usually considered when other commoner causes of polycythaemia have been excluded. It must be suspected when several members of a family have a raised PCV. Diagnosis can be confirmed by plotting the oxygen dissociation curve and finding it shifted to the left. At least 20 different types of abnormal Hb with high oxygen affinity have been described (Stephens, 1977).

Symptoms of 'hyperviscosity' are not a feature of these patients and they do not seem particularly prone to stroke (Bellingham, 1976).

In contrast to patients with other types of polycythaemia, c.b.f. is not reduced. Wade et al (1980) measured c.b.f. in six members of a family with Hb Yakima. Their mean grey matter flow was found to be 99 ml/100 g/min with a mean PCV of 0.513 which was higher than the 68 ml/100 g/min of an age matched control group and very much higher than the 59 ml/100g/min of a control group matched for age and PCV. This high flow compen-

sates for the high affinity of the abnormal Hb for oxygen. It is interesting that a high flow is possible despite the high blood viscosity. The PCV and viscosity are elevated from infancy and it is possible that the cerebral circulation has adapted by developing more collateral vessels which would tend to reduce peripheral resistance.

In the absence of symptoms of hyperviscosity and without any definite evidence of an increased risk of occlusive vascular disease in patients with high oxygen affinity Hb, attempts to reduce PCV are not indicated.

Polycythaemia of high altitude

An increase in Hb and PCV occurs as a normal physiological response to hypoxia in people moving to high altitude. In most individuals this is a moderate response but in some it is excessive and they develop a polycythaemia which may be extremely severe; Hb exceeding 25 g/dl and PCV exceeding 0.80. The reasons for the development of extreme polycythaemia are complex and as yet not fully understood. Superadded respiratory disease is one factor but genetic factors also play a role.

Chronic mountain sickness (Monge's disease) has prominent neurological symptoms with headaches, lethargy, tinnitus, vertigo and vomiting. However, it is not possible to give any reliable epidemiological statistics on the prevalence of occlusive vascular disease and stroke in high altitude residents. People at high altitude undoubtedly may suffer cerebral infarction but on current evidence one cannot say whether the incidence rates are more than in a similar population at sea level. The difference is unlikely to be great since the inhabitants of mountainous regions have only a small amount of degenerative arterial disease, with less hypertension, poorer diet, and less sedentary lives. As the work of Tohgi et al (1978) indicates, a high PCV alone may not be dangerous but becomes so when combined with other risk factors.

Cerebral blood flow has been measured on several occasions in those living at high altitude. The situation is complex because while hypoxia tends to increase c.b.f. there is also a marked hyperventilation producing hypocapnia and tending to reduce c.b.f. Both Marc-Vergnes et al (1973) and Sorensen et al (1974) found a low c.b.f. in polycythaemic residents of La Paz, Bolivia (3750 m). In most acclimatised individuals there is obviously no case for reducing PCV. However, in those individuals who develop early symptoms of cerebrovascular disease or chronic mountain sickness the correct treatment is to transport them promptly to a lower altitude and to reduce the PCV, although for social reasons this is often impossible.

THE PARAPROTEINAEMIAS

In these conditions an abnormal band is seen on serum protein electrophoresis. This represents excess production of a single immunoglobulin, by a clone of abnormal cells. Most cases of paraproteinaemia have either multiple myeloma or macroglobulinaemia. These patients often have anaemia, bleeding problems and symptoms suggestive of hyperviscosity; all these features may involve the cerebral circulation.

Some degree of anaemia is almost invariable; usually the Hb is between 7 and 10 g/dl. The reticulocyte count is low and defective red cell production is typical. Bleeding may contribute to the anaemia. Sometimes the plasma volume is grossly expanded, producing a misleadingly low PCV (Kopp et al, 1969). The red cells are usually normocytic and normochromic and spontaneous rouleaux formation occurs, hindering the estimation of red cells.

A bleeding tendency is common and may be the presenting feature. Epistaxis and bleeding from the gums is most frequent but retinal, intracerebral and subarachnoid haemorrhage, haematuria, melaena and bleeding venepuncture sites may occur (Cohen et al, 1966). Several factors contribute to this bleeding tendency. Thrombocytopenia occurs and even when platelet numbers are satisfactory they may not function normally, possibly as a result of the effects of the abnormal protein on their membrane (Perkins et al, 1970). Inhibition of fibrin polymerisaton has been demonstrated (Lackner et al, 1970) but other factors are also involved. Bleeding is particularly liable to occur

when cryoglobulins are present. Removal of the abnormal proteins by plasmapheresis may be used to correct the bleeding abnormality (Preston et al, 1978a).

Many of the clinical features of patients with a paraproteinaemia are attributable to changes in blood viscosity and have been termed the hyperviscosity syndrome (Fahey et al, 1965). Headache, mental lethargy and drowsiness may occur. Visual symptoms are common. There is retinal venous congestion, ranging from slight engorgement to marked tortuosity and ballooning with a characteristic 'sausage-string' appearance of the veins. Retinal exudates and retinal or vitreous haemorrhages are seen. Venous thrombosis occurs in some cases as do papilloedema and a type of macular degeneration (Solomon, 1965; McCallister et al, 1967). Symptoms suggestive of vertebro-basilar ischaemia are also prominent, especially intermittent feelings of dysequilibrium. It is interesting to speculate why the retinal and vertebro-basilar territories are more frequently involved than the anterior and middle cerebral artery territories and why the coronary circulation is less commonly affected. The explanation is likely to involve the size of the vessels and the differing character of pulsatile flow in the different anatomical sites.

Some patients may deteriorate with increasing disorientation and depression of conscious level and may suffer seizures (Nutter & Kramer, 1965). Both cerebral haemorrhage (Logothetis et al, 1960; Solomon et al, 1965; Cohen et al, 1966) and cerebral infarction may occur (MacKay et al, 1956; Matzke et al, 1964; Abramsky & Slavin, 1974). In some cases small intracerebral vessels have been observed to be occluded with atypical thrombi. These contain an excess of acidophilic material and may represent protein precipitates (Marshall & Malone, 1954; Butler & Palmer, 1955).

In paraproteinaemia, plasma viscosity may be grossly elevated especially in the macroglobulinaemias where the molecular weight may exceed one million (O'Reilly & MacKenzie, 1967). Such abnormal plasma often behaves in a non-Newtonian manner with a viscosity of approximately 20 m.N.m^{-2} at high shear rates rising to 100 m.N. m^{-2} at low shear rates (Dintenfass & Rozenberg, 1967). The plasma viscosity may also rise unduly steeply with falling temperature (Dintenfass, 1971).

Patients with an IgA myeloma may also have a very high plasma viscosity because of the tendency to form high molecular weight complexes (Tuddenham et al, 1974). IgA trimer is found in patients with IgA myeloma with hyperviscosity syndrome but not in those patients with this myeloma but without symptoms.

The abnormal proteins increase whole blood viscosity not only by raising the plasma component but also by producing aggregation of blood cells. Some proteins are more likely to produce aggregation than others, for example, it is a feature of IgG_3 myeloma (Somer, 1975). These aggregates will tend to raise blood viscosity particularly at low shear rates and will further impede flow through the microcirculation.

The anaemia which commonly accompanies paraproteinaemia will have a compensatory effect on whole blood viscosity. The PCV has such a profound effect on blood viscosity measurements that despite a high plasma viscosity and cellular aggregation, whole blood viscosity measured *in vitro* may not appear abnormal. Furthermore, the reduced oxygen carrying capacity of the anaemic blood will tend to increase c.b.f. in order to maintain oxygen delivery to the brain. Humphrey et al (1980a), have measured c.b.f. in paraproteinaemic patients, comparing them with age-matched control and anaemic groups. The whole blood viscosities and c.b.f. values were similar to those of the normal subjects. The paraproteinaemic patients had significantly higher plasma and whole blood viscosity, the same oxygen carrying capacity but significantly lower c.b.f. than the anaemic controls. None of the patients had a severely elevated plasma viscosity, otherwise even lower flow values might have been obtained.

Treatment of paraproteinaemia

The underlying long-term haematological problem requires appropriate radiotherapy and chemotherapy. We are concerned here with the treatment of hyperviscosity crises and situations threatening the cerebral circulation.

Plasmapheresis can remove large amounts of paraprotein and can effectively reduce plasma viscosity. Approximately 80 per cent of IgM is in the circulation so that a single plasmapheresis is most effective in these patients. However, with IgG myeloma only 40 per cent of the abnormal protein is in the vascular compartment and more than one treatment is required.

In patients presenting with a bleeding problem plasmaphoresis is likely to be more beneficial than blood transfusion (Preston, 1980). Removing the paraprotein may help restore platelet function and fibrin polymerisation.

Blood transfusion is potentially hazardous on two counts. Firstly, increasing the number of cells without removing the abnormal protein may increase viscosity to dangerous levels. Secondly, paraproteinaemic patients may have grossly expanded blood volumes, often in proportion to the increase in viscosity (Tuddenham & Bradley, 1974; Russell & Powles, 1978). In these circumstances blood transfusions may lead to circulatory overload and left ventricular failure.

There is good evidence that plasmapheresis improves patients symptomatically (Solomon, 1965; Somer, 1975; Preston, 1980). However, it is not without its risks and should be reserved for crises. The mainstay of management is control of the underlying haematological abnormality.

Hyperfibrinogenaemia

Fibrin is an important constituent of thrombi and there is increasing suspicion that a raised concentration of its immediate precursor fibrinogen increases the chance of occlusive vascular disease.

The plasma concentration of fibrinogen (normally 2–4 g/l) is raised in patients with transient ischaemic attacks (Ott, 1975) and in patients with established cerebrovascular disease (Pilgeram, 1974). It is also raised in patients with angina (Nicolaides et al, 1977), myocardial infarction (Pilgeram, 1968) and peripheral vascular disease (Dormandy et al, 1973). The evidence indicates that the plasma level is continuously elevated but with a further, superimposed increase at the time of an occlusive vascular event.

Fibrinogen may exert its harmful effect in ways other than by enhancing coagulation. It has been shown to increase platelet stickiness (Salzman, 1971). It can affect the flow properties of the blood in several different ways; because of its large size (mol.wt. 400 000), it raises plasma viscosity (Eastham & Morgan, 1965); it enhances red cell aggregation, especially at low flow rates and therefore raises whole blood viscosity (Usami & Chien, 1973).

Thomas et al (1979) measured c.b.f. in a group of 8 patients with a raised fibrinogen (mean of 5.22 g/l) and found it to be significantly reduced at 50.6 ml/100g/min when compared with control patients. After treatment with clofibrate 1g twice daily for 6 weeks the fibrinogen had fallen to 3.98 g/l and c.b.f. had risen to 63.3 ml/100 g/min, a level no different from control values. There was no change in PCV or Pco_2 between the measurements and the improvement was attributed to a reduction in viscosity.

A raised fibrinogen should be suspected if the ESR is elevated, especially if the plasma globulins are normal. As fibrinogen rises above 4.5 g/l there is almost a linear relationship with the sedimentation rate. There are many factors which either singly or in combination tend to be associated with a raised fibrinogen:

1. increasing age
2. pregnancy and contraceptive pill
3. haemorrhage and trauma including surgery
4. infection
5. malignancy
6. diabetes
7. arterial disease
8. smoking.

An attempt to reduce fibrinogen levels seems indicated, especially in people judged to be at risk from occlusive vascular disease. The underlying cause must be diagnosed and treated appropriately whenever possible. However, one is often faced with a patient with arterial disease and with no other cause for high fibrinogen. In the acute situation fibrinogen can be reduced promptly and most effectively by arvin, derived from the venom of the Malayan pit viper (Bell et al, 1968; Sharp et al, 1968). However, unless properly controlled there is a risk of haemorrhage especially when used peri-operatively and after about six weeks allergic reactions are common. As indicated above, clofibrate may also reduce an elevated fibrinogen but its use has now been restricted because of its possible carcinogenic effects. There is some evidence that inositol nicotinate favourably influences abnormal plasma fibrinogen levels (Aylward, 1979).

ANAEMIAS

Iron deficiency anaemia

There is good epidemiological evidence that anaemia protects against occlusive vascular disease (Elwood et al, 1974). In anaemia there is an increase in blood flow to compensate for the reduction in oxygen carrying capacity (Scheinberg, 1951; Heyman et al, 1952; Gottstein, 1965) and it is possible that it is this factor which protects against vascular occlusion.

Patients with anaemia may complain of feelings of faintness, dizziness and rushing noises in the ears but there is a poor correlation with the severity of the anaemia; many people with a haemoglobin of 7 g/dl or less have no cerebral symptoms. Angina or intermittent claudication are more common (Pickering & Wayne, 1934). When anaemia and vascular disease coexist and when there is a stenosis of an intracerebral vessel the compensatory mechanisms may fail from time to time and symptoms of transient focal cerebral ischaemia develop. Under these circumstances the cerebral symptoms may respond to treatment of the anaemia (Siekert et al, 1960).

With very low Hb (less than 6 g/dl), retinal ischaemia may occur with flame-shaped haemorrhages, cotton-wool exudates and even papilloedema (Trujillo et al, 1972). These changes are much more likely if the anaemia is accompanied by a thrombocytopenia (Rubenstein et al, 1968).

Some patients with iron deficiency anaemia secondary to chronic blood loss may develop a marked thrombocytosis — over $1000 \times 10^9/l$. These patients may develop cerebral ischaemia and hemiparesis (Knizley & Noyes, 1972). Treatment with iron usually corrects the thrombocytosis as well as the anaemia. It is important to exclude the possibility that the patient is in the iron-deficiency phase of polycythaemia rubra vera.

In severe acute haemorrhage, e.g., from the gastro-intestinal tract, cerebral and retinal problems are more often seen because of the associated factors of low blood volume and hypotension; furthermore there are none of the adaptations to chronic anaemia, such as the left shift of the oxygen dissociation curve produced by increased concentration of 2,3 diphosphoglycerate (Torrance et al, 1970). The elderly, in whom compensatory mechanisms are less efficient, are particularly vulnerable and they may have watershed territory infarction or an infarct distal to an arterial stenosis. The retina is again at risk (Pears & Pickering, 1960). Blindness may occur several days after the haemorrhage although the fundus appears normal initially. However, the veins eventually became engorged, haemorrhages occur and papilloedema develops with subsequent optic atrophy. In the cerebral type of blindness which develops with normal pupillary reflexes and with normal fundi, the site of the ischaemia is likely to be the occipital poles and parieto-occipital regions.

Prompt treatment of acute haemorrhage with plasma expanders followed by fresh blood is essential. However, the indications for transfusion in chronic anaemia are few and the potential complications are many (Isbister, 1980). The underlying cause of the iron-deficiency is identified and corrected.

Pernicious anaemia

Patients with pernicious anaemia do not seem any more prone to cerebrovascular problems than those with iron deficiency. Despite the macrocytosis and the theoretical possibility that passage through the micro-circulation might be impeded, c.b.f. has been found to be high (Scheinberg, 1951). When the Hb falls below 6 g/dl retinal ischaemic changes are frequently observed.

Sickle cell anaemia

Cerebrovascular events are very common in sickle cell anaemia (Greer & Schotland, 1962; Portnoy & Herion, 1972). Life expectancy in Hb SS disease is reduced and many of the patients who suffer stroke are young and without significant atheroma. Both hemisphere and brain stem events may occur and individuals often experience recurrent episodes

with a progressive residual disability. Occlusion of arteries of all sizes from internal carotid downwards may occur at the time of a sickle cell crisis but haemorrhage, both intracerebral and subarachnoid may also occur (Greer & Schotland, 1962). People with sickle cell trait (Hb AS) suffer sickling crisis only rarely and consequently cerebral events are also unusual.

A defect in the Hb S molecule renders it relatively insoluble when oxygen tension is reduced, producing the 'sickle-shaped' distortions of the erythrocytes. Sickling is likely to occur when the local Po_2 falls below 60 mmHg. A crisis is possible during dehydration, infection, injury, surgery or pregnancy.

The sickle cells are more rigid than normal and have difficulty passing through the microcirculation. Flow is impeded, hypoxia and acidosis increase and further sickling occurs. Small terminal vessels may be seen to be occluded by aggregates of many sickled cells (Diggs, 1965). Partial or complete occlusion of major vessels occur during crises and may be followed by development of collaterals (Stockman et al, 1972). Between crises overall c.b.f. may be high, in keeping with the low Hb (Heyman et al, 1952).

In addition to the rheological problems, platelet function and haemostasis may be disrupted. Thrombocytosis is extremely common in sickle cell anaemia due in part to the extensive splenic infarction. Platelet activity may be enhanced with reduced platelet survival (Haut et al, 1973). Impaired fibrinolytic activity has also been demonstrated (Mahmood, 1969).

Patients with sickle cell-Hb C disease are less anaemic than those with SS disease and they generally have fewer complications. However, retinal problems are more common in SC than SS disease. This is unlikely to be just because they tend to live longer. A rheological cause is likely because ocular problems are commoner with higher Hb (Lehmann & Huntsman, 1974). In particular, the incidence of retinitis proliferans varies with the Hb; it is infrequent when the Hb is low but occurs in over 70 per cent of SC patients with Hb exceeding 12.5 g/dl. Intra-ocular haemorrhage may occur in over 10 per cent of SC patients while it is unusual in SS disease (Konotey-Ahulu, 1974).

Paroxysmal nocturnal haemoglobinuria

Unlike some of the other acquired haemolytic anaemias, paroxysmal nocturnal haemoglobinuria (PNH) is associated with a high risk of occlusive cerebrovascular disease. The thrombotic events usually occur following attacks of increased haemolysis and it is tempting to suggest that thrombogenic substances are produced when the erythrocytes fragment. However, other factors must come into play because of the low risk of thrombotic events in some haemolytic disorders.

Cortical venous thrombosis with extension to the major sinuses is the most common serious complication (Scott et al, 1938; Johnson et al, 1970; Davies-Jones et al, 1980). After an initial stage of headache, nausea and vomiting, focal and generalized fits may occur with hemiparesis, loss of consciousness and death. Treatment may be attempted with anticonvulsants, heparin and steroids but may be unsuccessful. Large artery occlusion has also been reported (Ham & Horack, 1941).

THE LEUKAEMIAS

Cerebral haemorrhage is very frequent in patients with leukaemia while cerebral infarction is unusual (Williams et al, 1959). Haemorrhage is quite a common component of the initial presentation, of relapses and of the terminal event. As many as 50 per cent of children dying from acute leukaemia show evidence of cerebral haemorrhage (Groch et al, 1960).

There are several reasons for an increased risk of intracranial bleeding. Leukaemic infiltrations may distort and weaken the blood vessel walls (Leidler & Russell, 1945; Moore et al, 1960). However, it is uncommon for bleeding to occur at only one site. Usually, there is multifocal intracranial bleeding as part of a generalised bleeding tendency (Groch et al, 1960; Pochedly, 1975). Several factors are involved.

A thrombocytopenia of less than $20 \times 10^9/l$ is often found in the presence of bleeding, although it is not uncommon for bleeding to occur with platelets over $100 \times 10^9/l$. The reduction in platelets may be due to leukaemic infiltration of the bone marrow, to depressed production as a result of chemotherapy or to excess consumption as part of disseminated intravascular coagulation.

The risk of bleeding correlates well with the number of white cells (Groch et al, 1960; Moore et al, 1960). There is a very much greater chance of haemorrhage when the white count exceeds $300 \times 10^9/l$.

Soon after the start of a course of chemotherapy disseminated intravascular coagulation may occur, probably as a result of thromboplastins released from large numbers of damaged white cells. The granules of the promyelocyte are rich in thromboplastins (Gralnick & Abrell, 1973) and patients with promyelocytic leukaemia are especially prone to disseminated intravascular coagulation and cerebral haemorrhage.

In their huge series of 1864 patients with leukaemia, Williams et al (1959) found only two cases of massive cerebral infarction. This is almost certainly an underestimate and with computerised tomography more infarcts would be detected. Flow through the microcirculation may be seriously impaired by large numbers of white cells and patients may have symptoms suggestive of hyperviscosity (Preston et al, 1978b). All types of leukaemia with very high white counts may have the hyperviscosity syndrome. With only a moderate increase in white cells, symptoms are most likely to occur in myeloid leukaemias because of the large size of the cells.

The tendency for viscosity to rise as a result of the high white count is counteracted to some extent by the severe anaemia that is so frequent in leukaemia. However, if the patient is transfused, viscosity may rise dangerously and cerebral infarction may be precipitated (Davies-Jones et al, 1980). Leucophoresis has been advocated in patients with white counts exceeding $200 \times 10^9/l$ who are judged to be at risk from hyperviscosity problems (Preston et al, 1978b). Symptoms of headache, lethargy, depressed alertness and visual disturbances can be promptly relieved on lowering the white cell count by this method.

BLEEDING DISORDERS

Intracranial haemorrhage, either post-traumatic or spontaneous, is the main neurological problem in patients with a bleeding disorder. Expert haematological assistance is essential if the correct diagnosis is to be made and the best treatment given. In inexperienced hands the clotting factor concentrates that are now available may introduce a thrombogenic component to the patient's problems. The haemostatic mechanism can be disturbed by local problems such as trauma and infection, by thrombocytopenia or thrombasthenia or by one of the coagulation defects.

In a patient presenting with intracranial haemorrhage, the history may provide valuable haematological information and if the patient is unable to give the necessary information a relative must be interviewed. Patients with a serious congenital coagulation disorder usually know it and can indicate the variety. There may be other affected relatives. There may be a history of excess bruising, purpura, epistaxis, menorrhagia and excessive blood loss following dental extraction, venepuncture, trauma and surgery. Recent drug treatment may have included aspirin or an anticoagulant. The possibilities of alcohol abuse and liver disease must also be considered.

The clinical features and some simple investigations may promptly aid classification of the disorder. Platelet abnormalities may be detected by the platelet count and bleeding time. Other tests of platelet function are usually unnecessary. Clotting factor deficiencies may be detected by:

1. Prothrombin time. This is prolonged with deficiencies of fibrinogen (I) prothrombin (II) or factors V, VII and X.

2. Partial thromboplastin time. This is abnormal when there is a reduction in fibrinogen or factors V, VIII (haemophilia), IX (Christmas Disease), X, XI, and XII.

3. Thrombin clotting time. This is abnormal if there is a reduction in the quantity or quality of fibrinogen.

PLATELET ABNORMALITIES

Thrombocytopenia.

Thrombocytopenia should not be diagnosed purely on a single platelet count below $150 \times 10^9/l$. Spontaneous bleeding is uncommon when the platelets exceed $40 \times 10^9/l$ but post-traumatic haemorrhage may be serious. With under $20 \times 10^9/l$ platelets, spontaneous bleeding is not uncommon. If there are associated problems such as disseminated intravascular coagulation, leukaemia, aplastic anaemia or infection, spontaneous and profuse haemorrhage is more likely for any given platelet count.

A reduction in the platelet count may result from impaired production from the bone marrow, increased consumption as in disseminated intravascular coagulation or increased breakdown as in hypersplenism. The possibility of a drug producing marrow suppression must always be considered.

Patients with idiopathic thrombocytopenic purpura are particularly at risk from intracranial haemorrhage in the early stages of the disease (Davies-Jones et al, 1980). At this time and for several weeks they should be advised to avoid activities, (e.g., coitus) which raise blood pressure.

Treatment includes controlling the underlying cause whenever possible. Steroids and platelet-rich plasma may be necessary in the presence of haemorrhage. Splenectomy has to be resorted to in some cases, particularly those with hypersplenism. Prophylactic treatment with platelet-rich plasma is indicated in patients with low platelet counts after head injury.

Qualitative platelet defects

The possibility of a qualitative platelet defect should be considered when a patient with a prolonged bleeding time has a normal platelet count. There may be impaired platelet aggregation, adhesion or release-reaction.

The rare congenital varieties are not usually associated with intracranial bleeding. In contrast, the much commoner, acquired varieties may be the cause of serious haemorrhage. The possibility that it is drug-induced must be considered. Aspirin, phenylbutazone, carbenicillin and high molecular weight dextran are known to be responsible and many others are likely to be found. Impaired platelet function may occur in uraemia, scurvy, paraproteinaemias, polycythaemia and myelofibrosis. Treatment involves firstly correcting the underlying problem whenever possible; secondly, infusions of platelet-rich plasma; finally, steroids and plasmapheresis in patients with para-proteinaemia.

Thrombotic thrombocytopenic purpura

Although this is an uncommon disorder it is important neurologically because the brain is almost invariably involved (Silverstein, 1968; Aita, 1973). The small arteries and capillaries are occluded by an eosinophilic material containing little fibrin but numerous platelets. There are several similarities to the haemolytic uraemic syndrome of childhood. An immunological disturbance is likely because there is often a history of recent infection, immunisation, penicillin or sulphonamide treatment or of a collagen vascular disease (Antes, 1958).

The diagnosis should be suspected in a patient in whom neurological features are prominent but accompanied by thrombocytopenia with petechial haemorrhages plus a microangiopathic haemolytic anaemia with fragmented, misshaped and contracted erythrocytes. In the early stages the patient may complain of headache, nausea and vomiting and his relatives report some mental changes. The focal features that develop later depend on the sites of small vessel occlusion. Retinal haemorrhage, papilloedema, visual field defects and other cranial nerve signs are common. Hemiparesis, hemisensory disturbances or ataxia may occur; marked fluctuation in the signs is a feature. Patients are usually pyrexial with a mild jaundice, lymphadenopathy and splenomegaly; some joints may become swollen and painful; stupor and coma may supervene.

Apart from the thrombocytopenia and fragmented, distorted erythrocytes there is an anaemia with many reticulocytes, leucocytosis, elevated bilirubin and blood urea and reduced haptoglobin level. Only in a minority is there evidence of significant disseminated intravascular coagulation with fibrinolysis.

The response to treatment may be poor. Several therapeutic approaches, some of them contradictory, have been tried: platelet inhibitors, heparin (Bernstock & Hirson, 1960), steroids, splenectomy (Rodriguez et al, 1957), platelet-rich plasma, fresh blood (Rubenstein, 1959) and exchange transfusion (Bukowski et al, 1976). On the assumption that thrombotic thrombocytopenic purpura is an immunological disease, plasma exchange may prove to be the most appropriate therapy (Davies-Jones et al, 1980).

Thrombocytosis

Thrombocytosis can be said to be present if the platelet count is consistently above $400 \times 10^9/l$. It may predispose to both thrombosis and haemorrhage.

There are several important and common causes: following haemorrhage, trauma, surgery; in some cases of iron deficiency anaemia; in polycythaemia, myelosclerosis and leukaemia; in some malignancies and infections, post-splenectomy and in hyposplenism. There is also an idiopathic variety (essential thrombocythaemia). Thrombotic events are particularly common in polycythaemic and post-splenectomy types. Haemorrhagic events are frequent in essential thrombocythaemia. Paradoxically, bleeding is more likely when the platelet count exceeds $1000 \times 10^9/l$. Perhaps the bleeding time is prolonged because platelets produced in such numbers are malformed and fail to function normally.

Neurological complications are common in essential thrombocythaemia (Ozer et al, 1960). Temporary loss of vision from retinal platelet embolism is not unusual and may respond to aspirin and dipyridamole (Davies-Jones et al, 1980). Transient hemisphere ischaemia may occur (Levine & Swanson, 1968) or cerebral infarction (Spach et al, 1963).

The underlying cause should be sought and the appropriate corrective measures begun. Busulfan or radioactive phosphorus are effective in reducing the platelet count in myeloproliferative disorders but there is usually some delay before they act. In the interim, antiplatelet agents like aspirin and dipyridamole should be used and for urgent cases thrombophoresis may be available (Colman et al, 1966).

CLOTTING FACTOR DEFICIENCIES

Haemophilia

Cerebral haemorrhage is an extremely common cause of death in haemophilia; Biggs (1977) found intracranial haemorrhage to account for almost 30 per cent of haemophiliac deaths. The mortality rate from a single bleed is still estimated to be about 30 per cent (Van Trotsenberg, 1975) despite freeze-dried preparations of Factor VIII and cryoprecipitate.

The haemorrhage may be intracerebral, subarachnoid, subdural or extradural. Those with very low Factor VIII levels (less than one per cent of normal) often have spontaneous bleeding. In those with higher levels (over two per cent of normal) an additional factor such as hypertension or trauma may be present. Haemophiliacs with hypertension should have their blood pressure carefully controlled. Patients who have bumped their heads should be encouraged to attend promptly for prophylactic treatment with freeze-dried Factor VIII concentrate. This may prevent the catastrophic bleeding that may occur over 24 hours after trauma (Eyster et al, 1978).

C.T. scanning facilities have greatly improved the non-invasive assessment of these patients. In some, surgical intervention is necessary to remove large haematomas. The Factor VIII levels can be measured and corrected by infusions and surgery undertaken without undue risk.

Christmas disease

These patients are also prone to intracranial haemorrhage. Factor IX-containing concentrates must be used for treatment and prophylaxis. Cryoprecipitate does not contain Factor IX and should therefore not be given.

Von Willebrand's disease

Fortunately, spontaneous intracranial bleeding is not a common complication of Von Willebrand's disease. However post-traumatic haemorrhage is a danger, and patients should be instructed to attend for prophylactic Factor VIII concentrate after head injury.

Other clotting factor deficiencies

Apart from the very rare congenital afibrinogenaemia (Flute, 1977), spontaneous intracranial haemorrhage is unusual in the other congenital factor deficiencies. However, post-traumatic haemorrhage is still a problem and the appropriate replacement therapy should be given prophylactically (Davies-Jones et al, 1980).

Haemorrhagic complications of liver disease

Patients with alcohol-induced liver disease have an increased incidence of subdural haematomas due, in part, to their more frequent head injuries. Spontaneous intracranial bleeding is not particularly common.

The liver is the site of production of many of the clotting factors and their synthesis may be seriously reduced in many hepatic disorders. Thrombocytopenia is also common and even when platelet numbers are normal, function may be impaired (Thomas, 1972).

Treatment should be with fresh plasma and vitamin K1. Clotting factor concentrates need to be used with the greatest care because of the risk of disseminated intravascular coagulation (Gazzard et al, 1974).

Anticoagulant treatment

Despite careful supervision of anticoagulant therapy there remain a number of cases of 'unavoidable' haemorrhage, some of them intracranial. Bleeding may occur even in those with 'perfect' laboratory control.

The optimal dose of an oral anticoagulant may be readily established by adjusting the prothrombin ratio to 2.5 or the thrombotest to 10 to 15 per cent of the control value. It is more difficult to control intravenous heparin therapy. Anticoagulation may be adequate if the whole blood coagulation time and the partial thromboplastin time with kaolin are twice control values or if the thrombin clotting time is between 25 and 100 seconds (control 10 to 15 s). However, there is a considerable fluctuation in an individual's requirements from day to day. High doses tend to be necessary initially but in most cases the dose can be reduced subsequently and still achieve the same effect.

If a patient on an oral anticoagulant is found to have a dangerously prolonged prothrombin time without any evidence of bleeding, reversal can usually be achieved by 10 mg of vitamin K1 orally. If bleeding is severe the patient should be given concentrates of vitamin K-dependent clotting factors plus 10 mg of vitamin K1 intravenously.

The effect of heparin may be reversed promptly by giving protamine sulphate intravenously. The precise dose of protamine may be determined using the heparin neutralisation test. If this is not promptly available one should proceed on the basis of how much heparin has been given, remembering that 1 mg protamine neutralises 1 mg (100 units) of heparin. This ratio is only necessary if heparin has just been injected. If injected 30 minutes before, only 0.5 mg protamine to 100 units heparin should be given and its effect measured by repeating the thrombin clotting time. It is sometimes necessary to give a further injection of protamine because heparin is cleared more slowly.

Disseminated intravascular coagulation

In this haemorrhagic disorder, there is excessive intravascular thrombus formation producing widespread ischaemia. Clotting factors and platelets are consumed and fibrinolysis is activated such that a haemostatic defect also occurs. This may be a much commoner cause for severe neurological damage than is often realised (Davies-Jones et al, 1980).

In most cases there is a mixture of microvascular obliteration and haemorrhage. In a minority the picture is an overwhelmingly haemorrhagic one. Usually, disseminated intravascular coagulation (DIC) originates elsewhere and then involves the brain. In fact the brain is extremely rich in thromboplastins and if brain damage is accompanied by some defect of the circulating coagulation inhibitors, generalised fibrin deposition may be initiated. Severe head injury, especially gunshot wounds (Goodnight et al, 1974) or cerebral abscess (Preston et al, 1974) may be responsible.

DIC is a well-recognised complication of the following:

1. septicaemia, especially from gram-negative organisms and meningococci
2. trauma and burns
3. surgery, particularly cardiopulmonary
4. severe obstetric complications
5. mismatched blood transfusion
6. malignancies, especially leukaemias but also mucin-secreting adenocarcinomas
7. diabetic ketoacidosis
8. immune-complex disorders
9. snake venom.

The usual process is for tissue damage to produce thromboplastin release. If this is particularly rapid and the inhibitory mechanisms fail there may be massive fibrin deposition. This triggers fibrinolytic mechanisms. Fibrin degradation products reduce platelet aggregation, inhibit thrombin and fibrin polymerisation and so have an anticoagulant effect. Secondary fibrinolysis tends to be particularly excessive in the young such that haemorrhage is the predominant problem.

The intravascular fibrin-platelet complexes are swept into the small peripheral vessels in the microcirculation, some of which they occlude. The brain and kidney are particularly common sites because of their generous share of the cardiac output. At autopsy the cerebral cortex may contain numerous blocked blood vessels with surrounding haemorrhages. Any part of the brain may be involved but the emphasis of damage is often in the watershed areas. The fibrin deposits may not occlude a vessel completely and flow may be impeded temporarily to a degree that impairs neuronal function without cell death. Fibrinolysis may lead to improved flow and restored function.

The possibility of DIC should be considered when a sick patient suddenly develops focal or scattered neurological signs. The CT scan may be misinterpreted as showing multiple metastases. For the reasons cited a marked fluctuation in the clinical signs is typical. An excellent neurological recovery may occur with appropriate treatment even in apparently hopeless cases (Davies-Jones et al, 1980).

The clinical suspicion may be confirmed by finding raised concentrations of fibrin degradation products, a low platelet count and very low fibrinogen. The blood film may show fragmented and misshapen red cells, presumably from mechanical damage on being forced through the fibrin mesh. The prothrombin, thrombin and partial thromboplastin times are prolonged.

Management should be in conjunction with a

skilled haematologist and may be most effective even in a desperately ill patient. In addition to treatment of the underlying cause, patients will require infusions of platelets and coagulation factors plus attempts to limit the thrombotic process with heparin, trasylol or epsilon amino-caproic acid.

Haematological assessment of a patient with cerebrovascular symptoms

The history may provide an invaluable clue to an underlying haematological disorder. There may have been a prior tendency to petechiae, bruising or excessive bleeding. Previous thrombotic events may have occurred either spontaneously, peri-operatively or following infection or trauma. It should be established whether there has been a recent infection, trauma, surgery or obstetrical problem, whether an underlying malignancy is a possibility or if the patient has been on any drugs capable of producing marrow toxicity.

Physical examination may reveal evidence of anaemia, jaundice, plethora or of a bleeding tendency. There may be splenomegaly or lymphadenopathy.

Some simple and widely available laboratory tests may reveal the haematological diagnosis. It is prudent to repeat some of them not only to confirm any abnormality but also to detect any change from day to day. The following are recommended:

1. Hb, PCV and red cell indices
2. blood film and differential white cell count
3. platelet count
4. sedimentation rate and, if elevated, plasma protein electrophoresis
5. fibrinogen and, if fibrinolysis is a possibility, fibrin degradation products
6. blood urea and bilirubin
7. a 'coagulation screen', if there is a bleeding tendency (an equally precise 'thrombosis screen' is yet to be developed)
8. specialised whole-blood and plasma viscosity

measurements may be helpful when there is an increase in PCV or white cell count, when fibrinogen is high or when there is a paraproteinaemia. A satisfactory method for measuring red cell flexibility is badly needed.

Therapeutic possibilities

Modifying the nature of the blood may prove to be the most hopeful avenue for therapy in both the prevention and management of stroke. Attempts at flow improvement may include reducing blood viscosity. There is no dispute about the need for fluid replacement in hypovolaemia with haemo-concentration. Isovolaemic haemodilution with dextran in stroke has been reported to be of value (Gilroy et al, 1969; Gottstein et al, 1976) but a controlled trial is necessary because some doubt its place, except in those with definite polycythaemia. A controlled trial is also necessary to assess the protective effect against stroke of reducing PCV and maintaining it in the low normal PCV range.

Removal of unwanted formed elements and plasma proteins is a logical approach. Phlebotomy may be essential in some cases of polycythaemia (Pearson & Wetherley-Mein, 1978); plasmaphe-resis in paraproteinaemias (Preston et al, 1978a), leucophoresis in leukaemia (Preston et al, 1978b) and thrombopheresis in thrombocytosis (Colman et al, 1966). Defibrination may be achieved acutely with arvin (Bell et al, 1968) and attempts to moderate fibrinogen levels chronically may prove to be beneficial. Thrombolytic therapy with strep-tokinase or urokinase may be worth re-exploring despite early discouraging results (Meyer et al, 1965). Attempts to limit thrombus formation by using heparin, oral anticoagulants and inhibitors of platelet function are discussed elsewhere.

In patients in whom there is a bleeding tendency, the type of deficiency must be accurately diagnosed and the appropriate replacement therapy given. Close cooperation with a haematologist is strongly advised.

REFERENCES

Abramsky O, Slavin S 1974 Neurologic manifestations in patients with mixed cryoglobulinemia. Neurology 24:245–249

Aita J A 1973 Neurologic involvement of thrombotic thrombocytopenic purpura. Nebraska State Medical Journal 58:76–78

Antes E H 1958 Thrombotic thrombocytopenic purpura: a review of the literature with report of a case. Annals of Internal Medicine 48:512–536

Aylward M 1979 Hexopal in Raynaud's Disease. Journal of International Medical Research 7:484–491

Barabas A P, Offen D N, Meinhard E A 1973 The arterial complications of poly cythaemia vera. British Journal of Surgery 60:183–187

Bell W R, Pitney W R, Goodwin J F 1968 Therapeutic defibrination in the treatment of thrombotic disease. Lancet 1:490–493

Bellingham A J 1976 Haemoglobins with altered oxygen affinity. British Medical Bulletin 32:234–238

Bernstock L, Hirson C 1960 Thrombotic thrombocytopenic purpura. Remission on treatment with heparin. Lancet 2:28–29

Berthrong M, Sabiston D C 1951 Cerebral lesions in congenital heart disease; review of autopsies of 162 cases. Bulletin of the Johns Hopkins Hospital 89:384–406

Biggs R 1977 Haemophilia treatment in the United Kingdom from 1969 to 1974. British Journal of Haematology 35:487–504

Bouhoutsos J, Morris T, Chavatzas D, Martin P 1974 The influence of haemoglobin and platelet levels on the results of arterial surgery. British Journal of Surgery 61:984–986

Bukowski R M, Hewlett J S, Harris J W 1976 Exchange transfusions in the treatment of thrombotic thrombocytopenic purpura. Seminars in Haematology 13:219–232

Burch G E, De Pasquale N P 1963 Phlebotomy. Archives of Internal Medicine 111:687–695

Burge P S, Johnson W S, Prankerd T A 1975 Morbidity and mortality in pseudopolycythaemia. Lancet 1:1266–1269

Burrows B, Earle R H 1969 Course and prognosis of chronic obstructive lung disease. New England Journal of Medicine 280:397–404

Butler K R, Palmer J A 1955 Cryoglobulinaemia in polyarteritis nodosa with gangrene of extremities. Canadian Medical Association Journal 72:686–688

Card R T, Weintraub L R 1971 Metabolic abnormalities of erythrocytes in severe iron deficiency. Blood 37:725–732

Chievitz E, Thiede T 1962 Complications and causes of death in polycythaemia vera. Acta Medica Scandinavica 172:513–523

Cohen R J, Bohannon R A, Wallerstein R O 1966 Waldenstrom's macroglobulinaemia. American Journal of Medicine 41:274–284

Colman R W, Sievers C A, Pugh R P 1966 Thrombocytopheresis: a rapid and effective approach to symptomatic thrombocytosis. Journal of Laboratory and Clinical Medicine 68:389–399

Cottrill C M, Kaplan S 1973 Cerebral vascular accidents in cyanotic congenital heart disease. American Journal of Diseases of Children 125:484–487

Cranley J J, Fogarty T J, Krause R J, Strasser E S, Hafner C D 1963 Phlebotomy for moderate erythrocythaemia. Journal of the American Medical Association 186:206–210

Davies-Jones G A B, Preston F E, Timperley W R 1980 Neurological complications in clinical haematology. Blackwell, Oxford

Dawson A A, Ogston D 1970 The influence of the platelet count on the incidence of thrombotic and haemorrhagic complications in polycythaemia vera. Postgraduate Medical Journal 46:76–78

Diggs L W 1965 Sickle cell crises. American Journal of Clinical Pathology 44:1–19

Dintenfass L 1971 Blood microrheology: viscosity factors in blood flow ischaemia and thrombosis. Butterworths London

Dintenfass L, Rozenberg M 1967 Some observations on the viscosity of blood in various diseases. Angiologica 4:116–127

Dormandy J A, Hoare E, Colley J, Arrowsmith D E, Dormandy T L 1973 Clinical haemodynamic, rheological and biochemical findings in 126 patients with intermittent claudication. British Medical Journal 4:576–581

Eastham R D, Morgan E H 1965 Plasma viscosity in clinical laboratory practice. Journal of Medical Laboratory Technology 22:70–73

Elwood P C, Waters W E, Benjamin I T, Sweetnam P M 1974 Mortality and anaemia in women. Lancet 1:891–894

Eyster M E, Gill F M, Blatt P M, Hilgartner M W, Ballard J O, Kinney T B 1978 Central nervous system bleeding in haemophiliacs. Blood 51(6):1179–1188

Fahey J L, Barth W F, Solomon A 1965 Serum hyperviscosity syndrome. Journal of the American Medical Association 192:464–467

Ferencz C 1960 The pulmonary vascular bed in tetralogy of Fallot. 1. Changes associated with pulmonic stenosis. Bulletin of the Johns Hopkins Hospital 106:81–99

Flute P T 1977 Disorders of plasma fibrinogen synthesis. British Medical Bulletin 33:253–259

Gazzard B G, Lewis M L, Ash G, Rizza C R, Bidwell E, Williams R 1974 Coagulation factor concentrate in the treatment of the haemorrhagic diathesis of fulminant hepatic failure. Gut 15:993–998

Gilroy J, Barnhart M I, Meyer J S 1969 Treatment of acute stroke with dextran 40. Journal of the American Medical Association 210:293–298

Goodnight S H, Kenoyer G, Rapaport S I 1974 Defibrination after brain tissue destruction. A serious complication of head injury. New England Journal of Medicine 290:1043–1047

Gottstein U 1965 Physiologie und Pathophysiologie des Hirnkreislaufs. Die Medizinische Welt 15:715–726

Gottstein U, Seldmeyer I, Heuss A 1976 Treatment of Acute Cerebral Ischaemia with Low Molecular Dextran. Results of a retrospective study. Deutsche Medizinische Wochenschrift 101:223–227

Gralnick H R, Abrell E 1973 Studies of the procoagulant and fibrinolytic activity of promyelocytes in acute promyelocytic leukaemia. British Journal of Haematology 24:89–99

Greer M, Schotland D 1962 Abnormal haemoglobin as a cause of neurologic disease. Neurology, Minneapolis 12:114–123

Groch S N, Sayre G P, Heck F J 1960 Cerebral haemorrhage in Leukaemia. Archives of Neurology 2:439–451

Ham G C, Horach H M 1941 Chronic hemolytic anaemia with paroxysmal nocturnal hemoglobinuria. Archives of Internal Medicine 67:735–745

Harman J B, Ledlie E M 1967 Survival of polycythaemia vera patients treated with radio-active phosphorus. British Medical Journal 2:146–148

Harrison B D W, Davis J, Madgwick R G, Evans M 1973 The effects of therapeutic decrease in packed cell volume on responses to exercise of patients with polycythaemia secondary to lung disease. Clinical Science and Molecular Medicine 45:833–847

Harrison M J G, Mitchell J R A 1966 The influence of red blood cells on platelet adhesiveness. Lancet 2:1163–1164

Haut M J, Cowan D H, Harris J W 1973 Platelet function and survival in sickle cell disease. Journal of Laboratory and Clinical Medicine 82:44–53

Heyman A, Patterson J L, Duke T W 1952 Cerebral circulation and metabolism in sickle cell and other chronic anaemias with observations on the effects of oxygen inhalation. Journal of Clinical Investigation 31:824–828

Humphrey P R, du Boulay G H, Marshall J et al 1979 Cerebral blood-flow and viscosity in relative polycythaemia. Lancet 2:873–876

Humphrey P R, du Boulay G H, Marshall J et al 1980a Viscosity, cerebral blood flow and haematocrit in patients with paraproteinaemia. Acta Neurologica Scandinavica 61:201–209

Humphrey P R, Michael J, Pearson T C 1980b Management of relative polycythaemia: studies of cerebral blood flow and viscosity. British Journal of Haematology 46:427–434

Humphrey P R, Michael J, Pearson T C 1980c Red cell mass, plasma volume and blood volume before and after venesection in relative polycythaemia. British Journal of Haematology 46:435–438

Isbister J P, Klarkowski D 1980 Adverse reactions to blood transfusion. Anaesthesia and Intensive Care 8:111

Johnson R V, Kaplan S R, Blailock Z R 1970 Cerebral venous thrombosis in paroxysmal nocturnal haemoglobinuria. Neurology, Minneapolis 20:681–686

Kannel W B, Gordon T, Wolf P A, McNamara P 1972 Hemoglobin and the risk of cerebral infarction: the Framingham study. Stroke 3:409–420

Kiraly J F, Feldmann J E, Wheby M S 1976 Hazards of phlebotomy in polycythaemic patients with cardiovascular disease. Journal of American Medical Association 236:2080–2081

Knizley H, Noyes W D 1972 Iron deficiency anaemia, papilloedema, thrombocytosis and transient hemiparesis. Archives of Internal Medicine 129:483–

Konotey-Ahulu F I D 1974 The Sickle cell diseases. Archives of Internal Medicine 133:611–619

Kopp W L, MacKinney A A Jr, Wasson G 1969 Blood volume and hematocrit value in macroglobulinemia and myeloma. Archives of Internal Medicine 123:394–396

Lackner H, Hunt V, Zucker M B, Pearson J 1970 Abnormal fibrin ultrastructure polymerization and clot retraction in multiple myeloma. British Journal of Haematology 18:625–636

Lawrence J H, Berlin N I 1952 Relative Polycythemia — The polycythemia of stress. Yale Journal of Biology and Medicine 24:498–505

Lehmann H, Huntsman R G 1974 Man's haemoglobins. North Holland Publishing Company, Amsterdam and Oxford

Leidler F, Russell W O 1945 The brain in leukaemia. A clinico-pathological study of twenty cases with a review of the literature. Archives of Pathology 40:14–33

Levine J, Swanson P D 1968 Idiopathic thrombocytosis. A treatable cause of transient ischemic attacks. Neurology, Minneapolis 18;711–713

Logothetis J, Silverstein P, Coe J 1960 Neurological aspects of Waldenstrom's macro globulinaemia. Archives of Neurology 3:564–573

McCallister B D, Bayrd E D, Harrison E G, McGuckin W F 1967 Primary macroglobulinemia. American Journal of Medicine 43:394–434

MacKay I R, Ericksen H, Motulsky A G, Volwiler W 1956 Cryo- and macroglobulinemia. Electrophoretic, ultracentrifuged and clinical studies. American Journal of Medicine 20:564–587

Mahmood A 1969 Fibrinolytic activity and sickle-cell crises. British Medical Journal 1:52–53

Marc-Vergnes J P, Blavo M C, Coudert J, Antezana G, Dedieu P, Durand J 1973 Cerebral blood flow and metabolism in high altitude residents. Stroke 4:345–345

Marshall R J, Malone R G S 1954 Cryoglobulinaemia with cerebral purpura. British Medical Journal 3:279–280

Matzke J, Clausen J, Guttler F 1964 Significance of paraproteinaemia in patients with primary neurologic symptoms. Acta Neurologica Scandinavica 40:269–284

Meyer J S, Gilroy J, Barnhart M E, Johnson J F 1965 Therapeutic thrombolysis in cerebral thrombo-embolism: randomised evaluation of intravenous streptokinase. In: Millikan C H, Siekert R G, Whisnant J P (eds) Cerebral vascular diseases, transactions of the 4th Princeton conference. Grune and Stratton, New York p 200

Moore E W, Friereich E J, Shaw R K, Thomas L B 1960 The central nervous system in acute leukaemia. Archives of Internal Medicine 105:451–467

Nicolaides A N, Horbourne T, Bowers R, Kidner P H, Besterman E M 1977 Blood viscosity, red-cell flexibility, haematocrit and plasma fibrinogen in patients with angina. Lancet 2:943–945

Nutter D O, Kramer N C 1965 Macrocryogelglobulinaemia. American Journal of Medicine 38:462–469

O'Reilly R A, MacKenzie M R 1967 Primary macroglobulinaemia. Archives of Internal Medicine 120:234–238

Ott E 1975 Klinischer Verlauf and Risikofaktoren bei zerebralen transitorisch — ischaemischen Attacken. Wiener medizinishe Wochenschrift 125:374–376

Ozer F L, Raux W E, Miesch D E, Levin W C 1960 Primary hemorrhagic thrombocythemia. American Journal of Medicine 28:807–823

Paulson O B, Henriksen L, Smith O B 1979 The effect of hemodilution on cerebral blood flow and blood gases in patients with polycythemia. Acta Neurologica Scandinavica 60 Suppl 72:588–589

Pears M A, Pickering G W 1960 Changes in the fundus oculi after haemorrhage. Quarterly Journal of Medicine 29:153–178

Pearson T C, Glass U H, Wetherley-Mein G 1978 Interpretation of measured red cell mass in the diagnosis of polycythaemia. Scandinavian Journal of Haematology 21:153–162

Pearson T C, Wetherley-Mein G 1978 Vascular occlusive episodes and venous haematocrit in primary proliferative polycythaemia. Lancet 2:1219–1229

Pearson T G, Wetherley-Mein G 1979 The course and complications of idiopathic erythrocytosis. Clinical and Laboratory Haematology 1:189–196

Perkins H A, MacKenzie M R, Fudenberg H H 1970 Hemostatic defect in dysproteinaemias. Blood 35:695–707

Pickering G W, Wayne E J 1934 Observations on angina pectoris and intermittent claudication in anaemia. Clinical Science 1:305–325

Pilgeram L O 1968 Turnover rate of autologous plasma fibrinogen ^{14}C in subjects with coronary thrombosis. Thrombosis et Diathesis Haemorrhagica 20:31–43

Pilgeram L O 1974 Abnormalities in clotting and thrombolysis as a risk factor for stroke. Thrombosis et Diathesis Haemorrhagica 31 : 245–264

Pochedly C 1975 Neurologic manifestations in acute leukaemia. Symptoms due to increased cerebro-spinal fluid pressure and haemorrhage. New York State Journal of Medicine 75 : 575–580

Portnoy B A, Herion J C 1972 Neurologic manifestations in sickle-cell disease with review of literature and emphasis on prevalence of hemiplegia. Annals of Internal Medicine 76 : 643–652

Preston F E 1980 Hyperviscosity and other complications of paraproteinaemia. Journal of Clinical Pathology 32, Supplement 13 : 85–89

Preston F E, Cooke K B, Foster M E, Winfield D A, Lee D 1978a Myelomatosis and the hyperviscosity syndrome. British Journal of Haematology 38 : 517–530

Preston F E, Malia R G, Sworn M J, Timperley W R, Blackburn E H 1974 Disseminated intravascular coagulation as a consequence of cerebral damage. Journal of Neurology, Neurosurgery and Psychiatry 37 : 241–248

Preston F E, Sokol R J, Lilleyman J S, Winfield D A, Blackburn E K 1978b Cellular hyperviscosity as a cause of neurological symptoms in leukaemia. British Medical Journal 1 : 476–478

Rich A R 1948 Hitherto unrecognized tendency to development of widespread pulmonary vascular obstruction in patients with congenital pulmonary stenosis (tetralogy of Fallot). Bulletin of the Johns Hopkins Hospital 82 : 389–401

Rodriguez H F, Babb D F, Perez Santiago E, Costas-Dirieux J 1957 Thrombotic thrombocytopenic purpura; remission after splenectomy. New England Journal of Medicine 257 : 983–985

Rosenthal A, Button L N, Nathan D G, Meittinen O S, Nadas A S 1971 Blood volume changes in cyanotic congenital heart disease. American Journal of Cardiology 27 : 162–167

Rubenstein M A 1959 Unusual remission in a case of thrombotic thrombocytopenic purpura syndrome following fresh blood exchange transfusion. Annals of Internal Medicine 51 : 1409–1419

Rubenstein R A, Yanoff M, Albert D M 1968 Thrombocytopenia, anemia and retinal hemorrhage. American Journal of Ophthalmology 65 : 435–439

Russell J A, Powles R L 1978 The relationship between serum viscosity, hypervolaemia and clinical manifestations associated with circulating paraprotein. British Journal of Haematology 39 : 163–175

Salzmann E W 1971 Role of platelets in blood-surface interactions. Federation Proceedings 30 : 1503–1509

Scheinberg P 1951 Cerebral blood flow and metabolism in pernicious anaemia. Blood 6 : 213–227

Scott R B, Robb-Smith A H T, Scowen F F 1938 The Marchiafava-Micheli syndrome of nocturnal haemoglobinuria with haemolytic anaemia. Quarterly Journal of Medicine 7 : 95–114

Sharp A A, Warren B A, Panton A M, Allington M J 1968 Anticoagulant therapy with a purified fraction of Malayan pit-viper venom. Lancet 1 : 493–499

Siekert R G, Whisnant J P, Millikan C H 1960 Anaemia and intermittent focal cerebral arterial insufficiency. Archives of Neurology 3 : 386–390

Silverstein A 1968 Thrombotic thrombocytopenic purpura. The initial neurologic manifestations. Archives of Neurology 18 : 358–362

Sorensen S C, Lassen N A, Severinghaus J W, Coudert J, Zamora M P 1974 Cerebral glucose metabolism and cerebral blood flow in high altitude residents. Journal of Applied Physiology 37 : 305–310

Smith J R, Landaw S A 1978 Smokers' Polycythemia. New England Journal of Medicine 298 : 6–10

Solomon A 1965 Neurological manifestations of macroglobulinemia. In : Brain R, Norris F (eds). The remote effects of cancer on the nervous system. Grune and Stratton New York, p 112–123

Somer T 1975 Hyperviscosity syndrome in plasma cell dyscrasias. Advances in Microcirculation 6 : 1–55

Spach M S, Howell D A, Harrison J S 1963 Myocardial infarction and multiple thrombosis in a child with primary thrombocytosis. Pediatrics 31 : 268–276

Stephens A D 1977 Polycythaemia and high affinity haemoglobins. British Journal of Haematology 36 : 153–159

Stockman J A, Nigro M A, Mishkin M M 1972 Occlusion of large cerebral vessels in sickle-cell anaemia. New England Journal of Medicine 287 : 846–849

Swales J D, Evans D B 1969 Erythraemia in renal transplantation. British Medical Journal 2 : 80–83

Thomas D J 1977 The establishment of an intravenous method for measuring cerebral blood flow and its application to the study of the effects of high haematocrit on flow. MD Thesis University of Birmingham

Thomas D J et al 1977a Cerebral blood-flow in polycythaemia. Lancet 2 : 161–163

Thomas D J et al 1977b Effect of haematocrit on cerebral blood-flow in man. Lancet 2 : 941–943

Thomas D J et al 1979 Prevention of stroke — The viscosity factor. In : Meyer J S, Lechner H, Reivich M (eds) Cerebral vascular disease 2. Excerpta Medica, Amsterdam, p 211–215

Thomas D P 1972 Abnormalities of platelet aggregation in patients with alcoholic cirrhosis. Annals of New York Academy of Science 201 : 243–250

Tohgi H, Yamanouchi H, Murakami M, Kameyama M 1978 Importance of the hematocrit as a risk factor in cerebral infarction. Stroke 9 : 369–374

Torrance J, Jacobs P, Restrepo A, Eschbach J, Lenfant C K, Finch C 1970 Intraerythrocytic adaptation to anaemia. New England Journal of Medicine 283 : 165–169

Trujillo M H, Desenne J J, Pinto H B 1972 Reversible papilledema in iron deficiency anemia. Two cases with normal spinal fluid pressure. American Journal of Ophthalmology 4 : 378–380

Tuddenham E G, Whittaker J A, Bradley J, Lilleyman J S, James D R 1974 Hyperviscosity syndrome in IgA multiple myeloma. British Journal of Haematology 27 : 65–76

Usami S, Chien S 1973 Optical reflectometry of red cell aggregation under shear flow. Bibliotheca Anatomica 11 : 91–97

Van Trotsenburg L 1975 Neurological complications of haemophilia. In : Brinkhous K M, Hemker H C (eds) Handbook of haemophilia. Excerpta Medica, New York, ch 25, p 389

Videback A 1950 Polycythaemia vera; Course and prognosis. Acta Medica Scandinavica 138 : 179–187

Wade J P H 1981 Studies on the relative importance of blood viscosity and oxygen carriage in determining cerebral blood flow in primary and secondary polycythaemia. MD Thesis University of Cambridge

Wade J P H, du Boulay G H, Marshall J et al 1980 Cerebral blood flow, haematocrit and viscosity in subjects with a high oxygen affinity haemoglobin variant. Acta Neurologica Scandinavica 61:210–215

Wedemeyer A L, Lewis J H 1973 Improvement in hemostasis following phlebotomy in cyanotic patients with heart disease. Journal of Pediatrics 83:46–50

Weinreb N J, Shih C F 1975 Spurious polycythemia. Seminars in Hematology 12:397–407

Williams H M, Diamond H D, Craver L F, Parsons H 1959 Neurological complications of lymphomas and leukemias. Thomas, Springfield, Illinois, ch 3, p 44

Willison J R, Thomas D J, du Boulay G H et al 1980 Effect of high haematocrit on alertness. Lancet 1:846–848

18

Dementia in cerebral arterial disease

J. M. S. Pearce

When considering the patient suspected of dementia attributed to cerebrovascular disease, the physician is faced with several major issues of definition and with basic considerations of clinico-pathological correlation.

What does he mean by dementia? Is the term to be used loosely for a general decline in communication, faulty judgements and poor memory? Is dementia to be used to describe aberrations of behaviour, irrespective of the patient's response to psychometric tests? Should the term be restricted to certain diseases in which progressive mental decline is a prominent feature, e.g., general paralysis or Alzheimer's disease?

Should dementia be diagnosed only in the presence of demonstrated brain atrophy on a CT scan, or should some biochemical hallmark be insisted upon — if there were a reliable one. It is obvious that pathological evidence of brain atropy and electron microscopic features of various diseases cannot be used routinely for clinical purposes. This highlights the clinician's dilemma since to date there exist no precise criteria, which either singly or collectively allow an accurate demarcation.

Although in years gone by arteriosclerotic dementia, cerebrovascular dementia and cerebral arteriosclerosis were terms widely applied to elderly patients with waning mental faculties, recent studies have rightly led to the profoundest scepticism of these labels, lacking as they do reliable evidence of the underlying pathological process. Whereas it is true that the brains of many demented subjects show infarcts, softenings or lacunes, it is unwarranted to presume that these wholly explain the demented state, since identical lesions may be found also in non-demented subjects. The question arises: is it necessary to have a minimum area or volume of infarcted tissue to produce dementia, or is it the site of the infarct(s) that is the deciding factor? Or, is the presence of old infarction irrelevant to the clinical picture of mental deterioration?

If it were assumed that cerebral infarction *per se* is not related to the presence of dementia could proximal large vessel disease in carotid or vertebral arteries and the aortic arch be responsible for the syndrome by reduction of brain perfusion over a prolonged period? Similarly, in the hypertensive patient in whom deep small lacunes are common, can these tiny lesions be responsible, without large hemisphere infarcts? If vascular changes are dismissed, or if it were supposed they play only a contributory role in the genesis of dementia, then it follows that the complex mixture of Alzheimer's disease and the degree of diffuse atrophy due to ageing alone are the likely causal factors. Yet, the definition of these two processes is equally difficult and at least as imprecise as the accurate apportionment of blame which applies to cerebrovascular disease.

In this chapter I shall try to weigh the existing evidence and describe the clinical picture, investigation and treatment of those demented patients who have cerebral vascular disease.

PATHOLOGY OF MULTI-INFARCT DEMENTIA

The obsolete term cerebral arteriosclerosis implied that dementia was due to arterial disease. Opinion has swung against this concept and it is now acknowledged that when dementia results from cerebrovascular disease it is not the changes in the arteries but the infarction of the brain which is responsible for this process; hence the term multi-infarct dementia (Hachinski et al, 1974). Atherosclerosis does not cause slowly progressive dementia nor is there evidence that it contributes to the aetiology of Alzheimer's parenchymal degeneration during this period of life. The description of multi-infarct dementia assumes that multiple infarcts in the brain can lead to a global decline in brain function as it affects memory, personality, behaviour, mood and the powers of reasoning and intelligence.

Many brain infarcts are caused not by intracerebral but by extracranial vascular disease, due to either thrombosis or embolism. Primary sources of atheromatous plaques may lie in the aorta or in the great vessels of the neck, or the heart. Thrombosis on an atheromatous plaque may be either primary or secondary to proximal lesions. Once a thrombus has developed it may spread by anterograde or retrograde extension. The development of infarction depends on the adequacy of the collateral circulation through the circle of Willis and through the pial vessels of the cortex. The efficiency of this anastomotic mechanism depends on the patency, perfusion pressure and flow through other feeding vessels and on the blood viscosity affecting flow.

Atherosclerosis with thromboembolism is the commonest finding, but a variety of inflammatory disorders including giant cell arteritis, neurosyphilis and collagen vascular diseases may be the underlying pathological process each with its distinctive pathology. Embolic material can originate both from neck vessels and from the endocardium. Atrial fibrillation, mural thrombus superimposed on myocardial infarction, bacterial endocarditis and septicaemic processes are sources of embolism which should not be neglected. Rarer types of emboli include fat, amniotic fluid, air and degenerative material from atrial myxoma. In all these instances multiple areas of infarction are the end result; they may involve the deep grey matter areas of the basal ganglia, the internal capsule, cerebellum and pons, as well as the cerebral cortex. Massive episodes of hypoperfusion of the cerebral circulation may similarly give rise to extensive infarction following cardiac arrest or episodes of anoxia from respiratory arrest or from carbon

monoxide poisoning. Dementia may follow the gross brain damage resulting from these causes. Hypoperfusion or anoxia may cause infarction in the watershed territories between the end arteries of the major anterior, middle and posterior cerebral arteries, resulting in a distinctive appearance of zonal cortical necrosis.

Patterns of vascular occlusion

Primary occlusive thrombosis develops at or adjacent to a site of atherosclerotic stenosis which has reduced the arterial lumen, usually by more than 75 per cent. Thrombosis of the arteries within the brain is rare with the exceptions of the basilar artery or when secondary to vasculitis or oral contraceptives. Pathological evidence shows that infarction due to atheroma, arteritis or to cardiac embolism, results from permanent or transient vascular occlusion *beyond* the circle of Willis. This results from the fact that perforating arteries that enter the brain are devoid of collaterals of a size sufficient to compensate for occlusion of the lumina of the major feeding vessel. Thus the size of the infarct correlates well with the length of intra-arterial thrombus.

There are three common types of embolic material: atheromatous, platelet and mixed (red and white thrombus) emboli. Cholesterol and fibrinous debris constitute the atheromatous emboli through spontaneous or traumatic rupture of the plaque. Platelet emboli are usually small in size and are carried distally into the retinal or cerebral arteries for a brief period and then may fragment into tiny peripheral vessels. Mixed emboli may be small or large and they block small or large extracranial or intracranial arteries, resulting in cerebral infarction. In general, embolic infarcts are purpuric or red; thrombotic ones are pale.

Hypertension accelerates the progression of atheromatous disease and also produces a characteristic pattern of hypertensive vascular disease. This is much the commonest cause of multi-infarct dementia. Initially hypertrophy of the media and hyalinisation occur, but the small perforating end arteries eventually form multiple micro-aneurysms of Charcot-Bouchard type, (Ross Russell, 1963). They may rupture or thrombose causing small areas of necrosis from tiny infarcts. The rupture releases blood and the cavities are seen microscopically to contain haemosiderin. At autopsy they are seen as multiple small spaces or lacunes (*état lacunaire*) which measure one to five millimetres in diameter in most cases. They are characteristically located in the internal capsule, thalamus, basal ganglia and basis pontis. These lacunes are responsible for a number of transient ischaemic attacks in the hypertensive subject, though their number suggests many are clinically silent. They can also mimic a small cerebral infarct and when they result in a number of small strokes the characteristic picure of pseudo-bulbar palsy with or without dementia will result from bilateral involvement of the corticospinal pathways. It should be stressed that this small vessel disease with multiple tiny infarcts is much more important in the production of mental symptoms than is the isolated occurrence of large infarcts in one hemisphere or in the brain stem.

Attempted clinico-pathological correlation

It should be emphasised that both arterial disease and cerebral infarcts are common in patients who have had no evident clinical signs of intellectual failure. Corsellis (1976) observed that 'many people who were not demented in life are found to have severely degenerated and stenosed cerebral vessels'. Difficulties in interpretation occur both at a pathological and at a clinical level. It is impossible for a pathologist to define patterns of brain infarction from which he can reliably deduce the presence of dementia in life. Similarly, dysphasic disorders may make it clinically impossible to recognise an underlying dementia. Further, a variety of amnesic syndromes reflecting lesions in the thalamus, mammillary bodies and hippocampi, may produce such complex patterns of disordered thought, behaviour and memory that the existence of dementia may be unrecognisable. Lastly, since the gross pathological changes and the characteristic senile plaques and neurofibrillary tangles of Alzheimer's disease are so common in presenile and senile periods, it is inevitable that the pathologist will encounter Alzheimer's disease coexisting with cerebral infarction.

When the entire vascular tree is examined in demented and non-demented patients of similar age, atheromatous involvement of both cerebral and extracerebral vessels is found in roughly the same amount in the two groups, according to Corsellis & Evans (1965). Worm-Petersen & Pakkenberg in a study of 108 cases concluded that the atherosclerotic involvement of basal vessels did not play a decisive role in the manifestations of dementia in old age.

By contrast, the changes of Alzheimer's disease are diffuse, affecting much of the entire cortical mantle. The brain weight is reduced, ventricles show symmetrical enlargement (hydrocephalus *ex vacuo*) and cortical gyri are narrowed and sulci enlarged. Histologically, Alzheimer's disease is characterised by the well-known abundance of senile plaques and neurofibrillary tangles (Alzheimer) and granulovacuolar degeneration in the cortical ribbon, especially marked in the hippocampi of the temporal lobes. One or two coincident cerebral softenings are not uncommon, but these may also be seen in non-demented subjects. Thus, in the well-established case, differentation of Alzheimer's disease from multi-infarct dementia is apparent on naked eye examination of the brain. When the conditions coexist, or when the amount of cerebral infarction is only of questionable significance, more precise measurement is necessary. In Alzheimer's disease Roth et al (1967) found dense concentrations of plaques (greater than 11 per high powered field) whereas low plaque counts (0 to 5 per high powered field) were found in normal ageing brains and also in affective psychoses and in so-called arteriosclerotic dementia. The high plaque counts in Alzheimer's disease predict the occurrence of dementia with about 80 per cent certainty. Such high concentrations of Alzheimer's neurofibrillary tangles are found only in Alzheimer's disease although occasional neuronal tangles are seen in the elderly and in low concentration in other miscellaneous cerebral infective and degenerative disorders.

Roth and his colleagues (1967) have shown that the majority of demented subjects show a total of greater than 50 ml of cerebral softening. Below this limit dementia is found infrequently, even in elderly subjects. There is however no evidence that cerebral vascular disease can induce or modify the development of plaque or tangle formation.

CLINICAL FEATURES

The diagnosis of dementia itself is notoriously prone to error. A recent study by Ron et al (1979) from the Maudsley Hospital has shown that the diagnosis of dementia was wrong in up to 20 per cent of subjects after prolonged follow-up and reassessment. Some, but not all of these, proved to have depressive pseudo-dementia. There appear to be no pathognomonic clinical features of multi-infarct dementia.

Diagnosis is in effect a statement of probability based on clinical and investigative phenomena, but it should be borne in mind that there is a considerable margin of error, and ultimately there is no definitive marker, even in some instances after extensive patholgical studies.

Nonetheless Hachinski et al (1974) made a valuable contribution in describing the syndrome. They proposed that multiple infarcts could produce a condition in which dementia was the dominant symptom. In addition to dementia there are focal neurological signs and symptoms, a stepwise deterioration in the clinical course of the illness and often hypertension. They rightly commented that this was a small group. Its delineation was thought to be important because hypertension can be controlled and in selected cases anticoagulation or surgery may be indicated. The importance of recognising this syndrome is the possibility of treatment. Attempts to investigate each case of dementia are eminently worthwhile, because they disclose 10 to 15 per cent of patients in whom some reversible disease process is present. These include instances of meningiomas, subdural haematomas and communicating hydrocephalus as well as instances of neurosyphilis, vitamin B12 and thyroxine deficiency.

It is difficult to ascertain the proportion of demented patients in whom vascular disease is significant. Of 258 cases with dementia studied by Sourander & Sjogren (1970) 132 were of Alzheimer's type, 54 had other organic encephalopathies and 72 were considered due to cerebrovascular disease — a relatively small group.

The mode of onset is a valuable clue. Patients with an insidious onset and slow progression with prominent memory loss and later lack of judgement with parietal lobe signs are likely to fall into the Alzheimer class. (Pearce, 1980). By contrast, sudden episodes of small TIAs or strokes are the hallmark of multi-infarct dementia. In practice these are multiple and in most patients based on established hypertension with characteristic changes in the retinae, heart and kidneys. Fisher (1968) lucidly summarises the situation: 'in brief, cerebrovascular dementia is a matter of strokes large and small'.

Multiple large softenings in the cortex and adjacent white matter are only rarely the cause of vascular dementia. In most patients multiple small infarcts are associated with hypertension and lacunes. This is accompanied by sudden episodes of hemiparesis, dysarthria, dysphasia and ultimately by the appearance of bilateral corticospinal tract signs. When these affect the facial muscles, there is spastic weakness which may be symmetrical, slowness of alternating movements of the tongue and a brisk jaw jerk. Not uncommonly primitive reflexes around the mouth — pouting, sucking and a glabellar tap sign are present with forced grasp reflexes in the hands and feet.

The resulting facial involvement may produce an impassive mask-like face which is commonly mistaken for Parkinsonism (Pearce, 1974). Bilateral pyramidal affection of the limbs produces slowness of movement, a shuffling short-stepped gait (marche à petit pas) which is frequently mistaken for Parkinsonian gait. Careful clinical examination will invariably disclose the pyramidal pattern of weakness and the typical clasp-knife spasticity with hyperactive tendon reflexes and extensor plantar responses. Upper motor neurone involvement of the bulbar muscles produces a typical pseudo-bulbar palsy. This is easily recognised from the resulting spastic dysarthria, slow movements of the tongue and perhaps the hallmark of the syndrome — pathological explosive laughter and crying. Whether this reflects true emotional lability or simply an overflow of normal emotions by facilitation of the release mechanism controlling them, is a matter of speculation.

The well-developed case with multiple strokes or transient ischaemic attacks, hypertension and a pseudo-bulbar palsy is characteristic (Pearce & Miller, 1973). The occurrence of dementia is by no means invariable in such patients, but when it does occur it can be reasonably ascribed to the underlying destruction of brain tissue by multiple infarcts.

The onset of vascular dementia seldom occurs after a first stroke. If it appears to do so, a more careful history or a C.T. scan will show signs of a previous incident. Cognitive impairment may fluctuate. Short periods of drowsiness, apathy or a greater tendency to fall, to misuse words or to have more than usual difficulty in dressing or eating may betoken minor ischaemic incidents. Recovery is initially complete, but succeeding attacks leave greater mental residua.

Nocturnal wanderings, delirium and clouding of consciousness are more common than in Alzheimer's disease. Further TIAs or frank hemiparesis are self-evident. In many cases analysis of the residual mental syndrome poses problems of nosology. Dysphasia makes it hard to assess intellect. The amnesia of temporal lobe lesions may invalidate the assessment of dementia. The gross preservation of personality traits, humour and extroversion in some patients suggests that what we call 'dementia' is in fact the summation of a number of focal defects of higher mental function and that there is no true loss of some general intellectual level of cognition.

Similar conjectures can be derived from Alzheimer's disease even though a 'global impairment' is more characteristic. Accurate distinction from psychological study alone is seldom possible.

Depression may complicate or simulate early dementia. Thus when the patient's performance improves after antidepressants we must not be deceived into thinking that pseudo-dementia was the diagnosis and a cure achieved: many will relapse three or four years later with unmistakable cerebral atrophy and dementia.

Prognosis

All forms of irreversible dementia diminish life expectancy. Of patients admitted to a psychiatric hospital, one third of those with 'arteriosclerotic dementia' had died within six months and three-quarters had perished in two years (Roth, 1955). Much depends on the severity and duration of the hypertension; effective modern hypotensive drugs may have improved these survival rates. Death arises more from coronary heart disease than further strokes.

Better social supportive services at home, improved nutrition and diversionary activities play important roles in survival.

This picture which, although distinctive, is relatively uncommon should be separated from the demented patient who has had perhaps a single stroke but in whom the other features described are lacking. If such a patient is demented, the attribution of the dementia to vascular disease is unwarranted.

Investigation

The first aim is to confirm that the patient is suffering from dementia. Clinical assessment supplemented by psychological tests in selected cases is necessary to separate dementia from transient sub-acute amnesic states, from focal cerebral lesions with dysphasia and is most important in excluding patients with affective psychoses and depressive pseudo-dementia.

Clinical and psychometric assessment is supplemented by CT scanning and angiography in appropriate cases but even then certain subjects in whom depression is the presenting feature of an early dementia may need an empirical trial of antidepressant drugs.

The second aim is the systematic exclusion of systemic diseases, endocrine disease, occult infection as well as the demonstration of possible space-occupying lesions or communicating hydrocephalus. A suitable plan of investigation is shown in Table 18.1.

In a large number of cases the clinical issue resolves itself into the separation of vascular dementia with multiple infarcts from patients with parenchymatous cerebral degeneration of Alzheimer type. The picture of the hypertensive subject with multiple episodes of cerebral ischaemia and signs of pseudo-bulbar palsy is clear enough evidence of a vascular basis. By contrast the history of an insidious impairment of memory, and a variety of subtle dyspraxic and dysphasic signs are characteristic of Alzheimer's disease. It should be stressed that this forms the majority of patients under consideration.

Table 18.1 Scheme for investigation of dementia

Investigation	Possible results
Blood count and film	Anaemia and macrocytosis of vitamin B$_{12}$ or folate deficiency
ESR	Collagen vascular disorders etc.
Chest radiography	Bronchial neoplasm, cardiac lesions
Plasma urea	Azotaemia
Liver function tests	Hepatocellular failure
VDRL, TPI, TPHA	Neurosyphilis
Serum B$_{12}$ and Schilling test	Vitamin B$_{12}$ deficiency
Red cell folate	Folate deficiency
Serum T3, T4, TBG	Hypothyroidism
Skull radiograph	Pineal shift, calcified mass, erosion of posterior clinoids or bone in space-occupying lesion
c.s.f.	Chronic meningitides, or neurosyphilis
e.e.g.	Slowing in primary cerebral atrophies and metabolic encephalopathies; focal change in space-occupying lesion
e.c.g.	Arrhythmias, rheumatic and ischaemic heart disease, other sources of embolism
Angiography*	Carotid and cerebral vascular stenoses, occlusions. Subdural haematoma; tumours
C.T. scanning	Central and cortex atrophy. Other focal lesions, infarcts, tumours, haematomas, etc.

*In selected cases

Specialised neurological investigations

Air encephalography

This has now been rendered obsolete by C.T. scanning.

The electroencephalogram (e.e.g.) in most demented subjects will show diffuse reduction of alpha activity in the occipital regions, with a generalised slowing of the basic resting record and with more or less symmetrical runs of theta and delta activity. A focal slow-wave abnormality may suggest an infarct, and a progressing slow-wave focus on serial e.e.g.s is suggestive of a progressive space-occupying lesion. It has been claimed that bifrontal slow-wave abnormalities are suggestive of vascular dementia, but in general the e.e.g. is a poor diagnostic tool in separating vascular from parenchymatous cerebral degeneration. It seldom adds significantly to the clinical findings. Electroencephalogram findings do not correlate with ventricular size on C.T. scans (Roberts et al, 1978).

C.T. scanning

One of the great advantages of C.T. scanning is that it has now been used in large numbers of so-called normal subjects, so that good control data should be available for purposes of comparison with pathological states. This was seldom achieved in previous investigations with air studies. There is a very striking increase in measurements of ventricular size and of cortical atrophy in normal subjects above the age of 60 (Figs. 18.1. 18.2). The

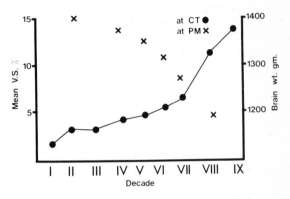

Fig. 18.1 Normal brain ageing — ventricular perimetry and brain weight post-mortem (after Barron et al, 1976 135 CTs and von Braunmuhl, 1957).

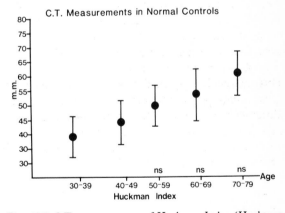

Fig. 18.2 C.T. measurements of Huckman Index (Huckman 1975) (mm) in normal control subjects (personal series).

occurrence of a mild degree of ventricular enlargement and of cortical atrophy is therefore not a reliable index of dementia. Jacoby et al (1980a) screened a group of healthy elderly volunteers, excluded previous neurological and psychiatric illness yet found 8 of 50 subjects with ventricles enlarged beyond that expected for their age group.

Enlargement of the ventricles is not necessarily related to psychometric performance in either the aged non-demented subject or in patients suffering from dementia. However, in general terms there is a relationship between brain atrophy and the clinical diagnosis of dementia. Huckman et al (1975) found only one normal scan in a group of 57 demented patients compared with 8 scans from 20 controls. Jacoby & Levy (1980) found a greater degree of atrophy in a group of 40 patients with senile dementia of Alzheimer's type than in 50 controls. However there was considerable overlap. Discriminant function analysis was carried out by the same workers using various indices of both ventricular dilatation and cortical atrophy. The optimal prediction produced in this analysis incorporated all the variables of the scan and assigned 83 per cent of cases to their correct group. However 17 per cent were incorrectly assigned.

Attempts have been made to use the C.T. scan to differentiate Alzheimer's disease from vascular dementia. Radue et al (1978) found only 40 per cent agreement between clinical and radiological diagnosis. This included 10 out of 19 false positive diagnoses of vascular dementia. It is rare to find C.T. scan abnormalities in patients with TIAs who have no physical signs. Most patients with multi-infarct dementia also have roughly normal scans, since the lesions are probably too small and deeply placed to show. It is not known how small an infarct must be to be invisible, nor what proportion of brain parenchyma has to be destroyed, in an area, to change the attenuation value on the scan. Enhancement by Conray 420 and by Xenon inhalation may add to our understanding of the potentially viable tissue at the periphery of cerebral infarcts.

Relationship of CT scanning to cognitive impairment

Jacoby & Levy (1980a) report earlier studies suggesting that atrophy was more related to age than to the degree of intellectual decline. Their own studies showed in a sample of dements only a few weakly significant correlations with measurements of ventricular enlargement but not with cortical atrophy. The more severely the patient was demented the greater was the degree of enlargement of the ventricles.

Exceptions have been seen to this rule and the scan cannot be used to diagnose the presence of dementia nor can the severity or pattern of loss of mental function be correlated with the C.T. results. The most important use of the technique is to show unsuspected intra-cranial lesions other than infarcts or atrophy. Unsuspected subdural haematomas, gliomas and meningiomas may be revealed. A further important use is to detect communicating hydrocephalus. This can be suspected from the C.T. scan when there is gross ventricular enlargement, often three or four times the normal size for the patient's age, with an absence of cortical atrophy. However the C.T. scan findings in this respect will not reliably separate communicating hydrocephalus from gross hydrocephalus *ex vacuo*, nor can it predict the results of ventriculo-atrial shunting. What it will do is to indicate those patients with gross hydrocephalus in whom 24 hour intracranial pressure monitoring is necessary. With the use of this valuable technique, the presence of nocturnal pressure peaks and plateau waves will indicate a significant dynamic disorder of c.s.f. pressure in a proportion of patients which will often predict a good response to ventriculo-atrial shunting.

In cerebrovascular disease old or new infarcts or haemorrhages will be disclosed in many patients, but in the most important group of hypertensive subjects where the infarcts are multiple, deep and small, the C.T. scan may be normal.

Cerebral blood flow studies

It has been recognised since the 1950s that there is a decrease in the total hemisphere blood flow in dementia from various causes. Disturbances of regional blood flow particularly in the frontal and temporal lobes have been emphasised. Regional cerebral blood flow can be measured by inhalation of [133]Xenon or by intracarotid [133]Xenon injections alone or prior to angiography. Technical details and theoretical considerations of the various methods are discussed by Crawley (1979) and by Thomas & Jones (1979).

Hachinski et al (1975) studied 24 patients with dementia, whom they had assigned on an 'ischaemic clinical score' into either a multi-infarct or a primary degenerative dementia. In both groups of patients there was a decreased proportion of rapidly clearing brain tissue, largely grey matter. Cerebral blood flow per 100 g of brain per minute was normal in the primary degenerative group but was reduced in the multi-infarct group. There was no close correlation between the degree of dementia and cerebral blood flow in the primary degenerative group but an inverse relationship existed in the vascular group. Assessment of the reactivity of blood vessels to reduction in P_aCO_2 was also measured and was normal in both groups.

Earlier, Ingvar et al (1968) found a reduction in hemisphere flow and in the relative amount of grey matter in senile and presenile dementia, the reduction being proportional to the degree of dementia. However the patients were probably a mixed group and interpretation is difficult. Similarly, Simard et al (1971) found reduced blood flow in presenile and senile dementia, and O'Brien & Mallett (1970) measured cortical perfusion rates in demented subjects and found that the primary neuronal degenerations showed normal findings whereas the cerebrovascular cases showed reduced blood flow. Again however the material was mixed. The study of Hachinski et al (1975) confirmed that a significant reduction in blood flow was confined to the multi-infarct group. There was correlation between the mean hemisphere flow and the degree of dementia in this group; but no close relationship between the decrease in c.b.f. and ventricular size or mental deterioration was shown by Melamed et al (1978).

The interpretation of the reduced blood flow is open to conjecture. The normal reactivity of cerebral vessels to CO_2 indicates that it is not a generalised loss of reactivity that is responsible for the low flow. Infarcted tissue is underperfused rather than not perfused. The vessels are capable of supplying more blood, but the metabolic demand of necrotic neurones is decreased. There remains the therapeutically important possibility that a cerebral infarct contains not only metabolically inert tissue but also an appreciable zone of chronically underperfused cerebral neurones which under optimal conditions could be capable of recovering normal metabolic function.

More recent studies of the relationship between regional oxygen utilisation and c.b.f. in multi-infarct dementia have been reported by Lenzi et al (1977). They used an intravenous modification of ^{133}Xenon inhalation, and shortly afterwards regional oxygen extraction was assessed by the continuous ^{15}Oxygen inhalation technique. This can show regions where flow exceeds metabolic need (luxury perfusion); and regions where metabolic need exceeds flow (ischaemia). They showed a low flow in multi-infarct dementia, which appeared adequate for the local metabolic demand. Flow matched oxygen extraction. They failed to show areas of high metabolism with low flow, and concluded that attempts to improve the prognosis would be better aimed at preventing further infarcts than at attempting to improve flow with vasodilators.

Regional blood flow studies and tests of vascular reactivity have therefore shed light on this complex subject but their place in clinical management is a small one, and they remain a research technique. This will undoubtedly be extended in the future by the use of the tomographic positron scanner which will improve imaging and quantitation of regional pathophysiology.

Cerebral angiography

This long-established technique has no place in the established case of presenile or senile dementia of Alzheimer type. Clinical and psychometric diagnosis supplemented by the gross C.T. scan findings suffice in almost all these cases to exclude potentially reversible vascular lesions. Though angiography is still vital in the assessment of patients with cerebral ischaemia, its application in multi-infarct dementia is very limited. Most of these subjects have hypertensive small vessel disease which is not shown reliably by angiographic studies.

Nonetheless there are occasional instances where carotid or subclavian stenoses play a contributory role in these patients, a state suggested by vascular bruits in the neck or by discrepancies between the brachial arterial pressures. The occurrence of dementia in patients with signs of large vessel disease in most instances will prove to be incidental. If they are not severely demented and are having transient ischaemic attacks in the presence of carotid or subclavian stenosis, then angiography either by direct puncture or percutaneous catheterisation should be carried out. The performance of these procedures should however be clearly seen to be directed towards the demonstration and reversal of a vascular stenosis to prevent TIAs and ultimately strokes. It is unlikely that vascular surgery will modify dementia in these subjects. Further the patient with severe multi-infarct dementia will often be unsuitable for angiography or vascular surgery.

The assessment of the demented patient is in every instance made on an individual basis, and 'routine' performance of undirected laboratory tests are to be avoided. The tests must be influenced by the presence of intercurrent illness and by the patient's general health. Serious incapacity, from for example, advanced respiratory failure, coronary heart disease or malignancy would make extensive investigations wholly inappropriate once easily treatable causes of dementia were excluded. Equally however, age alone should not prevent adequate assessment.

MANAGEMENT

Medical evaluation has a number of separate aims:

1. Confirmation that the clinical symptoms are due to dementia and not to an amnesic syndrome, depressive pseudo-dementia or other organic mental states.

2. Documentation of the mental and physical state of the patient; in most instances this should include objective tests of higher mental function performed preferably by a clinician but supplemented in certain cases by a psychologist and a speech therapist.

3. Investigation to exclude remediable systemic causes mentioned in Table 18.1.

4. The assessment and treatment of coincident medical conditions such as anaemia, urinary infection, prostatism, cardiac and respiratory failure.

5. A clinical correlation of all these features combined with a social assessment aiming at reintegration of the patient at home or their subsequent care in hospital.

In many instances this overall plan will necessitate admission to hospital, although much of the investigative work can be done as an outpatient. Early problems in management will be concerned with deciding the prognosis, and ensuring adequate surveillance of the patient and of his drug treatment. This is particularly important in control of hypertension. In the early stages employment may continue, depending on the nature of the job and the severity of the patient's disabilities, both physical and mental. Care and supervision of the patient at home become necessary at a later date. Recruitment of the Social Services and Welfare Officers is helpful, and attendance at a Day Centre may do much to relieve the family for a substantial part of the week and enable them to continue at work. Symptomatic treatment involves the *simplification* of all drug therapy and the exclusion of any long-standing treatments which are not vitally necessary for other medical conditions. Nocturnal sedation with chloral, benzodiazepines or phenothiazines may be necessary for the restless patient prone to wander at night. Daytime treatment with phenothiazines may be of value in selected cases when daytime wandering and toxic confusional episodes are troublesome. They should however be kept under close review and all such drugs should be used in minimum dosage and stopped when the symptoms are no longer pressing.

A number of drug therapies aimed at more specific treatment of dementia have been suggested, but none has proved convincingly successful.

Cerebral vasodilators

Like many other therapeutically blind alleyways, vasodilators have been used for many years on the naive assumption that dilatation of cerebral blood vessels is possible and will increase neuronal function and hence clinical performance. Many enthusiastic reports abound but are based almost invariably on uncontrolled or poorly monitored investigations. The beneficial effect of careful supervision and psychological monitoring implicit in these drug trials has often been overlooked.

Cyclandelate (Cyclospasmol) was used in a double-blind crossover trial by Fine et al (1970) in 40 elderly subjects with arteriosclerotic dementia. Significant improvements were claimed in orientation, communication and socialisation. Young et al (1974) claimed improvements in memory, apraxia and ability to cope with every day life in a group of arteriosclerotic dements. There is a suggestion that the drug increases cortical perfusion rates.

Hydergine, a combination of several hydrogenated ergot alkaloids has been used in double-blind trials. Claims for improvement in mood, attitude and self care as well as the relief of certain physical symptoms have been made by Banen (1972). Improvement in cognitive function has been less consistently reported, but Rao & Norris (1972) noted improvement in alertness and memory as well as in the e.e.g. Hydergine is claimed to act by improving cell metabolism, oxygen uptake and possibly by reducing oedema in astrocytes.

Naftidrofuryl (Praxilene) is another vasodilator for which benefit has been claimed (Judge & Urquhart, 1972; Gerin, 1974). These results were based on double-blind trials in geriatric patients, often severely demented. The improvements were on more subtle aspects of motivation and cognitive function, but changes in mobility and physical independence were not significant. Merory et al (1978) showed that tinofedrine given intravenously increased cerebral blood flow by 28 per cent, but clinical value in preventing infarcts has not been shown.

Anticoagulants

The role of anticoagulants in the treatment of transient ischaemic attacks is still unresolved. Early trials claimed reduction in attacks of monocular blindness and in cerebral ischaemic incidents, but subsequent double-blind trials (e.g., Pearce et al, 1965) failed to show any convincing benefit. There have been several shortcomings in all of the trials so far, dependent upon the shortage of adequately controlled and comparable groups of patients, the duration of follow-up in the trials and the complexities of comparing TIAs in patients without stroke with those in whom TIAs have followed a stroke. Brust (1977) has extensively reviewed the literature on the subject, and it appears that no substantial claim for improvement in the rate of reinfarction or mortality can be based on existing data. There have been no formal controlled trials of anticoagulants in patients suffering from multi-

infarct dementia, and indeed since most of these subjects are hypertensive, anticoagulants would be contraindicated in many of these patients.

Hyperoxygenation

Hyperbaric oxygen, 100 per cent concentration and 2.5 atmospheres of pressure, was used in a group of 13 elderly demented patients by Jacobs et al (1969). Significant improvements on psychological test scores and ward behaviour was claimed. Similar findings have been reported in less severely affected patients by Edwards & Hart (1974). The immediate duration of improvement was short, and this physically cumbersome method of treatment would seem unlikely to have any long-term application, though it is of considerable theoretical interest. Improvement does imply that there is a population of neurones which is viable, but functioning at less than optimal level because of inadequate oxygen uptake or availability.

Antiplatelet drugs

There are numerous studies which have shown that platelets tend to be hyperaggregable in patients with atherosclerosis and therefore in those with transient ischaemic attacks. It follows that drugs which might inhibit platelet clumping may be useful in the prevention of cerebral ischaemic episodes and cerebral infarction. The drugs include aspirin, indomethacin, sulphinpyrazone and dipyridamole.

Aspirin and non-steroidal anti-inflammatory drugs (NSAI) inhibit the formation of cyclic endoperoxides derived from arachidonic acid. Thromboxane A_2 (Fig. 18.3) is derived from platelets and causes aggregation of these elements. By contrast, prostacyclin (PGI_2) arises in blood vessels and is a potent inhibitor of platelet clumping. The search for a safe prostacyclin or a closely related compound which is easily administered has considerable therapeutic potential.

The results of clinical trials are discussed elsewhere in the book, and the subject has been reviewed recently by Fields (1979). The Canadian MRC trial (and the United States collaborative study) have suggested a reduction of 48 per cent in the incidence of stroke as a result of taking aspirin

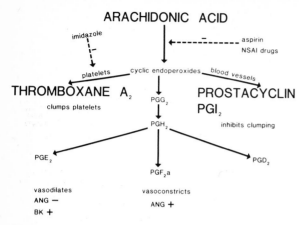

Fig. 18.3 Metabolic derivations of arachidonic acid in blood vessels and platelets.

but not sulphinpyrazone, but this benefit was curiously confined to males. Since the pathology of multi-infarct dementia is mainly dependent on the presence of lacunes from arteriolar micro-aneurysms, it would seem unlikely that antiplatelet therapy would play a significant role in this form of vascular occlusion, though only comprehensive controlled studies would resolve this issue.

Vascular surgery

Vascular surgeons now proclaim with confidence that carotid endarterectomy is standard surgical procedure for localised extracranial internal carotid arterial disease and is effective in preventing strokes. The procedure aims to remove stenotic obstruction to flow, but more important to remove sources of cerebral emboli. The American joint study of extracranial arterial occlusion has shown

that the best results are obtained in patients with TIAs with complete recovery and stable neurological status. Bilateral carotid stenoses should be treated surgically on the side appropriate to the symptoms, but a period of at least four weeks should elapse after the last clinical episode and surgery on the opposite side is unnecessary if the patient remains symptom free (Fields, 1977).

It is now technically possible to bypass a middle cerebral occlusion by anastomosis of the superficial temporal artery to distal or cortical branches of the middle cerebral artery. Most published reports have not been controlled, and despite impressive individual results much more information is needed to decide on the indications and potential role of this interesting surgical advance (McDowell, 1977). It has no present routine application.

CONCLUSION

In the clinical context of dementia in middle and late life vascular disease does not figure prominently. Multi-infarct dementia is a real entity with characteristic clinical and investigative findings as described but its existence is often difficult to prove. The need for adequate investigation and clinical assessment is stressed. Most current forms of therapy are valueless. Although there is considerable potential for treatment, the most important means of preventing the development and retarding the progression of multi-infarct dementia is the early recognition and strict control of hypertension.

REFERENCES

Banen D 1972 An ergot preparation (hydergine) for relief of symptoms of cerebrovascular insufficiency. Journal of the American Geriatrics Society 20:22–24

Barron S A, Jacobs L, Kinkel W R 1976 Changes in size of normal lateral ventricles during aging determined by computerized tomography. Neurology 26:1011–1013

Brust J C M 1977 Transient ischaemic attacks: natural history and anticoagulation. Neurology (Minneapolis) 27:701–707

Corsellis J A N 1976 In: Blackwood W, Corsellis J A N (eds.) Greenfield's Neuropathology, 3rd edn. Arnold, London, p 797–8

Corsellis J A N, Evans P H 1965 Proceedings of the 5th International Congress of Neuropathology, p 546

Crawley J C W 1979 Recent technical developments in the Xenon 133 inhalation technique for cerebral blood flow measurement. In: Greenhalgh R M, Rose F C (eds.) Progress in stroke research 1. Pitman, London. ch. 34, p 319–329

Edwards A E, Hart G M 1974 Hyperbaric oxygenation and the cognition functioning of the aged. Journal of the American Geriatrics Society 22:376–379

Fields W S 1977 Transient cerebral ischaemic attacks. In: Zulch K J, Kaufman W, Hossmann K A (eds.) Brain and heart infarct. Springer-Verlag, Berlin, p 281–287

Fields W S 1979 Platelet-suppressive therapy in cerebral ischaemia. In: Greenhalgh R M, Rose F C (eds.) Progress in stroke research 1. Pitman, London. ch 23, p 204–206

Fine E W, Lewis D, Villa-Landa I, Blakemore C B 1970 The effect of cyclandelate on mental function in patients with arteriosclerotic brain disease. British Journal of Psychiatry 117:157–161

Fisher C M 1968 In: Toole J F, Siekert R G, Whisnant J P (eds.) Cerebral vascular disease: 6th Princeton conference. New York. p 232

Gerin J 1974 Double-blind trial of naftidrofuryl in the treatment of cerebral arteriosclerosis. British Journal of Clinical Practice 28:177–178

Hachinski V C, Lassen N A, Marshall J 1974 Multi-infarct dementia. A cause of mental deterioration in the elderly. Lancet 2:207–209

Hachinski V C et al 1975 Cerebral blood flow in dementia. Archives of Neurology 32:632–637

Huckman M S, Fox J, Topel J 1975 The validity of criteria for evaluation of cerebral atrophy by computerised tomography. Radiology 116:85–92

Ingvar D H et al 1968 General and regional abnormalities of cerebral blood flow in senile and presenile dementia. Scandinavian Journal Clinical and Laboratory Investigations suppl. 102 p XIIB

Jacobs E A, Winter P M, Alvis H J, Small S M 1969 Hyperoxygenation effect on cognitive functioning in the aged. New England Journal of Medicine 281:753–757

Jacoby R, Levy R 1980 CT scanning and the investigation of dementia. Journal of the Royal Society of Medicine 73:366–369

Jacoby R J, Levy R, Dawson J M 1980 Computed Tomography in the elderly. British Journal of Psychiatry 136:249–255

Judge T G, Urquhart A 1972 Naftidrofuryl — a double blind cross-over study in the elderly. Current Medical Research and Opinion 1:166–172

Lenzi G L, Jones T, Moss S, Thomas D J 1977 The relationship between regional oxygen utilization and cerebral blood flow in multi-infarct dementia. Acta Neurologica Scandinavica Supplement 56 (64):248–9

McDowell F H 1977 The extracranial–intracranial bypass study. Stroke 8:545

Melamed E, Lavy S, Siew F. Bentin S, Cooper G 1978 Correlation between regional cerebral blood flow and brain atrophy in dementia. Journal of Neurology, Neurosurgery and Psychiarty 41:894–899

Merory J, Du Boulay G H, Marshall J, Morris J, Ross Russell R W, Symon L, Thomas D J 1978 Effect of tinofedrine (Homburg D8955) on cerebral blood flow in multi infarct dementia. Journal of Neurology, Neurosurgery and Psychiatry 41:900–902

O'Brien M D, Mallett B L 1970 Cerebral cortex perfusion rates in dementia. Journal of Neurology, Neurosurgery and Psychiatry 33:497–500

Pearce J M S, Gubbay S S, Walton J N 1965 Long-term anticoagulant therapy in transient cerebral ischaemic attacks. Lancet 1:6–9

Pearce J M S 1974 The extrapyramidal disorder of Alzheimer's disease. European Neurology 12:94–103

Pearce J, Miller E 1973 In: Clinical aspects of dementia. Ballière Tindall, London. ch 3, p 31–33

Pearce J M S 1980 Dementia. Medicine 31:1617–1620

Radue E W, Du Boulay G H, Harrison M J G, Thomas D J 1978 Comparison of angiographic and CT findings between patients with multi-infarct dementia and those with dementia due to primary neuronal degeneration. Neuroradiology 16:113–115

Rao D B, Norris J R 1972 A double-blind investigation of hydergine in the treatment of cerebrovascular insufficiency in the elderly. John Hopkins Medical Journal 130:317–324

Roberts M A, McGeorge A P, Caird F I 1978 Electroencephalography and computerised tomography in vascular and non vascular dementia in old age. Journal of Neurology, Neurosurgery and Psychiatry 41:903–906

Ron M A, Toone B K, Garralda M E, Lishman W A 1979 Diagnostic accuracy in presenile dementia. British Journal of Psychiatry 134:161–168

Roth M 1955 The natural history of mental disorder in old age. Journal of Mental Science 101:281–301

Roth M, Tomlinson B E, Blessed G 1967 The relationship between quantitative measures of dementia and degenerative changes in the cerebral grey matter of elderly subjects. Proceedings of the Royal Society of Medicine 60:254–258

Russell R W R 1963 Observations on intracerebral aneurysms. Brain 86:425–442

Simard D, Olesen J, Paulson O B, Lassen N A, Skinhoj E 1971 Regional cerebral blood flow and its regulation in dementia. Brain 94:273–288

Sourander P, Sjogren H 1970 In: Wolstenholme G, O'Connor M (eds.) Ciba Symposium; 'Alzheimer's disease and related conditions'. Churchill, London p 145–165

Thomas D J, Jones T 1979 The combined use of the intravenous ^{133}Xenon technique and the $^{15}O_2$ inhalation method. In: Greenhalgh R M, Rose F C (eds.) Progress in stroke research 1. Pitman, London ch 45 p 330–339

Von Braunmuhl A 1957 In: Lubarsch O, Henke F, Ross R (eds) Handbuch der Speziellen Pathologischen Anatomie und Histologie 13:347. Berlin. (Cited by McMenemey, 1963)

Worm-Petersen J, Pakkenberg H 1968 Atherosclerosis of cerebral arteries, pathological and clinical correlations. Journal Gerontology 23:445–449

Young J, Hall P, Blakemore C 1974 Treatment of the cerebral manifestations of arteriosclerosis with cylandelate. British Journal of Psychiatry 124:177–180

19

Less common varieties of cerebral arterial disease

R. W. Ross Russell

CONGENITAL ARTERIAL ABNORMALITIES

Absence of one or both internal carotid arteries is a rare congenital defect; only about 25 cases have been recorded (Turnbull, 1962; Hills & Sament, 1968). The condition may be discovered by chance in infants dying from other malformations. In later life patients may present with haemorrhage from dilated collateral arteries or from a coexistent berry aneurysm, or with multiple lower cranial nerve palsies caused by pressure from a greatly enlarged basilar artery. Absence of the carotid canals may be detected radiologically. Hypoplasia of the internal carotid arteries on one or both sides is also a rarity; familial cases have been reported by Austin & Sears (1971). It affects the whole length of the artery except for the proximal two centimetres. It too is associated with malformation of the Circle of Willis, berry aneurysm, or abnormal collateral channels, and the condition only usually comes to light during investigation of intracerebral or subarachnoid haemorrhage (Lhermitte et al, 1968; Smith et al, 1968).

Congenital arterial looping and kinking; carotid arteriomegaly

Looping and tortuosity of the internal carotid artery may be found at any age (for review see Desai & Toole, 1975). In children the condition has a prevalence of 15 per cent and is undoubtedly congenital in origin since the fetal carotid artery is normally tortuous at the point where it is crossed by the glossopharyngeal nerve. In adults tortuosity and coiling become exaggerated as a result of degenerative arterial disease and the prevalence rises to 25 per cent (Weibel & Fields, 1965). Kinking or angulation of the artery with narrowing of the lumen is regarded as an acquired condition affecting a previously tortuous artery.

Any relationship between these extracranial abnormalities and cerebral ischaemia is uncertain but possible mechanisms have been suggested. Tortuous arteries may become kinked or occluded during movements of the neck (Bauer et al, 1961). The endothelium of the kinked segment may become damaged and act as a nidus of thrombus formation; during kinking flow may be temporarily arrested and the carotid sinus may be distended causing reflex hypotension and bradycardia (Sarkavi et al, 1970). Other clinical features found in association with carotid loops included hypoglossal palsy, pulsatile tinnitus, and attacks of headache and vertigo.

It is difficult to assess the clinical relevance of tortuosity in individual patients. In one report for instance (Metz et al, 1961) there were slightly more ischaemic episodes in patients with tortuosity of the carotid artery than in normal patients. In another (Bauer et al, 1961) the frequency of carotid and vertebral tortuosity in patients with clinical cerebrovascular disease was 25 per cent, the same frequency as in a random sample. It is probable that tortuosity is only rarely a primary cause of symptoms in adults but a syndrome in childhood has been described with seizures, transient hemiparesis, hemianopia, and dysphasia in association with looping of the internal carotid artery on the appropriate side usually just below the base of the skull (Sarkavi et al, 1970).

The condition can be treated surgically by resection of the redundant loop. This has been claimed to abolish transient attacks (Vollmar et al,

1976). Other reports take a more sceptical view of the value of surgery (Perdue et al, 1975).

Enlargement and lengthening are frequently seen in large and medium sized arteries affected by atherosclerosis and hypertension. In the innominate artery this causes a redundant loop and may be noticed as prominent pulsation over the head of the clavicle in the right side. It is often mistaken for an aneurysm.

Rarely a general arterial ectasia has been described in young children (Ochsner et al, 1977). Its pathological basis is dysplasia and disruption of elastic tissue and it may present as massive pulsating carotid swellings on each side of the neck.

Fibromuscular dysplasia

Fibromuscular dysplasia, a condition first recognised in the renal arteries, is now known to involve a variety of small and medium-sized arteries throughout the body. Affected vessels exhibit alternate segments of stenosis and ectasia, the narrowed segments having a constant and sharply localised 'string of beads' appearance. Microscopically the medial coat is either thick and fibrotic or thinned. The thinned regions show a loss of elastic tissue (mural aneurysm) and the muscle coat may be entirely absent. There are no changes of atherosclerosis.

The condition affects two to three centimetre lengths of the mid-cervical portion of the internal carotid artery usually at the level of the second cervical vertebra. The proximal internal carotid artery is normal and points of branching are characteristically spared. (Fig. 19.1). Narrowing of the lumen is a constant feature but complete obstruction is most unusual (Frens et al, 1974); in 75 per cent of cases the condition is bilateral. The vertebral artery may also be involved in its extracranial course. Intracranial fibromuscular dysplasia is rare and is usually limited to the osseous or cavernous portions of the internal carotid artery (Rimaldi et al, 1976).

The condition is most frequently found in women over the age of 55. In one-third of the cases it comes to notice as a chance finding on angiography for an unrelated condition. The remaining two-thirds of patients have a variety of cerebrovascular symptoms — transient ischaemic attacks

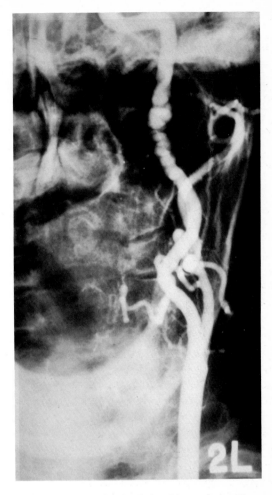

Fig. 19.1 Fibromuscular dysplasia of internal carotid artery. The patient, a woman aged 60, presented with carotid transient ischaemic attacks. A carotid bruit was present. (Courtesy of Professor G. du Boulay).

40 per cent; subarachnoid haemorrhage 36 per cent; cerebral infarction 24 per cent (Osborn & Anderson, 1977). The frequency of berry aneurysm in radiological reports is 25 per cent (Houser & Baker, 1968).

Fibromuscular dysplasia must be distinguished from two other conditions. The first is *circular spastic contraction* which may take one of two forms. The first is one or more band-like constrictions narrowing the lumen by 10–20 per cent. The second is a tubular type of stenosis affecting usually the entire length of the internal carotid artery and narrowing the lumen by 50 per cent. Neither of these conditions is usually associated with vascular disease or with significant obstruction to blood flow. The appearance may be produced by trauma such as the sub-intimal injection of contrast medium at angiography. Frequently the abnormality is a temporary one and is said to respond to vasodilators (Houser & Baker, 1968). The second condition is *stationary arterial waves*, often an incidental angiographic appearance sometimes found with retarded blood flow in the carotid artery. It produces regular corrugations of the artery wall with only slight narrowing and is distinguished from fibromuscular dysplasia by the absence of dilated segments. Some authors interpret stationary arterial waves as another type of artifact of contrast injection and state that they may disappear on a second injection (New, 1966).

Aneurysms of the cervical carotid artery

Dissecting aneurysm of the cervical portion of the artery is an unusual cause of occlusion in youth and middle age. Although in some cases dissection may follow trauma it may also occur spontaneously. Many patients have an underlying arterial dysplasia which may be cystic medial necrosis of the aorta (Marfan syndrome), Ehlers-Danlos syndrome or pseudoxanthoma elasticum. There have been a number of reports of abnormal amounts of mucopolysaccharide within the arterial wall and of degeneration of elastica. Some authors stress the frequency with which fibromuscular dysplasia is found on the contralateral side and there is also a possible link with contraceptive medication (Ehrenfeld & Wylie, 1976). Dissection begins as an intimal tear a short distance above the origin of the internal carotid artery. Blood enters a false lumen within the media or between the medial and adventitial coats and tracks upwards to the skull base.

The condition may affect young or middle-aged patients of either sex. There is severe unilateral headache with facial, ocular or neck pain with or without an oculosympathetic palsy. Transient cerebral ischaemia, amaurosis fugax or completed stroke may all occur. If the symptoms are repetitive then they are probably due to embolism of mural thrombus. On arteriography the carotid artery may show irregular narrowing throughout its cervical course (string sign) or may show a tapering occlusion (Ojemann et al, 1972). The origin of the

dissection may be visible as the contrast medium tracks into the wall of the artery. (Fig. 19.2).

In some patients partial dissection has been observed to progress to complete occlusion. In others a second arteriogram after some weeks may show a normal vessel, the intramural haematoma having probably reabsorbed.

Various surgical treatments have been recommended. Excision of the affected segment with vein grafting may be possible in some patients but usually the dissection extends upwards as far as the base of the skull where resection is not possible. In patients with recurrent transient ischaemia in whom a good distal carotid stump pressure (greater than 65 mm) is found, carotid ligation may be performed to reduce the risks of further embolism. Some patients have been treated by external-internal carotid artery bypass but intraluminal

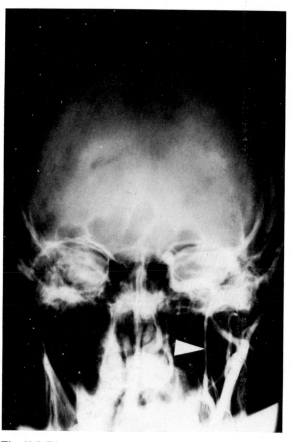

Fig. 19.2 Dissecting aneurysm of left internal carotid artery in the neck. The artery is narrowed up to the base of skull (string sign). (Courtesy of Professor G. du Boulay).

forced dilatation using a balloon catheter is not recommended because of the risk of embolism. Because of the generally favourable prognosis and the possibility of spontaneous resolution conservative treatment is to be preferred in the majority of patients.

A related condition has been described as 'idiopathic regressing arteriopathy' (Mokri et al, 1979). This presents as unilateral cephalgia spreading to the neck and mastoid region with episodes of cerebral ischaemia. A long attenuated segment of the cervical internal carotid artery is seen on angiography but if the study is repeated after a few days or weeks the abnormality may have disappeared. The cause of this condition is unknown; in some cases there may be a spontaneous dissecting aneurysm which heals spontaneously. In others vascular spasm may be responsible. If surgical exploration is undertaken the artery may appear normal.

Other aneurysms of the cervical carotid artery are rare. If a saccular aneurysm arises near the origin of the artery transient cerebral ischaemia may occur due to embolism (Schwartz et al, 1962) or to obstruction of the artery during head turning (Countee et al, 1979). Fusiform aneurysm or irregular outpouching of the artery may occur near the origin following radiation treatment for thyroid disease.

Saccular aneurysms most commonly occur just below the skull base and have been described in relation to pharyngeal pyogenic infection, to trauma or to syphilitic infection. (Fig. 19.3). Transient or permanent cerebral ischaemic attacks are probably due to embolism to the middle cerebral artery and there may also be pain and ocular sympathetic palsy. The aneurysm may also present as a lump in the pharynx causing hoarseness and dysphagia (Margolis et al, 1972). Recurrent embolism may necessitate carotid ligation with or without transcranial bypass. Other patients complain of headache, tinnitus or symptoms of lower cranial nerve palsies, and in some the condition may be symptomless.

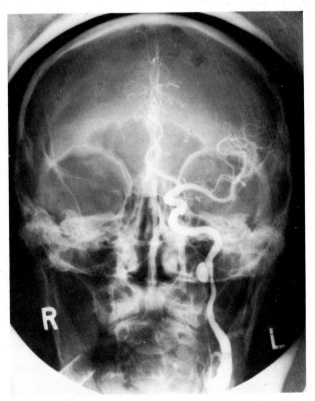

Fig. 19.3 Saccular aneurysm of left internal carotid artery just below the skull base. The patient, man aged 60, presented with transient cerebral ischaemia. (Courtesy of Professor W. I. McDonald).

Infraclinoid carotid aneurysm

The cavernous portion of the carotid artery is a frequent site for small berry aneurysms which may be an incidental finding on angiography or at autopsy. At this point the artery is extra-dural and although the aneurysm may rupture into the cavernous sinus massive subarachnoid haemorrhage is exceptional. The aneurysm may arise at the origin of the small hypophyseal branch vessel and although originally saccular is may slowly expand to distent the sinus taking up the original artery wall as it does so and stretching the nerves on the lateral wall of the sinus (Barr et al, 1971). The aneurysm may eventually come to occupy much of the floor of the middle fossa.

Patients are almost always elderly women and they present with a painful unilateral cavernous sinus syndrome. The pain may be severe, it has a constant boring quality and is felt behind the eye, in the forehead and root of the nose. There follows after a variable period an ophthalmoplegia involving the sixth then third and fourth cranial nerves (Meadows, 1961). The pupil is usually smaller on the affected side due to damage to the sympathetic fibres around the carotid artery; its reactions to light and accommodation are reduced or absent (efferent pupillary defect). Some disturbance of facial sensation over the first two divisions of the trigeminal nerve is often present and the corneal reflex is reduced although seldom absent. Proptosis is slight and vision normal except in the case of giant aneurysms which may compress the ipsilateral nerve or the side of the chiasma (Peiris & Russell, 1980). Plain X-rays of the skull may be normal or may show erosion of the anterior clinoid process and sella turcica. The wall of the aneurysm itself may be calcified and may erode the superior orbital fissure and middle fossa. Orbital venograms show obstruction of the cavernous sinus; CT scanning may show a circular enhancing lesion; carotid angiography is diagnostic.

If untreated the aneurysm slowly enlarges although pain usually improves after some weeks. Ophthalmoplegia may persist or recover partially. For intractable pain the carotid artery may be ligated in the neck and in some patients the aneurysm may be isolated by a trapping procedure or by embolisation. All these methods of treatment carry a considerable risk of hemiplegia in elderly patients, a risk which may be lessened by extra-intracranial anastomosis performed as a preliminary to surgery.

Basilar aneurysm

Although less frequent than on the anterior part of the Circle of Willis berry aneurysms may occur on the posterior cerebral arteries at the point of bifurcation of the basilar artery, on the vertebral artery or on any of its branches, especially on the posterior inferior cerebellar artery. The presenting symptom is subarachnoid haemorrhage and is discussed in Chapter 12. The basilar artery is occasionally involved in dissecting aneurysm (Alexander et al, 1979) and is also the site of an unusual type of vascular ectasia or fusiform aneurysm often, though not invariably, found in association with extensive atheroma and hypertension (Alajouanine et al, 1948). A similar generalised vascular ectasia may affect the carotid arteries. There is extensive dilatation and lengthening of the basilar artery which becomes serpiginous and extends laterally into the cerebello-pontine angle to compress the lower cranial nerves on one side. Thrombosis occurs in successive layers on the luminal surface and may finally occlude the artery. The clinical presentation is diverse; many patients present with symptoms of transient vertebrobasilar ischaemia in brain stem and posterior cerebral territories. Attacks of hemiparesis may simulate carotid TIA (Hirsch & Gonzales, 1979). Headache and neck pain are prominent and may be made worse by head movement. A special diagnostic feature is the involvement of cranial nerves mainly the seventh and eighth and including attacks of hemifacial spasm (Denny-Brown & Foley, 1952).

In addition these large aneurysms act as mass lesions and simulate posterior fossa tumours usually in the cerebello-pontine angle or foramen magnum regions. There may be progressive ataxia, spastic quadriplegia, and pseudobulbar palsy from compression of the brain stem by the aneurysm (Fig. 19.4). Any of the cranial nerves from third to twelfth may also be involved (Yaskin & Alpers, 1944). Raised intracranial pressure and organic dementia are also reported (Michael, 1974). Cerebrospinal fluid examination normally shows a

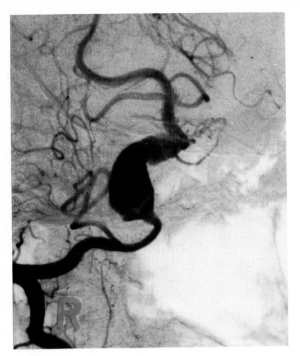

Fig. 19.4 Fusiform aneurysm of the basilar artery. The patient, a male aged 25, had attacks of vertebrobasilar ischaemia followed by a pontine infarction. (Courtesy of Dr P. Gautier-Smith).

raised protein content with or without xanthochromia. Vertebral angiography is diagnostic but may underestimate the size of the aneurysm because of thrombus within the lumen. The prognosis is poor, death occurring from basilar occlusion or haemorrhage within two years of diagnosis in the great majority of patients.

Aortic arch syndrome (pulseless disease)

Occlusion of the origins of the major brachiocephalic arteries gives rise to distinctive symptoms due to progressive reduction in blood flow to the territories of the external and internal carotid and subclavian arteries. The disease as a rule evolves very slowly and may be present for many years before blood flow to the brain is affected. During the slow development of narrowing of the major extracranial artery a point is reached at which there is restriction of blood flow. This does not occur until 80–90 per cent of the lumen has been occluded. Under these circumstances the reduction in blood flow is offset by an increased flow in the remaining arteries and vasodilatation of intracerebral resistance vessels so that the total cerebral blood flow may be little affected. If however the remaining arteries are also diseased other homeostatic mechanisms may come into operation such as the development of collateral channels to bypass the occlusion. These usually involve muscular branches of thyro-cervical, costo-cervical and vertebral trunks. The effectiveness of collateral flow is illustrated by reportes of symptomless patients with occlusion of three or even four of the main extracranial arteries (Vitek et al, 1972).

When there is restriction of blood flow in the external carotid territory a temporary and reversible insufficiency similar to intermittent claudication can arise as the result of increased metabolic tissue demand, e.g., in the jaw muscles when the patient chews.

By contrast, cerebral metabolism requires a relatively constant blood supply but if the perfusion pressure is low and the resistance vessels maximally dilated there is little homeostatic reserve in the system and any minor fall in blood pressure may cause temporary cerebral ischaemia.

Although there are many causes of the aortic arch syndrome the symptomatology is uniform and varies only in degree and duration (Ross & McKusick, 1953). Episodes of vertigo, confusion or lightheadedness are the commonest complaints and are present in over half the patients; there may be actual loss of consciousness or true seizures. Some patients experience episodes of hemiparesis, dysarthria, deafness, tinnitus or rarely an unusual type of drop attack without change in consciousness but with incontinence of urine (Currier et al, 1954). Intense occipital headache and claudicating pain in the jaw on eating are commonly reported. Visual symptoms are often present, may affect one or both eyes and may be provoked by sudden standing or by physical exercise. When the defect is uniocular it signifies a reduction in blood flow to one eye but in bilateral or altitudinal field loss the mechanism may be ischaemia of the occipital cortex (Russell, 1973).

Ischaemic pain in the arms on exercise is an unusual symptom although pallor and coldness may be noted on examination. Chronic ischaemia in the external carotid territory may lead to facial atrophy, ulceration of the scalp, palate or nasal septum. In the brain there may be memory loss, progressive intellectual impairment and dementia, with focal signs suggesting bilateral parieto-occipital lesions (Russell, 1973). This region is the arterial borderzone where all three vascular territories meet and where the perfusion pressure is at its lowest. The region tends to be selectively involved in patients with attacks of extreme hypotension.

Chronic ocular ischaemia may occur and cause progressive visual impairment with low pressure retinopathy, scattered retinal and vitreous haemorrhages, slowing of blood flow in the small veins of the retina, optic atrophy, peripheral microaneurysms and arterial attenuation (Knox, 1965). The peripapillary anastomosis described by Takayasu (1908) is seen only in severe cases.

The principal findings on examination are reduced or absent pulsations in the head, neck and arms. The brachial pressures are reduced or unrecordable as is the pressure in the ophthalmic artery. Spontaneous pulsations are sometimes visible in the retinal arteries. Vascular bruits around the neck or scapula may be detected. In spite of occlusion of the subclavian arteries blood flow to the arms may be normal at rest but fails to show the expected increase on exercise (Held et al, 1973). There may also be evidence of aortic regurgitation, aortic dilitation, renal artery stenosis and ischaemic changes in the legs. Angiography may show segmental dilatation and stenosis of the aorta with occlusion at the origin of the great vessels (Strachan, 1966). In some patients the subclavian arteries are preferentially affected; in others both carotid and subclavians show occlusive changes (Fig. 19.5).

Various types of arterial pathology may be responsible. Many of the early cases occurred in young oriental women and showed histological evidence of *low grade arteritis* of unknown cause. The artery wall is thickened due to fibrous proliferation and there is mononuclear infiltration and occasional giant cells. Fibrinoid change or eosinophils are absent (Danaraj et al, 1963). Some patients show predominant involvement of the descending aorta and in some there is concurrent tuberculous infection. In another variety of aortic disease recently reported from Sri Lanka and South India there are focal exudative inflammatory

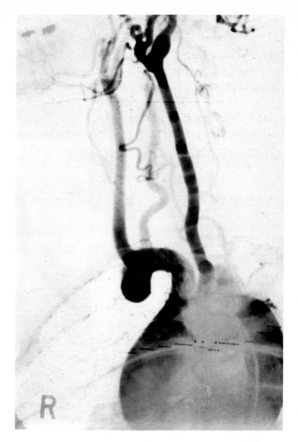

Fig. 19.5 Aortic arch syndrome (Takayasu's arteritis). Bilateral occlusion of the subclavian arteries in an Indian woman aged 30 with ten year history of episcleritis and polymyalgia.

lesions centred on the elastica of the aorta, carotid and subclavian arteries. Overlying the lesions are areas of mural thrombus. The symptoms in these patients are due to a recurrent embolism in the carotid, subclavian or vertebrobasilar territories and the disease is usually found in young adults of either sex (Peiris, 1979).

A fibrous hyperplastic type of *atheroma* accounts for many of the less florid examples of pulseless disease seen in India or in Europe (Dalal, 1973). *Syphilitic aortitis* with or without aneurysm formation is now rarely encountered but *giant cell arteritis* is probably the commonest non-atheromatous condition affecting the aorta and occluding the origins of the subclavian arteries; (see Fig. 19.11) less commonly the carotid arteries are also involved. This affects elderly patients who present with chronic brachial ischaemic pain in exercise.

In the younger age group, including some patients reported from the Orient, there is evidence of a systemic disorder which may precede arterial occlusion by some years. The features are fever, anaemia, pleurisy, haemoptysis, arthralgia, Raynaud's syndrome and erythema nodosum. The sedimentation rate is markedly raised (Strachan, 1966). It is suggested that this variety is due to a hypersensitivity angiitis to vascular elastic tissue. Corticosteroid treatment is recommended for these patients. Atheromatous and non-inflammatory types of aortic arch syndrome may be amenable to reconstructive surgical procedures.

Moya-moya disease

The term refers to a radiological appearance caused by the enlargement of many small collateral channels (pseudoangioma) bypassing obstruction in the terminal carotid artery. This unusual variety of cerebrovascular disease occurs chiefly in female infants and in young adults and is characterised by narrowing or occlusion of both internal carotids and the major branches of the Circle of Willis and by the development of a fine vascular anastomotic network involving both the perforating and pial arteries. In the later stages other collateral channels are formed utilising the orbital and ethmoidal branches of the external carotid as well as leptomeningeal and transdural anastomoses. The cervical portion of the internal carotid artery is narrowed (Fig. 19.6 A & B).

The disease was at first thought to be confined to Japanese (Kudo, 1968) and is certainly much commoner in the Orient. However, it has now been described in many parts of the world in Caucasian and Negro patients. Familial cases have also been reported (Sogaard & Jorgensen, 1975). The cause is unknown; some writers suggest a form of acquired arteritis related to nasopharyngeal infection or trauma, others a congenital malformation or persistence of an embryonic vascular pattern (Levesque et al, 1974). The majority of pathological reports favour an acquired, non-inflammatory type of arteriopathy arising over a long period. The potential for collateral development of this type may be related to age since serial angiography may show progression of the lesion in children whereas in adults the condition is usually stable (Fig. 19.7).

In a recent report of pathological findings in one patient (Coakham et al, 1979) there was extensive dilatation of small pial arteries over the surface of the brain; the occluded vessels appeared thin and white and, on microscopy, were filled with cellular connective tissue. They also showed thickening of the elastica with excessive infolding. There were no features of old thrombosis or recanalisation. The anastomotic vessels had the characteristic of capillaries or veins with some development of elastic tissue but no muscularis.

The symptoms vary according to age. Infantile forms account for 70 per cent of cases in the literature. In children the disease presents with repeated episodes of cerebral ischaemia, hemiparesis, dysphasia, headache or mental retardation. Occasionally there are seizures or involuntary movements (Susuk & Takaku, 1969). In older children the episodes become fewer but mental retardation may persist. A fatal outcome is exceptional. In adults the presentation is with subarachnoid or sometimes intracerebral haemorrhage (Higashi et al, 1974) (Fig. 19.8). Basal anastomoses are less prominent but ethmoidal and meningeal anastomoses may be extensive. Carotid stenosis rarely extends below the level of the third cervical vertebra (Picard et al, 1974).

In Western Europe and America a similar angiographic pattern of collateral vessel development may be seen in children with acute hemiplegia or in older patients with occlusive atheromatous or thromboembolic disease involving the terminal carotid artery (Solomon et al, 1970). Other possible causes are neurofibromatosis, X-ray therapy, basal meningitis, Marfan's syndrome and stenotic tumours (Taveras, 1969). In the great majority of cases however no underlying cause has been established and the condition appears to be unrelated to the chronic inflammatory arteritis described in Takayasu's disease.

Traumatic thrombosis of the carotid, vertebral and subclavian arteries

Carotid thrombosis may be caused by direct trauma as in laceration, missile injury, attempted strangulation or skull fracture near the carotid canal (Milligan & Anderson, 1980). Thrombosis forms at the point of injury and propagates upwards. In

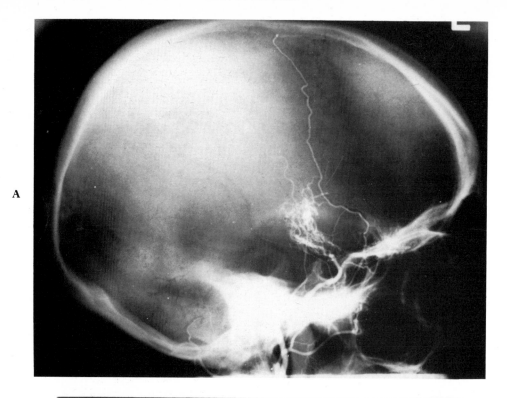

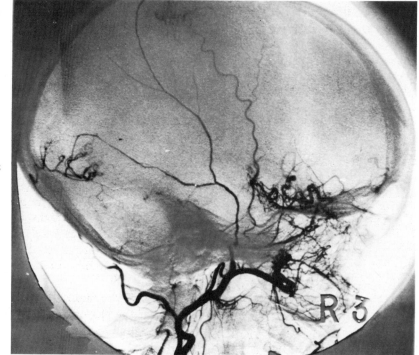

Fig. 19.6 Distal carotid occlusion, male aged 25, with bilateral pyramidal signs and mental retardation. (A) Moya-moya appearance on internal carotid angiography. (B) Extensive spontaneous external-internal collateral development. (Courtesy of Dr R. S. Kocen).

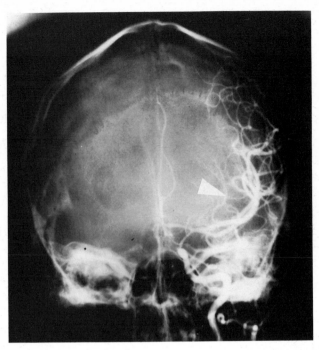

Fig. 19.7 Distal carotid occlusion — occlusion with involvement of terminal internal carotid and origin of anterior and middle cerebral arteries. The striate arteries are enlarged (arrowed). (Courtesy of Dr M. J. G. Harrison).

fatal cases it may involve the ophthalmic artery, the Circle of Willis and its main branches (Caldwell & Hadden, 1948). The internal carotid artery may also be injured during tonsillectomy or by penetrating injuries to the tonsillar fossa or soft palate in children (Fairburn, 1957). A more difficult diagnostic problem is posed by those cases resulting from indirect trauma, which need not be very

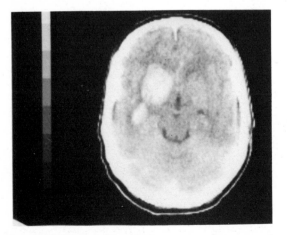

Fig. 19.8 Distal carotid occlusion — spontaneous capsular haemorrhage on man aged 30 with distal carotid occlusion.

severe. A typical history is a motor cycle injury where the patient is thrown from the vehicle landing on the point of the shoulder. As a result of sudden stretching during violent lateral neck flexion or extension of the head the internal carotid artery may develop a transverse tear 2–3 cm above its origin (Hughes & Brownell, 1968). Extravasation of blood into the arterial wall and carotid sheath occurs and the intimal injury acts as a nidus for mural intravascular thrombosis which may then propagate upwards and downwards. Propagation does not normally extend beyond the carotid siphon and for that reason the brain may escape injury. However, should the thrombus extend into the middle or anterior cerebral arteries or should embolism occur before all blood flow through the artery is arrested then cerebral infarction may result.

Traumatic thrombosis of the *internal carotid artery* should be suspected when signs of cerebral or retinal ischaemia suddenly develop some hours after injury. (Fig. 19.9 A & B). The patients are young men and there may be other injuries including facial abrasion, bruising of the neck, fracture of the jaw, clavicle or first rib. In the 16

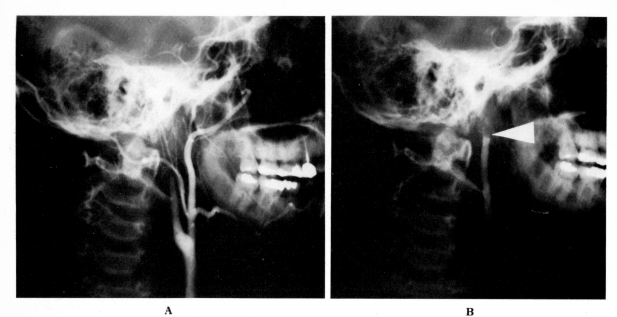

A   B

Fig. 19.9 Traumatic carotid thrombosis — male aged 25 six hours after indirect neck injury. (A) Common carotid angiogram showing occlusion of internal carotid artery. (B) Later film showing site of occlusion below base of skull (arrowed). (Courtesy of Dr K. Tonge).

cases reviewed by Hockaday (1959) motor involvement of the arm and leg was equally severe in 10, in 4 the arm was more severely affected and in 2 the leg. Immediate angiography is advisable to confirm the condition and to exclude other intracranial lesions. If occlusion is complete there is little to be gained by exploring the artery but if flow is continuing and if the thrombus is visible within the lumen the artery may be ligated to prevent cerebral embolism. Immediate anticoagulation treatment using heparin intravenously is advisable.

The *vertebral arteries* may also be damaged in acute or chronic trauma to the cervical spine (Schneider & Schemm, 1961). There are three vulnerable points: (1) at the intervertebral foramina, (2) at the atlantoaxial joint when there is subluxation leading to stretching and angulation of the artery, (3) at the atlanto-occipital joint where the condyle slides forward over the groove in the lamina of the atlas. Thrombosis with distal embolism to basilar and posterior cerebral arteries has been reported following chiropractic manipulation of the neck (Easton & Sherman, 1977) and dissection of the vertebral artery has also been reported in these circumstances (Bladin & Merony, 1975). Vertebral thrombosis is a rare sequel of Yoga or other gymnastic contortions (Hanus et al,

1977). Vertebral artery injury may also cause intermittent vertebrobasilar insufficiency, the artery being obstructed as a result of extension or rotation of the neck or by atlantoaxial subluxation or fracture dislocation (Ford, 1952). Medullary infarction may follow whiplash injury to the neck (Levy et al, 1980). Atlantoaxial subluxation is a frequent complication of severe rheumatoid arthritis affecting the cervical spine (Schneider & Crosby, 1959; Kao et al, 1974) and death from vertebral artery thrombosis has been reported in this condition (Webb et al, 1968).

In patients with cervical rib or congenital fibrous band the *subclavian artery* may be stretched and angulated as it crosses the first rib. During movements of the arm the artery may become compressed between the first rib and clavicle and chronic trauma may result in a local area of fibrosis and intimal damage sometimes with formation of an aneurysm. Mural thrombosis in this segment of artery gives rise to distal embolism with occlusion of digital and palmar arteries and to attacks of pain due to ischaemia in the muscles of the arm. On rare occasions the thrombus may propagate in the reverse direction to involve the origin of the vertebral arteries and on the right side the brachiocephalic trunk. Cerebral embolism may then occur in the territory of the vertebral or right carotid arteries (Gunning et al, 1964). It has also been shown by the Doppler ultrasonic technique that in this condition there may be periods of reverse blood flow in the subclavian arteries creating a potential for reflux of embolic material to the ostia of the cerebral vessels (Prior et al, 1979).

Acute arteritis of extracranial and cerebral arteries

Inflammation of the tonsils, retropharyngeal tissues and regional lymph nodes may spread to the walls of the carotid artery in the neck. A number of such cases were reported in children in the pre-antibiotic era but are now rare (Litchfield, 1938). The first indication of *carotid thrombosis* is usually the occurrence of a transient or permanent hemiplegia often with headache and convulsions; these cerebral effects are due to distal propagation or embolisation of thrombus. At an earlier stage angiography may show an irregularity of the lumen in relation to the infected lymph gland or narrowing of the whole internal carotid and its branches (Fig. 19.10 A & B) (Bickerstaff, 1964). *Congenital rubella* may also involve the extracranial arteries causing intimal fibrosis, muscular proliferation and diffuse cellular infiltration (Stebhens, 1972). A few instances of acute hemiplegia in apparently healthy infants (usually male) or in children with congenital heart disease have been caused by internal carotid artery thrombosis without an obvious source of infection (Bickerstaff, 1964).

In severe virus infection with *Coxsackie A9* or in *varicella-zoster encephalitis* the sudden appearance of hemiplegia in the course of the infection may indicate either thrombosis of the carotid artery or diffuse intracerebral arterial inflammation. Most cases occur in children with disordered immune mechanisms. (Roden et al, 1975).

In septic *cavernous sinus thrombosis*, a sequel to pyogenic infections of the face, there may be occlusion or narrowing of the intracavernous portion of the carotid artery with multiple emboli in the branches of the anterior or middle cerebral arteries (Mathew et al, 1971). In *Pneumococcal or meningococcal meningitis* the intracerebral branches of the carotid or vertebral arteries in the subarachnoid space and on the pial surface of the brain are surrounded by inflammatory exudate. Histological evidence of arteritis is described in fatal cases with fibrin deposition in the lumen, foci of pan-arteritis and phlebitis, and patchy cerebral infarction (Cairns & Russell, 1946). Cerebral ischaemia is rarely recognised clinically in the acute stage since

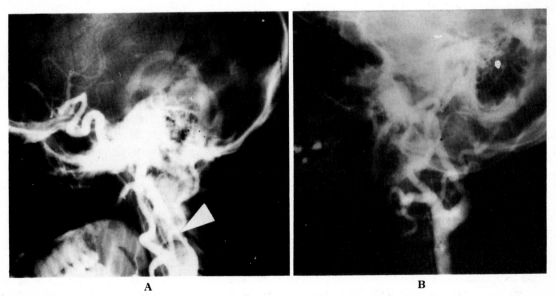

A   B

Fig. 19.10 Acute carotid arteritis. Child aged six with acute tonsillitis and tonsillar glandular suppuration who developed acute right hemiparesis. (A) The internal carotid artery is narrowed near its origin (arrowed). (B) Six weeks later the arterial lumen is restored. (Courtesy of Dr J. Mendez).

the clinical state of the patient is dominated by the features of acute meningitis. When antibiotic treatment has been used the acute inflammatory reaction in the artery wall may progress to fibrinoid necrosis and at a later stage to a proliferative fibrous endarteritis. Progressive narrowing of the vascular lumen may then lead to ischaemia in the territory of one of the carotid branches, usually the middle cerebral artery.

CHRONIC ARTERITIS

Chronic inflammation and fibrosis of the meninges at the base of the brain frequently involves the Circle of Willis and its major branches as well as the adjacent cranial nerves. In *tuberculous meningitis* miliary tuberculous nodules may be detected histologically within the walls of both arteries and veins, the outer coats being most severely affected (Blackwood, 1958). *Syphilitic arteritis* affects large and medium-sized meningeal vessels causing inflammatory infiltration of the middle and outer coats with a secondary fibrosis. The medial coat is thin and a fusiform aneurysm may form although rupture is rare; the elastic lamina is intact. The intima shows fibroblastic and later collagenous thickening (endarteritis obliterans) with eccentric narrowing of the lumen and sometimes thrombosis (Blackwood, 1958). *Mucor mycosis* is a rare fungus infection which may cause a localised meningitis by spread from the nasal sinuses. Most patients are severe diabetics or have an immunological abnormality. Inflammatory cells may invade the cerebral cortex and the walls of the arteries leading to thrombosis and to extensive infarction (Kurrein, 1954). *Aspergillus* infection may have similar effects but vasculitis is less severe. *Candidiasis* may involve leptomeningeal vessels leading to infarction, petechial haemorrhages and rarely mycotic aneurysm.

The angiographic changes in the various forms of chronic meningitis are similar and have been especially well studied in tuberculous meningitis in the Far East where the disease is still prevalent. Narrowing or occlusion of the distal internal carotid and the proximal segment of anterior and middle cerebral arteries are described. Smaller branches may also be affected. Various patterns of collateral circulation may be seen according to the site of occlusion; the collateral vessels may be the striate arteries (moya-moya type), transdural internal-external carotid anastomoses, and pial anastomoses (Mathew et al, 1970).

The diagnosis of chronic infective arteritis of the cerebral vessels rests on the recognition of its two major components, meningitic and vascular, together with detection of any source of infection in the sinuses or chest. The disease usually affects young patients at an age when degenerative arterial disease is uncommon. The occurrence of headache, fever, personality change, seizures, cranial nerve palsies or signs of raised intracranial pressure in the days or weeks before the onset of hemiplegia is an indication of preceding basal meningitis, and the diagnosis is confirmed by the finding of inflammatory cellular reaction and positive serological tests in the cerebrospinal fluid. The causative organism may be visible on a stained smear of c.s.f.

The ischaemic cerebral symptoms, being caused by thrombosis of the inflamed vessel, are usually abrupt in onset and vary in severity according to size of the infarcted zone. Any of the main carotid or basilar branches may be occluded. Provided that appropriate treatment is given for the primary infection the degree of recovery is often greater than would be expected in ischaemic stroke secondary to atheromatous disease.

A non-specific *granulomatous periarteritis* confined to the cavernous segment of the internal carotid artery was first described by Tolosa (1954). The carotid artery may show a localised stenosis and the adventitial coat is thickened. The condition presents in adult patients as a painful cavernous sinus syndrome involving the third to sixth cranial nerves and responds rapidly to steroids. Visual impairment is rare and ischaemic cerebral symptoms do not occur. The cause is unknown.

TROPICAL INFECTIONS

The cerebral vascular complications of *malaria* occur almost exclusively in infections due to *Plasmodium falciparum*. Cerebral malaria is a diffuse encephalopathy due to disseminated small vessel occlusion by clumps of pigment and by infected erythrocytes. Hypoxia from the decreased oxygen-carrying capacity of the infected erythrocytes may be a further factor in severe infections. Disseminated intravascular coagulation and vasogenic oedema are also important. There is endothelial oedema and proliferation as well as multiple petechial haemorrhages. Cerebral oedema and multiple small areas of softening are responsible for the neuro-psychiatric symptoms of intense headache, confusion, depressed consciousness, toxic delirium and seizures which make up the clinical picture. Focal neurological signs due to major vessel occlusion occur much less frequently (Musoke, 1966).

In fatal cases of *typhus* and *scrub typhus* disseminated acute vasculitis of small intracerebral vessels is described with pervascular typhus nodules. Focal symptoms of cerebral vascular occlusion are rare (Stebhens, 1972).

COLLAGEN DISEASES

Polyarteritis nodosa

Polyarteritis nodosa is a widespread destructive inflammatory disorder of small arteries and arterioles sometimes also involving larger vessels. It tends to heal by granulation and fibrosis with occasional aneurysm formation. The cause is thought to be a hypersensitivity reaction to a variety of antigenic stimuli (Miller & Daley, 1946).

The disease principally affects visceral, renal, and pulmonary arteries but those of the brain and spinal cord may also be involved (Rose & Spencer, 1957). Estimates of the frequency of cerebral involvement vary widely from 8–60 per cent. Both intracerebral and pial branches and occasionally major cerebral arteries may be affected and may have a beaded appearance due to multiple aneurysms (Facon et al, 1960; Ford & Siekert, 1965). Pathologically there are foci of cortical necrosis surrounded by an acute inflammatory reaction with eosinophilia and sometimes with giant cells. Areas of haemorrhage are frequently found. C.n.s. involvement is said to be commoner in children and to run a relapsing course with long tract brain stem and cranial nerve signs. The clinical picture may be confused with multiple sclerosis (Weiseberg et al, 1975).

About one third of patients show clinical symptoms of c.n.s. involvement throughout the course of the illness (Parker & Kernohan, 1949). The symptoms are extremely variable; sometimes multiple small vascular occlusions predominate and sometimes haemorrhage. The symptom most commonly recorded is sudden hemiparesis or hemianopia (15 to 20 per cent) sometimes with an organic confusional state or with headache and seizures. At other times the clinical picture may suggest a slowly evolving cerebral abscess or glioma (Roger et al, 1955). Diabetes insipidus and choreic involuntary movements are also recorded. Rupture of aneurysms is not common but subarachnoid haemorrhage is the presenting feature in five per cent of cases (Ford & Siekert, 1965).

A further third of patients show neurological features only in the terminal illness. These are usually related to severe hypertension and consist of headache, seizures, hypertensive encephalopathy, brain stem signs and subarachnoid haemorrhage (Roger et al, 1955). At autospy multiple haemorrhages in the hemispheres and brain stem may be found (Haft et al, 1955). Treatment consists of corticosteroids in a dose sufficient to control the symptoms and reduce the sedimentation rate to normal. Large amounts may be required and side effects are common. In some patients it may be possible to control the disease by administration of corticosteroids on alternate days. The addition of azathioprine or cyclophosphamide may allow the condition to be controlled by a smaller dose of steroids.

Systemic lupus erythematosus

Involvement of the blood vessels of the c.n.s. is common in systemic lupus erythematosus, occurring in three-quarters of fatal cases (Johnson & Richardson, 1968). A wide variety of clinical effects result from small ischaemic lesions in the hemispheres, basal ganglia and brain stem. The vascular lesion consists of necrotic and proliferative change affecting arterioles and capillaries. Fibrin is found within and outside the vessel indicating an increased permeability (Gold & Yahr, 1960). Small haemorrhages may also occur (Glaser, 1952). True vasculitis with cellular infiltration of the vessel wall is not a feature. The pathological changes are distinct from those of polyarteritis nodosa but are similar to those of acute rheumatic fever, hypertensive encephalopathy and thrombotic thrombocytopenic purpura. Microemboli consisting of fragments of bland thrombus from heart valves (verrucose endocarditis) may also cause retinal and cerebral arterial occlusion. Deposits of circulating immune complexes in the renal vessels are a characteristic feature of systemic lupus but immunofluorescence studies of the cerebral cortex have been negative; the choroid plexus however may show diffuse deposits of gammaglobulin.

Clinical evidence of c.n.s. involvement in systemic lupus erythematosus occurs in half or more of the patients (Feinglass et al, 1976; Lee et al, 1977; Appenzeller & Williams, 1979). The symptoms are often transient, usually occur late in the disease but may appear at any time. Headache, generalised seizures and mental change are the most regular symptoms. Psychiatric symptoms vary from a mild affective disorder to a confusional state or to a florid psychosis with hallucinations and dementia. Less common presenting features include cranial nerve palsies (chiefly oculomotor) pseudo-bulbar palsy, hemiparesis, hypothalamic symptoms, transverse myelitis and subarachnoid haemorrhage (Hazelton et al, 1980; Lee et al, 1977). Vision may be affected in a number of ways; by occlusion of the central retinal artery, by optic neuritis or by cortical visual defects (Brandt et al, 1975; Hackett et al, 1974). Involuntary movements of choreic type may be the presenting symptom particularly in young patients and are usually accompanied by mental changes (Donaldson & Espiner, 1971).

The diagnosis of cerebral lupus rests on finding characteristic immunological changes or evidence of the disease in other organs. These consist of alopecia, nasopharyngeal ulceration, arteritis, pleuritis or pericarditis, proteinuria and haemolytic anaemia. There is no specific test for the disease although a raised antinuclear factor in peripheral blood is frequently found. This correlates poorly however with clinical cerebral involvement. Increased DNA binding activity and a chronic false positive serological test for syphilis may also occur. In cerebral lupus e.e.g. changes are present in 70–90 per cent but are non-specific. C.s.f. is abnormal in one-third of patients, usually showing a raised protein; complement levels may be reduced but the test is at present insufficiently reliable. Arteriography occasionally shows a major vessel occlusion but is more often normal.

Changes in cerebral blood flow and metabolism demonstrable by positron emission tomography using ^{15}Oxygen have been claimed in a high proportion of patients with systemic lupus erythematosus, some with no cerebral symptoms. Regions of reduced flow or increased oxygen extraction may be demonstrated and the regression of these abnormalities on repeated testing is said to be a useful index of response to treatment (Pinching et al, 1977).

The prognosis for cerebral lupus has greatly improved in recent years. At one time high doses of corticosteroids were recommended to control the acute cerebral symptoms (500–3000 mg hydrocortisone per day). At present much smaller doses are used in combination with immunosuppression, azathioprine being the drug of choice (Hughes, 1979). Although severe renal impairment carried a high mortality, cerebral lupus now has a relatively good prognosis, the five year survival rate being 80 per cent.

Giant cell arteritis

In this type of arteritis there is a granulomatous reaction involving arteries of all sizes from the aorta downwards (Armsworth & Gresham, 1961; Crompton, 1959). Extracranial scalp arteries derived from the external carotid and vertebral are the most regularly affected (Wilkinson & Russell, 1972).

Pathologically there is subintimal cellular proliferation with a chronic inflammatory reaction of giant cell type centred on the elastic tissue which is largely destroyed. The arterial wall is thickened, the lumen is greatly narrowed and thrombosis may occur.

Although the cervical portion of the vertebral artery is constantly involved and the cervical part of the internal carotid may also be affected the intracranial segments of both carotid and vertebral arteries are practically free from arteritis, possibly because they contain only small amounts of elastic tissue (Wilkinson, 1972). Microscopic granulomas have occasionally been found in the middle cerebral artery branches (Greenfield, 1951) but in the reported cases of cerebral infarction in giant cell arteritis there has been either complete occlusion of the internal carotid artery usually with thrombosis (Macmillan, 1950) or evidence of cerebral embolism.

The disease is almost unknown under the age of 60, affects both sexes equally and runs a chronic course of from one to ten years. Involvement of the scalp vessels and of the maxillary and facial branches of the external carotid accounts for the principal symptoms of headache, scalp tenderness, trismus, pains in the jaw, tongue and throat. The scalp arteries are nodular, thickened and tender to palpation. They remain pulsatile in the early stages but later the pulse may disappear. The patchy nature of the disease is shown on angiography which reveals segments of irregular narrowing. The most important complication is ischaemia or infarction of the optic nerve or inner retina or of the oculomotor nerves. This is due to spread of arteritis to affect the ciliary arteries and other branches within the orbit.

The coronary arteries may be involved and there is a small mortality in the first few weeks from myocardial infarction. The aorta may show a progressive enlargement and there are occasional early deaths from aortic dissection. A fusiform aneurysm of the aorta may slowly develop. Giant cell arteritis may also cause occlusion at the origin of the subclavian arteries producing ischaemic pain in the muscles of the upper limbs on exercise (Fig. 19.11).

In contrast to the visual symptoms which may occur in up to 25 per cent of patients symptoms of cerebral involvement are most unusual (Fisher, 1959). They consist of one or more sudden episodes of carotid TIA often accompanied by an organic confusional state in senile patients. There have also been a number of reports of ischaemic episodes or completed strokes in the brain stem territory (most often the lateral medullary syndrome) or in both occipital lobes. This can be traced to embolism from a source of thrombosis in the vertebral and carotid arteries (Wilkinson & Russell, 1972). The diagnosis of arteritis is suggested by a preceding headache, scalp pain, muscle pains, ischaemic optic neuritis, tenderness of the scalp arteries or the carotid artery in the neck (Hamilton et al, 1971). The sedimentation rate and serum alkaline phos-

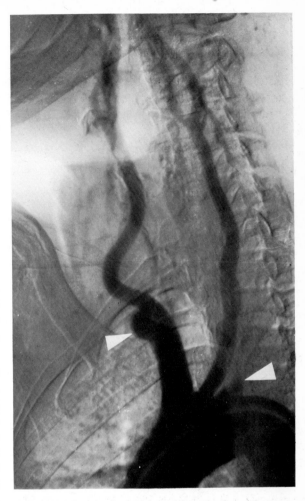

Fig. 19.11 Giant cell arteritis — bilateral subclavian artery occlusion (arrowed) in a female patient aged 60 with upper limb claudication and positive temporal artery biopsy. (Courtesy of Dr Edward Housley).

phatase (liver fraction) are constantly elevated, and these tests should be routine in all elderly patients with ischaemic stroke. Confirmation of the diagnosis by biopsy of the scalp artery is advisable although false negative results are not uncommon due to patchy involvement.

Treatment consists of corticosteroids given immediately and in high dose (60–80 mg/day). After a few days these are slowly reduced to a level sufficient to keep the sedimentation below 30 mm/one hour. Treatment should be started as soon as the diagnosis is suspected because of the risk of permanent visual loss. There is good evidence that steroids prevent visual complications although loss of vision may still occur during the first 48 hours of treatment. Once treatment has begun loss of vision is not a long term risk and after six months it is reasonable to reduce steroids to a level which controls headache and muscle pain. Long term follow-up studies show that once the acute stage is passed life expectancy is normal for age although some patients, approximately 30 per cent, require to take a small dose of steroids indefinitely (Graham et al, 1981).

Granulomatous angiitis

A pathological entity distinct from systemic giant cell arteritis is the rare condition of giant cell granulomatous angiitis of the central nervous system. This disease, the cause of which is unknown, occurs at any age and in either sex and runs a progressive course to a fatal outcome in a few weeks or months (Nurick et al, 1972). The symptoms of headache, memory loss, seizures, blurred vision and impaired consciousness combined with features of an organic psychosis appear to be due to diffuse ischaemia affecting chiefly the grey matter of both cerebral hemispheres. In some patients there are disturbances of eye movement, pupillary abnormalities, and facial sensory loss indicating brain stem involvement. The cerebrospinal fluid which is under raised pressure usually contains an excess of mononuclear cells and protein. The electroencephalogram is diffusely abnormal and carotid angiography either shows no abnormality or segmental regions of small vessel irregularity. CT scanning shows multiple hypodense lesions in the hemispheres (Faer et al, 1977). Corticosteroids may lead to temporary improvement.

Pathologically the lesions may be confined to intracerebral blood vessels; unsuspected visceral arteritis may be found in a minority of cases. There is necrosis of the walls of small leptomeningeal and intracerebral arteries and veins which are infiltrated with chronic inflammatory cells. The brain shows foci of ischaemic necrosis with or without haemorrhage (Hughes & Brownell, 1966).

Behcet's disease

Although its cause is unknown this condition is regarded by many as a variety of vasculitis caused directly or indirectly by immunopathogenic mechanisms (circulating immune complexes). Involvement of the nervous system occurs in 10 to 20 per cent of patients. The most regular pathological findings are perivascular meningeal infiltration with lymphocytes, plasma cells and macrophages. There are multiple small foci of infarction in grey and white matter especially in the brain stem. Regions of demyelination may also occur, e.g., in optic nerves. The blood vessels themselves may show hyaline degeneration of the media and thrombosis may occur in arteries or veins. Elastic degeneration may effect the aorta and cause aneurysm formation. Occlusion may affect carotid and subclavian arteries at their origins and Behcet's disease is a rare cause of the aortic arch syndrome (Shimizu et al, 1979).

The main clinical features are recurrent oral and genital ulceration with ocular lesions — severe uveitis, retinal vasculitis and papilloedema. Other less common manifestations are arthritis, erythema nodosum, thrombophlebitis, skin and gastrointestinal ulceration. The onset of neurological complications is usually sudden and suggestive of vascular occlusion. A great variety of abnormalities are described, the commonest being hemiparesis or quadriparesis, pseudo-bulbar palsy combined with brain stem signs, e.g., nystagmus and gaze palsy. There may also be seizures and an organic confusional state. Progressive obliteration of the retinal arteries frequently leads to blindness. Headaches are a prominent feature and c.s.f. cellular reaction is constant (O'Duffy & Goldstein, 1976).

The disease pursues a relapsing course with progressive disability. Treatment is by cytotoxic drugs especially cyclophosphamide in low dose or by immunosuppression using azathioprine supplemented by corticosteroids.

Rheumatic fever

There are many reports in the older literature of cerebral complications in acute rheumatic fever (Winkelman & Eckel, 1932). In fatal cases the brain is swollen and shows numerous perivascular haemorrhages and focal areas of cell loss. The arterioles and capillaries show endarteritis with proliferative, hyaline, and fibrotic changes in the walls. These changes are non-specific and are found in other severe infections. The primary damage may be a widespread hypersensitivity angiitis with abnormal permeability of the vessel wall (Costero, 1949). Early symptoms consist of restlessness and delirium with meningism and sometimes chorea. This may lead on to impairment of consciousness and finally death in coma. Hyperpyrexia is usual but not invariable.

Although fibrin-platelet vegetations are frequently found on the heart valves and although occasional patients with embolic obstruction of the retinal arteries have been described in chorea (Hearn & Roper-Hall, 1961), there is general agreement that the vascular changes found in fatal cases of rheumatic fever are unlikely to be due to embolism alone.

Rheumatoid athritis

There are a few reports of cerebral vasculitis in association with rheumatoid disease. In some instances this is a generalised systemic vasculitis and in others the changes are confined to the central nervous system. The severity of inflammatory changes varies; there may be profuse cellular infiltration and fibrinoid medial necrosis similar to polyarteritis nodosa in small intracerebral arteries and producing multiple cortical infarcts. In other patients the changes are less acute and consist of mononuclear cuffing with intimal proliferation and fibrous scarring. Areas of haemorrhage may also occur. Deposition of immunoglobulin and complement has been demonstrated in the walls of involved arteries (Watson et al, 1977).

Clinical features are diverse. Most patients have severe rheumatoid disease often with polyneuritis and many have received corticosteroid treatment. Reported neurological symptoms include focal hemisphere infarction, hemisphere haematoma, and brain stem infarction. The vertebral arteries may also suffer as a result of spontaneous atlanto-axial dislocation (Ramos & Mandybar, 1975).

Scleroderma

In contrast to other forms of collagen disease, involvement of the cerebral arteries in scleroderma is exceptionally rare. Occasional case reports have appeared of cerebral infarction secondary to stenosis and occlusion of the terminal carotid artery with thrombosis of the major branches (Lee & Haynes, 1967). The carotid artery shows marked medial fibrosis and thickening due to proliferation of normal collagen fibres. Smaller arteries show medial and intimal hyperplasia with fibrinoid necrosis and some cellular infiltration.

METABOLIC DISEASES

Diabetes mellitus

The effect of diabetes on the occurrence of ischaemic vascular symptoms during life and on arterial pathology after death has long been a matter for debate; for many years it was held that degenerative vascular disease was no different in diabetics and non-diabetics. More recently it has been conclusively shown in a population study that ischaemic symptoms occur at a significantly younger age in diabetics than in a matched control group and that the probability of ischaemic symptoms is related to the blood sugar level (Keen et al, 1965). It is also established that the mortality from occlusive vascular disease is twice as high in diabetics as in non-diabetics (Entmacher et al, 1964) and that the prevalence at autopsy of cerebral infarction and lacunar infarction (focal encephalomalacia) is significantly greater in the brains of diabetics than in others (Alex et al, 1962). On the other hand cerebral haemorrhage does not show any increased prevalence at autopsy and hypertension occurs with significantly greater frequency only in diabetics over the age of 70 (Freedman et al, 1958).

Occlusive vascular disease in diabetic patients comprises two main types, *macrovascular* and *microvascular*. The first is usually found in older patients with mild rather than severe diabetes and consists of non-specific atherosclerosis affecting elastic and muscular arteries throughout the body, particularly those of the heart, brain, and lower limbs. Pathologically the changes differ only from those of atherosclerosis in non-diabetics in being more severe and beginning at a younger age. There is also a tendency for atherosclerosis to occur in smaller arteries and in the brain; the striate arteries supplying the basal ganglia, normally free from atheroma, may be involved.

Macrovascular disease shows great geographical variations, tending to be less severe in oriental than in westernised countries. These differences are not fully understood and cannot be explained by variations in other associated factors such as blood pressure, cholesterol or cigarette smoking. When diabetes occurs in premenopausal women there is loss of the relative immunity from vascular disease normally seen in this group and the incidence rates for females equal or exceed those for males (Keen & Jarrett, 1979). In the cerebral circulation macrovascular atheroma affects arteries of all sizes from the internal carotid and the vertebral down to the secondary branches of the three major cerebral arteries and the larger intracerebral penetrating arteries. As in non-diabetics, occlusion occurs as the result of thrombosis at the site of atheromatous lesions and most commonly affects the internal carotid artery in the neck, the vertebral or basilar artery and the middle cerebral artery near its origin.

The microangiopathy of diabetes shows specific features. Pathologically it occurs throughout the body and affects small arterioles and capillaries which exhibit patchy hyalinisation of the walls with accumulation of PAS-positive material in the subintima. There is a variable amount of fibrous and cellular proliferation. Capillary walls are thickened by the accumulation of glycoprotein in the basement membrane. Microvascular disease is responsible for three of the most important diabetic complications — retinopathy, nephropathy and neuropathy. These often coexist in the same patient (triopathy). In the brain microvascular change affects intracerebral arteries, size 50 to 150 microns, most commonly in the basal ganglia, pons and subcortical white matter. These vessels have no intercommunications and occlusion produces a small deep infarct or encephalomalacia (lacune) similar to those found in hypertensive and senile brains. The symptomatology of lacunes is described elsewhere. Microangiopathy also affects the vasa nervorum of the cranial nerves and is responsible for the oculomotor or abducens palsy commonly occurring in diabetic patients (Asbury et al, 1970).

A recent large prospective study has shown that microvascular disease is related to the duration of diabetes and occurs equally in males and females (Pirart, 1977). There is no clear correlation with the severity of the disease as measured by the degree of hyperglycaemia on presentation but there is a strong correlation with poor diabetic control. This latter finding has received recent confirmation from experimental animal work; rats rendered diabetic and maintained at different levels of hyperglycaemia developed microvascular complications similar to those seen in man, in inverse proportion to the degree of control. Regression of microangiopathy has also been shown when control is improved (Fox et al, 1977).

These findings have given a fresh impetus to treatment of diabetic patients. There is renewed emphasis on stricter control of blood glucose using frequent or sometimes continuous insulin injection and aided by monitoring of blood glucose by the patient and by estimation of haemoglobin A1c, a useful index of long-term hyperglycaemia. There is already evidence that improved control of blood sugar significantly lessens the degree of retinopathy (Job et al, 1976; Tchobroutsky, 1978).

Weight reduction may be desirable as an adjunct to achieving normal glycaemia especially in obese maturity-onset diabetics. For severely affected younger patients there is a move away from drastic carbohydrate restriction towards a relatively high carbohydrate diet consisting of unrefined carbohydrates and with a low fat and high fibre content.

If a lipid abnormality is present and persists in spite of dietary and diabetic control the type of hyperlipidaemia is determined and specific therapy given (see below). Hypertension and extracranial arterial stenosis are treated as in a non-diabetic patient, In diabetic ketoacidosis there may be marked dehydration and haemoconcentration with increased blood viscosity; this carries some additional risk of cerebral infarction from arterial or venous thrombosis. A further complication is intravascular coagulation which may also occur in diabetic coma. Modern management of coma emphasises the importance of early and adequate fluid and electrolyte replacement with the addition of heparin to combat intravascular coagulation.

Hyperlipidaemia

Although there is strong evidence from prospective studies that subjects with elevated serum cholesterol are at increased risk from myocardial infarction the association between lipid levels and stroke is less definite. The Framingham prospective study shows that an elevated serum cholesterol (over 335 mg/dl) carries a slightly increased risk of brain infarction only in men under the age of 50 (see Chapter 1). When in combination with other risk factors, such as hypertension and smoking, cholesterol levels may become more significant. The assessment of the significance of hypercholesterolaemia is complicated by the fact that the patient with an elevated serum cholesterol may either be at the upper end of a normal distribution curve or may be a heterozygote for familial hypercholesterolaemia, a condition with a prevalence rate of about 1 in 500. These two conditions may carry a different prognosis and may be clinically indistinguishable but familial cases tend to show tendon xanthomata and have pronounced eyelid xanthelasma.

Many reports of lipid levels in patients with established cerebrovascular disease have been published although most can be criticised on the grounds of varying diagnostic criteria, lack of homogeneity, imperfectly matched control groups and arbitrary levels of lipid normality. Most workers have found no difference in *cholesterol* levels between patients with any type of cerebrovascular disease and controls (Meyer et al, 1959; Cumings et al, 1967; Ballantine et al, 1974). On the other hand Hayman et al (1961) who studied a stroke group including patients with hypertension, heart disease and diabetes found a significant elevation of serum cholesterol compared with the healthy controls. The mean cholesterol level for all patients was 227 mg/dl and for controls 205 mg/dl. In recent years *HDL cholesterol* has also been studied. Rossner et al (1978) found normal serum cholesterol but low HDL cholesterol concentrations in a group of young patients with ischaemic cerebrovascular disease. A recent Italian study also showed a significant decrease in HDL cholesterol in men with ischaemic brain disease (34.72 ± 1.1). Women showed no such difference (Sirtori et al, 1979).

Other lipid abnormalities have also been investigated. Jakobson (1967) found no difference between 52 patients and controls with respect to *triglycerides* although the level in the control group was unusually high. On the other hand, Fogelholm & Aho (1973) studied 213 patients under 50 with cerebral infarction, most of whom had angiography. They found a significant rise in triglycerides in men between 40 and 50 and in women between 30 and 50. The group contained an excess of young women, some taking the contraceptive pill, an agent known to increase triglyceride levels. An increase in triglycerides was also found in patients of both sexes with transient ischaemic attacks by Crepaldi et al (1980).

Thus the consensus of opinion at the present time is that of the two main types of lipid abnormality prebetalipoproteinaemia (having markedly elevated triglycerides and a modest increase in cholesterol) shows the stronger link with stroke and with premature peripheral vascular disease. A number of latent diabetic patients are probably included in the prebetalipoproteinaemia group which also shows a greater incidence of heart disease than normal subjects but not as great as that found in betalipoproteinaemia. There is no explanation for the lesser correlation between betalipoproteinaemia and stroke except that coronary artery disease develops at a younger age and that in cerebral arterial disease hypertension predominates as a risk factor.

Considerable controversy surrounds the question of *therapy* and the level at which hyperlipidaemia should be treated. It is worth noting that the mortality rates at different levels of cholesterol in serum have been calculated and these indicate little change in mortality in the range 159–250 mg/dl but a more definite increase at higher levels (Slack, 1979). There are a number of dietary and drug regimes which can reduce elevated blood lipids and it is customary to advise treatment in patients with established cerebral arterial disease or TIA who have cholesterol levels over 250 mg/dl, especially if other risk factors such as hypertension are present. There is however little evidence that reducing blood lipids will diminish the size of existing arterial lesions or improve symptoms (Acheson & Hutchinson, 1972), although skin xanthomata and hard retinal exudates may regress, and some patients show angiographic evidence of an increase in arterial lumen diameter.

For prebetalipoproteinaemia a reduction in lipid level ranging from 10–15 per cent may be achieved by diet and weight reduction and this seems the most satisfactory method of treatment for this group. Clofibrate, which decreases hepatic synthesis and increases faecal excretion of cholesterol, has been the subject of a large clinical trial in the primary prevention of ischaemic heart disease in men with moderate and severe hypercholesterolaemia. The treated group, followed for a number of years, had fewer myocardial infarctions than controls but a significantly greater mortality from other causes, mostly malignant disease (WHO trial, 1978; VA Cooperative Study, 1973). The reason for this is at present unknown. It is also uncertain whether other drugs known to reduce cholesterol such as nicotinic acid or probucol will have a similar effect.

For betalipoproteinaemia cholestyramine which increases the faecal excretion of bile acids is used, with or without restriction of dietary saturated fat and cholesterol. Young relatives should be screened to detect any lipid abnormality since it is in childhood that long-term preventive treatment is most likely to be effective.

Homocystinaemia

Homocystinaemia is a rare inborn error of metabolism due to a deficiency of the enzyme cystathionine synthetase. Homocystine accumulates in plasma and tissues and may be detected in the urine. The main features are ectopia of the lens, a moderate degree of mental defect, skeletal deformities and cutaneous flushing. There is a strong tendency to progressive cardiovascular disease and a high incidence of thromboembolism which occur within the first year of life. One-third of patients die before the age of 30 (Carson et al, 1965).

Pathological changes affect arteries of all sizes and include medial degeneration, intimal fibrosis and hyperplasia. Thrombosis may occlude the carotid artery and is followed by fibroelastic organisation (Schimke et al, 1965).

Experimental homocystinaemia in animals causes loss of vascular endothelium, a rise in platelet consumption and thrombosis and it is suggested that arterial thrombi are secondary to endothelial injury. It has been shown that a reduction of plasma homocystine by pyridoxin stops the excessive consumption of platelets. Dipyridamole has the same effect (Harker et al, 1974).

INHERITED DISORDERS INVOLVING THE CEREBRAL VASCULAR SYSTEM

In *pseudo-xanthoma elasticum*, inherited as an autosomal recessive trait, characteristic skin lesions are found in association with visual loss, gastrointestinal haemorrhage, coronary, peripheral and cerebral vascular disorders. Patches of loose wrinkled skin are found on the neck or flexural folds. The retina shows dark angioid streaks radiating from the disc and pigmentary and haemorrhagic lesions at the macula are responsible for progressive visual loss. The retinal appearances are caused by degeneration in Bruch's membrane and similar changes affect the media and internal elastic lamina of the aorta and muscular arteries throughout the body (Robertson & Shroeder, 1959). Patients with pseudo-xanthoma may have hypertension, widening of the aorta, aneurysm formation and medial calcification (Igbal et al, 1978). In the cerebral circulation fragmentation of the elastic layer may affect the middle cerebral artery and internal carotid artery with accelerated atherosclerosis. Cerebral or subarachnoid haemorrhage may occur (Dixon, 1951) and there may be multiple small areas of cerebral infarction involving white matter (Messis & Budzilovich, 1970).

The *Ehlers-Danlos syndrome* is an uncommon disorder of connective tissue possibly due to defective deposition of collagen fibres. There are a number of different genetic types (including an X-linked variety) in some of which the enzymatic defect has been identified (e.g., deficiency of lysylhydroxylase and procollagen protease). The usual mode of inheritance is autosomal dominant. Three clinical types are described — classical, varicose and arterial (Barabus, 1967). On pathological examination all arteries show abnormal collagen deposition in the media, small medial haemorrhages and increased amounts of acid mucopolysaccharide. Brain arteries show in addition medial defects leading to aneurysm formation (Imahori et al, 1969). The classical features of the disease are fragile and hyperextensible skin and subcutaneous tissues, abnormal mobility of joints and aneurysm formation, varicose veins and cardiac anomalies. Affected subjects are liable to dissection of the aorta, rupture of various arteries and to gastro-intestinal haemorrhage (Beighton,

1970). In the cerebral circulation patients are reported with multiple intracranial aneurysms causing subarachnoid haemorrhage (Rubenstein & Cohen, 1964). There is also a tendency to spontaneous carotico-cavernous fistula producing a pulsating exophthalmos (Graf, 1965), to diffuse ectasia of the internal carotid artery (Fig. 19.12) and to aneurysms of the superficial temporal artery (Imahori, 1969). Because of the fragility of arterial wall, angiography carries an increased risk in this condition.

The *Marfan syndrome* is a related disorder of mesenchymal development having its main expression in the cardiovascular and muscular skeletal systems. The mode of inheritence is autosomal dominant. Affected arteries show fragmentation of the elastic elements with distortion and degeneration of muscle fibres, replacement fibrosis and accumulation of pools of mucoid metachromatic material within the wall. Skeletal features include arachnodactyly, funnel deformity of the chest, high arched palate and increased joint mobility (Parish, 1960). Cardiovascular abnormalities are present in 25 per cent of cases and are very varied, the commonest being aortic dilatation, dissecting aneurysm, aortic reflux, dilatation of the pulmonary artery, atrial septal defect, cardiac dysrhythmias and dextroversion (Sinclair et al, 1960). Coarctation of the aorta is also an associated feature and these patients may present with subarachnoid haemorrhage from a berry aneurysm on the Circle of Willis. The chief importance of the syndrome is as a cause of aneurysmal enlargement or dissection on the extracranial carotid arteries; the common, external and internal segments can be affected (McKusick, 1966). Such patients have been treated surgically (Hardin, 1962).

Angiokeratoma corporis diffusum (Fabry's disease) is a rare familial disorder due to deficiency of alpha-galactosidase. It is characterised by cutaneous lesions of vascular type, progressive renal disease and paroxysmal attacks of severe pain in the extremities (Wise et al, 1962). Cerebral vessels are frequently affected and show deposits of glycolipid in the media of small arteries in the leptomeninges. Larger arteries may show dilatation. There are scattered small areas of infarction in the hemispheres and brain stem (Kahn, 1973). Symptoms due to cerebral vascular occlusion and

to renal failure occur in the third to fifth decade. Basilar artery aneurysm is a rare complication (Maisey & Cosh, 1980).

Neurocutaneous syndromes

Under this heading are included a group of inherited developmental anomalies of brain, skin and retina, some associated with mental retardation. In *neurofibromatosis* (von Recklinghausen's disease) which is inherited as an autosomal dominant trait, most of the clinical features relate to bony dysplasia and to tumours of the nervous system. Vascular symptoms are rare but narrowing or ectasia of aorta, renal, coeliac or mesenteric arteries is decribed (Tomsick et al, 1976). There is proliferation of Schwann cells within the arterial wall and secondary fibrosis.

In the cerebral circulation the vascular dysplasia may affect the carotid artery which shows alternating segments of stenosis and dilatation (Hilal, 1974). Occlusions may also affect the distal internal carotid, proximal middle cerebral and anterior cerebral arteries with the development of extensive collaterals of pseudo-angiomatous type. In some of the reported cases previous X-ray therapy given for optic nerve glioma may have influenced the vascular appearances. Symptoms related to vascular disease may occur in young adults who present with hemiparesis and epilepsy, less commonly with subarachnoid haemorrhage or transient ischaemic attacks. There may be marked hypertension from involvement of the renal arteries (Pellock et al, 1980).

Patients with *tuberose sclerosis* tend to develop multiple cerebral tumours usually in relation to the ependymal lining of the ventricles or in the retina. They also show facial angiofibromas, angiomyolipomas of the kidney, white 'ash-leaf' cutaneous patches on the trunk and subungual fibromas. Patients present with epilepsy and mental retardation. Though vascular conditions are uncommon angiography may reveal dysplasia of the cerebral arteries with excessive tortuosity and segments of stenosis or ectasia (Hilal, 1974).

In the rare *epidermal naevus syndrome*, a type of neurocutaneous dysgenesis, congenital naevi are found in association with skeletal, neural, ocular, renal and cardiac defects.

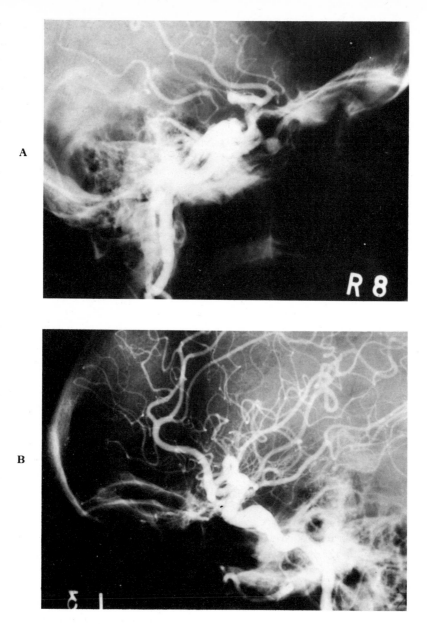

Fig. 19.12 Ehlers-Danlos syndrome. (A) Spontaneous right carotico-cavernous fistula in a female patient aged 50 with long history of spontaneous arterial fragility. (B) Left internal carotid ectasia in same patient. (Courtesy of Dr D. J. Thomas).

There may be intracerebral bleeding from angiomatous malformation or infarction from carotid occlusion (McAuley et al, 1978).

IATROGENIC ARTERIAL DISEASE
Oral contraceptives
An association between oral contraceptive agents and cerebral infarction has been suspected since 1965 (Illis et al, 1965) when an increase was noted in the number of strokes occurring in young women. Bickerstaff & Holmes (1967) found a fivefold increase in the incidence of stroke in young women in their practice after 1964 when the use of contraceptives became widespread. In an individual patient the risk of stroke increases over twentyfold (Jick et al, 1978). Further retrospective

studies established a definite statistical link between venous thrombembolism and oral contraceptives (Inman & Vessey, 1968). The American Collaborative Group for Study of Stroke in Young Women (1975) issued its findings in a group of 598 women aged 15 to 44 with cerebral vascular disease compared with age-matched controls. There were 140 thrombotic events, 59 in women taking the contraceptive pill, 81 in non-users. It was calculated that women on oral contraceptives had a fourfold increase in the risk of stroke and that this risk was independent of other factors such as smoking and blood pressure although both these factors were also much more prevalent in the stroke group. It appears that the thrombotic tendency is related to the oestrogen content of the preparation (Inman et al, 1970). In this context it is also notable that there is a twofold increase in stroke in men receiving high dose oestrogen for prostatic carcinoma (Blackwood et al, 1970). Pathogenesis is not yet clear; a number of coagulation changes have been shown to follow oestrogen ingestion including a rise in plasma antiplasmin, plasmogen and fibrinogen and a decrease in serum antithrombin activity (Howie et al, 1970). Platelet adhesiveness also increases (Caspary & Peberdy, 1965).

There are no specific clinical features which distinguish this type of stroke. Angiography may show occlusion of the internal carotid artery or a major cerebral branch and the appearances often suggest embolism rather than thrombosis-in-situ (Enzell & Lindemalm, 1973). The arteries do not appear unduly atheromatous and it is suggested that emboli may originate in the pulmonary veins. The increased incidence of haemorrhagic as distinct from thrombotic cerebrovascular disease may possibly be related to the effect of oral contraceptives in raising blood pressure (Weir et al, 1971). No significant association has been found between oral contraceptives and fatal subarachnoid haemorrhage (Inman, 1979).

An association between dissection of the internal carotid artery and oral contraceptives has also been suggested.

Drug addiction

There is increasing evidence of a connection between chronic drug abuse and cerebral vasculitis.

Citron & colleagues (1970) published 14 fatal cases showing widespread fibrinoid vascular necrosis with thrombosis in many cerebral arteries. Intracerebral arteries are the most affected but the larger arteries may show irregular constriction and dilatation on angiography (Lognelli & Buchhert, 1971). The clinical presentation is an acute focal cerebral infarction; in most cases patients are young male chronic drug addicts. As a rule drugs such as heroin or amphetamine have been administered by intravenous injection but there are also reports of occlusion of larger vessels in relation to lysergic acid, a derivative of the ergot alkaloids with powerful vasoconstrictor properties (Lieberman et al, 1974).

Effect of irradiation

There are a number of reports of damage to blood vessels following the therapeutic use of X-rays and such changes have also been produced experimentally.

The immediate changes of exposure of cerebral tissue to X-rays are an acute inflammatory vasculitis and meningitis with neuronal damage. After a latent period of seven to twelve months further proliferative changes became evident in vascular tissues and in astrocytes. The small arteries appear to show the greatest change, notably a marked fibrinoid infiltration of the subintima and various degrees of cellular infiltration with lipid-containing histiocytes. Fragmentation of elastic tissue, fibrosis, mural thrombosis and recanalisation are also evident. Large arteries including carotids and aorta also show inflammatory changes or fibrosis with extensive premature atherosclerosis. Induration of the tissues of the neck and atrophy of the skin may be present (Bladin & Royle, 1977). Small multiple aneurysms in the cervical carotid arteries may be seen many years after irradiation for thyroid carcinoma, and may lead to mural thrombosis (Fig. 19.13). Some of the cerebral changes are undoubtedly a result of multiple vascular occlusions, but these are thought unlikely to account for all the damage, which shows a predilection for subcortical white matter in brain stem and spinal cord in a pattern not seen in vascular disease. Extensive development of collat-

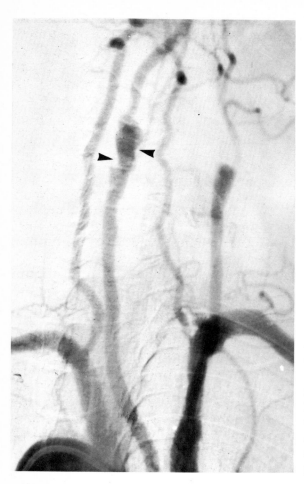

Fig. 19.13 Irradiation carotid damage. Localised ectasia and ulceration of internal carotid artery (arrowed) in 55 year old man with TIA. The thyroid had been irradiated 25 years before.

eral vessels of Moya moya or transdural type has been described.

The clinical presentation results from the combined effects of irradiation necrosis of the brain and blood vessels; affected patients have usually been irradiated for pituitary tumour (Peck & McGovern, 1966) or lymphoma (Zeman, 1968). A specifically vascular presentation is unusual. One report describes a patient who developed, six months after cobalt treatment for Hodgkin's disease, transient ischaemic attacks followed by a stroke. Foam cell arteritis and multiple ischaemic areas were found at autopsy and the terminal carotid and its main branches showed irregular narrowing (Kagan et al, 1971).

OTHER VARIETIES OF CEREBRAL VASCULAR DISEASE

Migraine

It is often stated that the prodromal phase of migraine is due to focal cerebral ischaemia, a consequence of arterial spasm affecting particularly the posterior cerebral artery and that the subsequent headache is due to a more generalised state of vasodilatation mainly in the carotid system.

There is strong evidence for changes in blood flow during the migraine attacks and a number of workers have found a reduction in flow during the *migraine prodrome* over the affected hemisphere (Simard & Paulson, 1973) or over both hemispheres (Sakai & Meyer, 1978). However, the amount by which blood flow is reduced (20–50 per cent) would not necessarily cause cerebral dysfunction; furthermore a reduction in blood flow may not be the primary event — it could also be a homeostatic adjustment to a state of reduced cerebral metabolism.

Angiographic studies during the aura of migraine have been made on very few occasions. Some have shown a reduction in arterial calibre and in the filling of the internal carotid artery system during the migraine aura (Dukes & Vieth, 1964). Other studies find no evidence of vessel narrowing but reflux into the basilar system (Skinhoj, 1973).

The evidence that vascular narrowing is caused by spasm is based on unconfirmed observations in a few patients that amylnitrite or CO_2 inhalation rapidly abolish the visual aura (Marcussen & Wolff, 1950). Simard & Paulson (1973) could not however increase the reduced blood flow found during the migraine aura by CO_2 inhalation.

During the *headache phase* most patients show a somewhat increased cerebral perfusion (Norris et al, 1975) although in some studies the cerebral blood flow has been normal. CT scanning has shown low density regions between attacks usually affecting white matter in the posterior part of the hemisphere. There is also said to be an unexpectedly high prevalence of cerebral atrophy in those who have suffered life-long migraine (Hungerford et al, 1976).

The various clinical and pharmacological factors which have been found to provoke migraine attacks suggest that migraine may be a complex state of inherited neurovascular instability which shows an abnormal reactivity to circulating vasoactive amines. At the onset of the attack there is an increase in plasma serotonin which falls rapidly as the headache develops (Anthony et al, 1968). In a susceptible subject an injection of reserpine, which reduces plasma serotonin, will provoke an attack and this can be relieved by a further injection of intravenous serotonin (Kemball et al, 1960). Harper et al (1977) suggest that there is a primary defect in the blood/brain barrier with increased permability allowing circulating amines and prostaglandins to cross the barrier and act on the cerebral resistance vessels.

Although traditional descriptions have emphasised the role of vascular spasm it may be noted that a reversible state of oedema of the vessel wall is consistent with the observed cerebral blood flow changes and is a more satisfactory explanation of some of the angiographic findings. The evolution of a migraine attack which tends to spread from the occipital to the parietal lobe to involve more than one vascular territory is not like the effects of vascular occlusion as generally understood.

Longlasting permanent neurological defects following migraine

Migraine is a common disorder and permanent and prolonged neurological sequelae are extremely rare; it is not always easy to be certain of a causal relationship in an individual patient between migraine and a cerebral vascular lesion. The most convincing instances are those affecting known migraineurs where the prolonged deficit begins during a severe attack of migraine; other patients may develop a deficit which resembles a migraine aura but does not come on during an attack. It is usually unwise to invoke migraine as a cause of otherwise unexplained vascular events in patients with chronic or recurrent headache although some authorities regard migraine as responsible for many unexplained transient ischaemic attacks in middle age even in the absence of headache (Fisher, 1980).

However, a variety of prolonged vascular syndromes do occur in association with migraine and require to be distinguished from degenerative varieties of vascular disease. In *hemiplegic migraine* a typical migrainous headache is succeeded by an episode of hemiparesis with or without dysphasia which clears slowly and completely over four to ten days. The diagnosis can be made with confidence only when there is a history of a previous attack affecting one or other side. There is usually a strong family history (Whitty, 1953). Carotid angiography during the phase of hemiparesis is usually normal and has been said to provoke further attacks.

In *ophthalmoplegic migraine* the headache is succeeded by a third or sixth nerve palsy clearing over some weeks and sometimes leaving a residual cycloplegia. As in hemiplegic migraine, the patient is usually a child or young adult with a past and family history of similar headaches. The cause of the ophthalmoplegia is thought to be oedema of the cavernous portion of the carotid artery and a narrowed segment may be seen angiographically. Biopsy in a single case showed oedema of the arterial wall (Walsh & O'Doherty, 1960).

In rare instances a migraine aura fails to recover, local infarction occurs and a permanent deficit remains. This has been recorded in the *retina* (Graveson, 1949), in the *optic nerve* (McDonald & Sanders, 1971), and in the *middle cerebral artery* territory (Dorfman et al, 1979) but occurs most frequently in the *posterior cerebral artery* where the trunk or one of the main branches, such as the calcarine artery, may be occluded. (Fig. 19.14 A & B). Sometimes a major artery is occluded (Rascol et al, 1979); at other times there is reduced capillary perfusion over a localised area (Kaul et al, 1974). Initially the visual field defect may be dense and involve the whole half-field but some degree of recovery is the rule. Residual defects are most commonly small homonymous paracentral scotomas close to the fixation point but usually sparing central visual acuity (Polyak, 1957). Such a case has recently been examined by positron scanning (Bousser et al, 1980). The findings were similar to those of a cerebral infarct, the occipital area on the affected side showing reduced metabolism and a blood supply more than adequate for metabolic requirement (luxury perfusion). The adjoining temporal lobe showed reactive hyperaemia.

There is only one well-documented case examined pathologically (Polyak, 1957). The appearances many years after permanent migrainous

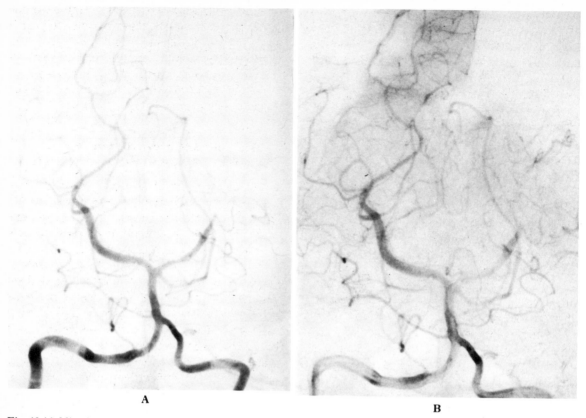

Fig. 19.14 Migraine. (A) Occlusion of the left posterior cerebral artery in a woman aged 30 following a severe attack of migraine. (B) Absence of capillary filling in the left posterior cerebral artery territory. (Courtesy of Professor G. du Boulay).

hemianopia were typical of localised cerebral infarction. Other instances of permanent hemisphere or brainstem infarction occurring in migrainous patients are recorded by Connor (1962).

Cerebral atheroembolism

Atheromatous lesions in large arteries have a tendency to ulcerate and to discharge semi-fluid contents into the lumen of the vessel. The resulting emboli consisting of fragments of thrombus, collagenous intima, and cholesterol esters in crystalline form are carried in the microcirculation where they lodge in small arterioles. Many observations of such emboli have been made in the retinal arteries and have shown that they tend to impact at bifurcations of small arterioles, diameter 20–100 microns. A single embolus may obstruct the lumen but more commonly tends to lodge across the vessel where the flat cholesterol crystal

offers little resistence to blood flow. Cholesterol emboli are usually multiple and tend to persist for a few weeks in retinal arterioles. They may then disappear entirely or leave behind a short segment of arterial sheathing. Pathologically this consists of a foreign body giant cell reaction causing thickening and opacification of the wall.

Atheroembolism is indicative of advanced ulcerating atheromatous lesions; such lesions most often occur in the descending aorta or its major branches and since atheroma is almost universal in elderly subjects it is not surprising that cholesterol emboli may be found at autopsy in the small peripheral arterioles of the viscera or lower limbs in 16 per cent of hypertensive males (Gore & Collins, 1960).

Involvement of the brain by atheromatous embolism is uncommon since ulcerating atheroma tends to be less extensive in the proximal aorta and carotid arteries than in the abdominal aorta. Reported instances have all had extremely severe arterial disease often aggravated by hypertension, diabetes, hyperuricaemia or syphilis (Elliot et al, 1964). Because of the small size of the emboli and the well-developed pial collaterals cerebral infarction is only likely to occur when large numbers of emboli reach the brain. Histological examination of the brain may show many penetrating and leptomeningeal arteries stuffed full of accumulated embolic material. The infarcts are small and multiple, bilateral, sometimes haemorrhagic. They are most frequently found in subcortical regions in the arterial borderzones (Beal et al, 1980).

The clinical diagnosis of cerebral atheroembolism is seldom made during life. The symptoms usually consist of brief attacks of focal neurological disturbance but some patients present as a fluctuating organic dementia with confusion, drowsiness, disorientation and memory loss. Seizures, either focal or general, occur more frequently than in other varieties of vascular disease. The onset of symptoms is sometimes provoked by such measures as manipulation of the neck, coughing or straining, arterial surgery or the administration of anticoagulants.

Physical signs are not prominent but transient hemiparesis, hemisensory disturbance or dysphasia may indicate a small subcortical softening in the middle cerebral territory. Dysarthria, diplopia, vertigo or hemianopia are indicative of a similar event in the vertebrobasilar field.

Visual disorientation (a bilateral disturbance of visual localisation and attention, with abnormalities of ocular motor pursuit) has been described and is caused by bilateral lesions of the parietal occipital borderzones between middle and posterior cerebral arterial territories. In addition to cerebral involvement patients usually also show evidence of visceral or peripheral microemboli (Russell, 1979). Systemic symptoms of episodic abdominal pain due to pancreatitis, cholecystitis or duodenal ulceration may occur and haematuria and renal failure are prominent. Painful papular nodules on the fingers may indicate occlusion of digital arterioles.

In severely arteriopathic elderly or demented patients there is little that can be done. If the condition is supected at a younger age or if symptoms are unilateral the appropriate investigation is arch aortography since if a single

discharging atheromatous lesion is identified in the carotid artery it may be removed surgically. It is possible but as yet unproved that long term preventive treatment of factors known to predispose to atheroma, such as hypertension and hyperlipidaemia, may retard the progress of the disease to this advanced stage.

Stroke related to pregnancy or the puerperium; occult thromboembolism

Acute hemiplegia in the last four weeks of pregnancy or in the puerperium has often been recorded but until recently was regarded as invariably due to cerebral venous thrombosis. Recent studies show that the majority of such cases are arterial in origin. Cross et al (1968) described 31 such patients of whom 16 were pregnant (mostly in the third trimester) and the remainder puerperal (most from 1 to 16 days post partum). All had a hemiparesis and six had seizures. More than half the patients had occlusion of a major cerebral artery such as the internal carotid or middle cerebral shown at angiography or autopsy. Three fatal cases showed thrombosis of the internal carotid artery but no significant artery wall disease, source of embolism or venous occlusion (Adams & Graham, 1967).

A further 21 patients were recorded by Fisher (1971). Some of these had previous features of migraine or thrombophlebitis. One third of puerperal patients showed cerebral arterial occlusion or stenosis. All angiograms on pregnant patients were normal.

A recent and comprehensive report on this subject comes from Rascol et al (1980) who described 15 patients and separated them into a number of groups. Four patients had typical eclampsia including seizures, coma and severe hypertension but angiography showed multiple intracerebral occlusions of small arteries with inconstant filling defects in larger vessels. The appearances may have been caused by disseminated intravascular coagulation. The authors also describe a second group of patients having intense headache but with no hypertension or proteinuria. Angiography in these showed multiple distal arterial occlusions and a remarkable multifocal segmental narrowing affecting intracranial arteries

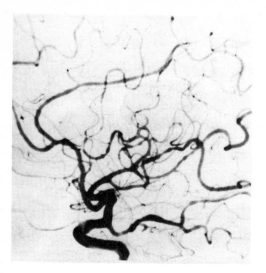

Fig. 19.15 Puerpural vascular occlusion. Multiple regions of arterial stenosis. The patient, aged 25, developed severe headache and vomiting and seizures one month after normal delivery. A repeat angiogram seven months later was normal. (Courtesy of Dr Andre Rascol).

of all sizes (Fig. 19.15). The condition was completely reversible within a few weeks and occurred in patients who had not received ergot alkaloids. The third group of three patients showed a focal cerebral deficit within three weeks of a normal pregnancy. Each showed a local arterial occlusion possibly due to embolism. No venous occlusions were demonstrated. In the fourth group there were three patients who had inflammatory arterial disorders similar to systemic lupus but localised to the brain. The relationship to pregnancy is uncertain. The patients showed focal cerebral deficits and spontaneous abortion occurred. Immunological abnormalities were demonstrable in blood and the illness persisted after pregnancy.

It seems that there are many factors which may combine to cause stroke in this group of patients. There is little evidence of premature atherosclerosis, hyperlipidaemia or inflammation but there may be an abnormal tendency to thrombosis. By analogy with the thrombogenic effect of contraceptive medication it is suggested that increased levels of oestrogen may be responsible.

Apart from the special risks of pregnancy and contraceptive medication a small group of pre-menopausal women develop occlusive cerebrovascular disease often involving the internal carotid artery or its middle cerebral branch. In some the attack may follow unusual exertion (Fisher, 1971) and in some a relationship to migraine has been suggested (Fisher, 1980). These patients seldom show coronary artery disease but they may develop venous thrombi or thrombi in peripheral systemic arteries. Some may be examples of *paradoxical embolism* which is probably commoner than is generally realised (Johnson, 1951), since 28 per cent of hearts have an unclosed foramen ovale (Fig. 19.16). Any condition such as pulmonary embolism which may cause the pressure in the pulmonary circulation to rise to a level at which the interatrial pressure gradient is reversed may cause right to left shunting and venous thrombi from the iliac or femoral veins may pass into the systemic arterial circulation. Septal defects of this kind can be closed surgically. Other cardiac conditions which may be difficult to detect but may give rise to cerebral embolism include ventricular aneurysm, prolapsed mitral valve, atrial myxoma and paroxysmal atrial fibrillation.

There are other reports of patients with a *generalised thrombotic tendency* developing over years and causing a progressive dementia, bilateral hemisphere signs and cortical blindness. The thrombotic tendency involves arteries and veins throughout the body; platelets and coagulation factors are normal but platelet survival is decreased indicating accelerated thrombogenesis (Torvik et al, 1971). Occult embolism from a source of thrombosis in the heart or in the proximal aorta may account for some puzzling cases of cerebrovascular occlusion in young patients in whom a diagnosis can only be reached after angiocardiography and arch aortography. A series of patients of this kind with multiple cerebral emboli originating from aortic thrombosis but without evidence of arteritis has been recently reported from Sri Lanka (Peiris, 1979).

It is customary in patients who suffer repeated minor strokes and in whom no underlying abnormality either cardiovascular, haematological or hormonal can be found, to use anticoagulant treatment, apparently with good effect in some cases (Fisher, 1971). A history of heavy cigarette smoking is often present in patients with occult

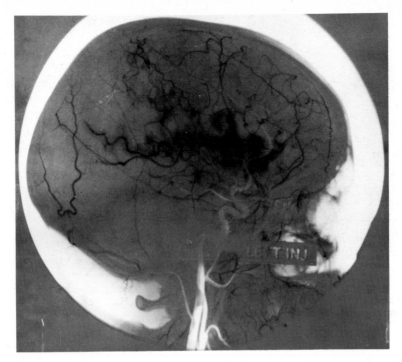

Fig. 19.16 Occult thromboembolism. Extensive small arterial occlusion in a woman aged 21 in middle cerebral territory possibly due to multiple cerebral embolism. (Courtesy of Dr Graham Wilson).

thromboembolism and it is advisable to proscribe the cigarette habit entirely in this context.

Cerebral fat embolism

The condition of cerebral fat embolism should be considered when impaired consciousness and neurological signs appear at an interval after fracture of a long bone. The duration of the latent period is usually 12 to 48 hours and the first symptoms are respiratory distress, fever, tachycardia and a petechial rash characteristically over the chest. Neurological distrubances can take various forms, the commonest being impaired consciousness, seizures and focal signs such as dysphasia, hemiparesis or conjugate ocular deviation. Attacks of decerebrate rigidity may also occur. The mortality is 10 to 20 per cent and the brains of fatal cases show marked cerebral swelling and multiple petechiae, especially in the white matter of the centrum semiovale and the internal capsule but also in the brain stem, cord and cerebellum. At a later state the changes are those of multiple small infarcts. Intravascular fat may be demonstrated on frozen sections especially

in cortical penetrating arteries (Kamenar & Burger, 1980).

Diagnosis is confirmed during life by observation of fat emboli in the retinal arteries or by renal or skin biopsy to show intravascular fat globules. Reliance should not be placed on the presence of globules in the urine, c.s.f. or blood.

The pathogenesis is not fully understood and differs from the effects of other types of emboli. It has also proved difficult to reproduce the changes experimentally. Secondary factors, such as acutely raised venous pressure from pulmonary hypertension, disseminated coagulopathy and the effect of hypotension or hypoxia may play a significant part. Although the emboli consist of neutral fat it is possible that toxic fatty acids may be released by the action of circulating lipase.

If the patient survives four days after the onset of symptoms the prognosis is generally favourable although residual mental impairment and visual field defects are reported (Thomas & Agyar, 1972). Massive corticosteroid treatment is recommended to combat brain swelling and the clearance of microemboli from the circulation may be aided by intravenous infusion of heparin and five per cent ethanol.

Vascular hemiplegia in children

Acute hemiplegia in children and adolescents is rare but when it does occur it may be of unusual severity and may be followed by a substantial motor deficit, by epilepsy and by mental retardation. Under the age of six permanent dysphasia does not occur with unilateral infarction. In general the mortality is low but bad prognostic features include age under two years and prolonged or repeated seizures at the onset.

Except in the rare mesodermal dysplasias such as Marfan's disease, or in metabolic abnormalities such as homocystinuria, acute childhood cerebral vascular disease is not due to intrinsic arterial disease and its occurrence should prompt a search for an underlying cause such as a systemic infection, cardiac abnormality or trauma. In the first few months of life cerebral infarction may complicate severe respiratory or pharyngeal infection especially in debilitated or dehydrated infants. It has been traditionally ascribed to cortical venous thrombosis but some cases are due to pyogenic carotid arterial thrombosis with extension of thrombus or to cerebral embolism.

In toddlers direct trauma to the tonsillar fossa, usually due to a fall while sucking a pencil, has been a cause of carotid thrombosis and hemiplegia on many occasions. Indirect trauma to the carotid artery in the neck is unusual but the vertebral artery may be injured during gymnastic exercises especially if there is a congenital abnormality of the upper cervical spine (Fraser & Simbler, 1975). In specific infections such as tuberculous meningitis where chronic endarteritis affects the basal cerebral arteries, cerebral infarction may occur in the course of the illness. Subacute bacterial endocarditis should also be suspected when signs of neurological deficit are accompanied by evidence of meningeal infection. Children with cyanotic heart disease are especially prone to cerebral venous thrombosis, infective or non-infective, as well as to cerebral abscess. A combination of right to left shunting and polycythaemia is responsible. Other blood diseases such as sickle cell disease, thrombocytopenic purpura, thrombocytosis and leukaemia may also present with focal cerebral signs of vascular origin either from thrombosis or haemorrhage.

In some children no underlying cause can be found and it is possible that developmental abnormalities are playing a part. Looping of the carotid artery just below the skull base is a congenital abnormality usually found incidentally in young children. It may rarely be associated with transient ischaemic attacks and has been treated by resection. A variety of other carotid abnormalities have been described in childhood hemiplegia, the frequency being 65 to 80 per cent. The commonest finding is carotid artery occlusion at the base of the brain with extensive collateral development (moya-moya syndrome). Distal carotid occlusion may also be found without collateral development and in some patients the artery may appear attentuated throughout its length. Other angiographic abnormalities found in childhood hemiplegia are multiple distal branch occlusions of intracerebral vessels and a curious cork-screw pattern of terminal arteries (Golden, 1978). The cause is unknown but some may be related to low grade meningeal infection or to an abnormality of development. Dissecting aneurysms of the intracerebral arteries have also been recorded (Manz et al, 1979).

Venous sinus thrombosis

Thrombosis of a cerebral venous sinus may occur spontaneously (bland, marantic thrombosis) or may be a sequel to local sepsis, as in purulent thrombophlebitis of the cavernous sinus which sometimes followed orbital cellulitis in the pre-antibiotic era. Septic thrombosis of this kind is now seldom seen and the following description is of spontaneous thrombosis.

The sinus most frequently involved is the superior longitudinal (sagittal) sinus sometimes in combination with other sinuses (transverse, sigmoid, straight, petrosal) or the major cerebral veins, such as the superior or inferior cerebral veins and the internal cerebral vein.

Patients with spontaneous thrombosis fall into two main groups — an infantile group where thrombosis may occur during a systemic illness especially where dehydration or malnutrition is present, and an adult group where the majority of cases occur during the puerperium. Venous sinus thrombosis may also follow thrombophlebitis migrans, ulcerative colitis or head injury (Kalbag & Woolf, 1967), or during pregnancy (Lavin et al, 1978).

Puerpural thrombosis mostly affects primipara and occurs one to three weeks after delivery. The sagittal sinus is most often involved and the most prominent early symptom is headache, sometimes intense and accompanied by depressed consciousness, stupor or delirium. Seizures, either focal or generalised, are a regular feature and may be followed by a postictal hemiparesis sometimes alternating from side to side.

An unusual type of hemiparesis affecting first the leg and later ascending to involve the arm and face is thought to indicate spread of thrombosis from the sinus to involve the major veins draining the posterior frontal cortex. Progression from hemiplegia to tetraplegia may indicate extension of thrombosis into the internal cerebral vein.

In some patients where the thrombus is more posteriorly situated in the sagittal sinus the symptoms point to biparietal rather than to bifrontal lesions. The syndrome of visual disorientation may occur; this comprises of an inability to localise visual stimuli in either field, bilateral visual inattention and defective oculomotor fixation and pursuit (Martin, 1944).

Sinus thrombosis may prevent the normal absorption of the cerebrospinal fluid in to the sagittal sinus and may then give rise to raised intracranial pressure. The clinical features are headache, drowsiness, papilloedema, abducens palsy and slight neck stiffness. Lumbar puncture reveals fluid under increased pressure which may be bloodstained; the protein and lymphocyte contents are sometimes elevated.

Chronic thrombosis of the lateral sinus may be a sequel of mastoid infection or glomus jugulare tumour. It is thought to be of serious significance only when the thrombus extends into the torcula. The clinical features are then those of sagittal sinus thrombosis.

The diagnosis of sinus thrombosis can usually be made on clinical grounds but may be confirmed by carotid angiography which shows failure of filling of a segment of venous sinus. CT scanning at an early stage may show parasagittal low-density lesions due to oedema and later infarction.

The principles of treatment in cerebral sinus thrombosis are to limit extension of the thrombus by anticoagulation, to treat raised intracranial pressure and cerebral oedema with dexamethasone and to control seizures with anticonvulsants. In addition any local infection will require appropriate antibiotic administration and in children dehydration may necessitate intravenous fluid replacement.

REFERENCES

Acheson J, Hutchinson E C 1972 Controlled trial of clofibrate in cerebral vascular disease. Atherosclerosis 15:177

Adams J H, Graham D I 1967 Twelve cases of fatal cerebral infarction due to arterial occlusion in the absence of atheromatous stenosis or embolism. Journal of Neurology, Neurosurgery & Psychiatry 30:479

Alajouanine T, Le Beau J, Houdart R 1948 La symptomologie tumorale des volumineux aneurysms des artères vertebrales et basilaires. Revue Neurologique 80:321

Alexander C B, Burgery P C, Goree J A 1979 Dissecting aneurysm of the basilar artery. Stroke 10:294–9

Anthony M, Hinterberger H, Lance J W 1968 The possible relationship of serotonin to the migraine syndrome. In: Friedman A P (ed) Research and clinical studies in headache. Karger, Basal and New York

Appenzeller O, Williams R C 1979 Cerebral lupus erythematosus. Annals of Internal Medicine 90:430

Armsworth R W, Gresham G H 1961 Giant cell arteritis with rupture of the aorta. Journal of Pathology and Bacteriology 82:203

Asbury A K, Aldredge H, Hershverg R, Fisher C M 1970 Oculomotor palsy in diabetes mellitus: a clinico-pathological study. Brain 93:555

Austin J H, Sears J C 1971 Familial hypoplasia of both internal carotid arteries. Archives of Neurology 24:1–10

Ballantyne D, Groshart K W G, Ballantyne J P, Young A, Lawrie T D B 1974 Relationship of plasma lipids and lipoproteins to cerebral atherosclerosis and ecg findings. In: Third international symposium of atherosclerosis, West Berlin. Springer-Verlag, Berlin and New York

Barabus A 1967 Heterogeneity of the Ehlers-Danlos syndrome. British Medical Journal ii:612

Barr H W K, Blackwood W, Meadows S P 1971 Intracavernous carotid aneurysms — a clinical pathological report. Brain 94:607

Bauer R, Sheehan S, Meyer J S 1961 Arteriographic study of cerebrovascular disease. Archives of Neurology 4:119

Beal M F, Williams R S, Fisher C M, Richardson E P 1980 Cholesterol embolism as a cause of transient ischaemic attacks and cerebral infarcts. Neurology 30:443

Beighton P 1970 The Ehlers-Danlos syndrome. Heinemann, London

Bickerstaff E R 1964 Aetiology of acute heimplegia in childhood. British Medical Journal ii:82

Bickerstaff E R, Holmes J M 1967 Cerebral arterial insufficiency and oral contraceptives. British Medical Journal i:726

Blachard C E, Doe R P, Mellinger G T, Byar D P 1970 Incidence of cardiovascular disease and death in patients receiving diethyloestradiol for carcinoma of prostate. Cancer 26:249

Bladin P F, Merory J 1975 Mechanism of cerebral lesions in trauma to high cervical portion of the vertebral artery — rotation injury. Proceedings of Australian Association of Neurologists 12:35–41

Bladin P F, Royle J 1978 Post-irradiation extracranial cerebrovascular disease. Clinical and Experimental Neurology 14:8

Bousser M G, Baron J C, Iba-zizen M T et al 1980 Migrainous cerebral infarction: a tomographic study of CBF and oxygen extraction fraction with the $_{15}$oxygen inhalation technique. Stroke II:145–48

Brandt K D, Lessell S, Cohen A S 1975 Cerebral disorders of vision in S.L.E. Annals of Internal Medicine 83:163

Cairns H, Russell D S 1946 Cerebral arteritis and phlebitis in pneumococcal meningitis. Journal of Pathology and Bacteriology 58:649

Caldwell H W, Hadden F C 1948 Carotid artery thrombosis; report of 8 cases due to trauma. Annals in Internal Medicine 28:1132

Carson N A J, Dent C E, Field C M B 1965 Homocystinuria: a clinical and pathological review of 10 cases. Journal of Paediatrics 66:565

Caspary E A, Peberdy M 1965 Oral contraception and blood platelet adhesiveness. Lancet i:1142

Citron B P, Halpern M, McCarron M, Lundberg G D, McCormic R, Pincus T J, Tatter D, Halveback B J 1970 Necrotising angiitis associated with drug abuse. New England Journal of Medicine 283:1003

Coakham H B, Duchen L W, Scaravilli F 1979 Moya Moya disease: clinical and pathological report of a case with associated myopathy. Journal of Neurology, Neurosurgery and Psychiatry 42:289–97

Costero I 1949 Cerebral lesions responsible for death of patients with active rheumatic fever. Archives of Neurology and Psychiatry 62:48

Countee R W, Vijayanathan T, Barrase C 1979 Cervical carotid aneurysm presenting as recurrent cerebral ischaemia with head turning. Stroke 10:144–6

Crepaldi G, Marlini S, Barocchi M R et al (1980) Lipids and Atherosclerosis in TIA. Special program on preventive medicine. N.R.C. Rome

Crompton M R 1959 Visual changes in temporal arteritis. Brain 82:377

Cross J N, Castro P O, Jennett W B 1968 Cerebral strokes associated with pregnancy and the puerperium. British Medical Journal iii:214

Cumings J N, Grundt I K, Holland J T, Marshall J 1967 Serum lipids and cerebrovascular disease. Lancet ii:194

Currier R D, De Jong R N, Bole G C 1954 Pulseless disease: central nervous system manifestations. Neurology (Minneapolis) 4:818

Dalal P M 1973 Aortic arch syndrome. In: Spillane J D (ed) Tropical neurology. Oxford University Press

Danarj T J, Wong H O, Thomas M A 1963 Primary arteritis of the aorta causing renal artery stenosis and hypertension. British Heart Journal 25:153

Denny-Brown D, Foley J M 1952 The syndrome of basilar aneurysm. Transactions of the American Neurological Association 77:30

Desai B, Toole J F 1975 Kinks, coils and carotids: A review. Stroke 6:649–53

Dixon J M 1951 Angioid streaks and pseudoxanthoma elasticum with aneurysm of the internal carotid artery. American Journal of Ophthalmology 34:1322

Donaldson I M, Espiner E A 1971 Disseminated lupus erythematosus presenting as chorea gravidarum. Archives of Neurology 25:240

Dorfman L J, Marshall W H, Enzmann D R 1979 Cerebral infarction and migraine — clinical and radiological correlations. Neurology 29:317–22

Dukes H T, Vieth R G 1964 Cerebral arteriography during migraine prodrome and headache. Neurology 14:636–9

Easton J D, Sherman D G 1977 Cervical manipulation and stroke. Stroke 8:594–6

Ehrenfeld W K, Wylie E J 1976 Spontaneous dissection of the internal carotid artery. Archives of Surgery 111:1294–1300

Elliott R S, Kanjuh V I, Edwards J E 1964 Atheromatous embolism. Circulation 30:611

Enzell K, Lindemalm G 1973 Cryptogenic cerebral embolism in women taking oral contraceptives. British Medical Journal iv:507

Facon E, Mestes E, Georgesco T 1960 Polyarteritis nodosa with lesions particularly in large cerebral arteries. Revue Neurologique 103:147

Faer M J, Mead J H, Lynch R D 1977 Cerebral granulomatous angiitis. American Journal of Roentgenology 129:413–7

Fairburn B 1957 Thrombosis of internal carotid artery after soft palate injury. British Medical Journal ii:750

Feinglass E J, Arnett F C, Dorsch C A et al 1976 Neuropsychiatric manifestations of systemic lupus erythematosus. Medicine (Baltimore) 55:323

Fisher C M 1959 Ocular palsy in temporal arteritis. Minnesota Medicine 42:1258

Fisher C M 1971 Cerebral ischaemia — less familiar types. Clinical Neurosurgery 18:267

Fisher C M 1980 Late-life transient cerebral ischaemia of obscure nature — migrainous accompaniment? In: Castaigne P, L'Hermitte F, Gautier J-C (eds) Cerebrovascular disease, 2nd Salpêtrière conference. Balliere, Paris. p 293–322

Fogelholm R, Aho K 1973 Ischaemic cerebrovascular disease in young adults. 1. Smoking habits, use of oral contraceptives, relative weight, blood pressure and electrocardiographic findings. Acta Neurologica Scandinavica 49:415

Ford F R 1952 Syncope, vertigo and disturbances of vision resulting from intermittent obstruction of the vertebral artery. Bulletin of Johns Hopkins Hospital 91:168

Ford R G, Siekert R G 1965 Central nervous system manifestations of periarteritis nodosa. Neurology (Minneapolis) 15:114

Fox C J, Darby S C, Ireland J T, Sonksen P H 1977 Blood glucose control and glomerate capillary basement membrane thickening in experimental diabetes. British Medical Journal ii:605

Fraser R A R, Zimbler S M 1975 Hind brain stroke in children caused by extracranial vertebral artery trauma. Stroke 6:153–8

Freedman P, Moulton R, Spencer A G 1958 Hypertension and diabetes mellitus. Quarterly Journal of Medicine 27:293

Frens D B, Petrjam J, Anderson R, Leblanc H J 1974 Fibromuscular dysplasia of the posterior cerebral artery: report of a case and review of the literature. Stroke 5:161

Glaser G H 1952 Lesions of the central nervous system in disseminated lupus erythematosis. Archives of Neurology and Psychiatry 67:745

Gold A P, Yahr M D 1960 Childhood lupus erythematosus: a clinical and pathological study of the neurological manifestations. Transactions of the American Neurological Association 85:96

Golden G S 1978 Strokes in children and adolescents. Stroke 9:169–71

Gore I, Collins D P 1960 Spontaneous atheromatous embolization. American Journal of Clinical Pathology 33:416

Graf C J 1965 Spontaneous carotid–cavernous fistula. Archives of Neurology 13:662

Graham E, Holland A, Avery A, Russell R W R 1981 Prognosis in giant cell arteritis. British Medical Journal 282:269–71

Graveson G S 1949 Retinal arterial occlusion in migraine. British Medical Journal ii:838

Greenfield J G 1951 Discussion of some less common cerebrovascular diseases. Proceedings of the Royal Society of Medicine 44:855

Gunning A J, Pickering G W, Robb Smith A H T, Russell R W R 1964 Mural thrombosis of the subclavian artery and subsequent embolism in cervical rib. Quarterly Journal of Medicine 33:133

Hackett E R, Martinex R D, Larson P F, Paddison R M 1974 Optic neuritis in systemic lupus erythematosus. Archives of Neurology 31:9

Haft H, Finneson B E, Cramer H, Fiol R 1957 Polyarteritis nodosa as a source of subarachnoid haemorrhage and spinal cord compression. Journal of Neurosurgery 14:608

Hamilton C R, Shelley W M, Tumulty P A 1971 Giant cell arteritis including temporal arteritis and polymyalgia rheumatica. Medicine 50:1

Hanns S H, Homer T D, Harter D H 1977 Vertebral artery occlusion complicating Yoga exercises. Archives of Neurology 34:574–5

Hardin C A 1962 Successful resection of carotid and abdominal aneurysms in two related patients with Marfan's syndrome. New England Journal of Medicine 267:141

Harker L A, Slichter S J, Scott R, Ross R 1974 Homocystinaemia vascular injury and arterial thrombosis. New England Journal of Medicine 291:537

Harper A M, Mackenzie E T, McCulloch J, Pritchard J D 1977 Migraine and blood-brain barrier. Lancet ii:1034–6

Hazelton R A, Reid A C, Rooney P J 1980 Cerebral lupus erythematosus: case report and evaluation of diagnostic tests. Journal of Neurology, Neurosurgery & Psychiatry 43:357

Hearn G W, Roper-Hall M J 1961 Obstruction of central retinal artery associated with chorea. British Medical Journal ii:684

Held K, Jipp P, Schreier A 1973 Natural history and muscle blood flow of patients with occlusion of the subclavian arteries and aortic arch syndrome. In: Meyer J S, Lechner H, Reivich M, Eichhorn O (eds) Cerebral vascular disease: Sixth Salzburg conference. Stuttgart: Thieme

Heyman A, Nefzger M D, Estes E H 1961 Serum cholesterol in cerebral infarction. Archives of Neurology 5:46

Higashi K, Hatano M, Maza T 1974 Disease with abnormal intracranial network complicated with intracerebral haematoma. Journal of Neurology, Neurosurgery and Psychiatry 37:365

Hilal S K 1974 Arterial occlusive disease in infants and children. In: Newton T H, Potts D G (eds) Radiology of the skull and brain, Vol 2. C. V. Mosby, St Louis. p 2286–2309

Hills J, Sament S. 1968 Bilateral agenesis of the internal carotid artery associated with cardiac and other anomalies. Neurology (Minneapolis) 18:142

Hirsch L F, Gonzales C F 1979 Fusiform basilar aneurysm simulating carotid TIAs. Stroke 10:598–601

Houser O W, Baker H L 1968 Fibromuscular dysplasia and other uncommon diseases of the cervical carotid artery: angiographic aspects. American Journal of Roentgenology 104:201

Howie P W, Mallinson A C. Prentice C R M, McNicol G 1970 Effect of combined oestrogen–progestogen oral contraceptives, oestrogen and progestogen on antiplasmin and antithrombotic activity. Lancet ii:1329

Hughes G R V 1979 Systemic lupus erythematosus: treatment and prognosis. British Medical Journal ii:1019

Hughes J T, Brownell B 1966 Granulomatous giant-cell arteritis of the central nervous system. Neurology (Minneapolis) 16:293

Hughes J T, Brownell B 1968 Traumatic thrombosis of internal carotid artery in the neck. Journal of Neurology, Neurosurgery & Psychiatry 31:307–14

Hungerford G D, du Boulay G H, Zilkha K J 1976 Computerised tomography in patients with severe migraine. Journal of Neurology, Neurosurgery & Psychiatry 39:990–4

Igbal A, Ater M, Lee S H 1978 Pseudoxanthoma elasticum: a review of neurological complications. Annals of Neurology 4:18

Illis L, Kocen R S, McDonald W I, Mondkar V P 1965 Oral contraceptives and cerebral arterial occlusion. British Medical Journal ii:1164

Imahori S, Bannerman R M, Graf C J, Brennan J C 1969 Ehlers-Danlos syndrome. American Journal of Medicine 47:967–77

Inman W H W, Vessey M P 1968 Investigation of death from pulmonary coronary and cerebral thrombosis and embolism in women of child-bearing age. British Medical Journal ii:193

Inman W H W, Vessey M P, Westerholm B, Engelund A 1970 Thromboembolic disease and the steroidal content of oral contraceptives: a report to the Committee on Safety of Drugs. British Medical Journal ii:203

Inman W H W 1979 Oral contraceptives and fatal subarachnoid haemorrhage. British Medical Journal ii:1468

Jakobsen T 1967 Glucose tolerance and serum lipid levels in patients with cerebrovascular disease. Acta Medica Scandinavica 182:233

Jick H, Rothman K J, Porter J 1978 Oral contraceptives and non fatal stroke in healthy young women. Annals of Internal Medicine 89:58

Job D, Eschwege E, Guyot-Argemtor C, Aubry J P, Tchobroutsky G 1976 Effect of multiple daily insulin injections on the course of diabetic neuropathy. Diabetes 25 : 463–9

Johnson B I 1951 Paradoxical embolism. Journal of Clinical Pathology 4 : 316

Johnson R T, Richardson E P 1968 The neurological manifestations of systemic lupus erythematosus. Medicine 47 : 337

Kagan A R, Bruce D W, Di Chiro G 1971 Fatal foam cell arteritis of the brain after irradiation for Hodgkin's disease. Angiography and Pathology. Stroke 2 : 232

Kahn P 1973 A histopathological study of three cases of Anderson-Fabry disease. Journal of Neurology, Neurosurgery & Psychiatry 36 : 1053

Kalbag R M, Woolf A L 1967 Cerebral venous thrombosis. Oxford University Press

Kamenar E, Burgery P C 1980 Cerebral fat embolism : a neuropathological study of a microembolic state. Stroke 11 : 477–84

Kao C C, Messert B, Winkler S S, Turner J H 1974 Rheumatoid atlantoaxial dislocation : pathogenesis and treatment. Journal of Neurology, Neurosurgery and Psychiatry 37 : 1069

Kaul S N, Du Boulay G H, Kendall B E, Russell R W R 1974 Relationship between visual field defect and arterial occlusion in the posterior cerebral circulation. Journal of Neurology, Neurosurgery and Psychiatry 37 : 1022

Keen J, Jarrett R J 1979 WHO Study of vascular disease in diabetes. Diabetic Care 2 : 187

Kemball R W, Friedman A P, Vallejo E 1960 Effect of serotonin in migraine patients. Neurology (Minneapolis) 10 : 107

Knox D L 1965 Ischaemic ocular inflammation. American Journal of Ophthalmology 60 : 995

Kudo T 1968 Spontaneous occlusion of the Circle of Willis, a disease apparently confined to Japanese. Neurology (Minneapolis) 18 : 485

Lavin P J M, Bone I, Lamb J T, Swinburne L M 1978 Intracranial venous thrombosis in first trimester of pregnancy. Journal of Neurology, Neurosurgery and Psychiatry 41 : 776

Lee J E, Haynes J M 1967 Carotid arteritis and cerebral infarction due to scleroderma. Neurology (Minneapolis) 17 : 18

Lee P, Urowitz M B, Brookman A M et al 1977 Systemic lupus erythematosus. Quarterly Journal of Medicine 46 : 181

Levesque M, Lefevre J, Legre J 1974 Infantile forms of the syndrome of progressive stenosis of branches of the polygon of Willis. Journal of Neuroradiologique 1 : 55

Levy R L, Dugan T M, Bernat J T, Keating T 1980 Lateral medullary syndrome after neck injury. Neurology 30 : 788

Lhermitte F, Gautier J C, Derouesne C, Buirand B 1968 Ischaemic accidents in the middle cerebral artery territory. Archives of Neurology 19 : 248

Lieberman A N, Bloom W, Kishore P S, Luin J S 1974 Carotid artery occlusion following ingestion of L.S.D. Stroke 5 : 213

Litchfield H R 1938 Carotid artery thrombosis complicating retropharyngeal abscess. Archives of Paediatrics 55 : 36

Lognelli G T, Buchhert W A 1971 Angiitis in drug abusers. New England Journal of Medicine 284 : 112

Macmillan G C 1950 Diffuse granulo-arteritis with giant cells. Archives of Pathology 49 : 63

Maisey D N, Cosh J A 1980 Basilar artery aneurysm in Anderson–Fabry disease. Journal of Neurology, Neurosurgery and Psychiatry 43 : 85–7

Manz H J, Vester J, Lavenstein B 1979 Dissecting aneurysm of the cerebral arteries in childhood. Virchow's Archives of Pathology, Anatomy and Histology 384 : 325

Marcussen R M, Wolff H G 1950 Studies of headache. Archives of Neurology and Psychiatry 63 : 42–51

Margolis M T, Stein R L, Newton T H 1972 Extracranial aneurysm of internal carotid artery. Neuroradiology 4 : 78–89

Martin J P 1944 Venous thrombosis in the central nervous system. Proceedings of the Royal Society of Medicine 37 : 383–6

Mathew N T, Abraham J, Taori G M, Gopalakrishna V I 1971 Internal carotid artery occlusion in cavernous sinus thrombosis. Archives of Neurology 24 : 11

McAulay D L, Isenberg D A, Gooddy W 1978 Neurological involvement in the epidermal naevus syndrome. Journal of Neurology, Neurosurgery and Psychiatry 41 : 466

McDonald W I, Sanders M D 1971 Migraine complicated by ischaemic papillopathy. Lancet ii : 521

McKusick V 1966 Heritable disorders of connective tissue. St. Louis : C V Mosby

Meadows S P 1951 Intracranial aneurysms. In : Feiling A (ed) Modern trends in Neurology. Butterworth : London

Messis C P, Budzilovich G N 1970 Pseudoxanthoma elasticum : a report of an autopsied case with cerebral involvement. Neurology 20 : 703–9

Metz H, Murray-Leslie R M, Bannister R G, Bull J W D, Marshall J 1961 Kinking of the internal carotid artery in relation to cerebrovascular disease. Lancet i : 424

Meyer J S, Waltz A G, Hess J W, Zak B 1959 Serum lipid and cholesterol levels in cerebrovascular disease. Archives of Neurology (Chicago) 1 : 303

Michael W F 1974 Posterior fossa aneurysms simulating tumours. Journal of Neurology, Neurosurgery and Psychiatry 37 : 218

Miller H G, Daley R 1946 Clinical aspects of periarteritis nodosa. Quarterly Journal of Medicine 15 : 255

Milligan N, Anderson M 1980 Conjugal disharmony as a hitherto unrecognised cause of strokes. British Medical Journal 281 : 421–2

Mokri B, Sundt T M, Houser O W 1979 Idiopathic regressing arteriopathy. Archives of Neurology 36 : 677–80

Musoke L K 1966 Neurological manifestations of malaria in children. East African Medical Journal 43 : 561

New P J F 1966 Arterial stationary waves. American Journal of Roentengenology 97 : 488

Norris J W, Hachinski C, Cooper P W 1975 Changes in cerebral blood flow during a migraine attack. British Medical Journal iii : 676–7

Nurick S, Blackwood W, Mair W P G 1972 Giant cell granulomatous angiitis of the central nervous system. Brain 95 : 133

Ochsner J L, Hughes J P, Leonard G L, Mills W C 1977 Elastic tissue dysplasia of the internal carotid artery. Annals of Surgery 185 : 684–91

O'Duffy J D, Goldstein N P 1976 Neurological involvement in seven patients with Behcet's disease. American Journal of Medicine 61 : 170

Osborn A G, Anderson R E 1977 Angiographic spectrum of cervical intracranial fibromuscular dysplasia. Stroke 8 : 617–26

Parish J G 1960 Hereditable disorders of connective tissue. Proceedings of the Royal Society of Medicine 53:515

Parker H L, Kernohan J W 1949 Central nervous system in periarteritis nodosa. Mayo Clinic Proceedings 24:43

Peck F C, McGovern F R 1966 Radiation necrosis of the brain in acromegaly. Journal of Neurosurgery 25:536

Peiris J B, Russell R W R 1980 Giant aneurysms of the carotid system presenting as visual field defects. Journal of Neurology, Neurosugery and Psychiatry 43:1053–64

Pellock J M, Kleinman P K, McDonald B M, Wixson D 1980 Childhood hypertensive stroke with neurofibromatosis. Neurology 30:656–9

Perdue G D, Barreca J P, Smith R B, King O W 1975 Significance of elongation and angulation of the carotid artery: a negative view. Surgery 77:45–52

Picard L, Andre J M, Roland J, Arnould G, Lepoire J, Crouzet G, Djindjian R 1974 Moya-moya syndrome of the adult. Transient forms. Journal Neuroradiologique 1:69

Pinching A J, Travers R L, Hughes G V R et al 1978 Oxygen-15 brain scanning for detection of cerebral involvement in systemic lupus erythematosus. Lancet i:898

Pirart J 1977 Diabète et complications degeneratives. Diabète et metabolisme 3:97–107

Polyak S 1957 The vertebral visual system. University of Chicago Press

Prior A L, Wilson L A, Gosling R G et al 1979 Retrograde cerebral embolism. Lancet ii:1044–7

Ramos M, Mandybar T I 1975 Cerebral vasculitis in rheumatoid arthritis. Archives of Neurology 32:271–5

Rascol A, Cambier J, Guirand B et al 1979 Cerebral ischaemic accidents during migraine attacks. Revue neurologique 12:867

Rascol A, Guirand B, Manelfe C, Clanet M 1980 Late migrainous accompaniments and a case of unexplained cerebral attacks. In: Castangne P, Lhermitte F, Gautier J C (eds) Cerebrovascular accidents during pregnancy and post partum. Deuxième Conférences de la Salpêtrière. Cerebrovascular diseases. J-B Balliere, Paris. p 85–130

Robertson M A, Schroder J S 1959 Pseudoxanthoma elasticum. American Journal of Medicine 27:433

Roden V J, Canter H E, O'Connor D M et al 1975 Acute hemiplegia of childhood associated with Coxsackie A9 virus infection. Journal of Pediatrics 86:56–8

Roger H, Poursines Y, Roger J 1955 Les aspects neurologiques de la periarterite nodeuse. Revue Neurologique 92:430

Rose G A, Spencer H 1957 Polyarteritis nodosa. Quarterly Journal of Medicine 26:43

Rossner S, Kjellin K G, Mattinger K L et al 1978 Normal serum cholesterol but low HDL Cholesterol concentration in young patients with ischaemic cerebrovascular disease. Lancet i:577–9

Ross R S, McKusick V 1953 Aortic arch syndromes. Archives of Internal Medicine 92:701

Rumaldi E, Harris W O, Kopp J E, Legier J 1976 Intracranial fibromuscular dysplasia: report of two cases. Stroke 7:511–6

Russell R W R 1973 The posterior cerebral circulation. Journal of the Royal College of Physicians 7:331

Russell R W R 1979 Atheroembolism in cerebral ischaemia. In: Greenhalgh R M, Rose F C (eds) Progress in Stroke Research. Pitman Medical, Tunbridge Wells. p 40–3

Sakai F, Meyer J S 1978 Regional cerebral haemodynamics during migraine and cluster headaches measured by the [133]Xenon Inhalation method. Headache 18:122–32

Sarkavi N B S, Holmes J M, Bickerstaff E R 1970 Neurological manifestations associated with internal carotid loops and kinks in children. Journal of Neurology, Neurosurgery and Psychiatry 33:194

Schimke R N, McKusick V A, Huang T, Pollack A D 1965 Homocystinuria. Studies of 20 families with 38 affected members. Journal of the American Medical Association 193:711

Schneider R C, Crosby E C 1959 Vascular insufficiency of brain stem and spinal cord in spinal trauma. Neurology (Minneapolis) 9:643

Schneider R C, Schemm G W 1961 Vertebral artery insufficiency in acute and chronic spinal trauma. Journal of Neurosurgery 18:348

Schwartz C J, Mitchell J R A, Hughes J T 1962 Transient recurrent cerebral episodes and aneurysm of the carotid sinus. British Medical Journal i:770

Shimizu T, Ehotich G E, Inaba G, Hayashi K 1979 Behcet's disease. Seminars in arthritis ans rheumatism 8:223

Simard D, Paulson O B 1973 Cerebral vasomotor paralysis during migraine. Archives of Neurology 29:207–9

Sinclair R J G, Kitchin A H, Turner R W D 1960 The Marfan syndrome. Quarterly Journal of Medicine 29:19

Sirton C R, Gidefraneschi G, Gritti I et al 1979 Decreased HDL-cholesterol levels in male patients with TIA. Atherosclerosis 32:205–11

Skinhoj E 1973 Haemodynamic studies within the brain during migraine. Archives of Neurology 29:95–8

Slack J 1979 In: Guyer B M, Wood C (eds) Lipids and heart disease. Myers Laboratory: Bristol. p 39

Smith K R, Nelson J S, Dolley J M 1968 Bilateral hypoplasia of the internal carotid arteries. Neurology (Minneapolis) 18:1149

Sogaard I, Jorgensen J 1975 Familial occurrence of bilateral intracranial occlusion of internal carotid arteries. Acta Neurochirurgica 31:245–52

Solomon G E, Hilal S K, Gold A P, Carter S 1970 Natural history of acute hemiplegia of childhood. Brain 93:107

Stebhens W E 1972 Pathology of the cerebral blood vessels. C V Mosby: St. Louis

Strachan R W 1966 Prepulseless and pulseless Takayasu's arteritis. Postgraduate Medical Journal 42:464

Susak J, Takaku A 1969 Cerebrovascular moya-moya disease. Archives of Neurology 20:288

Takayasu M A 1908 A case with peculiar changes of the central retinal vessels. Acta Societatis Japonicae 12:554

Taveras J M 1969 Multiple progressive intracranial arterial occlusions; a syndrome of children and young adults. American Journal of Roetgenology 106:235

Tchobroutsky G 1978 Relation of diabetic control to development of micro-vascular complications. Diabetologia 15:143–52

Thomas J E, Agyar D R 1972 Systemic fat embolism. Archives of Neurology 26:517–23

Tomsick T A, Lukin R R, Chambers A A, Benton C 1976 Neurofibromatosis and intracranial arterial occlusive disease. Neuroradiology 11:229–34

Torvik A, Endresen G K M, Abrahamsen A F, Godal H C 1971 Progressive dementia caused by an usual type of generalised small vessel thrombosis. Acta Neurologica Scandinavica 47:137–50

Turnbull L 1962 Agenesis of the internal carotid artery. Neurology (Minneapolis) 12:588

V A Cooperative Study 1973 Treatment of cerebrovascular disease with clofibrate. Stroke 4:684–93

Vitek J V, Halsey J H, McDowell H A 1972 Occlusion of all four extra-cranial vessels with minimum clinical symptomatology. Stroke 3:462

Vollman J, Nadjafi A S, Stalker C G 1976 Surgical treatment of kinked internal carotid arteries. British Journal of Surgery 63:847–50

Waisburg H, Meloff K L, Buncic R 1975 Polyarteritis nodosa complicated by multiple sclerosis like syndrome. Canadian Journal of Neurological Sciences 1:250

Walsh J P, O'Doherty D S 1960 A possible explanation of the mechanism of ophthalmoplegic migraine. Neurology (Minneapolis) 10:1079

Watson P, Fekete J, Deck J 1977 Central nervous system vasculitis in rheumatoid arthritis. Canadian Journal of Neurological Sciences 4:269–72

Webb F W S, Hickman J A, Brew D St J 1968 Death from vertebral artery thrombosis in rheumatoid arthritis. British Medical Journal ii:537

Weibel J, Fields W S 1965 Tortuosity, coiling and kinking of the internal carotid artery. Neurology (Minneapolis) 15:7

Weir R J, Briggs E, Mack A, Taylor L, Browing J, Naismith L, Wilson E 1971 Blood pressure in women after one year of oral contraceptives. Lancet i:467

Whitty C W M 1953 Familial hemiplegic migraine. Journal of Neurology, Neurosurgery and Psychiatry 16:172

WHO Clofibrate Trial 1978 A cooperative trial in the primary prevention of ischaemic heart disease using clofibrate. British Heart Journal 40:1069–118

Wickremasinghe H R, Peiris J B, Thanabadu P N, Sheriffdeen A H 1978 Transient emboligenic aorto-arteritis. Archives of Neurology 35:416–22

Wilkinson I M S 1972 The vertebral artery: extracranial and intracranial structure. Archives of Neurology (Chicago) 27:392

Wilkinson I M S, Russell R W R 1972 Arteries of the head and neck in giant cell arteritis. Archives of Neurology 27:378

Winkelman N W, Eckel J L 1932 The brain in acute rheumatic fever non-suppurative meningoencephalitis rheumatic. Archives of Neurology and Psychiatry 28:844

Wise D, Wallace H J, Jellinek E H 1962 Angiokeratoma corporis diffusum. Quarterly Journal of Medicine 31:177

Yaskin H E, Alpers B J 1944 Aneurysm of the vertebral artery. Report of a case in which the aneurysm simulated a tumour of the posterior fossa. Archives of Neurology and Psychiatry 51:271

Zeman W 1968 Article. In: Minckler J (ed) Pathology of the nervous system, vol. 1. McGraw-Hill: New York

20

Stroke prevention

H. J. M. Barnett

Death from stroke is declining as attested by the figures from many countries. The current rate of decline approximates to five percent per year. Although the evidence indicates that there may be no decline in deaths from ischemic heart disease, the reduction occurs both in ischemic and in hemorrhagic fatal strokes (Soltero et al, 1978; Statistics Canada, 1954–1980; Haberman et al, 1978; Sigurjonsson, 1974). Stroke prevention has become a realistic goal for the practising physician.

Any concerted effort to reduce the incidence of stroke requires that the *varieties of stroke* be identified and that the *threatening symptoms of stroke* be recognized. Treatment programmes available for one type of threatening stroke may be contraindicated for another. All programmes require critical scrutiny as do all potential treatments. This chapter will summarize the varieties of stroke and threatened stroke so as to indicate their relative importance and will discuss the medical treatment programmes that might be available or promising in each variety.

THE VARIETIES OF STROKE

In considering therapy the relative incidence of the varieties of stroke must be kept in focus. They are represented in Table 20.1. The first set of figures is from the careful clinical records of the Mayo Clinic, analyzed for the years 1945 to 1954 (Whisnant et al, 1971). The second group of figures are Framingham data obtained from a prospective community study of a stable population (Kannel et al, 1965). The third set of figures is compiled from published data from the Harvard Stroke Registry (Mohr et al, 1978). This was a prospective study of patients hospitalized in Boston hospitals utilizing newer methods including C.T. scanning to ascertain accurate diagnosis.

The striking difference between the early and the latest study is the upsurge in numbers of strokes attributed to *lacunar infarction* and to *emboli from the heart*. Better recognition is the explanation for the increase in each. The Boston group, led by C. Miller Fisher, have delineated the clinical syndromes of lacunar infarction and these have become increasingly common diagnoses (Fisher, 1965a; Mohr et al, 1978; Fisher & Curry, 1965; Fisher, 1965b; Fisher, 1967; Fisher & Cole, 1965). The rise from 3 percent to 19 percent of strokes attributed to heart disease is explained in part by technological advances: prolonged E.C.G. monitoring, wall-motion studies and echocardio-

Table 20.1 The changing incidence of the varieties of stroke reflects a growing awareness of lacunar infarction, an improvement in the ability to recognize cardiac disorders and an increased ease of recognition of smaller hemorrhages with the C.T. scan (per cent)

	Athero-thrombosis	Lacunes	Cardiac embolism	Intracranial hematoma	Aneurysm AVM	Unknown or other
Mayo Clinic 1945–1954 (n = 548) (Whisnant et al, 1971)	75	—	3	10	5	7
Framingham 1954–1974 (n = 90) (Kannel et al, 1965)	57	5	16	5	12	5
Harvard Stroke Registry 1975–1978 (n = 694) (Mohr et al, 1978)	46	19	19	10	6	—

graphy assuring a more accurate assessment of the heart.

C.T. scanning permits the diagnosis of intra-cerebral hematoma to be made without equivoca-tion. Deaths due to intracerebral hemorrhage are declining but there has been a rise in the numbers of small, nonfatal and previously unrecognized intracerebral hematoma (Ropper & Davis, 1980). Thus the figure of 10 percent is the same for the early and late studies.

The varieties of threatened stroke

A reversible retinal or hemisphere event that persists for 24 hours or less by custom is called a *transient ischemic attack (TIA)*; that which lasts more than 24 hours and then recovers completely is a *reversible ischemic neurological disability (RIND)*, and the persistent deficit with incomplete disability is called a *partial nonprogressing stroke (PNS)*. From the point of view of pathogenesis it is reasonable to regard all these conditions as a continuum; all are precursors of major strokes; taken together they form the clinical spectrum of conditions to be treated with whatever measures are available to prevent the final disaster of a disabling stroke. The C.T. scan also suggests that rigid boundaries between these conditions are artificial; depending on size and location, some lesions responsible for either TIA, RIND or PNS will not be detected by C.T. imaging, but in other patients lesions producing any of these conditions may be associated with a C.T. abnormality sug-gesting infarction (Nelson et al, 1980).

Table 20.2 outlines the conditions which give rise to TIA, RIND and PNS, in thrombotic and embolic stroke. Accurate information is not avail-able to give a quantitative estimate of the impor-tance of each condition but the order in which they

Table 20.2 Pathogenetic mechanisms of threatened stroke

Artery-to-artery emboli
Cardiac emboli
Lacunar infarction
Hemodyamic factors
Mechanical interference with arteries
Coagulation abnormalities
Thrombocytosis
Nonarteriosclerotic vasculopathies
Cerebral venous and sinus thrombosis

are listed is a close approximation. Artery-to-artery embolic events from atherothrombosis appear to be equal in incidence to all the others combined.

Table 20.3 is a classification of the commoner varieties of cardiac conditions giving rise to cerebral embolization which are capable of producing transient events varying from TIA to PNS as well as permanent stroke.

The more important cardiac lesions which will lead to cerebral embolization are shown in the left-hand column and the probable nature of the embolic material in the right-hand column.

Table 20.3 Cardiac lesions producing cerebral embolic events

Cardiac condition	Nature of embolus
1. Myocardial infarction	Mural thrombi
2. Postinfarction aneurysms and akinetic segments	Stasis thrombi
3. Postinfarction atrial fibrillation	Atrial thrombi
4. Mitral stenosis with or without fibrillation	Atrial or auricular thrombi
5. Atrial fibrillation of any cause	Atrial thrombi
6. Mitral regurgitation with atrial mural 'jet lesions'	Small mural thrombi
7. Bacterial endocarditis	Valvular mycotic thrombi
8. Nonbacterial thrombotic endocarditis	Valvular thrombi
9. Prolapsing mitral valve	Valvular thrombi, atrial thrombi
10. Mitral annulus calcification	(?) Degenerate valve fragments
11. Calcific aortic stenosis	(?) Degenerate valve fragments
12. Atrial myxoma	Neoplastic fragments, (?) attached thrombi
13. Prosthetic heart valve	Attached thrombi

A classification, according to arterial size, of the disorders of nonarteriosclerotic and nontraumatic origin which produce cerebral ischemic events, mostly with some degree of thrombus formation, some with hemorrhage (especially those marked *).

Whereas all of these atherothrombotic, cardiac and miscellaneous conditions may present with TIA, they do so with varying frequency. At the one extreme are the mural thrombi associated with myocardial infarctions which commonly are silent until major strokes occur. At the other extreme are the arteriosclerotic ulcers and stenoses in the

Table 20.4 Nonarteriosclerotic angiopathies capable of causing TIA and stroke

Particularly of the large arteries
 1. Fibromuscular dysplasia
 2. Dissecting aneurysm of aorta
 3. Spontaneous dissections of the carotid and vertebral-basilar system
 4. Takayasu's arteritis (Pulseless disease)
 *5. Moya Moya disease
 6. Radiation fibrosis of carotid artery

Particularly of the smaller arteries and arterioles
 *7. Collagen-vascular disease
 8. Temporal (giant-cell) arteritis
 9. Granulomatous angiitis
 10. Meningovascular syphilis
 11. Allergic vasculitis
 *12. Congophilic angiopathy
 13. Vasculitis with homocystinuria
 *14. Vasculopathy resulting from drug abuse
 15. Vasculitis with Behcet's disease
 *16. Vasculopathy from elastic tissue abnormality (Ehlers Danlos syndrome; pseudoxanthoma elasticum

extracranial arteries; TIA or RIND presage an embolic stroke from these lesions in about 50 percent of such cases (Mohr et al, 1978).

Within the framework of these types of *stroke* and these varieties of *threatening stroke*, measures that are available or suggested for *stroke prevention* will be discussed. Table 20.5 indicates the important risk factors that have been identified in respect to risk for stroke.

Table 20.5 Important risk factors for stroke

 1. Hypertension
 2. Diabetes
 3. Hyperlipidemia
 4. Cardiac abnormalities
 5. Cigarette smoking
 6. Increased hematocrit
 7. Intermittent claudication
 8. Estrogen contraceptive medication
 9. Bruits in the neck
10. TIA
11. Previous stroke
12. Heredity

RISK FACTORS AND THEIR MANAGEMENT

Hypertension is the most significant risk factor in stroke occurrence. In Canada between 1953 and 1978 a 51 percent reduction in stroke affecting those 65 years of age or under has been identified from the Vital Statistics Division of the Health Protection Branch. It is not possible to state categorically that improved hypertensive management has been the cause of this striking reduction but it coincides with a similar decline (88 percent) in deaths attributed to hypertension. This reduction in deaths attributed to hypertension may be an overestimate but other evidence of very substantial reduction is on record (Haberman et al, 1979).

Blood pressure elevation in the Framingham Study emerged as the strongest independent contributor to atherothrombotic stroke risk (Kannel et al, 1976). The authors have stated that 'some degree of hypertension is an almost ubiquitous finding in the background of stroke victims'. Risk of stroke is present with systolic as well as diastolic elevations and is proportional to the level of blood pressure at any age and in either sex. There is no decrease noted in the adverse influence of elevated diastolic blood pressure with advancing age. The original opinion that postmenopausal women tolerate hypertension better than men has not been substantiated. The Veterans Administration Study indicated no particular advantage in the control of milder hypertension but the numbers involved were small (Veterans Administration National Heart, Lung and Blood Institute Study Group for Cooperative Studies on Antihypertensive Therapy 1977).

The five-year hypertension and detection and follow-up program in the United States randomly assigned patients to two treatment groups, one of which received antihypertensive therapy administered at special centres and the other group of patients received therapy from their usual community sources (Hypertension Detection and Follow-Up Program Cooperative Group 1979). The results showed substantial difference in stroke incidence between individuals afflicted with mild (defined as a diastolic pressure between 90 to 104 mmHg, as well as moderate (between 105 to 114 mmHg) and severe (a diastolic pressure of 115 plus) hypertension.

The effect of antihypertensive treatment on stroke recurrence has been studied in two series of hypertensive patients presenting with cerebral infarction. In one group (Carter, 1970) of 99 patients in a randomized four-year study, 26.5 percent of the treated and 46 percent of the untreated patients died; 14 percent in the treated group had nonfatal recurrences compared with 22 percent of the untreated cases. In another study (Beevers et al, 1973) all patients were treated but with varying degrees of success in achieving satisfactory blood pressure levels. Recurrent stroke occurred in 55 percent in whom poor control was achieved; recurrences were substantially reduced (16 percent), in those in whom good control was achieved and maintained.

The message is clear: no level of hypertension is permissible because of the increased risk of stroke. Even after a cerebral ischemic event blood pressure must be controlled and kept normal.

Diabetes mellitus is a risk factor for stroke (Hutchinson & Acheson, 1975a). The majority of published studies indicate a two to three-fold increase in diabetes in patients with stroke compared with its occurrence in the normal population. Silverstein & Doinger (1963) recorded the highest incidence of diabetes mellitus (32 percent). Their series was of patients with angiographic evidence of occlusive vascular disease; in another study of major stroke involving 276 patients 27 percent had diabetes, although one in three were not so diagnosed prior to the ictus (Bental & Pillar, 1972). The usual published figures are somewhat below these higher numbers but the Framingham analysis identified impaired carbohydrate tolerance as an important contributor to stroke risk, noting that its importance is greater in women than in men (Kannel, 1976).

By comparison with these figures for diabetes mellitus in major stroke, the incidence in the 585 TIA and partial stroke cases entered into The Canadian Cooperative Study was 11 percent. In diabetics, stroke due to cardiac emboli, intracerebral hemorrhage, subarachnoid hemorrhage and aneurysm rupture varies from 12 to 16 percent. Estimates of the incidence of diabetes in the population at large vary between 3 and 12 percent, so that it is not possible to state with certainty that diabetes contributes to risk except in major ischemic stroke.

Patients with higher blood sugars are at greater risk for stroke (Kannel, 1976). It might be inferred therefore, that strokes would be more common in patients whose diabetes was difficult to regulate or who were careless about diabetic regulation. This is not clearly established. Recent studies indicate that hyperglycemic individuals have more widespread and serious infarction than do normoglycemic individuals. This observation has been corroborated in experimental animal studies (Pulsinelli et al, 1980).

It is not known with certainty that diabetics who suffer a stroke or transient ischemic attack survive longer with rigid diabetic regulation than without it. One study did not find any effect on long-term survival from stroke in 24 diabetics compared with nondiabetic patients (Robinson et al, 1959). A major controversy exists as to whether the use of oral hypoglycemic agents or insulin is the preferred treatment. Evidence exists suggesting that some oral hypoglycemic agents are atherogenic (The University Group Diabetes Program 1970); other evidence indicates that insulin-treated diabetics are at greater risk of stroke (Garcia et al, 1973). Further discussion of this problem is beyond the scope of this chapter.

The facts suggest that diabetes should be detected early and regulated as well as possible to minimize the stroke.

Blood lipids: Accelerated atherogenesis has been demonstrated in the coronary arteries and in the aorta in association with an increase in blood lipids. High serum cholesterol and triglycerides are found in very significant numbers of males with myocardial infarction. In the cerebral circulation the association is less apparent but can be found in men under 55 with raised serum cholesterol, cholesterol-rich betalipoprotein and triglyceride-rich prebetalipoprotein (Kannel, 1976). These Framingham data indicated that 'blood lipids are best considered as an ingredient of a stroke profile, and in the absence of other contributors to risk, the influence of lipids is feeble'. No data are available to point to a reduced risk of stroke in either sex submitted to lipid-reducing measures. The ratio of high-density to low-density lipoprotein may also be of importance. A recent study in patients with normal levels of total cholesterol and triglycerides and with only slight elevations of very low density lipoprotein indicated that the stroke risk is increased in these patients when there is a reduction in the level of high-density lipoprotein (Rossner et al, 1978). The possibility exists that high-density lipoprotein is protective, preventing low density lipoprotein from entering endothelial cells. This area of research will be watched with interest.

The logical recommendation appears to be that dietary intake of fat should be held at moderate levels.

Cardiac abnormalities play a significant role in increasing stroke risk. An increased cardiothoracic ratio and left ventricular enlargement in the e.c.g., intraventricular conduction defects, nonspecific ST and T wave abnormalities are all associated with increased risk of stroke and are independent of the influence of hypertension in increasing the risk of atherothrombotic stroke (Wolf et al, 1973; Wolf et al, 1978). A number of cardiac rhythm disorders such as atrial fibrillation contribute to thromboembolism and are important risk factors (Hinton et al, 1977).

It is essential that all patients threatened with stroke are investigated and treated for any relevant cardiac disorder.

Cigarette smoking is less pronounced as a risk factor for stroke than it is for coronary artery disease. Nevertheless it emerged as an important risk factor in the Framingham Study (Shurtleff, 1974) and in other reports (Paffenbarger & Wing, 1969). Men who were heavy smokers developed three times as many strokes as did nonsmokers; this was not found for women. The impact increased with the number of cigarettes smoked per day and waned with advancing age. Cigarette smoking has an effect on endothelial cells and therefore could promote thrombogenesis in subjects afflicted with atheroma (Stoel et al, 1981). The mortality figures for heart disease in individuals who have stopped smoking begin to approach those of nonsmokers (Doyle et al, 1964; Kannel et al, 1968) and intermittent claudication is known to decrease with cessation of smoking. It is not known what benefit follows the cessation of smoking in persons with TIA, RIND or PNS. Data are lacking but the inference might be made that it will prove beneficial when the information is gathered.

Cigarette smoking should be abandoned in all patients with threatened stroke.

Increased blood viscosity as found in polycythemia, macroglobulinemia and sickle cell disease is associated with increased risk of stroke. Recent evidence indicates that the risk begins to increase at the upper limits of what has been considered normal hematocrit range (Kannel et al, 1972). Increased blood viscosity appears to be the undesirable result of increased hematocrit and the level of c.b.f. is inversely proportionate to the hematocrit (Thomas, 1979).

The evidence is sufficiently strong that phlebotomy is indicated to maintain the hematocrit at levels within the accepted 'normal range'.

Intermittent claudication is evidence of atherosclerosis in major arteries and is present in 7 to 12 percent of patients with cerebral ischemia (Silverstein & Doinger, 1963; Friedman et al, 1968). It is thus a marker for atherosclerosis (Gordon & Kannel, 1972).

Estrogen therapy. Several studies, including the Collaborative Group for the Study of Stroke in Young Women, have shown that the relative risk for stroke in women taking contraceptive estrogen therapy is increased (Vessey & Doll, 1969; Heyman et al, 1969; Collaborative Group for the Study of Stroke in Young Women 1973). The data from the latter study suggested that smoking potentiates the risk imposed by contraceptive usage. The relative risk has been estimated to increase 4 to 11 times over that of women not on the pill, and is related particularly to those contraceptives with a higher dose of estrogen. A woman without other contributory factors can be reassured that in absolute terms the individual risk is very small (Schoenberg et al, 1970).

Women who smoke cigarettes, who have a history of classical migraine, thromboembolic disease, hypertension or other risk factors should seek an alternative form of contraception.

Asymptomatic carotid bruits are associated with an increased risk of stroke (Kagan et al, 1976; Wolf et al, 1979; Heyman et al, 1980). The risk is not greater in the territory of the artery which is the site of the bruit than it is for the side contralateral to the bruit or for the posterior circulation. Bruits are commoner in females but the risk of stroke in women is less than in men. Patients with asymptomatic carotid bruits have an increased risk from heart disease as well as stroke. Careful longterm studies of patients with asymptomatic carotid bruits and stenosis have cast serious doubt on the practice followed in some centres of performing angiography and prophylactic endarterectomy.

Convincing data about subgroups at particular risk are needed.

As long as the bruit or stenosis is not symptomatic, the best treatment for these patients is careful management of other risk factors.

Transient ischemic attacks carry a risk for stroke. The magnitude of this has been calculated from a variety of sources. The early calculations were made from the control groups in the anticoagulant drug trials (Millikan et al, 1971; Baker et al, 1968; Acheson et al, 1964). A 5 to 7 percent risk of stroke per year is a usual estimate. An additional 5 to 6 percent probability of death per year has been noted, mostly from myocardial infarction.

In a study of 198 patients diagnosed over a 15 year period as having TIA and followed up for a minimum of 5 years, a total of 72 strokes occurred. Slightly less than half of these patients were given anticoagulants for most of this time; the other half did not receive anticoagulant therapy. Of the 72 strokes, 15 occurred in the first month, 37 in the first year and at a rate varying between 4 and 8 percent per year thereafter. The conclusion was reached that stroke risk is greatest in the first three months after the onset of TIA. It should be noted that the total numbers in the study are small, that the pathogenesis of the TIA and stroke are not stated (i.e., whether some were cardiac and some of lacunar origin) and that the study was done before the recognition of lacunar and cardiac embolic strokes was as certain as it is today. Unlike other published studies the risk for females was higher than for males. While the conclusion that the highest risk is in the first two to three months after TIA onset may prove to be correct, more data are needed before this can be accepted finally and without any reservation.

A group of patients who experienced amaurosis fugax with bright retinal embolic plaques have been submitted to longterm follow-up (Pfaffenback & Hollenhorst, 1973). Of 208 cases followed for a total of 7 years, the risk of death was 54 percent and the majority of the deaths were from myocardial infarction and stroke. The data from the group of 289 cases not treated with aspirin in the Canadian Collaborative Stroke Study provides information on patients threatened with non-atherothrombotic stroke, since this was the particular variety selected for the trial (Barnett 1979b).

Table 20.6 indicates that there was a 13 percent overall likelihood of stroke and death in the first year, a 22 percent cumulative likelihood of stroke and death by the end of the second year, and a 30 percent likelihood of stroke and death by the end of the third year. The risk for males is higher and for females lower at each time interval.

Table 20.6 Prognosis of threatened stroke of atherothrombotic origin in 289 cases with average follow-up 26 months.

| | Stroke or death — percent | | |
	All	Male	Female
One year	13	14	11
Two years	22	24	16
Three years	30	35	16

The question of an increased risk of stroke with frequent rather than few attacks has been the subject of several studies (Baker et al, 1968; Marshall, 1964). It is written, quite commonly, that 'crescendo TIAs' represent a higher risk of stroke than few or infrequent attacks. This is an unsubstantiated speculation for which more data are required. Multiple TIAs in a large hospital population study were related, not unexpectedly, to the occurrence of further TIAs, but a single TIA placed the patient at increased risk for the more important end-point of early infarction (Conneally et al, 1978).

Repeated attacks may cease spontaneously. The risk of future stroke is not eliminated because of cessation of attacks. The fact that attacks do cease spontaneously is important when giving consideration to the possible benefit of treatment; cessation of attacks cannot always be attributed to treatment nor can it be regarded with complacency.

Previous stroke imposes a great risk for further stroke. The rates given in the literature cover a wide range but are drawn from studies with varying duration of follow-up, accounting for estimates on recurrence rates as low as 19 percent and as high as 53 percent (Hutchinson & Acheson, 1975b). Marquardsen (1969), calculating the number of recurrences observed for 100 patient years, has determined recurrence rates in published series ranging from 8 to 11 per 100 patient years. In his own series the annual rate of recurrence was fairly constant for 10 years after the first stroke averaging 8.9 percent per year for males and 10.6 percent per year for females but without a statistically significant difference between the two sexes. In the absence of death from other causes, he estimates that 75 percent of patients will have a recurrent stroke within 15 years.

ANTISPASMODICS, VASODILATOR AND VASOACTIVE DRUGS

A variety of preparations with vasodilator or 'vasoactive' capabilities have been marketed for 20 years and claimed to be of value in the treatment of patients with transient ischemia and cerebral arteriosclerosis. Critical study of the evidence does not substantiate claims that have been made for their efficacy. The commonest fault in the reported clinical trials has been the failure to study large enough numbers of cases to indicate a convincing difference between those treated and those untreated. Since end-points occur in approximately 10 percent of symptomatic patients per year, a convincing evaluation of the drugs used in these trials to bring about a 50 percent stroke reduction would require between 500 and 1000 cases, followed for no less than three and ideally for four to five years. No such study has been carried out and most studies have involved only 30 or 40 patients followed for a few months.

The definition of cases entered into these trials has been inexact. They have been patients afflicted with symptoms of nonspecific origin such as dizziness, forgetfulness, dementia and a variety of psychological symptoms. In many series, batteries of neuropsychological tests have been claimed to show improvement in the treated but not the untreated groups. These are dubious end-points from which to conclude that these agents are beneficial in stroke prevention or in doing anything of consequence for patients afflicted with symptomatic cerebral vascular disease. The alleged relief from a variety of vague symptoms has not been impressive. Benefit has been inferred in some instances because of reported improvement in cerebral blood flow measurements. No trial has involved symptoms which can be described without equivocation as acceptable examples of TIA, RIND or PNS. None of the reported trials has claimed the elimination of definite TIAs nor the prevention of stroke in any population of patients.

The rationale for the use of these drugs has never been sound. With the exception of patients with hypertensive crises, complicated migraine and recent subarachnoid hemorrhage, vasospasm is not a significant mechanism in the production of TIA, RIND and PNS. A major symposium devoted to the appraisal of each one of these preparations came to the conclusion that their value has not been established (Tognoni & Garattini, 1979).

Vasodilators, antispasmodics and vasoactive drugs have no proven value in stroke prevention or therapy.

ANTITHROMBOTIC DRUGS

Thrombogenesis plays an important role in stroke and in the pathogenesis of threatened stroke. Tables 20.1 and 20.2 make it clear that there are varieties of stroke and threatened stroke in which the importance of thrombosis is less than in others; in some, thrombosis plays a minor and secondary role. Thus antithrombotic agents may be indicated in some varieties of stroke and threatened stroke but in others their rationale as primary treatment or prophylaxis will be less convincing. Antithrombotic therapy is imperfect and must be coupled with risk factor management; a continuing active search for new drugs and improved programs is required. Thrombolysins, anticoagulants and platelet antiaggregants have been utilized and will be discussed in turn:

(a) *Thrombolysins* have been shown to be capable of removing thrombi in recently occluded carotid arteries (Fletcher & Alkjaesig, 1980). The tendency to convert an ischemic infarction into a hemorrhagic lesion by the opening up of the occluded artery has resulted in an unacceptably high morbidity and mortality rate. This has led to the virtual abandonment of this treatment in cerebral arterial disease until such time as better control of this bleeding tendency can be realized (Meyer et al, 1964). For the present any further use of these preparations must be regarded as experimental. Urokinase is under investigation and if the hazards of hemorrhage can be overcome, it may have therapeutic potential (Hanaway et al, 1976).

(b) *Anticoagulants* Heparin and coumadin derivatives have been utilized since the early 1950s when the role of thrombosis in TIA symptomatology was first recognized. If one demands strict scientific evidence derived from methodologically-sound studies as the criterion for their use, it must be admitted at once that this type of evidence has not been forthcoming. Heparin therapy has not been evaluated in controlled studies to establish its potential in stroke prevention. The trials of the coumadin-type drugs were not executed with attention to most of the stringent criteria now regarded as essential. They were concluded before the discipline of strict clinical trials had been established. Firm decisions about their overall value cannot be reached without equivocation in the absence of further trials.

The outstanding faults that emerge from a review of the studies that were done may be listed as follows:

(i) *Sample sizes* were too small. The study of treatment in chronic disease with few end-points per year requires large numbers of cases to yield significant results.

(ii) The *controls* were seldom adequate. Very few of the studies required random selection of the treatment and control groups. Often the method of selecting the control group was not specifically recounted. They appear for the most part to have been patients available for convenient comparison because they did not receive anticoagulant treatment for a variety of unspecified reasons.

(iii) Strict and predetermined definitions of *entry criteria* were seldom stated. A heterogeneous variety of partial and threatened stroke cases, involving some varieties in which thrombogenesis is of less significance, and some varieties with different prognostic significance were included. Much of the present understanding of the different varieties of threatened stroke had not been clarified so that the anticoagulant trials involved patients belonging to the 'genus' of threatened stroke rather than to particular 'species'.

(iv) The *end-points* were not stated clearly in advance in a number of the studies.

(v) *Risk factor influence* had not been well delineated at the time of the trials. No consistent policy in the handling of risk factors including their identification, possible exclusion or baseline treatment was required.

(vi) Other methodological principles were breached that could be described as less important, but collectively they would violate the demanding standards of a proper treatment trial. This would include the prerequisite for *completeness of follow-up*, avoidance of *contaminating therapy* and exclusion of patients with *co-morbid conditions* that would not be expected to survive the duration of the trial.

Flaws in the anticoagulant trials are not spelled out with a view to criticizing their conduct, but to examine the reasons why anticoagulant usage remains controversial and uncertain. In many instances their use depends on clinical judgment, the anecdotal experience of the individual practitioner, and, it must be admitted, the lack of satisfactory alternative therapy.

Before describing conditions in which anticoagulants might be reasonably considered, certain principles must be followed to govern their usage:

(i) The patient must be reliable; an adequate laboratory to check the prothrombin time must be available and the patient must live in an area where a physician skilled in their use is available.

(ii) Uncontrolled or uncontrollable hypertension precludes their usage, as does evidence of serious liver disease and most blood disorders.

(iii) Gastrointestinal bleeding within two years of their administration makes this hazardous, as does the need to administer most non-steroidal anti-inflammatory drugs.

(iv) Unless C.T. scanning is available, lumbar puncture is advisable.

Heparin should be administered by continuous infusion. Intermittent subcutaneous injection is less likely to yield predictable absorption and leads to more complications. Bleeding occurs most commonly when the partial thromboplastin time exceeds 60 seconds and it should be maintained between 50 and 60 seconds. A prothrombin time one-and-a-half times the control value is necessary with coumadin therapy. Bleeding complications mount rapidly if the prothrombin time exceeds twice the control value. The occurrence of hematoma and bleeding after two years of treatment may reflect reduced alertness and the adoption of a casual approach to what has become an accustomed and familiar treatment.

Anticoagulants in atherothrombosis: threatened stroke, progressing stroke and completed stroke

(a) **TIA** — Reviews of the major studies of anticoagulants in TIA have been published recently (Genton et al, 1977; Easton & Sherman, 1980). It is important to recall that more than 15 years have elapsed since the last randomized trial of anticoagulants in TIA was published, signifying that none has been designed in the past 20 years. Only four studies of a randomized nature and six nonrandomized studies are available. None of the randomized studies of TIA patients yielded benefit in stroke prevention (Baker, 1961; Baker et al, 1962; Pearce et al, 1965; Baker et al, 1966). The total number of patients in the treatment category from these four studies was a meagre 93 and the total in the four control groups only 85, with an average follow-up of 19 months and 21 respectively. The lack of benefit in stroke prevention could be the result of such a small sample size. Eight ischemic strokes occurred in the treatment and 10 in the control groups from the combination of these four studies. Results might have shifted in the direction of convincing benefit for treatment had the studies been larger and longer, but this is purely speculative. Fifteen deaths were recorded in the treated and 10 deaths in the control patients. Again this may have been skewed because of the small numbers. Most deaths were of cardiovascular origin but 6 were due to hemorrhage in those receiving anticoagulant compared with 1 fatal hemorrhage in the control group. Major bleeding episodes were reported in 13 treated patients compared with 4 control group patients.

Six nonrandomized studies have been published in which some control population was used for contrast. Four of the six have indicated benefit in stroke prevention but the claims must be accepted with caution (Genton et al, 1977). The reasons for assignment to 'treatment' and to 'no anticoagulant therapy' are not known and the comparability of the two contrasting groups is quite uncertain. The fifth study involved 21 patients given anticoagulant compared with 56 who did not receive it over a period of six weeks to four years (Toole et al, 1975). There were 6 strokes in the treated and 7 in the untreated group and of course no benefit was claimed. The sixth nonrandomized study involved 47 patients with carotid TIAs and 17 patients with vertebro-basilar TIAs who were compared with 75 patients with carotid and 47 with vertebro-basilar TIAs not given anticoagulants (Whisnant et al, 1978). There was no overall reduction in death but the stroke incidence was less in the treated cases. This benefit was reached within six months of beginning treatment and there was no difference thereafter between the treated and untreated patients. An overall benefit for death and stroke was claimed in subset analysis of the vertebro-basilar cases. The numbers were small, the selection process for treatment unknown and the variety of TIA admitted to the study not specified. Nine hemorrhages into the brain occurred in the patients receiving anticoagulant therapy, compared with 5 in those not receiving this treatment. No data on the levels of the prothrombin time at the times of these hemorrhages have been supplied.

It is clear that the data available on which to make recommendations for use of anticoagulants in stroke prevention in TIA cases are sparse and incomplete. The definitive study has not been done. TIAs are known to occur in flurries and to disappear spontaneously. The risk of serious hemorrhage increases with continued anticoagulant usage possibly because vigilance becomes reduced after prolonged use.

On an empirical basis it appears reasonable to consider administration of anticoagulants in TIA cases when platelet antiaggregants fail to stop the episodes, when TIAs progress to a minor stroke despite platelet antiaggregants, and when a surgical approach is unreasonable. A three or four month period on anticoagulants rather than indefinite usage seems wise.

(b) **Progressing stroke.** Two randomized (Baker et al, 1962; Carter, 1961a; Carter, 1961b) and two nonrandomized (Fisher, 1958; Millikan, 1965; Millikan, 1971; Siekert et al, 1963) studies of stroke-in-evolution are in the literature; the four studies have methodological weaknesses. The definition of progressing stroke is not precise; the selection process for entry is uncertain and relatively small numbers of patients were entered. The results are not conclusive but there is suggestive evidence favouring anticoagulant usage. The study of Baker et al (1962) led them to the conclusion that the progression of stroke might be retarded but the death rate was not affected.

Opinion is divided but many neurologists recommend anticoagulants in the form of heparin for progressing stroke followed by the substitution of coumadin derivatives within a few days. Three months of treatment appears a reasonable recommendation.

(c) **Completed stroke** — Seven randomized and two nonrandomized studies on this subject are available (Genton et al, 1977); one of the nonrandomized studies claims benefit but the data are not convincing. The consensus recommendation appears to be against the utilization of anticoagulants in completed stroke.

Anticoagulants in conditions with cardiac emboli

Utilizing modern diagnostic methods approximately one stroke in five is judged to arise from the heart and recurrence of cardiac emboli is common. These strokes are of thrombotic origin in most cases, so that antithrombotic treatment must be a major consideration in attempts to prevent them.

Within six weeks of a *myocardial infarction* the risk of cerebral embolization is approximately 5 percent when judged by clinical observation, but in postmortem examination 45 to 60 percent of fatal cases have evidence of systemic emboli, half of them in the cerebral circulation (Easton & Sherman, 1980). The timing of cerebral emboli from myocardial infarction is of consequence in the planning of therapy. Eighty-five percent occur in the first 4 weeks, with the highest number (33 percent) in the second week (Bean, 1938). Within the second and third months only 6 and 8 percent occur. Mural thrombi are found in 45 percent of fatal cases of myocardial infarction and are particularly prone to occur if the myocardial infarction is large, septal and associated with congestive heart failure. Thrombi are detectable at postmortem studies in 75 percent of postinfarction ventricular aneurysms.

Early studies by Wright et al (1954), the American Veterans' Administration (1973) and the trial supported by the British Medical Research Council (Report of the Working Party on Anticoagulant Therapy 1969) indicated a 25 percent reduction in stroke in the treated compared with the control patients given anticoagulants after a recent myocardial infarction. The entry criteria to these trials was the occurrence of a cardiac, not a cerebral lesion. No trial has been conducted to assess the benefit of anticoagulants in patients after myocardial infarction when the threat of stroke has been heralded by warning cerebral or retinal ischemic events.

It is difficult to recommend treatment with scanty information and because of the incomplete data cardiologists do not agree in this matter. Nevertheless anticoagulants are recommended in patients in whom myocardial infarction has occurred within three months in whom cerebral or retinal ischemic events have occurred, or if echocardiography and wall motion studies indicate a thrombus or an aneurysm. In the absence of such events, but when a myocardial infarction is large, involves the septum or is associated with congestive heart failure, anticoagulants are a reasonable recommendation. As a rule the duration of anticoagulants should not be more than three months.

It is controversial whether anticoagulants are more hazardous immediately after a cerebral infarction resulting from a mural thrombus compared with their use after a delay of two to three days. No hard data exist on which to base a firm judgement. Experimental evidence is conflicting (Moyes et al, 1957; Wood et al, 1958; Sibley et al, 1957), but what clinical information exists would not support a mandatory delay (Carter, 1957; Carter, 1965). If there is no evidence of blood in the C.T. scan nor in the c.s.f. and no sign of bacterial endocarditis, the early institution of anticoagulants for these patients is recommended.

Emboli from rheumatic heart disease

Rheumatic heart disease is declining sharply. Followed for a five-year period, 20 percent of patients with mitral stenosis develop systemic emboli and three out of five involve the brain. Fifty percent of patients coming to postmortem with mitral stenosis show emboli and of these 40 to 50 percent affect the brain. Once emboli occur, recurrence is encountered in 30 to 75 percent of patients, depending on the duration of follow-up. These recurrences occur within the first month in 40 percent and within the first year in 50 to 65 percent of cases (Easton & Sherman 1980).

Anticoagulant administration in rheumatic heart disease has not been subjected to careful scrutiny in properly randomized studies. The single study of this type in the literature is negative, but it involved only 12 patients in the treated and 16 patients in the control groups. Many retrospective studies and others with a variety of flaws in design suggest that the treatment is efficacious, with indications that emboli and recurrent emboli are reduced by 80 to 90 percent (Genton et al, 1977).

Recommendations are therefore based on incomplete knowledge but the information appears to justify long-term use of anticoagulants in mitral stenosis after one embolic event has occurred.

Emboli resulting from atrial fibrillation with and without mitral stenosis or recent myocardial infarction

Atrial fibrillation in conjunction with rheumatic heart disease is associated with a 17-fold increase in stroke risk and atrial fibrillation alone by a 5.6-fold increase (Wolf et al, 1978). A study of 333 patients with atrial fibrillation examined at post-mortem at the Massachusetts General Hospital indicated that this rhythm disorder was extremely important as a cause of emboli in heart disease. Even in the patients who had fibrillation without rheumatic or ischemic heart disease a substantial number experienced systemic emboli (Hinton et al, 1977).

Other cardiac arrhythmias are associated with increased risk of stroke. Of 100 patients with the sick sinus syndrome (sinoatrial node disorder) 16 had emboli, 15 in the type of the disorder characterized by intermittent bradyarrhythmia and tachycardia (Fairfax & Lambert, 1976). In a parallel study 7.3 percent of 41 patients with bouts of bradyarrhythmia associated with atrial fibrillation or atrial flutter suffered systemic emboli.

The question is raised, occasionally, about the desirability of anticoagulant protection against any possible thromboembolic complications of cardioversion, electrically reverting atrial fibrillation to sinus rhythm. The incidence of systemic embolization after cardioversion has been variously estimated at 1–5.3 percent with most reports between 1–2 percent (Lown, 1967; Abernathy & Willis, 1973). One large but nonrandomized prospective study of the incidence of embolism after successful cardioversion indicated a lower incidence (0.8 percent) in those receiving anticoagulants compared with a significantly higher incidence (5.3 percent) in those not treated with anticoagulants (Bjerkelund & Orning, 1969). Nevertheless, having in mind that this was not a randomized study, most authorities in the field, on the basis of their own experience, limit anticoagulants as a prelude to cardioversion to high risk patients, those with a prior history of recurrent emboli or to those with mitral stenosis.

On the basis of the pathological process but not on the basis of carefully conducted clinical trials, a recommendation can be made for the cautious administration of anticoagulants to all patients with rhythm disorders who have evidence of systemic embolization. Higher risk candidates for cardioversion should be anticoagulated prior to this treatment and for six months thereafter.

PLATELET ANTIAGGREGANTS

(a) Rationale

Platelet-initiated thrombosis is important in fast-flowing arterial systems. Experimental studies have determined that downstream embolization of platelet-fibrin material occurs from arterial injury (figure 20.1) (Zucker, 1947; Denny Brown, 1960; Honour & Russell, 1962). In TIA patients platelet-fibrin emboli are visible in the retinal arterioles (Fisher, 1959; Russell, 1961); they have been studied in the distal branches of the subclavian and carotid arteries (Gunning et al, 1964). Platelet-initiated thrombogenesis is stimulated by atheromatous-debris embolization (Warren & Vales, 1974).

Drugs altering platelet function have been identified and their usefulness in altering thrombogenesis has been substantiated in experiments with lesions injuring the large arteries and in lesions of the microcirculation (Barnett, 1974).

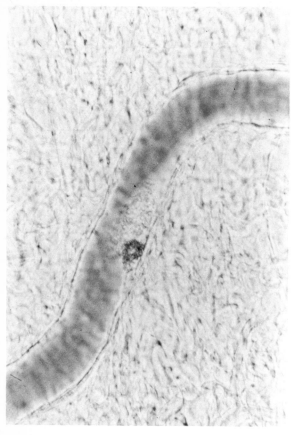

Fig. 20.1 Laser injury to endothelium of arteriole (dark area) induces platelet aggregation downstream (whitish clump). When platelet fibrin aggregations reach sufficient size, they can be observed passing downstream in this experimental model. (Reproduced by permission of Dr F. N. McKenzie from *Cerebrovascular Diseases*, P. Scheinberg (ed), Raven Press, 1976, p. 9.)

Case reports and small pilot studies have indicated the ability of aspirin and sulfinpyrazone to interfere with transient ischemic attacks. A number of controlled studies have been concluded and Table 20.7 indicates the results of the reported trials.

(b) Results of clinical trials

Most of the studies of platelet antiaggregant therapy involved too few patients to permit definitive conclusions. Nevertheless all that have been reported up to the present time support the benefit of aspirin. In the study which entered the most cases (585) with stroke-threatening symptoms, and followed them for the longest period of time, averaging 26 months (Canadian Cooperative Stroke Study Group, 1978), significant reduction in TIA, stroke or death was recorded (19 percent, $P < 0.05$). Omitting TIA from the analysis, a more striking reduction in stroke or death was apparent (31% $P < 0.05$). In sub-set analysis the benefit was for males, not for females. For males the reduction of stroke and death was 48 percent ($P < 0.005$) and for stroke and stroke-death was 49 percent ($P = 0.01$). Endarterectomy was discouraged for this group of patients during the conduct of the trial and the study included patients with vertebro-basilar as well as carotid artery symptoms. The early study of dipyridamole (Acheson et al, 1969), with negative results should not be accepted as the final statement on this drug. The small sample-size and reasonably short period of follow-up might have resulted in a negative conclusion whereas with a larger number of cases the trial might have been positive. The American aspirin study treated patients with carotid symptomatology and did not include patients who had vertebro-basilar symptoms nor those who had a lesion of the carotid artery amenable to surgery (Fields et al, 1977). Of the 178 cases, only 24 were in the study for 24 months and no significant reduction of stroke and death was apparent in the aspirin group. However when the combination of a reduction of TIA, stroke or death was assessed at the shorter period of six months, a difference between the treatment groups in favor of aspirin ($P < 0.01$) was noted.

The AMIS and PARIS studies were designed to test platelet antiaggregants in patients who had suffered recent myocardial infarction and secondary end-point observations were made on the stroke incidence in the placebo and treated groups (Aspirin Myocardial Infarction Study Research Group 1980, Persantine Aspirin Reinfarction Study Research Group 1980). In both studies the incidence of stroke in 36 and 41 months of follow-up respectively was 2 percent in the placebo group as compared to 1.1 and 1.2 percent for the aspirin-treated group. There was no added benefit for those on a combination of aspirin and dipyridamole in the PARIS study.

The Olsson study was without a placebo group (Olsson et al, 1980). All cases were given two months on coumadin drugs at the beginning and then randomized into a group to continue on

Table 20.7 Platelet antiaggregants in threatened stroke — randomized trials

Author	Entry criteria	Number	Treatment and dose/day	Average period of follow-up	End-points	Benefit
1. Acheson et al, 1969	TIA, RIND, stroke	T = 85 C = 84	Dipyridamole 400 mg 800 mg	14 months 11 months	TIA, stroke, death	Negative
2. Canadian Cooperative Study Group, 1978	TIA, RIND, PNS	T = 290 C = 295	ASA 1300 mg Sulfinpyrazone* 800 mg	26 months	Stroke, death	Positive — ASA
3. Fields et al, 1977	TIA, RIND, stroke	T = 88 C = 90	ASA 1300 mg	6 months	TIA, stroke, death	Positive — ASA
4. Reuther et al, 1980	TIA, RIND, PNS	T = 29 T = 29	ASA 1500 mg	24 months	TIA, stroke	Positive — ASA
5. AMIS Research Group, 1980	M.I.	T = 2267 C = 2257	ASA 1000 mg	36 months	(Stroke)†	Positive — ASA
6. PARIS Research Group 1980	M.I.	T = 1620 C = 406	ASA 972 mg, Dipyridamole 225 mg	41 months	(Stroke)†	Positive — ASA
7. Olsson et al, 1980	TIA, RIND	AC = 68‡ ASA + P = 67	ASA 1000 mg + dipyridamole 150 mg or coumadin	12 months	TIA, stroke	'Positive'§ ASA with dipyridamole

* Since sulfinpyrazone was no more effective than placebo, these two groups were combined in the analysis.
† See text. Patients randomized after myocardial infarction, to study recurrent M.I.
‡ No placebo group — AC = Anticoagulants; ASA + P = aspirin + persantine.
§ No single-therapy group.

anticoagulant or to enter the group receiving aspirin combined with dipyridamole. On the basis of the comparison made with historical controls, (an imperfect measure) the authors concluded that there was substantial benefit from both the coumadin treatment and the combined platelet anti-aggregant treatment.

(c) Usefulness in other varieties of TIA

None of the major trials discussed above was carried out to evaluate platelet-inhibiting drugs in other than TIA, RIND and PNS related to *atherothrombotic stroke*. It might be possible to infer that there is a usefulness in *cardiac embolic stroke* but very few data are available to support this hypothesis. A randomized, controlled trial has studied the prophylactic benefit of sulfinpyrazone in reducing the incidence of embolic stroke from mitral stenosis (Steele & Rainwater, 1980). Benefit was suggested in the active treatment group, in that thromboemboli occurred in only 2 of 78 patients given 800 mg of sulfinpyrazone per day compared with the incidence of 16 out of 76 patients given placebo. Shortened platelet survival

times were a prerequisite to inclusion in the study and 67 percent of the treated and 58 percent of the placebo cases were given anticoagulants for at least six months of the four year study.

Several small but well designed studies have been conducted in patients with *prosthetic heart valves* using dipyridamole combined with anticoagulants in an attempt to prevent emboli. The combination has been reported as superior to anticoagulants alone (Sullivan et al, 1971). The value of aspirin as adjunct therapy to anticoagulants was studied in a randomized double-blind trial involving 148 patients in whom a Starr Edward's aortic ball valve prosthesis had been inserted. Placebo was contrasted with one gram of aspirin per day, and in two years 12 emboli occurred in the placebo group (9.32 episodes per 100 patients per year) compared with 2 emboli in the aspirin group (1.76 episodes per 100 patients per year). Intracranial bleeding occurred twice in the aspirin and three times in the placebo group (Dale, 1977).

No statement can be made about the usefulness or lack of value of platelet antiaggregants in any of the other cardiac conditions which produce thromboemboli since no detailed studies have been done.

Patients with *thrombocytosis* and TIA have been subjected to aspirin treatment with dramatic cessation of events in a few anecdotal accounts. The occurrence of spontaneous and excess platelet aggregability in a number of these patients makes these results quite credible (Harrison et al, 1971; Mundall, 1972; Wu, 1978). Alternative treatment with busulfan (Myeleran) is equally effective (Levine & Swanson, 1968; Singer 1969).

As for the other varieties of TIA and threatened stroke listed in Table 20.2, less would be expected by way of benefit for most of them and other varieties of treatment would be more appropriate, considering their particular pathogenesis. Anti-hypertensive therapy is the treatment of prime importance in lacunar states. In hemodynamic abnormalities producing focal TIA their recognition and particular management is essential. Orthostatic hypotension may require some alteration in antihypertensive therapy and the installation of a cardiac pacemaker will be required in patients with serious bradyarrhythmia. When cerebral ischemic events are occurring in conditions recognized as due to or likely brought about by coagulation abnormalities, anticoagulants have a more rational basis than platelet antiaggregants. Some of the patients with nonarteriosclerotic arteriopathies and ischemic events (e.g., fibromuscular dysplasia) might benefit from aspirin. Others such as granulomatous angiopathy, giant-cell arteritis and Takayasu's disease will require steroids rather than antithrombotic agents.

(d) Optimum dosage

The optimum dosage of aspirin is unsettled. The clinical trials in stroke prevention were initiated before basic information was available regarding the mechanism of their antithrombotic activity. An average analgesic dose was utilized quite empirically and the trials have employed a dosage of approximately one gram per day (Table 20.7).

Aspirin is now known to inhibit the enzyme cyclooxygenase and thereby interferes with arachidonic acid metabolism. Arachidonic acid from the platelet membrane is converted through prostaglandin G_2 into thromboxane A_2. This unstable metabolite stimulates platelet aggregation and through the release reaction leads to the accumulation of such vasoconstricting substances as serotonin. The arachidonic acid of the endothelial cells in the vessel wall is metabolized by the same enzyme, cyclooxygenase, into prostacyclin (PGI_2). This compound is a powerful antagonist of platelet aggregation and by inhibiting serotonin release has a vasodilating effect (Moncada et al, 1979). The possibility presents itself that the aspirin-induced inhibition of cyclooxygenase, interfering with the production of prostacyclin as well as the thromboxanes might be an undesirable form of antithrombotic therapy, with the beneficial effect of platelet inhibition being counterbalanced by the undesirable effect of inhibiting prostacyclin production. A confusion of experimental data has accumulated in respect to this antagonistic effect of aspirin and the possibility of differential inhibition by reduced aspirin dosage. From what is known to date, firm decisions are difficult to make but a few of the important pieces of the puzzle may be summarized briefly:

(i) Bleeding time in men and women is prolonged by 300 mg per day of aspirin, but not by high doses, 3.9 g per day (O'Grady & Moncada, 1978).

(ii) Aspirin in some studies has been claimed to lead to a more prolonged inhibition of the platelet than of the endothelial cell both in rats and humans (Villa et al, 1979; Masotti et al, 1979).

(iii) In tissue culture, endothelial cells quickly recovered their aspirin-inhibited ability to synthesize prostacyclin after the low concentrations of this drug were removed by washing the cells (Jaffe & Wexler, 1979). These authors utilized these observations as the basis for a recommendation that aspirin, given as an antithrombotic agent, be limited to a dose schedule of once a day.

(iv) In conflict with these conclusions, radioimmunoassay measurements were made on platelet function and in vein biopsies from human volunteers after the administration of 150 to 300 mg of ASA. The inhibitory responses of both platelet and vessel wall cyclooxygenase were similar and both were affected for upwards of eight hours (Preston et al, 1981).

(v) Excessive dosage (200 mg/kg) of aspirin, 10 to 20 times the usual therapeutic dose, stimulated the thrombogenic process in rabbits (Kelton et al, 1978a).

(vi) High dosage of aspirin (3.9 g per day) was compared with placebo in a controlled study involving 36 women and 7 men subjected to total knee replacement (McKenna et al, 1980). A significant reduction in venous thromboembolism occurred in the aspirin group with this large dose in male and female subjects.

(vii) A daily dosage of 165 mg of aspirin prevented thrombi forming in the dialysis shunts of uremic patients (Harter et al, 1978). In this trial, the effect of moderate or high dosage was not tested and it must be noted that in uremia coagulation abnormalities are known to occur and an increase in circulating prostacyclin has been described.

(vii) Two case reports describe a congenital deficiency of cyclooxygenase (Malmsten et al, 1975; Pareti et al, 1980). Both patients exhibited a mild bleeding diathesis rather than a thrombotic tendency. In Pareti's case the deficiency was accompanied by absence of thromboxane and prostacyclin indicating that the pathophysiological process was comparable to aspirin administration.

The dose of aspirin must be determined in the end by clinical trials. The conflicting experimental and laboratory data make such a trial utilizing several dosage schedules a very reasonable consideration. In the meantime, all clinical data indicating benefit of aspirin in stroke prevention have come from trials in which 1.0–1.5 g per day has been used and this must remain the recommended dosage for the time being at least.

(e) The differential in responsiveness by sex

The nonresponsiveness of women in the Canadian, the American (Gent, 1979) and in a small Italian study soon to be reported (Candelise, 1980) came as a surprise. A similar observation was made in venous thrombosis utilizing aspirin prophylaxis after hip replacement (Harris et al, 1977). In dialysis shunts the incidence of thrombi was reduced with sulfinpyrazone and the benefit was confined to males (Kaegi et al, 1974). A retrospective analysis of rheumatoid arthritis patients who had utilized aspirin as their primary antiarthritic therapy for 15 years (Linos et al, 1978) indicated a reduction in cerebral and cardial ischemic episodes in the males but not in the females.

The reasons for the sex difference are not known. Several possibilities exist:

(i) Too few females may have been entered into the Canadian study to allow the valid analysis of a sex differential and the observation could have been a statistical artefact (Kurtzke, 1979). This is not a convincing argument and it overlooks all other corroborating data.

(ii) The difference may not be one of poor responsiveness to the drug of stroke-threatened women but an indication of a better prognosis enjoyed by women due to naturally-occurring mechanisms about which insufficient knowledge exists. Women fare better after TIA and other types of threatened strokes than do men. Dyken and his associates conducted a major collaborative inquiry into TIA characteristics and frequency in six participating hospitals in the United States (Conneally et al, 1978). In this study as well as in the review conducted by Kurtzke (1980) the threat to females with TIA was shown to be less serious than for males. Four percent of the females with TIA died each year compared with 12 percent of the male patients. Aspirin usage resulted in no improvement in the survival of females but there was benefit in males (Dyken, 1980).

The Canadian study is consistent with these prognostic observations: in the first year of follow-up stroke and death occurred in 13 percent of males and 11 percent of females; after the second year the cumulative stroke or death figures were 22 percent for males and 16 percent for females; after three years, 30 percent for males and 16 percent for females.

(iii) The sex-related variation in aspirin benefit might be related to the level of hormone activity. The responsiveness of younger women and men as well as the responsiveness of either sex in the older age group was not appreciably different. Nevertheless, thrombogenesis is known to be increased with testosterone and estrogen therapy.

(iv) There is experimental evidence which indicates sex-related differences in platelet and vessel wall reaction to aspirin therapy. Kelton has detected a significant reduction in the size of thrombi found in male rabbits compared to female rabbits treated with aspirin prior to identical endothelial injuries (Kelton et al, 1978b). The pretreated females were not different to the male and female control animals (Figure 20.2).

(v) Claims have been made that platelets from female subjects are more reactive than those of males (Johnston & Ramwell, 1974; Nordoy et al, 1978). This led to the suggestion that the sex differential might have been due to the presence of more active platelets in females. An experiment correcting for hematocrit differences between men and women by altering the amount of citrate used in collecting the blood specimens has now determined that the *in vitro* responsiveness to aggregating stimuli is the same in the two sexes (Kelton et al, 1980).

(vi) There are differences between the hydrolysis of aspirin in males and females as measured by the salicylic acid levels after aspirin ingestion. Acetylsalicylic acid esterase activity is less in women than in men (Menguy et al, 1972). Hemostatic plugs in humans are larger after aspirin therapy (Wester et al, 1978). In the aspirin-treated male rabbit these plugs are larger than in the female (Kelton et al,

1980). This evidence is interpreted as indicating that aspirin alters the efficiency of hemostasis so that more platelets are required to form an effective hemostatic thrombus. Since the platelet production of thromboxane-B2 is completely inhibited in both males and females, the sex difference in hemostatic plugs may be due to an altered interaction of aspirinized platelets with the vessel walls of males compared with females.

(vii) Template bleeding times in males are prolonged after low dose aspirin but not altered in females (Preston et al, 1981). Since this phenomenon is independent of the suppression of aggregation, the reason again might be due to a difference in reactivity in the vessel wall to injury between males and females.

It may be concluded that the accumulation of laboratory and clinical evidence provides considerable indirect support to the observation that stroke-threatened men respond more to platelet antiaggregant therapy in the form of aspirin than do stroke-threatened women. The difference in prognosis appears to be a biological phenomenon but responsiveness to drug is not the same for reasons not yet fully understood.

(f) Other platelet antiaggregants and combined antiaggregant therapy

Dipyridamole and sulfinpyrazone when administered alone have no demonstrable benefit for stroke-threatened patients. The combination of aspirin and sulfinpyrazone in the Canadian study might have been an advantage but the data did not allow this conclusion to be drawn. Theoretical reasons exist that dipyridamole and aspirin might have a synergistic effect on platelet function. Dipyridamole alters the platelet function by phosphodiesterase inhibition. Its combination with aspirin has been claimed to restore platelet survival times to normal in patients with symptomatic arterial disease in whom aspirin alone had no restorative effect and in whom dipyridamole alone affected an incomplete restoration (Harker & Slichter, 1974). Platelet thrombogenesis in electrically-injured pial arteries was not altered by aspirin nor by dipyridamole alone but was reduced when the two drugs were used in combination (Honour et al, 1977). Until the clinical trial now in progress

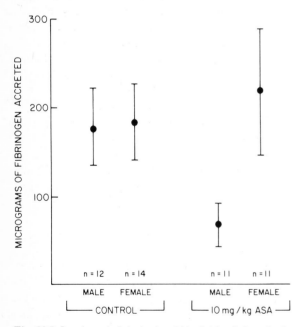

Fig. 20.2 Jugular vein injuries in rabbits initiated thrombosis of similar quantity in males and females. Pre-treatment with aspirin reduced the thrombus in male but not female rabbits. (Reproduced by permission of Dr J. G. Kelton and the journal 'Blood' — Kelton et al 1978.)

in North America is concluded the combined use of these two drugs must be regarded as empirical. Even then the possibility must be entertained that the dosage may be critical and that too much aspirin may counteract the benefit of dipyridamole (Moncada & Korbut, 1978). This enigma may not be resolved for a long time!

(g) Platelet abnormalities predictive of risk of stroke

Many studies have been carried out to determine whether any abnormalities of platelet function or whether any one of a variety of measurable platelet breakdown products will prove useful as predictors of threatened stroke. One of the major problems has been to determine whether the detected abnormalities are the result of the ischemic event or part of its cause. The studies have employed some tests which are difficult to duplicate with accuracy and have been carried out in a mixture of stroke-threatening situations, both in patients with arterial disease and in those with cardiac lesions. The time relationship to the ischemic events has not always been given in the reports and is of considerable importance in comparing results. The heterogeneity of the tests utilized and the particular conditions which have been studied make it difficult to generalize about their predictive value. A brief summary of the current status of this interesting problem is as follows:

(i) Patients with atherothrombotic TIA and stroke have platelets with an increased tendency to aggregate and to have increased circulating platelet aggregates which return to normal in 10 days to 6 weeks after the ischemic events (Dougherty et al, 1977).

(ii) Platelet factor 4 (PF_4) was found to be elevated within 14 days of a stroke in a group of 10 patients and within four weeks of TIA in a group of 11 patients compared with control subjects (Levine et al, 1981). This specific protein is released from the α granules of the platelets during aggregation, is the heparin-neutralizing factor and is believed to be an index of platelet activity.

(iii) Patients with mitral stenosis due to rheumatic heart disease who have experienced thromboembolism have been found to have a significantly higher incidence of reduced platelet survival times than do patients who have the same cardiac lesions without a history of embolic events (93 percent c.f. 31 percent) (Steele et al, 1974). None of these studies was done within two months of the last embolic event, so that the detected abnormality may reflect an increase in risk of thromboembolism.

(iv) Patients with mitral valve prolapse (MVP) may have a shortened platelet survival time. Thirty-three percent of 21 MVP patients without history of emboli had diminished platelet survival time (Steele et al, 1979), while in the same study the comparable figure for rheumatic heart disease (RHD) without history of emboli was 78 percent. The lower figure for MVP patients is consistent with the relative infrequency of embolization in MVP compared with RHD. Shortened platelet survival times were found more than three months after the ischemia in five MVP cases who suffered stroke with no other etiological factors detectable save for the cardiac lesion.

(v) Increased circulating platelet aggregates and hyperactive platelet coagulant activity have been detected in MVP patients with good evidence of systemic emboli (Walsh et al, 1980). When there was less convincing evidence of emboli less marked abnormalities were found in these tests, and when there was no evidence of embolization, the tests were normal or no more than minimally impaired.

(vi) Beta-thromboglobulin in the plasma, evidence of in-vivo platelet aggregation, was elevated in two groups of young persons with stroke — one group with associated MVP and one group without detectable MVP or other cause for the stroke (Scharf et al, 1981).

(vii) Platelet survival times were shortened in patients with older type substitute heart valves and the reduced survival time correlated with the history of thromboembolism (Weily et al, 1974).

(viii) Thrombocytosis, whether occurring alone or as part of polycythemia rubra, is a detectable platelet abnormality which clearly has predictive value for cerebral ischemia (Wu, 1978).

It is evident that further clarification of the role of platelet function and the measurement of platelet end-products is required before their predictive value as a risk of stroke is settled. However, as Dougherty et al (1977) have noted, the changes in platelet function, even if secondary to the primary disease, and even if temporarily present, may contribute in an important way to an increase in the clinical manifestations of a vascular event.

(h) Platelet antiaggregants and cerebral atherosclerosis

The role of platelets in atherogenesis has been identified (Ross & Glomset, 1976). Mitogenic factors released during aggregation at the site of endothelial lesions stimulate proliferation of smooth muscle cells in the arterial wall. The possible value of aspirin and other platelet antiaggregants in retarding development of atherosclerosis has become a subject of interest. Experimental thrombocytopenia has been shown to inhibit atheroma in the aortas of rabbits de-endothelialized by balloon catheters and fed an atherogenic diet (Moore et al, 1976). Aspirin did not inhibit the development of aortic atherosclerosis in the aortas of rabbits but it did decrease the size of the aortic plaques compared with the controls (Hollander et al, 1974). Later studies in primates reported significant reduction in the number of coronary arteries demonstrating atherosclerotic involvement when given aspirin in conjunction with an atherogenic diet and compared with controls fed the same diet but not given aspirin (Pick et al, 1979). The severity of aortic atherosclerosis was unaffected in this experimental model. Dipyridamole has been shown to prevent homocystinuric baboons from developing atherosclerosis (Harker et al, 1976).

Paradoxically, other evidence suggests that dipyridamole may have atherogenic properties, since rabbits on an atherogenic diet and dipyridamole were claimed to have enhanced atherosclerotic plaque formation compared to controls (Dembinska-Kiec et al, 1979). In a later experiment atheroma formation in New Zealand rabbits on a high fat diet was significantly inhibited with aspirin given in combination with dipyridamole while a distinct increase was observed in smooth muscle cell proliferation when dipyridamole was given alone (Koster et al, 1981).

More data are required before antiplatelet agents are prescribed in the hope of retarding atherosclerosis.

(i) The future of antithrombotic therapy

New and better drugs are required to perfect antithrombotic medication in stroke prevention. Patients in all trials have suffered stroke despite any given therapy including aspirin. Anticoagulants are sufficiently hazardous as to oblige investigators to develop substitutes as quickly as possible. Patients with advanced disease, as evidenced by multiple arterial lesions on angiography, and with widespread disease as evidenced by symptoms in both the carotid and vertebro-basilar territory, have not benefited from aspirin medication (Barnett, 1979a).

Failure of antiaggregant therapy in part may relate to the observation that prostacyclin is suppressed by aspirin and that prostacyclin production is diminished in human arterial walls which are the site of atheroma (D'Angelo et al, 1978; Sinzinger et al, 1978). Further prostacyclin studies will be followed with interest. In early clinical observations prostacyclin itself has proved to have a shortlived action whether given orally or intravenously. Interesting attempts are being made to increase its production in the body or to stimulate the production of a prostacyclin-like compound. Eicosapentaenoic acid is an analogue of eicosatetraenoic acid (arachidonic acid) It is found in caviar, oysters and in salt-water fish and partially blocks platelet function. It is said to be available to the vessel wall to make an antiaggregant substance that may be prostacyclin (Dyerberg & Bang, 1979; Dyerberg et al, 1978). Speculation exists that dietary habits which include heavy dependence on fish containing large quantities of this substance may protect Eskimos against vascular disease. The concept is exciting and some preliminary trials are to be watched with interest.

Recommendations about the usefulness of platelet aggregants in stroke prevention are to be regarded as preliminary. It would appear reasonable to recommend aspirin in men affected with symptoms of threatening stroke. It is empirical but common practice at the present time to recommend the combination of aspirin and dipyridamole for females. Continuation of episodes despite this treatment, or the acquisition of a neurological deficit, may be an indication for a period of two to three months of anticoagulant therapy. Surgical treatment will be discussed in Chapter 21 but its place is not on more certain ground than is the utilization of antithrombotic agents. Nevertheless in individual patients who are not in high risk categories for an operative procedure its use will be considered when antithrombotic agents have not eliminated symptoms and when extracranial arterial carotid lesions are appropriate to the symptoms. It will be carried out in conjunction with antiaggregant therapy.

REFERENCES

Abernathy W S, Willis P W 1973 Thromboembolic complications of rheumatic heart disease. Cardiovascular Clinics 5:131–175

Acheson J, Danta G, Hutchinson E C 1969 Controlled trial of dipyridamole in cerebral vascular disease. British Medical Journal 1:614–615

Acheson J, Hutchinson E C 1964 Observations of the natural history of transient cerebral ischaemia. Lancet ii:871–874

Aspirin Myocardial Infarction Study Research Group 1980 A randomized, controlled trial of aspirin in persons recovered from myocardial infarction. Journal of the American Medical Association 243:661–669

Baker R N 1961 An evaluation of anticoagulant therapy in the treatment of cerebrovascular disease. Report of the Veterans Administration Cooperative Study of atherosclerosis. Neurology 11:132–138

Baker R N, Broward J A, Fang H C et al 1962 Anticoagulant therapy in cerebral infarction. Report on cooperative study. Neurology 12:823–835

Baker R N, Ramseyer J C, Schwartz W S 1968 Prognosis in patients with transient cerebral ischemia. Neurology 18:1157–1165

Baker R N, Schwartz W S, Rose A S 1966 Transient ischemic strokes. A report of a study of anticoagulant therapy. Neurology 16:841–847

Barnett H J M 1974 Transient cerebral ischemia: Pathogenesis, prognosis and management. Annals of the Royal College of Physicians and Surgeons of Canada 7:153–173

Barnett H J M 1979a Recent intervention studies on platelet-suppressant drugs in cerebral ischemia: 1. Clinical aspects. In: Tognoni G, Garattini S (eds) Drug treatment and prevention in cerebrovascular disorders. Elsevier-North Holland, Biomedical Press, Amsterdam. p 369–386

Barnett H J M 1979b The pathophysiology of transient ischemic attacks. Therapy with platelet antiaggregants. Medical Clinics of North America 63:649–679

Bean W S 1938 Infarction of the heart. III Clinical course and morphological findings. Annals of Internal Medicine 12:71–94

Beevers D G, Hamilton M, Fairman M, Harpur J E 1973 Antihypertensive treatment and the course of established cerebral vascular disease. Lancet i:1407–1409

Bental E, Pillar T 1972 Symptoms and diseases accompanying arteriosclerotic cerebrovascular events. Geriatrics 27:142–146

Bjerkelund C J, Orning O M 1969 The efficacy of anticoagulant therapy in preventing embolism related to D.C. electrical conversion of atrial fibrillation. American Journal Cardiology 23:208–216

Canadian Cooperative Stroke Study Group 1978 A randomized trial of aspirin and sulfinpyrazone in threatened stroke. New England Journal of Medicine 299:53–59

Candelise L 1980 Personal communication

Carter A B 1957 The immediate treatment of cerebral embolism. Quarterly Journal of Medicine 26:335–348

Carter A B 1961a Anticoagulant therapy in progressing stroke. British Medical Journal 2:70–73

Carter A B 1961b Use of anticoagulants in patients with progressive cerebral infarction. Neurology 11:601–609

Carter A B, 1965 Prognosis of cerebral embolism. Lancet ii:514–519

Carter A B 1970 Hypotensive therapy in stroke survivors. Lancet i:485–489

Collaborative Group for the Study of Stroke in Young Women 1973 Oral contraceptives and increased risk of cerebral ischemia or thrombosis. New England Journal of Medicine 288:871–878

Conneally P M, Dyken M L, Futty D E, Poskanzer D C, Calanchini P R, Swanson P D, Price T R, Haerer A F, Gotshall R A 1978 Cooperative Study of hospital frequency and character of transient ischemic attacks: VIII. Risk factors. Journal of the American Medical Association 240:742–746

Dale J 1977 Prevention of arterial thromboembolism with ASA. American Heart Journal 94:101–111

D'Angelo V, Villa S, Myslieviec M, Donati M B, DeGatenao G 1978 Defective fibrinolytic and prostacyclin-like activity in human atheromatous plaques. Thrombosis and Haemostasis 39:535–536

Dembinska-Kiec A, Rucker W, Schonhofer P S 1979 Effects of dipyridamole in experimental atherosclerosis. Action of PGI_2, platelet aggregation and atherosclerotic plaque formation. Atherosclerosis 33:315–327

Denny Brown D 1960 Recurrent cerebrovascular episodes. Archives of Neurology 2:194–210

Dougherty J H Jr, Levy D E, Weksler B B 1977 Platelet activation in acute cerebral ischaemia: Serial measurements of platelet function in cerebrovascular disease. Lancet i:821–823

Doyle J T, Dawber T R, Kannel W B, Kinch S H, Kahn H A 1964 The relationship of cigarette smoking to coronary heart disease (the second report of the combined experience of the Albany N Y and Framingham Mass studies). Journal of the American Medical Association 190:108–112

Dyerberg J, Bang H O 1979 Haemostatic function and platelet polysaturated fatty acids in Eskimos. Lancet ii:433–435

Dyerberg J, Bang H O, Stoffersen E 1978 Eicosapentaenoic acid and prevention of thrombosis and atherosclerosis. Lancet ii:117–119

Dyken M L 1980 Antiplatelet aggregating agents in transient ischemic attacks and the relationship of risk factors: (Total experience of six medical centres). Fifth Colfarit Symposium, Mainz, W. Germany (in press).

Easton J D, Sherman D G 1980 Management of cerebral embolism of cardiac origin. Stroke 11:433–442

Fairfax A J, Lambert C D 1976 Neurological aspects of sinoatrial heart block. Journal of Neurology, Neurosurgery and Psychiatry 39:576–580

Fields W S, Lemak N A, Frankowski R F, Hardy R J 1977 Controlled trial of aspirin in cerebral ischemia. Stroke 8:301–316

Fisher C M 1958 The use of anticoagulants in cerebral thrombosis. Neurology 8:311–332

Fisher C M 1959 Observations of the fundus oculi in transient monocular blindness. Neurology (Minneapolis) 9:333–347

Fisher C M, 1965a Lacunes: Small, deep cerebral infarcts. Neurology (Minneapolis) 15:774–784

Fisher C M, 1965b Pure sensory stroke involving face, arm and leg. Neurology (Minneapolis) 15:76–80

Fisher C M, 1967 A lacunar stroke: The dysarthria-clumsy hand syndrome. Neurology (Minneapolis) 17:614–617

Fisher C M, Cole M 1965 Homolateral ataxia and crural paresis: A vascular syndrome. Journal of Neurology, Neurosurgery and Psychiatry 28:48–55

Fisher C M, Curry H B 1965: Pure motor hemiplegia of vascular origin. Archives of Neurology 13:30–44

Fletcher A P, Alkjaesig N 1980 Prophylactic and therapeutic uses of antithrombotic drugs in cerebrovascular disease. In: Siekert R G (ed) Cerebrovascular survey report for joint council subcommittee on cerebrovascular disease, NINCDS and National Heart and Lung Institute, Whiting Press Inc. Rochester, Minnesota, p 290–305

Friedman G D, Loveland D B, Ehrlich S P 1968 Relationship of stroke to other cardiovascular disease. Circulation 38:533–541

Garcia M., McNamara P M, Gordon T, Kannel W B 1973 Cardiovascular complications in diabetes. Advances in Metabolic Disorders (Early Diabetes) Supplement #2, p. 493–499

Gent M 1979 Recent intervention studies of platelet suppressant drugs in cerebral ischemia. Methodological aspects. In: Tognoni G, Garattini S (eds) Drug treatment and prevention in cerebrovascular disorders, Elsevier-North Holland, Biomedical Press, p. 437–448

Genton E, Barnett H M J, Fields W S, Gent M, Hoak J C 1977 Cerebral ischemia: The role of thrombosis and antithrombotic therapy. Stroke 8:150–175

Gordon T, Kannel W B 1972 Predisposition of atherosclerosis from head, heart and legs. The Framingham Study. Journal of the American Medical Association 221:661–666

Gunning A J, Pickering G W, Robb-Smith A H T, Russell R R 1964 Mural thrombosis of the internal carotid artery and subsequent embolism. Quarterly Journal of Medicine. New Series XXXIII #129:155–195

Haberman S, Capildeo R, Rose F C 1978 The changing mortality of cerebrovascular disease. Quarterly Journal of Medicine New Series XLVII #185:71–88

Haberman S, Capildeo R, Rose F C 1979 In: Greenhalgh R M, Rose F C (eds) Progress in stroke research, Pitman Medical, Kent, England, ch. 1

Hanaway J, Torack R, Fletcher A, Landau W 1976 Intracranial bleeding associated with urokinase therapy for acute ischemic hemispheral stroke. Stroke 7:143–147

Harker L A, Slichter S J 1974 Arterial and venous thromboembolism: Kinetic characterization and evaluation of therapy. Thrombosis et Diathesis Haemorrhatic (Stuttgart) 31:188–203

Harker L A, Ross R, Slichter S J, Scott C R 1976 Homocystine induced atherosclerosis — The role of endothelial cell injury and platelet response in its genesis. Journal of Clinical Investigation 58:731–741

Harris W H, Salzman E W, Athanasoulis C A, Waltman A C, DeSanctis R W 1977 Aspirin prophylaxis of venous thromboembolism after total hip replacement. New England Journal of Medicine 297:1246–1249

Harrison M J G, Marshall J, Meadows J C, Russell R W R 1971 Effect of aspirin in amaurosis fugax. Lancet ii:743–744

Harter H R, Burch J W, Majerus P W, Stanford N, Delmez J A, Anderson C B, Weerts C A 1978 Prevention of thrombosis in patients on hemodialysis by low-dose aspirin New England Journal of Medicine 301:577–579

Heyman A, Arons M, Quinn M, Camplong L 1969 The role of contraceptive agents in cerebral arterial occlusion. Neurology (Minneapolis) 19:519–524

Heyman A, Wilkinson W E, Heyden S, Helms M J, Bartel A G, Karp H R, Tyroler H A, Hames C G 1980 Risk of stroke in asymptomatic persons with cervical arterial bruits — a population study in Evans County, Georgia. New England Journal of Medicine 302:838–841

Hinton R C, Kistler J P, Fallon J T, Friedlich A L, Fisher C M 1977 Influence of etiology of atrial fibrillation on incidence of systemic embolism. American Journal of Cardiology 40:509–513

Hollander W, Kramsch D M, Franzblau C 1974 Suppression of atheromatous fibrous plaque formation by antiproliferative and anti-inflammatory drugs. Circulation Research Supplement #34/35:I131–I141

Honour A J, Russell R W R 1962 Experimental platelet embolism. British Journal of Pathology 43:350–362

Honour A J, Hockaday T D R, Mann J I 1977 The synergistic effect of aspirin and dipyridamole upon platelet thrombi in living blood vessels. British Journal of Experimental Pathology 58:268–272

Hutchinson E C, Acheson E J (eds) 1975a Other risk factors: cholesterol, diabetes mellitus, intermittent claudication and epilepsy. In: Strokes. Natural history; pathology and surgical treatment. W. B. Saunders Co. Ltd. Philadelphia, ch 10, p 211–213

Hutchinson E C, Acheson E J (eds) 1975b Natural history of stroke. In: Strokes. Natural history; pathology and surgical treatment, W. B. Saunders Co. Ltd. Philadelphia, ch 6, p 146–148

Hypertension Detection and Follow-Up Program Cooperative Group 1979 Five-year findings of the hypertensive detection and follow-up program. 1. Reduction in mortality of persons with high blood pressure, including mild hypertension. Journal of the American Medical Association 242:2562–2571

Jaffe E A, Weksler B B 1979 Recovery of endothelial cell prostacyclin production after inhibition by low doses of aspirin. Journal of Clinical Investigation 63:532–535

Johnston M, Ramwell P W 1974 Androgen mediated sex differences in platelet aggregation. Physiologist 17:256 (abstract)

Kaegi A, Pineo G F, Shimizu A G, Trivedi H, Hirsh J, Gent M 1974 The prevention of arteriovenous shunt thrombosis by sulfinpyrazone. New England Journal of Medicine 290:304–306

Kagan A, Popper J, Rhoads G G, Takeya Y, Kato H, Goode G B, Marmot M 1976 Epidemiologic studies on coronary artery disease and stroke in Japanese men living in Japan, Hawaii and California: Prevalence of stroke. In: Scheinberg P. (ed) Cerebrovascular disease, Raven Press. New York p 267–277

Kannel W B, Dawber T R, Cohen M E, McNamara P M 1965 Vascular disease of the brain — epidemiologic aspects: The Framingham study. American Journal of Public Health 55:1355–1366

Kannel W B, Castelli W P, McNamara P M 1968 Cigarette smoking and risk of coronary heart disease; epidemiological clues to pathogenesis. Framingham study. N.C.I. Mongr. #28:9–20

Kannel W B 1976 Epidemiology of cerebrovascular disease. In: Russell R (ed) Cerebral vascular disease, Churchill Livingstone, Edinburgh, ch 1 p 1–23

Kannel W B, Dawber T R, Sorlie P, Wolf P A 1976 Components of blood pressure and risk of atherothrombotic brain infarction. The Framingham study. Stroke 7:327–331

Kannel W B, Gordon T, Wolf P A, McNamara P M 1972 Hemoglobin and the risk of cerebral infarction: the Framingham study. Stroke 3:409–420

Kannel W B, Wolf P, Dawber T R 1978 Hypertension and cardiac impairments increase stroke risk. Geriatrics 33:71–83

Kelton J G, Carter C J, Santos A, Hirsh J 1980 Sex related differences in platelet function in vivo following aspirin administration. Circulation 62: supplement #III p 342 (abstract)

Kelton J G, Carter C J, Santos A, Hirsch J 1978a Thrombogenic effects of high-dose aspirin in rabbits. Relationship to inhibition of vessel wall synthesis of prostaglandin I_2-like activity. Journal of Clinical Investigation, 62:892–895

Kelton J G, Hirsh J, Carter C J, Buchanan M R 1978b Sex differences in the antithrombotic effects of aspirin. Blood 52:1073–1076

Kelton J G, Powers P, Julian J, Boland V, Carter C J, Gent M, Hirsh J 1980 Sex-related differences in platelet aggregation: Influence of hematocrit Blood 56:38–41

Koster J K, Tryka A F, H'Doubler P, Collin J J Jr. 1981 Effect of aspirin and dipyridamole upon atherosclerosis in the rabbit. Atherosclerosis 1:97 (abstract)

Kurtzke J F 1979 Controversy in neurology: The Canadian Study on TIA and aspirin. A critique of the Canadian TIA Study. Annals of Neurology 5:597–599

Kurtzke J F 1980 Epidemiology of cerebral vascular disease. In: Siekert R G (ed) Cerebral vascular survey report for joint council subcommittee on cerebral vascular disease, National Institute of Neurology and Communicative Disorders in Stroke and National Heart and Lung Institute, Bethesda Maryland, Office of Scientific and Health Reports. p 135–176

Levine J, Swanson P D 1968 Idiopathic thrombocytosis. A treatable cause of transient ischemic attacks. Neurology (Minneapolis) 18:711–713

Levine P H, Fisher M, Fullerton A L, Duffy C P, Hoogasian J J: Human platelet Factor 4: Preparation from outdated platelet concentrations and application in cerebral vascular disease. American Journal of Hematology (in press — April/81)

Linos A, Worthington J W, O'Fallon W, Fuster V, Whisnant J P, Kurland L T 1978 Effect of aspirin on prevention of coronary and cerebrovascular disease in patients with rheumatic arthritis. A long-term follow-up study. Mayo Clinic Proceedings 53:581–586

Lown B 1967 Electrical reversion of cardiac arrhythmias. British Medical Journal 29:469–489

Malmsten C, Hamberg M, Svensson J, Samuelsson B 1975 Physiological role of an endoperoxide in human platelets: Hemostatic defect due to platelet cyclooxygenase deficiency. Proceedings National Academy of Science 72# 4:1146–1450

Marquardsen J 1969 The natural history of cerebrovascular disease. Acta Neurologica Scandinavica Supplementum 45:90–188

Marshall J, 1964 The natural history of transient ischaemic cerebrovascular attacks. Quarterly Journal of Medicine 33:309–324

Masotti G, Poggesi L, Galanti G, Abbate R, Neri-Serneri G G 1979: Differential inhibition of prostacyclin production and platelet aggregation by aspirin. Lancet ii:1213–1216

McKenna R, Galante J, Bachmann F, Wallace D L, Kaushal S P, Meredith P 1980 Prevention of venous thromboembolism after total knee replacement by high dose aspirin on intermittent calf and thigh compression. British Medical Journal 280:514–517

Menguy R, Desbaillets L, Masters Y F, Okabe S 1972 Evidence for a sex linked difference in aspirin metabolism. Nature 239:102–103

Meyer J, Gilroy J, Barnhart M, Johnson J 1964 Anticoagulants plus streptokinase therapy in progressive stroke. Journal of the American Medical Association 189:373

Millikan C H 1965 Therapeutic agents current status: Anticoagulant therapy in cerebrovascular disease. In: Siekert R G, Whisnant J P (eds) Cerebral vascular diseases 4th Conference, Grune and Stratton Inc. New York, p 181–184

Millikan C H, 1971 Anticoagulant therapy in cerebrovascular disease. In: Cerebrovascular Survey Report. Subcommittee on Cerebrovascular Disease. N.I.N.C.D.S. pp 218–225

Millikan C H, 1971 Reassessment of anticoagulant therapy in various types of occlusive cerebrovascular disease. Stroke 2:201–208

Mohr J P, Caplan L R, Melski J W, Goldstein R J, Duncan G W, Kistler S P, Pessin M S, Bleich H L 1978 The Harvard cooperative stroke registry: A prospective registry. Neurology 28:754–762

Moncada S, Gryglewski R J, Bunting S, Vane J R 1976 An enzyme isolated from arteries transforms prostaglandin endoperoxides to an unstable substance that inhibits platelet aggregation. Nature 263:663–665

Moncada S, Korbut R 1978 Dipyridamole and other phosphodiesterase inhibitors act as antithrombotic agents by potentiating endogenous prostacyclin. Lancet i:1286–1289

Moore S, Friedman R J, Singal D P, Gauldie J, Blaschman M A, Roberts R S 1976 Inhibition of injury and induced thrombosclerotic lesions by antiplatelet serum in rabbits. Thrombosis and Haemostasis 35:70–81

Mundall J, Quintero P, von Kaulla K N, Harmon R, Austin J 1972 Transient monocular blindness and increased platelet aggregatibility treated with aspirin. Neurology 22:280–285

Moyes P D, Millikan C H, Wakim K G, Sayre G P, Whisnant J P 1957 Influence of anticoagulants on experimental canine cerebral infarcts. Proceedings of the Staff Meetings of the Mayo Clinic 32:124–130

Nelson R F, Pullicino P, Kendall B E, Marshall J 1980 Computed tomography in patients presenting with lacunar syndromes. Stroke 11:256–261

Nordoy A, Svensson B, Haycraft D, Hoak J C, Wiebe D 1978 The influence of age, sex and the use of oral contraceptives on the inhibitory effects of endothelial cells and PGI_2

(prostacyclin) on platelet function. Scandinavian Journal of Haematology 21:177–187

Olsson J E, Brechter C, Backlund H, Krook H, Muller R, Nitelius E, Olsson O, Tornberg A 1980 Anticoagulants vs. antiplatelet therapy as prophylactic against cerebral infarction in TIA. Stroke 11:4–9

O'Grady J, Moncada S 1978 Aspirin: a paradoxical effect on bleeding time. Lancet ii:780

Paffenbarger R S Jr, Wing A L, 1969 Chronic disease in former college students. X. The effect of single and multiple characteristics on risk of fatal coronary heart disease. American Journal of Epidemiology 90:527–535

Pareti F I, Mannucci P M, D'Angelo A, Smith J B, Sautebin L, Galli G 1980 Congenital deficiency of thromboxane and prostacyclin. Lancet i:898–900

Pearce J M S, Gubbay S S, Walton J N 1965 Longterm anticoagulant therapy in transient cerebral ischemic attacks. Lancet i:6–9

Persantine-Aspirin Reinfarction Study Research Group 1980 Persantine and aspirin in coronary heart disease. Circulation 62:449–461

Pick R, Chediak J, Glick G 1979 Aspirin inhibits development of coronary atherosclerosis in cynomalgus monkeys (macaca fascicularis) fed an atherogenic diet. Journal of Clinical Investigation 63:158–162

Pfaffenbach D D, Hollenhorst R W 1973 Morbidity and survivorship of patients with embolic cholesterol crystals in the ocular fundus. American Journal of Ophthalmology 75:66–72

Preston F E, Whipps S, Jackson C A, French A J, Wyld P J, Stoddard C J 1981 Inhibition of prostacyclin and platelet thromboxane A$_2$ after low-dose aspirin. New England Journal of Medicine 304:76–79

Pulsinelli W, Sigsbee B., Waldman S, Rawlinson D, Scherer P, Plum F 1980 Experimental hyperglycemia and diabetes mellitus worsen stroke outcome. Annals of Neurology 8:91 (abstract)

Report of the Working Party on Anticoagulant Therapy in Coronary Thrombosis to the Medical Research Council 1969. Assessment of short term anticoagulant administration after cardiac infarction. British Medical Journal 1:335–342

Reuther R, Dorndorf W, Loew D 1980 Behandlung transitorisch-ischamischer Attacken mit Azetylsalizylsaure. Munch. Med. Wschr. 122:795–798

Robinson R W, Cohen W D, Higano N, Meyer R, Lukowsky G H, McLaughlin R B 1959 Life table analysis of survival after cerebrothrombosis — 10 year experience. Journal of the American Medical Association 169:1149–1152

Ropper A H, Davis K R 1980 Lobar cerebral hemorrhages: Acute clinical syndromes in 26 cases. Annals of Neurology 8:141–147

Ross R, Glomset J A 1976 Pathogenesis of atherosclerosis. New England Journal of Medicine 295:369–377 and 420–425

Rossner S, Mettinger K L, Kjellin K G, Siden A, Soderstrom C E 1978 Normal serum-cholesterol but low HDL-cholesterol concentration in young patients with ischemic cerebrovascular disease. Lancet i:577–579

Russell R W R 1961 Observations on the retinal blood vessels in monocular blindness. Lancet ii:1422–1128

Scharf R E, Hennerici M, Bluschke V, Schneider W 1981 In vitro platelet activity in young patients with cerebral ischemia and mitral-valve prolapse. Thrombosis and Hemostasis (abstract — in press)

Schoenberg B S, Whisnant J P, Taylor W F, Kempers R D 1970 Strokes in women of childbearing age. A population study. Neurology 20:181–189

Shurtleff D 1974 Some characteristics related to the incidence of cardiovascular disease and death. The Framingham study. 18 Year follow up. Department of Health Education and Welfare, Washington

Sibley W A, Morledge J H, Lapham L W 1957 Experimental cerebral infarction: The effect of dicoumerol. American Journal of Medical Science 234:663–667

Siekert R G, Whisnant J P, Millikan C H 1963 Surgical and anticoagulant therapy of occlusive cerebrovascular disease. Annals of Internal Medicine 58:637–641

Sigurjonsson J 1974 Differences in mortality patterns of coronary heart disease and cerebrovascular lesions. Journal of American Geriatrics 22:241–245

Silverstein A, Doinger D E 1963 Systemic and local conditions predisposing to ischaemic and occlusive cerebrovascular disease. Journal of Mount Sinai Hospital, New York 30:435–450

Singer G 1969 Migrating emboli of retinal arteries in thrombocythemia. British Journal of Ophthalmology 53:279–283

Sinzinger H, Silberbauer K, Wagner O, Winter M, Auerswald W 1978 Prostacyclin — preliminary results with vascular tissue of various species and its importance for atherosclerotic involvement. Atherogenase 3:123

Soltero I, Liu K, Cooper R, Stamler J, Garside D 1978 Trends in mortality from cerebrovascular diseases in the United States, 1969 to 1975. Stroke 9:549–555

Statistics Canada 1954 Vital Statistics 1954. Catalogue #9004–505, December 1954, Queen's Printer, Ottawa, Canada

Statistics Canada 1980 Causes of death–1978. Catalogue 84–203. Queen's Printer, Ottawa, Canada.

Steele P, Rainwater J 1980 Favourable effect of sulfinpyrazone on thromboembolism in patients with rheumatic heart disease. Circulation 62:462–465

Steele P, Weily H S, Davies H, Genton E 1974 Platelet survival in patients with rheumatic heart disease. New England Journal of Medicine 290:537–539

Steele P, Weily H, Rainwater J, Vogel R 1979 Platelet survival time and thromboembolism in patients with mitral valve prolapse. Circulation 60:43–45

Stoel I, v/d Giessen W J, Zwolsman E, Quadt J F A, ten Hoor F, Verheugt F W A, Hugenholtz P G 1981 Effect of nicotine on prostacyclin production in human umbilical arteries. Arteriosclerosis 1:98 (abstract)

Sullivan J M, Harken D E, Gorlin R 1971 Pharmacologic control of thromboembolic complication of cardiac-valve replacement. New England Journal of Medicine 284:1391–1394

The University Group Diabetes Program 1970 A study of the effects of hypoglycemic agents on vascular complications in patients with adult-onset diabetes. Diabetes 19 (supplement #2): 747–830

Thomas D J 1979 The influence of blood viscosity on cerebral blood flow and symptoms. In: Greenhalgh R M, Rose F C (eds) Progress in stroke research, Pitman Medical, Kent England, ch 6

Tognoni G, Garattini S (eds) 1979 Drug treatment and prevention in cerebrovascular disorders. Elsevier-North Holland, Biomedical Press Amsterdam

Toole J F, Janeway R, Choi K, Cordell R, Davis C, Johnston F, Miller H S 1975 Transient ischemic attacks due to atherosclerosis. Archives of Neurology 32:5–12

Vessey M P, Doll R 1969 Investigation of relation between use of oral contraceptives and thromboembolic disease. A further report. British Medical Journal ii:651–657

Veterans Administration Hospital Investigators 1973 Anticoagulants in acute myocardial infarction. Results of a cooperative study. Journal of the American Medical Association 225:724–729

Veterans Administration National Heart, Lung and Blood Institute Study Group for Cooperative Studies on Antihypertensive Therapy 1977: Mild hypertension (Perry H M) Treatment of mild hypertension: Preliminary results of a two-year feasibility trial. Circulation Research 40:180–187

Villa S, Livio M, DeGaetano G 1979 The inhibitory effect of aspirin on platelet and vascular prostaglandins in rats cannot be completely dissociated. British Journal of Haematology 42:425–431

Walsh P N, Kansu T A, Corbett J J, Savino P J, Goldburgh W, Schantz N J 1980 Platelets, thromboembolism and mitral valve prolapse. Circulation 62:#III–276 (abstract)

Warren B A, Vales O 1974 Electron microscopy of the sequence of events in atheroembolic occlusion of cerebral arteries in an animal model. British Journal of Experimental Pathology 56:205–215

Weilly H S, Steele P P, Davies H, Pappas G, Genton E 1974 Platelet survival in patients with substitute heart valves. New England Journal of Medicine i:534–537

Wester J, Sixma J J, Geuze J J, VanDerVeen J 1978 Morphology of the early hemostasis in human skin wounds. Influence of acetylsalicyclic acid. Laboratory Investigation 39:298–311

Whisnant J P, Cartlidge N E F, Elvebach L R 1978 Carotid and vertebral-basilar transient ischemic attacks: Effect of anticoagulants, hypertension and cardiac disorders on survival and stroke occurrence — a population study. Annals of Neurology 3:107–115

Whisnant J P, Fitzgibbons J P, Kurland L T, Sayre G P 1971 Natural history of stroke in Rochester, Minnesota 1945 through 1954. Stroke 2:11–22

Whisnant J P, Matsumoto N, Elveback L R 1973 The effect of anticoagulant therapy on prognosis of patients with transient cerebral ischemic attacks in a community: Rochester, Minnesota 1955 through 1969. Mayo Clinic Proceedings 48:844–848

Wolf P A, Kannel W B, McNamara P M, Gordon T 1973 The role of impaired cardiac function in atherothrombotic brain infarction. The Framingham study. American Journal of Public Health 63:52–58

Wolf P A, Dawber T R, Thomas H E, Kannel W B, 1978 Epidemiologic assessment of chronic atrial fibrillation and risk of stroke. The Framingham study. Neurology (Minneapolis) 28:973–977

Wolf P A, Kannel W B, McNamara P M, Dawber T R 1979 Asymptomatic carotid bruit and risk of stroke. Stroke 10:96 (abstract)

Wood M W, Wakim K G, Sayre G P, Millikan C H, Whisnant J P 1958 Relationship between anticoagulants and hemorrhagic cerebral infarction in experimental animals. Archives of Neurology and Psychiatry 79:390–396

Wright I S, Marple C D, Beck D F 1954 Myocardial infarction: Its clinical manifestations and treatment with anticoagulants. A study of 1031 cases. Grune and Stratton, New York

Wu K K Y 1978 Platelet hyperaggregability and thrombosis in patients with thrombocythemia. Annals of Internal Medicine 88:7–11

Zucker M B 1947 Platelet agglutination and vasoconstriction as factors in spontaneous hemostasis in normal, thrombocytopenic, heparinized and hypoprothrombinemic rats. American Journal of Physiology 148:275–288

21

The surgical treatment of cerebrovascular disease

Norman Browse

The extracranial arteries which are concerned with the supply of blood to the brain and which are readily accessible to the surgeon comprise the aortic arch, the innominate artery, the common carotid arteries and the proximal parts of the internal carotid, subclavian and vertebral arteries on both sides.

When cerebral symptoms are caused by extracranial arterial disease the primary pathology is usually atherosclerosis with or without thrombosis; occasionally the underlying disease is a rarity such as fibromuscular dysplasia, Takayasu arteritis or spontaneous dissection (see Ch. 19).

Mechanisms

Extracranial cerebral vascular disease produces symptoms in three ways. First it may give rise to emboli which impact in the intracranial circulation to cause localised cerebral ischaemia. Secondly, multiple large-vessel disease may cause a reduction in total cerebral blood flow and the symptoms of generalised cerebral ischaemia. Thirdly, a stenosis at a critical point in one extracranial vessel may induce a reversal of the blood flow in another major vessel and in some circumstances may induce ischaemia in the territory of the latter (steal syndrome).

Emboli

Emboli from atherosclerotic plaques in large blood vessels may be of three types: platelet clumps, mixed thrombus and cholesterol.

Platelet clumps consist of aggregated platelets bound together with fibrin. In the initial stages there is little fibrin and the aggregation is reversible.

As the quantity of fibrin increases and the platelets change their structure the aggregate becomes more stable. These changes have profound clinical significance, for clumps of loosely aggregated platelets usually break up on impaction producing only transient symptoms, whereas more stable aggregates may lead to permanent vessel occlusion.

Red thrombus is not commonly found in the extracranial arteries because flow through these vessels is too rapid. Red thrombus, which is a mixture of blood cells within a fibrin mesh, tends to form in relatively stagnant conditions. However, when stasis occurs within atheromatous ulcers or beyond tight stenoses, red thrombus may form, break free or extend into the intracranial vessels to produce permanent obstruction.

Cholesterol emboli occur when the intima over an atheromatous plaque breaks down and allows the exposed contents of the plaque to spill into the blood stream. Plaques consist of insoluble fat globules and cholesterol crystals. When they impact in small blood vessels they may cause a permanent or temporary obstruction. Cholesterol crystals cause a marked reaction in the artery wall. In a retinal branch artery this reaction is easily recognisable (Hollenhorst, 1961).

The symptoms of emboli depend upon the site of impaction and the duration and extent of occlusion. The site of impaction is determined by the pattern of blood flow and the source of the embolus. As blood flow in major blood vessels is usually laminar, it is not surprising that a mural thrombus gives rise to repeated emboli in the same distal territory. Thus the same blood vessel within the eye or the same cerebral vessel may be repeatedly occluded. Repeated identical attacks of sudden onset are highly suggestive of recurrent emboli.

Emboli may also come from the cavities of the heart, the heart-valves or from plaques of atherosclerosis in other arteries. As in the carotid the extent of the atherosclerosis is variable; tight stenosis may be present for many years and never produce the conditions necessary for the development of emboli whereas a small ulcerated plaque which is causing little change in the diameter of the artery may be the source of repeated emboli. Thus the degree of obstruction to flow or the severity of stenosis may be of little importance.

The commonest *site* of embologenic atherosclerotic disease is the common carotid artery bifurcation. Although the disease affects the whole of the bifurcation it is invariably maximal in the first two centimetres of the internal carotid artery. Gross disease at this point takes the form of large deposits of atheroma producing haemodynamically significant stenoses or deep plaque ulceration. Emboli from this source may pass into the eye or into the brain.

A second common source of vessel wall emboli is the origin of the great vessels on the arch of the aorta. The artery most often affected by stenosing atherosclerosis is the origin of the left subclavian artery (Crawford et al, 1962). Disease in this artery is usually asymptomatic but it can cause the subclavian steal syndrome (see later) and may occasionally produce emboli which reach the hindbrain. More frequently, however, emboli from the subclavian artery pass into the arm to produce patches of ischaemia in the finger tips and Raynaud's phenomenon. Disease at the origins of the left and right common carotid arteries produces symptoms similar to carotid bifurcation disease.

The belief that almost all transient symptoms are caused by emboli is supported by the follow-up study of DeWeese et al (1973) who found that the majority of patients who were not cured by carotid endarterectomy had atypical symptoms.

Reduced cerebral perfusion

Because the brain is supplied by four large arteries, stenosis of one artery rarely causes a reduction of cerebral blood flow unless by chance this artery is isolated from the other three vessels by abnormalities of the Circle of Willis. A significant reduction of cerebral blood flow only occurs when at least two and usually three major arteries are occluded. It is not unusual to find patients living normal lives without any symptoms of cerebral ischaemia with both vertebral arteries and one carotid artery occluded. However, symptoms of a reduction of cerebral blood flow may appear if the one remaining patent artery becomes narrow. These may be focal from those parts of the brain most deprived of blood but there may also be symptoms of general cerebral ischaemia such as impaired alertness, memory and concentration.

Steal syndromes

Blood flows from regions of higher to lower pressures. If a situation arises in which there is a higher pressure in the Circle of Willis than at some point in the extracranial circulation blood flow may be reversed. Then an obstruction at the origin of the subclavian artery may reduce the pressure in the subclavian artery so that blood flows down the vertebral artery from the Circle of Willis rather than into the branches of the Circle (Contorni, 1960; Editorial, 1961). This reversed flow may be exacerbated when the muscle blood vessels of the arm dilate with exercise. Under these circumstances the arm is *stealing* blood from the vertebrobasilar circulation.

There are many varieties of steal syndrome. Blood may flow up the internal carotid artery and down the vertebral artery, or up one internal carotid artery and down the other but these are relatively rare. The left subclavian steal syndrome is the commonest because the proximal subclavian artery is a favoured site for atheroma.

Symptoms of a steal syndrome are vertigo, ataxia and dizziness, sometimes accompanied by visual disturbances caused by occipital cerebral cortex ischaemia. The patient may also notice pain in the muscles of the arm during arm exercise, equivalent to intermittent claudication in the legs, and coldness and pallor of the fingers.

The surgeon with a general vascular practice, dealing with all forms of extracranial vascular disease, will find that 95 per cent of the patients have symptoms related to atherosclerotic carotid artery bifurcation disease. The remaining five per cent are a mixture of patients with aortic arch and multi-vessel disease, the occasional steal syndrome and rarities such as fibromuscular dysplasia of the internal carotid artery and Takayasu arteritis of the great vessels. Thus, when any patient presents with cerebral or ocular symptoms possibly related to extracranial vascular disease, the most important sites to investigate are the bifurcations of the common carotid arteries.

INVESTIGATIONS

The suspicion of carotid artery disease is often confirmed by bruits over the origins of the great vessels or at the carotid bifurcation. A carotid artery bruit usually indicates significant disease of the internal carotid artery and a likely source of emboli. However the absence of a bruit does not exclude a possible source of emboli because ulcerating atheromatous plaques may have no effect on the diameter of the artery. Indeed they may make an artery wider. Consequently techniques which are designed to detect a reduction of flow through the carotid artery, such as oculoplethysmography, are not an accurate way of detecting disease which may be the source of emboli. Ultrasound scanning techniques, particularly the Duplex systems which combine Doppler imaging with B mode scanning, are more valuable and in the future they may be accurate enough to detect ulcerated plaques and minor abnormalities. At present the only completely reliable method for detecting artery wall disease, and defining its suitability for surgery, is arteriography.

There is always controversy about the best form of arteriography. It is generally advisable to visualise both carotid and both vertebral arteries. This requires an arch aortogram, a straightforward investigation, but not entirely without risk. Unfortunately an arch aortogram does not always give a good delineation of the carotid bifurcation so many centres practice carotid arteriography by direct puncture or selective catheterisation of the common artery especially when there are no features suggestive of more proximal disease. The best quality pictures of the carotid artery are obtained with carotid arteriography by direct puncture. The image can be magnified to reveal the fine details of the internal surface of the artery, including the hollows and cavities at the centre of an ulcerated atheromatous plaque.

When computer enhanced intravenous arteriography is freely available we will be able to obtain frequent arteriograms of the great vessels and carotid bifurcation and investigate asymptomatic disease without arterial puncture. This new technique may well displace the current forms of arteriography and all other popular non-invasive techniques of investigation, except those concerned with measurement of blood flow.

If emboli are thought to be the cause of a patient's symptoms, it is reasonable to assume that they come from any localised region of disease in the relevant artery. In my own practice I accept any degree of disease on the carotid arteriogram, however mild, as a possible source of emboli, provided the other great vessels are normal. The degree of stenosis, *per se*, is not relevant.

When the clinical problem is one of generalised cerebral ischaemia then it is essential to obtain an arteriogram which displays all the great vessels so that the significance and operability of disease at various sites can be assessed.

PRINCIPLES OF SURGICAL TREATMENT

Whatever the cause of the patient's symptoms, emboli or reduced perfusion, there are only two surgical techniques which can be applied to atherosclerosis; endarterectomy and bypass. Both techniques have one basic requirement, the artery above and below the diseased portion must be relatively healthy. For endarterectomy, the proximal artery need not be absolutely normal, but it is essential that the artery beyond the diseased area, i.e., the downstream part of the artery, is absolutely normal. If not, it is impossible to leave the end of the endarterectomy with a smooth non-thrombogenic surface.

Endarterectomy is the removal of the intima, subintimal atheroma and most of the media, leaving behind the external elastic lamina, which has a smooth inner surface, supported by the surrounding adventitia. Although this is a very thin layer of tissue it is strong enough to hold sutures and withstand arterial blood pressure, and rarely becomes aneurysmal.

It is not necessary for the vessels to be quite so healthy for a bypass operation, but the areas selected for both the take-off and the insertion of the bypass should be relatively healthy and must be widely patent. It is for these reasons that the knowledge gained from the accurate delineation of the degree and extent of the disease by arteriography is essential. None of the non-invasive techniques gives the surgeon a highly defined anatomical display of the problem, so none allows him to plan his operation precisely. Arteriography is essential before carotid endarterectomy because if it reveals disease spreading up the internal carotid artery towards the carotid foramen a satisfactory endarterectomy is impossible. Moderate or severe stenosis of the intracranial carotid siphon is also a contraindication to endarterectomy.

The advantage of endarterectomy is that it can be done through a simple arteriotomy and requires no foreign or additional material for its repair, other than simple stitches. A bypass performed with an autogenous vein or synthetic material requires a larger incision to display the vessel above and below the disease, and two arteriotomies for the two anastomoses. Bypass techniques are particularly useful for disease at the origins of the great vessels, but are rarely used for carotid bifurcation disease.

Patch procedures may be employed to widen narrow arteries. A few surgeons always use a patch after an endarterectomy, but the majority of experienced carotid endarterectomists find patches unnecessary. The use of any foreign material increases the risk of infection and aneurysm formation.

THE OPERATION

Carotid endarterectomy

The carotid bifurcation lies level with the hyoid cartilage, a centimetre or two below the angle of the jaw. The atheroma usually occupies the first two centimetres of the internal carotid artery as well as the termination of the common carotid artery and the first centimetre of the external carotid artery. The disease in the internal carotid artery rarely goes above the level of the jaw. If the arteriograph shows the disease ascending up the carotid artery towards the base of the skull, endarterectomy should not be attempted because the surgeon is likely to find that he cannot get proper control of the artery above the disease and will be unable to complete the upper end of the endarterectomy.

Carotid endarterectomy is *not* indicated when the internal carotid artery is totally occluded. In these circumstances there is likely to be thrombus in the artery right up to its entry into the Circle of Willis and any attempt to remove it could be extremely hazardous because pieces of the thrombus may be broken off and pushed on as emboli into the brain. The use of carotid endarterectomy for stroke secondary to acute occlusion of the carotid artery was often disastrous for this reason. Furthermore, in those cases when the artery was opened and the brain re-vascularised there was often a massive haemorrhage into the infarcted area.

The operation is performed through a longitudinal incision along the front edge of the sterno-cleido-mastoid muscle, centred over the carotid bifurcation. The artery is dissected free and isolated so that clamps can be placed on the common, internal, and external carotid arteries. These arteries must be handled carefully so that emboli are not dislodged.

Cerebral protection

When the endarterectomy is being performed the artery must be clamped and there is considerable dispute amongst surgeons about the best method of protecting the brain from ischaemic damage during the period of clamping. Although only 5–10 per cent of fit young men will have a stroke if the internal carotid artery is tied (McKissock et al, 1960), even the small risk is unacceptable in a preventive operation of this kind. There are three common approaches to this problem: to insert a temporary bypass (shunt) during the operation in all cases; to shunt those patients who have evidence of cerebral ischaemia after clamping; or to use no shunt but occlude the artery for the minimum length of time.

Routine shunting

Many surgeons insert a shunt at every operation (Thompson, 1979; Javid et al, 1979). Inserting and removing the shunt adds very little time to the operation but reduces the potential ischaemia time to two periods of 1 to 2 minutes. Because the shunt can get in the way of the endarterectomy, and if used improperly can damage the arteries, some surgeons reject it as a routine manoeuvre. Nevertheless the best published results of carotid endarterectomy come from surgeons who use shunting techniques regularly. Provided it is safe it is clearly the logical thing to do.

Monitoring with or without shunting

The measurement of stump pressure. In this technique the pressure is measured in the distal internal carotid artery after clamping. If the pressure is pulsatile and above 50 mmHg then it is almost certain that there is an adequate anatomosis at the Circle of Willis and that the whole of the brain is receiving an adequate blood flow (Boysen, 1973). If the pressure is below 50 mmHg then cerebral perfusion is likely to be inadequate and a shunt is inserted. This approach does not totally abolish postoperative strokes (Hays et al, 1972; Hertzer et al, 1978; Kelly et al 1979), for two reasons. First, not all postoperative strokes are caused by inadequate peroperative cerebral perfusion, and secondly a stump pressure above 50 mmHg at the beginning of clamping may not be maintained throughout the 10 or 15 minutes taken to perform the endarterectomy. It would be more logical to record the stump pressure throughout the operation but this would be impractical.

E.e.g. monitoring. As an alternative to stump pressure measurements some surgeons monitor the effect on the brain of any changes in cerebral circulation that occur during the operation with a continuous e.e.g. recording. If the e.e.g. remains normal when the arteries in the neck are clamped then the brain must be receiving an adequate circulation. If the e.e.g. is abnormal then a shunt must be inserted. (Harris et al, 1967; Baker et al, 1975; Callow et al, 1978). This form of monitoring does not interfere with the surgeon but does need extra apparatus and an extra technician. Boysen

(1973) has shown a good correlation between cerebral blood flow and e.e.g. activity; when the cerebral blood flow falls below 25 ml/100 g per min the amplitude of the e.e.g. waves diminishes and a shunt is indicated. In Boysen's study this occurred in 19 of 60 cases.

Clamping and operating under local anaesthesia is the most direct way of discovering the need for a shunt (Bland et al, 1970; Connolly et al, 1977) but has not found favour amongst most surgeons who prefer to do the operation with the patient fully anaesthetised.

Other methods. The other ineffectual techniques that have been advocated for protecting the brain from ischaemia are the use of very large doses of heparin (Kenyon et al, 1972), hyperbaric oxygen (Jacobsen et al, 1963), and the production of hypercapnia or hypertension during the operation (Bloodwell et al, 1968; Youmans et al, 1968; Ehrenfeld et al, 1970). There is little clinical evidence that any of these techniques have a worthwhile effect.

Every surgeon must choose between the routine use of a shunt or assessment for shunting during the operation with internal carotid artery stump pressure measurements, e.e.g. recordings, or operating under local anaesthesia. Any other approach is taking unnecessary risks. In my opinion it is logical and more practical to use a shunt on all occasions because none of the monitoring techniques discussed give an absolute guarantee that there is adequate cerebral perfusion throughout the operation. Furthermore, regular use of the shunt ensures that the surgeon is well practised in its use for the time when it is essential and a practised technique is vital. The effect of different forms of cerebral protection on the results of the operation is discussed in the Results section.

The endarterectomy

An adequate carotid endarterectomy removes all the disease in the internal carotid artery, leaving a smooth surface without any particles of atheroma or shreds of media which might provoke further thrombus and embolus formation, and then constructs a smooth junction between the endarterectomised artery and the normal distal artery so that there are no flaps of intima which can bend over into the lumen and provide a site for thrombosis and which might ultimately occlude the internal carotid artery or break free as an embolus. The upper end of the endarterectomy is the most critical part of the operation. Unless the surgeon sees the upper limit of the endarterectomy he cannot be certain there are no distal intimal flaps. If the endarterectomy is always continued up to normal intima there will be no flaps because thin normal intima is firmly adherent to the underlying media and will not split off when the blood flow is restored. If a plaque of atheroma is divided and part of it left behind it may easily dissect free and fold over when the blood flow is restored.

It is also important to ensure that the common carotid is of an adequate diameter, but there are frequently streaks of disease running down the whole length of the common carotid artery so it is often not possible to finish the lower (upstream) end of the endarterectomy in normal artery. Thick stenosing plaques must not be left in the common carotid artery but the chance of intimal flaps of minor disease causing thrombosis at the upstream side of an endarterectomy is extremely low.

Postoperative care

Wounds are usually closed with suction drainage and the patient observed carefully for 48 hours for neurological abnormalities. The anaesthetist, whilst giving adequate anaesthesia and relaxation during the operation, should adjust the anaesthetic so that the patient is awake within 15 minutes of the end of the operation to enable the surgeon to test the movement and sensation of the limbs. The simplest method of observing the patient for the next 24 hours is to use a standard head injury chart which reminds the nursing staff to assess the motor, sensory and reflex functions and the level of consciousness at regular intervals. If the patient

develops neurological signs during the post-operative period, having been normal at the time of awakening from the operation, it is customary to re-explore the neck to see if the artery has thrombosed, but it is most uncommon for re-explorations to have any worthwhile effect. In most cases, the artery is found to be pulsating and to be patent, findings which suggest that the symptoms were caused by further emboli.

RESULTS

It is important to define the object of an operation before assessing its result. Carotid endarterectomy has two objectives. The first is to prevent stroke in subsequent years. The second, less important, is to prevent the symptoms of transient ocular or cerebral ischaemic attacks.

Mortality

The majority of patients undergoing carotid endarterectomy are over the age of 60 and are suffering from generalised arterial disease. This means that some are hypertensive, some are diabetic and many have coronary artery disease and/or lower limb peripheral vascular disease. The causes of death can be divided into three groups, those directly related to the operation, those related to the generalised arterial disease and general causes associated with any operation. The causes of death directly related to the operation are complete stroke continuing to death and very rarely uncontrollable haemorrhage from the artery in the neck. The deaths related to the generalised arterial disease are usually from myocardial infarction, and the nonspecific deaths are caused by events such as pulmonary embolism and bronchopneumonia.

Table 21.1 gives the mortality rates of two

Table 21.1 Mortality of carotid endarterectomy with a shunt

Author	Indications	No. patients	No. operations	No. deaths	Patient mortality %	Procedure mortality %
Thompson (1979)	Frank stroke	296	358	20	6.8	5.6
	TIAs	575	737	7	1.2	0.9
	Asymptomatic bruit	132	167	0	0	0
Javid et al (1979)	Frank stroke	323	373	8	2.5	2.1
	TIAs	1205	1370	13	1.1	0.9
	Asymptomatic bruit	170	208	0	0	0

internationally recognised leading surgical groups in this field who use a shunt routinely. In both series the mortality rate for operations performed for TIAs is approximately one per cent. It is generally agreed that this is an acceptable mortality rate provided the surgeon is satisfied that the operation is reducing the incidence of subsequent stroke but it must be emphasised that this is not a proven or totally accepted fact. It must also be stressed that mortality rates of one per cent or less are obtained only by surgeons who regularly practise this operation and who have devoted their time and expertise to its study. In a study of the mortality rate of carotid endarterectomy performed in community hospitals, Easton & Sherman (1977) found a mortality rate of seven per cent. This is unacceptable.

Morbidity

The morbidity of carotid endarterectomy is of two types: cerebral complications such as stroke, and local complications in the neck such as haemorrhage, wound infection, nerve paresis, false aneurysm and true aneurysms.

Neurological defects can be divided into transient or permanent. There is no clearly accepted definition of the term transient. Duration of less than 6, 24 or 48 hours have each been used. Some defects recover only after three or four weeks, indicating a localised cerebral infarction.

Table 21.2 lists the incidence of transient and permanent neurological defects following carotid endarterectomy for TIAs of four large series. With one exception it can be seen that the incidence of transient defects is between 0.5–3.0 per cent and permanent defects between 1–5 per cent. Those surgeons with the largest series and a special interest in this field get the best results. Thompson (1979) reported a series of 323 patients undergoing 422 operations for transient cerebral ischaemia.

Two died (0.6 per cent), four operations were followed by transient cerebral effects (0.95 per cent) and six by permanent defects (1.4 per cent), an overall defect incidence of 2.4 per cent.

Effect on results of cerebral protection techniques

A number of published reviews have compared the results of uncontrolled studies from different surgeons in an attempt to assess the value of the different methods of cerebral protection already discussed. For example, Thompson (1979) cites 10 publications published between 1970 and 1978 which used 8 different methods and produced mortality rates ranging between 0.5–3.5 per cent and permanent defect rates from 0–7.7 per cent. It is impossible to draw firm conclusions from such dissimilar studies.

A better indication of the value of cerebral protection provided by shunting comes from studies on patients with bilateral disease. Table 21.3 gives the results of five series of operations in which the contralateral carotid artery was known to be occluded. This is the most testing situation met by the carotid endarterectomist. The incidence of deficits in those series which did not shunt was 8 per cent. When a shunt was used the incidence of deficits was 1 per cent. Although these figures strongly support the value of shunting they do not settle the question of whether it is best done on all patients or only on those in whom the stump pressure or the e.e.g. indicates its need.

Late results

If the risk of stroke in the untreated patient is 5 per cent per year (Whisnant et al, 1973; Toole et al, 1975) then a total neurological morbidity of 2–3 per cent is clearly acceptable and worthwhile provided the operation really does reduce the possibility of a stroke in the subsequent years.

Table 21.2 Cerebral complications of carotid endarterectomy for TIAs

Author	No. operations	Shunt	Neurological defects		Total
			Transient	Permanent	
Javid et al (1979)	1370	Yes	10 (0.7%)	8 (0.5%)	18 (1.3%)
Thompson (1979)	422	Yes	4 (0.95%)	6 (1.42%)	10 (2.37%)
Nunn et al (1975)	170	Yes	5 (2.9%)	4 (2.4%)	9 (5.3%)
DeWeese et al (1971)	187	No	17 (9%)	18 (10%)	35 (19%)

Table 21.3 Neurological deficits after carotid endarterectomy in the presence of a contralateral stenosis or occlusion

Author	Shunt	No. operations	No. and % deficits
Bloodwell et al (1968)	No	92	7 (7.6%)
Baker et al (1977)	No	34	3 (8.8%)
Patterson et al (1974)	Yes	23	0
Thompson et al (1976)	Yes	123	1 (0.8%)
Javid et al (1979)	Yes	94	1 (1%)

Sadly there are few *controlled* studies of the results of carotid endarterectomy, and most publications give only limited follow-up information.

De Weese et al (1973) reviewed 103 patients who had had a carotid endarterectomy at least five years previously. The mortality rate was approximately 10 per cent in the first year, and 5 per cent per year thereafter, so that 66 per cent were alive five years after the operation. Of the 35 patients who died, 25 died of myocardial infarction, 5 of cerebrovascular accidents and 5 of other unrelated causes. Only 10 of the 68 patients still alive had symptoms similar to those experienced before their operation. One patient had developed a severe neurological defect. Thus of the whole group of 103 patients, 78 (77 per cent) were cured of their symptoms and had not had a stroke by the time they died or were reviewed five years later, and only five patients died of stroke. Had the stroke rate been 5 per cent per year the predicted number of fatal strokes would have been 21.

Thompson (1966) reports a long-term follow-up of 151 patients operated on for transient cerebral ischaemia over an eight year period, some with a relatively short follow-up period. Twenty patients died, but only two of these deaths were caused by a stroke; one occurred several weeks after the operation and the other two years after the operation from occlusion of the contralateral carotid artery, which was known to be stenosed at the time of the operation. Of the 129 survivors 88 per cent had no further transient ischaemic attacks, 7 per cent had mild attacks and 2 per cent had strokes.

The figures of these two studies are remarkably similar and although they are not controlled, they certainly suggest that the incidence of stroke after carotid endarterectomy is far less than the 5 per cent per year believed to occur in the unoperated

patient (Whisnant et al, 1973) and suggest that the operation does achieve its prime objective.

Local neck complications

There are a multitude of minor complaints that can follow carotid endarterectomy but few are serious. On rare occasions there may be haemorrhage and false aneurysm formation but this can usually be cured surgically without risk of cerebral damage. Wound infection is a rarity and does not cause a serious problem provided there is no foreign material, such as a dacron patch, within the wound. Wound retractors may occasionally injure the hypoglossal or recurrent laryngeal nerves but the resulting paresis is usually transient. Many patients complain of a patch of numbness on the anterior aspect of the skin of the neck if a cutaneous branch of the cervical plexus has been divided during exposure of the artery. The incidence of complications after 1140 operations (Thompson, 1979) is set out in Table 21.4.

Table 21.4 Local complications of carotid endarterectomy Thompson 1979: 1140 Operations

	No.	%
Haematoma requiring drainage	8	0.7
False aneurysm	7	0.6
Tracheostomy	4	0.35
Wound infection	1	0.09

The general complications associated with all types of surgery are uncommon because the operation is a relatively minor procedure, short in duration (45–60 min), a small amount of trauma and not very painful. Patients are up and about the day after the operation and fit for discharge from hospital two or three days later.

The asymptomatic bruit

If it can be clearly demonstrated that patients with a bruit over the carotid bifurcation and evidence of a significant stenosis of the internal carotid artery have a higher incidence of stroke than a matched control group and if it is accepted that carotid endarterectomy reduces the incidence of stroke in patients with TIAs then it can be argued that asymptomatic bruits should be investigated and treated. At present not all of the information required to make this decision exists. There is some indication suggesting that patients with bruits have an increased risk of stroke and endarterectomy for asymptomatic bruits is already an accepted procedure in many American clinics. It has been claimed that operated patients have fewer strokes in the subsequent years than those treated conservatively but the difference is not great and the two groups are not strictly comparable. Two studies must be performed before surgery for asymptomatic bruits can be generally accepted. First there must be a careful, large, controlled study, with all other risk factors being taken into account, of the natural history of patients with carotid bruits. Then, if the patients with bruits are shown to have a greater incidence of stroke, there must be a long-term randomised controlled study of the effect of surgery. Only if this shows a statistically significant reduction of the incidence of strokes will operations on asymptomatic bruits be justified.

Surgical treatment for disease at the origin of the great vessels

When it was first appreciated that stenosis and/or ulceration in an artery could give rise to emboli it was assumed that it was essential to remove the lesion by endarterectomy. Thus the first operations practised for disease at the origin of the great vessels was open endarterectomy. These vessels lie in the superior mediastinum so the simplest approach to them is through a median sternotomy. This makes the procedure a major operation and all the early series had a high (15–20 per cent) mortality rate whether they were endarterectomies or bypasses from the aorta to the vessels in the neck (Crawford et al, 1969). As a result of this experience most surgeons gave up direct operations on the great vessels within the mediastinum unless there was no other possible approach. Fortunately the majority of patients have at least one patent large artery in the neck which can be used as the donor site for a bypass graft. Thus a healthy patent left common carotid artery can be used as a donor site for a carotid to carotid bypass or more often a carotid to subclavian bypass. The only requirement

for a cervical bypass operation is that the host artery be normal not only between the arch of the aorta and the site of graft attachment but also beyond this point because, if there is a stenosis beyond the take-off point of the graft, there might be preferential flow through the graft and a reduction of flow in the host artery beyond the graft. The introduction of these relatively non-traumatic bypass procedures reduced the mortality rate to 2.5 per cent (Crawford et al, 1969).

There are a variety of cervical bypass operations (Diethrich et al, 1967; DeBakey et al, 1965). The commonest is the left common carotid to the left subclavian bypass because left subclavian stenosis is the commonest site of great vessel disease. However if the left common carotid artery is not healthy then blood can be taken from the right subclavian artery or right common carotid artery, across the neck, to feed the left subclavian artery. Other combinations of bypasses are possible.

The only situation when there is no suitable donor artery within the neck is when the innominate artery is occluded and both the left common carotid and the left subclavian arteries are also diseased. If a cerebral revascularisation operation is indicated in these circumstances an innominate endarterectomy or bypass from the aorta is unavoidable. A bypass is the easier operation because it is simpler to side-clamp the ascending aorta, attach a dacron prosthesis to it, and route it into the neck to one or more of the neck arteries. Endarterectomy of the innominate artery is difficult if the disease extends into the aorta (Thevenet, 1979). It is unusual to have to use a shunt during these procedures but it may be necessary if the artery being operated on is the only source of blood supply to the brain.

Detailed long-term results of large series of these cervical bypass operations are not available but their mortality rate is low (3 per cent) and they appear to stay patent for many years with relief of symptoms. As with carotid endarterectomy there has been no controlled study of any of these operations, so whether they reduce the incidence of subsequent stroke is unknown. Operation seems worthwhile in the left subclavian steal syndrome where painful ischaemia of the digits and claudication of the forearm muscles as well as TIA may be relieved for many years.

Extracranial/intracranial anastomosis

The advent of microvascular surgery has made it possible to join branches of the superficial temporal artery to branches of the middle cerebral artery. Similar procedures have been devised to anastomose occipital to cerebellar arteries. The standard carotid operation has been performed for complete *internal carotid occlusion,* for distal *intracranial carotid stenosis,* and for *proximal middle cerebral occlusion or stenosis.* It may also be used as a preliminary measure in aneurysm or fistula surgery where ligation of the carotid artery may be necessary. The standard carotid operation is a simple procedure involving the dissection of the superficial temporal artery into a narrow pedicle. A small burr hole is made to expose a suitable branch of the middle cerebral artery and an end to side vascular anastomosis is performed with microvascular techniques under the dissecting microscope. The mortality rate for the operation is low (2 to 3 per cent), patency rates are high and cerebral blood flow studies have shown increased regional flow in some cases (Heilbrun et al, 1975).

Although many thousands of these operations have been performed, the indications and results are still difficult to evaluate. The majority of patients have undergone surgery following a TIA, prolonged reversible ischaemic deficit, or minor stroke when angiography has shown one of the arterial lesions listed above. However, the natural history of these conditions is not accurately known. In the case of carotid occlusion a retrospective study indicates a stroke rate of approximately 2 per cent a year (Furlan & Whisnant, 1979) but in the other groups information is not available. In patients with minor stroke, since some cerebral tissue has been infarcted the requirements for blood are reduced and c.b.f. measurements are of little help in assessing the need for revascularisation.

A randomised controlled trial of 1000 patients, followed for an average of five years and specifically designed to answer these questions, is at present in progress and the results should be available by the mid 1980s (Barnett et al 1980). In the meantime a rational approach is to restrict surgery to the much smaller group of patients who have continuing transient focal or general symptoms in the presence of one of the angiographic abnormalities described above. It is then easier in individual patients to judge the efficacy of the operation.

A chronic state of global under-perfusion leading to generalised cerebral dysfunction and to such symptoms as drowsiness, impairment of concentration and intellect or physical and mental lethargy may occasionally be encountered in patients with extensive multiple arterial occlusions. Provided that CT scanning shows that extensive infarction or atrophy is not present, and if extracranial vascular surgery is not feasible, there seem good reasons for transcranial revascularisation in this small group.

REFERENCES

Baker J D, Gluecklick B, Watson C W, Marcus E, Karnet V, Callow A D 1975. An evaluation of electroencephalographic monitoring for carotid surgery. Surgery 78:787–794

Baker W H, Dormer D B 1977. Carotid endarterectomy. Is an indwelling shunt necessary? Surgery 82:321–326

Barnett, H J M, Peerless, S J, McCormick C W 1980. A progress report on the EC/IC Bypass study. Stroke 11:137–40

Bland J E, Chapman R D and Wylie E J 1970. Neurological complications of carotid artery surgery. Annals of Surgery 171:459–464

Bloodwell R D, Hallman G L, Yeats A S, Cooley D A 1968 Carotid endarterectomy without a shunt, results using hypercarbic general anaesthesia to prevent cerebral ischaemia. Archives of Surgery 96:644–652

Boysen G 1973 Cerebral haemodynamics in carotid surgery. Acta Neurologica Scandinavica 49:Suppl. 52

Callow A D, Matsumoto G, Baker D, Cossman D, Watson W 1978 Protection of the high risk carotid endarterectomy patient by continuous electroencephalography. Journal of Cardiovascular Surgery 19:55–64

Connolly, J E, Kwaan J H M and Stemmer E A 1977 Improved results with carotid endarterectomy. Annals of Surgery 186:334–342

Contorni L 1960 Il circulo collaterale vertebro-vertebrale nell' obliteragione dell'arteria subclavia alla sua origine. Minerva Chirurgica 15:268

Crawford E S, DeBakey M E, Morris G C and Cooley D A 1962 Thrombo-obliterative disease of the great vessels arising from the aortic arch. Journal of Thoracic and Cardiovascular Surgery 43:38–53

Crawford E S, DeBakey M E, Morris G C, Howell J F 1969 Surgical treatment of occlusion of the innominate, common carotid and subclavian arteries. A 10 year experience. Surgery 65:17–31

DeBakey M E, Crawford E S, Cooley D A, Morris G C, Garrett H E, Fields W S 1965 Cerebral arterial insufficiency. Annals of Surgery 161:921–945

DeWeese J A, Rob C G, Satran R, Marsh D A, Joynt R J, Summers D and Nichols C 1973 Results of carotid endarterectomies for transient ischaemic attacks — five years later. Annals of Surgery 178:258–263

Diethrich E B, Garrett H E, Americo J, Crawford E S, El-Baya, M DeBakey M E 1967 Occlusive disease of the common carotid subclavian arteries treated by carotid subclavian bypass. Analysis of 125 bypass cases. American Journal of Surgery 114:800–808

Easton J, Sherman D G 1977 Stroke and mortality rate in carotid endarterectomy, 228 consecutive operations. Stroke 8:565–568

Editorial 1961. A new vascular syndrome: The subclavian steal. New England Journal of Medicine 165:912–913

Ehrenfeld W K, Hamilton F N, Larson C P, Hickey R F, Severinghaus J W 1970 Effect of CO_2 and systemic hypertension on downstream cerebral arterial pressure during carotid endarterectomy. Surgery 67:87–96

Furlan A J, Whisnant J P 1979 Long term prognosis following carotid artery occlusion. (Abstract) Stroke 10:105

Harris E J, Brown W H, Davy R N, Anderson W W, Stone D W 1967 Continuous electroencephalographic monitoring during carotid artery endarterectomy. Surgery 62:441–447

Hays R J, Levinson S A, Wylie E J 1972 Intraoperative measurement of carotid back pressure as a guide to operative management for carotid endarterectomy. Surgery 72:953–960

Heilbrum M D, Reichman O H, Anderson R E, Roberts J S 1975 Regional c.b.f. studies following superficial temporal middle cerebral artery anastomosis. Journal of Neurosurgery 43:706–716

Hertzer N R, Beven E G, Greenstreat R L, Humphries A W 1978 Internal carotid back pressure, intraoperative shunting, ulcerated atheromata and the incidence of stroke during carotid endarterectomy. Surgery 83:306–312

Hollenhorst R W 1961 Significance of bright plaques in the retinal arterioles. Journal of American Medical Association 178:23–29

Jacobson I, Bloor K, McDowall D G, Norman J N 1963 Internal carotid endarterectomy at two atmospheres of pressure. Lancet ii:546–548

Javid H, Julian O C, Dye W S, Hunter J A, Najifi H, Goldin M D, Serry C, Delana G A 1979 17 years experience with routine shunting in carotid artery surgery. World Journal of Surgery 3:167–177

Kelly J J, Callow A D, O'Donnell T F, McBride K, Ehrenberg, B Korwin S, Welch H, Gembarowicz M 1979 Failure of carotid stump pressures. Archives of Surgery 114:1361–1366

Kenyon J R, Thomas B W, Goodwin D P 1972 Heparin protection for the brain during carotid artery surgery. Lancet ii:153–154

Palubinskas A J, Perloff D, Newton T H 1966 Fibromuscular hyperplasia. An arterial dysplasia of increasing clinical importance. American Journal of Roetgenology 98:907–913

Patterson R H 1974 Risk of carotid surgery with occlusion of the contralateral carotid artery. Archives of Neurology 30:188–189

Ross Russell R W 1961 Observations on the retinal blood vessels in monocular blindness. Lancet ii:1422–1428

Thevenet A 1979 Surgical management of atheroma of the aortic dome and origin of supra aortic trunks. World Journal of Surgery 3:187–195

Thompson J E 1979 Complications of Carotid Endarterectomy and their prevention. World Journal of Surgery 3:155–165

Thompson J E, Katchner M M, Austin D J, Wheeling G G, Patman R D 1966 Carotid endarterectomy for cerebrovascular insufficiency. Follow up of 359 cases. Annals of Surgery 163:751–762

Toole J F, Janeway R, Choid K, Cordell R, Davis C, Johnston F, Miller H S 1975. Transient ischaemic attacks due to atherosclerosis. A prospective study of 160 patients. Archives of Neurology 32:5–12

Whisnant J P, Natsumato N, Elveback L R 1973 Transient ischaemic attacks in a community. Mayo Clinic Proceedings 48:194–198

Youmans J R, Kindt G W 1968 Efficacy of carbon dioxide in the treatment of cerebral ischaemia. Surgical Forum 19:425–429

22

Vascular diseases of the spinal cord

Malcolm Parsons

Clinical, radiological and pathological studies have disproved but not dispelled the traditional belief that vascular lesions of the cord are rare and that they are usually caused by syphilitic thrombosis of the anterior spinal artery. Syphilis and thrombosis of the anterior spinal artery are indeed rare but other vascular lesions are surprisingly common and their development and characteristics depend to a large extent on the anatomy of the blood supply of the spinal cord.

ANATOMY

The blood supply of the spinal cord is derived from the anterior and posterior spinal arteries and their radicular tributaries (Fig. 22.1). The *anterior spinal* is formed from branches of the vertebral arteries which unite somewhere above the 5th cervical segment, usually just beyond their point of origin. It runs the length of the cord in the anterior median fissure anastomosing with the posterior spinal arteries distally. In the embryo the artery is joined at every level by *radicular vessels* which lie on the anterior aspect of segmental nerves. Less than eight continue to make a significant contribution to the blood supply of the cord in adult life and their distribution is unpredictable. The most constant are the arteria magna of Adamkiewicz which usually lie on the left between T8 and L1, and vessels in the lower cervical and lower lumbar regions (Zulch & Kurth-Schumacher, 1970). On reaching the cord these vessels divide into ascending and descending branches which, by anastomosing with those above and below, form the anterior spinal artery. As these anastomoses are often far from perfect, the artery does not always

run an uninterrupted course and individual radicular vessels may be largely if not entirely responsible for the blood supply to long sections of the cord. Radiological studies have confirmed that there is an upward and downward flow in each segment towards the interface with the next (di Chiro & Fried, 1971).

The *posterior spinal* arteries are branches of the vertebral or posterior inferior cerebellar arteries. Smaller than the anterior spinal they remain separate and run on the posterior aspect of the cord medial to the dorsal roots. Their tributaries from the dorsal roots are also smaller but they are more numerous and there may be more than 20. The anterior and posterior spinal arteries unite in the sacral region and it has been shown that blood flows up the posterior spinal vessels in the distal part of the cord — i.e., that they are fed below by the anterior spinal artery (di Chiro & Fried, 1971).

The *central arteries* which run backwards from the anterior spinal into the anterior median fissure have been the subject of detailed microangiographic studies (Turnbull et al, 1966; Hassler, 1966). In the cervical and lumbar regions there may be eight or more per centimetre but in the thoracic region there may only be two in the same distance. Most only branch to one side and it is unusual for two consecutive vessels to branch in the same direction. These are end-arteries and there are no anastomoses but there is a considerable overlap between the territories of adjacent vessels (Fig. 22.2).

Within the pia lies a *coronal plexus* which branches into the surface of the cord to supply the substantia gelatinosa, a rim of white matter, part of the certicospinal tracts and much of the posterior columns. There is a considerable overlap between

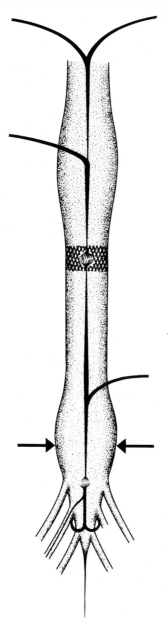

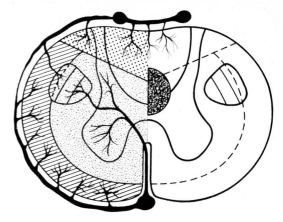

Fig. 22.2 The periphery of the cord is supplied by coronal vessels which do not form an effective anastomosis between the anterior and posterior spinal systems. The posterior spinal arteries supply the posterior third of the cord, and the remainder is supplied by central branches of the anterior spinal. The superficial fibres in the pyramidal tract, which supply the leg, are at the periphery of the anterior spinal territory and may be damaged in cervical spondylosis. If flow in all three systems is impaired e.g., by a dissecting aneurysm a central 'pencil' infarct (marked in black) may be found where their terminal branches meet.

enters coronal vessels which drain into posterior spinal veins, the disposition of which is very variable. Anteriorly, the lateral aspect of each half of the cord drains into coronal vessels, while the medial aspect is served by the central and anterior median veins. Radicular veins, like radicular arteries, are more numerous posteriorly, but the two do not run together (Gillilan, 1970).

APPLIED ANATOMY

The diverse and unpredictable manifestations of ischaemia of the spinal cord depend in large measure on the disposition of vessels and the presence or absence of a collateral circulation in the individual concerned. The *cervical region* is well protected for it receives blood from both vertebrals above and from various branches of the subclavian below. So good is this collateral circulation that it may be sufficient to bypass the stenosis in coarctation of the aorta, dilating until the cord is threatened by the very size of the vessels concerned. (Darwish et al, 1979).

The relatively small area supplied by the *posterior spinal artery* is also well protected for the twin vessels receive numerous tributaries. Infarcts caus-

Fig. 22.1 The anterior spinal artery is formed from branches of the vertebral arteries. It consists of a chain of vessels, often incompletely united, that anastomoses distally with the posterior spinal arteries. Vessels in this chain are supplied by radicular arteries, the number and position of which vary. The most important are the arteria magna of Adamkiewicz, which lies in the area of the diaphragm, (arrow) and vessels in the cervical and lumbar regions.

the territory supplied by the central and peripheral systems but the two are not directly connected (Turnbull et al, 1966).

Venous blood from the posterior half of the cord

ing segmental anaesthesia and areflexia with loss of deep sensation peripherally have, however, been described. (Hughes, 1970). In the distal part of the cord, where the posterior spinal arteries are perfused from below, lesions which impair the flow in the anterior spinal can cause a full thickness infarct. (Ferguson et al, 1975).

Below the cervical region sections of the anterior spinal artery which are isolated from those above and below may depend on a single radicular vessel for their supply, the coronal arteries being too slender to provide an effective anastomosis with the posterior spinal system. Occlusion of such radicular arteries can cause infarction of the anterior two-thirds of the cord including the pyramidal and spinothalamic tracts and the anterior horn cells. The upper limit of these infarcts is often far above the causative lesion, for radicular vessels divide into ascending and descending branches and damage will be most severe at the periphery of the territory involved. The boundary between the arteria magna and the vessel which supplies the upper thoracic cord is particularly vulnerable in this respect and ligation of an artery near the diaphragm sometimes causes transection of the cord at the 4th thoracic level (Fig. 22.1).

When the supply from several radicular arteries is reduced simultaneously as by a dissecting aneurysm *'watershed' infarcts* occur in depth as well as in length. At the interface described extensive destruction will occur but in adjacent areas there may be a central 'pencil' of necrosis. This is thought to represent the boundary between the central, coronal and posterior spinal arteries which, though able to prevent infarction near their points of origin, are unable to maintain an adequate circulation at the periphery of their territories. (Zulch & Kurth-Schumacher, 1970) (Fig. 22.2).

A *Brown Séquard syndrome* has been attributed to occlusion of a central artery for these vessels usually branch to one or other side of the cord (Rouques & Passelecq, 1957). Collateral circulation is impossible because these are end arteries but the territory they supply overlaps to such an extent that occlusion is usually silent. Such lesions may also be responsible for unilateral infarction of the posterior horn in the 'watershed' between the central and posterior spinal arteries (Zulch & Kurth-Schumacher, 1970).

ISCHAEMIC LESIONS

It is difficult to give a simple but accurate account of ischaemia of the spinal cord, for much of the information about this neglected subject comes from reports dealing with one or two patients, and the lesions observed were often caused by the interaction of two or more factors (e.g., stenosis and hypotension). To facilitate discussions the following topics will be considered:

Thrombosis
Emboli
Occlusion of radicular arteries
Iatrogenic lesions
Transient ischaemic attacks
'Intermittent claudication' of the cord
Chronic ischaemia
Venous thrombosis

Thrombosis

Thrombosis of the anterior spinal artery is widely regarded as the commonest cause of ischaemia of the spinal cord. Like thrombosis of the central arteries it is a serious condition for collaterals cannot provide an alternative blood supply. Even so the extent of the damage in reported cases is often out of all proportion to the vascular occlusion demonstrated, and with the disappearance of syphilis it has been suggested that thrombosis of the anterior spinal artery is a rare event (Garland et al, 1966). This accords with the finding of moderate or severe atheroma in the spinal vessels in 2.2 per cent of 1037 unselected autopsies when macroscopically detectable atheroma of the cerebral vessels was present in 39.3 per cent (Jellinger, 1967).

Stenosis of central and radicular vessels was even less common and the cord is usually spared when the aorta is occluded because of the development of a collateral circulation or because the thrombosis lies below the main radicular vessels. Thus Szilagyi et al (1978) did not encounter any neurological problems among 1089 patients with aortic thrombosis whereas eight of their 1724 patients with dissecting aneurysms became paraplegic. When, as sometimes happens, a paraplegic is found to have aortic occlusion it often transpires that the cord and the aorta were both damaged by emboli arising elsewhere (Cook, 1959). However, myelopathy due to thrombosis of vessels in or near the cord has been described in a variety of infections, collagen diseases and haematological or general medical disorders. These are listed in Table 22.1 but cannot

Table 22.1 Causes of thrombosis of spinal vessels

Infections
Syphilis (Adams & Merritt, 1944)
Tuberculous and pyogenic meningitis (Hughes, 1965)
Epidural abscesses (Grant, 1945)
Zoster (Hughes, 1965)
Schistosomiasis (Siddorn, 1978)
Trichiniasis (Barr, 1966)
Malaria (Reichert et al, 1934)

Collagen diseases
Disseminated lupus (Kewalramani et al, 1978)
Polyarteritis (Thenabadu et al, 1970)

Haematological disorders
Polycythaemia (Grunberg 1950)
Myeloma (Schott Cotte & Tommasi 1959)
Macroglobulinaemia (Peters et al, 1968)
Sickle cell trait (Wolman & Hardy, 1970; Ahmann et al, 1975)

General medical disorders
Diabetes (Ruhberg & Noble 1941)
Pregnancy (Barre & d'Andrade, 1938)
Sarcoid (Aszkanazy, 1952; Day & Sypert, 1977)
Radiotherapy (Judice et al, 1978)

be discussed in the space available. The accounts of myelopathy appearing during the treatment of a primary syphilitic infection (Lindemulder, 1931) in drug addicts (Judice et al, 1978) and in patients with a sickle cell trait are of particular interest.

Emboli

In 1882 Bastian drew an analogy between softening of the brain and softening of the cord, saying that 'far too large a share was attributed to inflammation' in the aetiology of myelopathy. Developing this idea he suggested that infarction was usually due to thrombosis and that 'emboli occurred with great rarity and were still more rarely recognised' because the vessels concerned were small subsidiary branches. Subsequent events have confirmed the importance of ischaemic lesions but suggest that it is emboli and not thrombi which are common.

Paraplegia due to emboli has been observed in a variety of disorders. Occlusion of the aorta in a patient with *rheumatic heart disease* and evidence of emboli elsewhere was described by Cook (1959).

In a similar patient with *subacute bacterial endocarditis* organisms were grown from the blood, the heart and the infarct (Harrington, 1925). Paraplegia due to emboli from an *atrial myxoma* has also been described on several occasions (Hirose et al, 1979) and infarction due to *cholesterol emboli* from an atheromatous aorta is well authenticated (Laguna & Craviota, 1973). The mechanism whereby fragments of *fibrocartilage* from the nucleus pulposus occasionally enter and occlude spinal arteries and/or veins has been discussed by Hubert et al (1974). Sudden paraplegia may also be caused by minor surgical procedures. Thus Wikler et al (1937) reported a transient Brown Séquard syndrome in a patient who evidently had *air emboli* and collapsed during an unsuccessful attempt to induce an artificial pneumothorax. More recently Gang et al (1977) found fragments of *gelatine sponge* in the spinal arteries of a patient with a renal carcinoma who became paraplegic after therapeutic embolisation of renal artery had been attempted.

The paraplegia of *decompression sickness* is also partly attributable to (nitrogen) emboli. Discussing this condition in the 1881 Croonian lecture Moxon noted that 30 of the 352 men working on one pier of the Mississippi bridge at St Louis were seriously affected, and that 12 died. Transient painless paraplegia was first reported by those who had been working at 60 ft and below that level there was an increase in the duration and severity of episodes, with involvement of the arms and sphincters. Obese people, new recruits and those who work for more than two hours are most vulnerable. Fifty per cent develop symptoms within two hours, and 90 per cent within 12 hours.

To explain his observations Moxon envisaged an increase in the cerebral blood flow to compensate for the rise in atmospheric pressure. This, he supposed, displaced spinal fluid into the canal where it compressed the arterioles of the cord. 'So overmuch activity of the cerebral circulation "he wrote" would tend . . . to interfere with the straight and narrow economy of the unfortunate end of the spinal cord. I think this is why very studious people get so delicate about the caudal end of their spinal cords'. Now it is known that bubbles of nitrogen are released into the blood, tissues and spinal fluid and act as emboli these ideas seem amusing, but Moxon did attempt to explain why 77 per cent of the neurological lesions are in the cord whereas a purely embolic disorder would primarily affect the brain. In fact the paraplegia is thought to be due to the release of gas bubbles in the spinal cord and experimental studies by Hallenbeck et al (1975) suggest that venous infarction due to obstruction of the vertebral plexus may occur.

This lucid account of decompression sickness and the circumstances under which it occurs has not prevented subsequent outbreaks, for during the building of the Budapest metro more than 100 cases were reported (Rozsahegyi, 1959). Indeed the number of people at risk is almost certainly rising for apart from naval and commercial divers there are now thought to be two million scuba divers (Strauss & Prockop, 1973). Flying at high altitudes can produce similar symptoms and flying after diving is particularly dangerous. The incidence of the condition obviously varies with the circumstances but 10 of the 20 divers questioned by Peters et al (1977) had had at least one episode in the previous two years and in four there was objective evidence of damage to the spinal cord.

Radicular arteries

Occlusion of a radicular artery on which a section of the cord depends for its blood supply is the commonest cause of an ischaemic myelopathy. Such episodes may be due to illness or injury, or may be iatrogenic. Thus, two of the 80 patients reported in one of the earliest papers on *dissecting aneurysms of the aorta* were paraplegic (Leonard, 1979). This figure accords with a recent estimate of 4 per cent (Leonard & Hasleton, 1979) but in a series described by Crawford et al (1970) 10 per cent of the patients had had transient weakness in the legs. In *herpes zoster*, where the basic lesion is infarction of the dorsal root ganglion, a patient may become paraplegic if the thrombus spreads to involve a major radicular vessel which happens to lie at the same level (Hughes, 1965). Paraplegia due to thrombosis of a radicular artery traversing a *psoas abscess* has also been reported (Hughes, 1965).

Spondylosis and scoliosis

The importance of ischaemia in the pathogenesis of the myelopathy associated with *cervical spondy-*

losis is debatable. According to Chakravorty (1969) the lower part of the cervical cord is supplied by vessels which enter between C4 and C6 (Fig. 22.1) — the levels at which degenerative changes are most common. These arteries are constricted by thickening of the peridural tissues in which they lie and the consequent ischaemia gradually causes loss of function of the cord which initially is reversible. A reduced flow in the anterior spinal artery accounts for the occasional finding of wasting of the small muscles of the hands, supplied by the first thoracic segment at the lower extremity of the territory perfused. It also explains why the legs are more severely affected than the arms, for fibres to the lower limbs lie on the outside of the pyramidal tracts at the periphery of the territory supplied by the central branches of the anterior spinal artery (Fig. 22.2). Foraminal decompression of roots and removal of the peridural fibrous tissue should relieve symptoms by restoring the blood supply, but this technique appears to be less impressive in practice than in theory.

Disc lesions at lower levels in the spine can also cause an ischaemic myelopathy. The paraplegia so easily precipitated by manipulation of the cord during operations on prolapsed *thoracic discs* is almost certainly produced in this way, for the sensory level may lie several segments above the point of compression (Logue, 1952 Case 11). Although it barely reaches the lumbar spine, the cord can also be damaged by a prolapsed *lumbar disc* in the condition known as *sciatique paralysante*. Here sciatic pain of exceptional severity is suddenly replaced — usually within days — by profound weakness and wasting. This has been attributed to compression of a radicular artery which, instead of supplying the trapped root alone as is usually the case, extends to supply the cord (Fig. 22.1). As a result the patient may also develop spasticity, loss of sphincter control and other evidence of cord damage for which a prolapsed disc far below the conus could not be directly responsible (de Sèze et al, 1957).

Paraplegia sometimes appears after operations to straighten the spine, and the *scoliosis* research society heard of 77 such incidents in 1970. The speed with which this weakness appears suggests that it is due to ischaemia, and preoperative angiograms show that a single artery supplies the cord between T4 and L2 in 25 per cent of patients. The importance of protecting this vessel cannot be over-emphasised (Hilal & Keim, 1972).

Tumours

The blood supply of the cord may be impaired by tumours in and around the spine; false localising signs and paraplegia which cannot be attributed to compression are often explicable on this basis. Thus Symonds & Meadows (1937) described wasting in the small muscles of the hands in patients with tumours near the foramen magnum, a finding that may be due to compression of the origin of the anterior spinal artery causing ischaemia in the distal part of the territory. Conversely Carrott et al (1959) noted a spastic paraplegia, loss of sphincter control and a level at the 10th thoracic segment in a patient with a meningioma compressing the first lumbar root. In this case the artery in question evidently ascended to supply the lower part of the cord. The tumour responsible for the paraplegia may lie outside the cord (Pennybacker, 1958) and in some cases the lesion is due to venous as opposed to arterial occlusion (Barron et al, 1959).

Trauma

Post-traumatic paraplegia may also be ischaemic in origin. Hughes (1964) reported a 62 year old woman who walked away from a road traffic accident in which she sustained fractured ribs and a haemothorax on the left. Four days later she became paraplegic. A myelogram was normal and it transpired that upper intercostal arteries were being compressed by a clot just below the subclavian artery where the wall of the aorta was torn. False localising signs may appear at the periphery of the ascending branch, as in a man with a fracture dislocation at T11/12 and a sensory level at T5 (Schneider & Crosby, 1959). Impaired flow in the proximal part of the anterior spinal artery could also account for the cord lesions reported in six children, born after difficult breech deliveries, who each had a paraplegia and a sensory level in the upper thoracic region (Ford, 1925). Neurological findings associated with atlanto-axial dislocation may be explained in the same way (Backs et al,

1955). Conversely, it has been suggested that the patient who becomes paraplegic after injury to the abdominal aorta sometimes has an ischaemic peripheral neuropathy as opposed to a myelopathy. In such cases weakness appears gradually, the patient complains of painful paraesthesia, all modalities of sensation are impaired, but the prognosis is good (Mozingo & Denton, 1975).

The injuries that cause ischaemic myelopathy are not necessarily severe. A 70 year old patient described by Hughes & Brownell (1964) was merely getting dressed when she suddenly developed pain in the neck and shoulders followed, within 24 hours, by tetraplegia. In this instance the anterior spinal artery thrombosis responsible was precipitated by serious cervical spondylosis, but there was nothing to account for an identical lesion in a 15 year old boy who felt his neck 'click' after yawning and stretching (Grinker & Guy, 1927). Such a lesion has even been reported in a two year old child four hours after being 'cuffed' on the face (Ahmann et al, 1975). There seems indeed to be a syndrome, precipitated by minor injury, in which infarction of the cord causes symptoms in the arms followed by weakness in the legs, sphincter paralysis and respiratory failure.

Iatrogenic paraplegia

As surgical, radiological and anaesthetic techniques become more complicated the incidence of iatrogenic paraplegia has increased. It has been reported after the repair of injuries caused by a machete (Henson & Parsons, 1967) and as a (bewildering) complication of various operations on the chest including thoracotomy for carcinoma of the bronchus (Thomas & Dwyer, 1950), thoracoplasty (Rouques et al, 1957) and sympathectomy (Hughes & MacIntyre, 1963). In such patients infarction is due to the fortuitous ligation of an intercostal artery on which a section of the cord depends for its blood supply.

Paraplegia after operations on the aorta is more common and more comprehensible. Operations on the abdominal aorta were once thought to be relatively safe for the arteria magna usually arises well above the level at which the clamp is applied, but when Szilagyi and his colleagues reviewed the subject in 1978, 44 cases of paraplegia due to such operations had been reported. The eight patients in their own series of 3164 were all in a sub-group of 1724 who had aneurysms and 83 per cent of those reported elsewhere had similar lesions. Operations on the thoracic aorta are obviously more hazardous and in several (relatively short) series the incidence of paraplegia has ranged from 0 to 17.6 per cent. Reviewing the subject in 1970, Crawford et al quoted a personal figure of 6.8 per cent. Emergency procedures on dissecting aneurysms in hypotensive patients are even more dangerous and increase the risk of paraplegia tenfold (Szilagyi et al, 1978). In aortic surgery success depends above all on the preservation of the important radicular vessels.

As it is important to preserve these vessels and impossible to predict their position, it seems logical to do angiograms before operating. Unfortunately such X-rays rarely provide information which is of practical value and, being time-consuming and potentially dangerous, they are not done as a routine. Instead reliance is placed on general measures to safeguard the blood supply of the cord. In particular the aorta is clamped as low down as possible to avoid the arteria magna and is manipulated gently to prevent the release of cholesterol emboli. Hypotension is avoided and the clamp released within 30 or at most 45 minutes. Shunts do not seem to be of value but there is general agreement that radicular vessels should be preserved or, if necessary, ligated well away from the aorta. The value of grafting vessels which have to be sacrificed on to the aorta is debatable (Crawford et al, 1970; Szilagyi et al, 1978).

Despite these precautions a few patients — notably those with extensive dissection or an arteria magna which arises at an exceptionally low level — do become paraplegic. Few of those whose legs are completely paralysed show any sign of improvement and 70 per cent soon die. Half of those in whom the paraplegia is incomplete make a full recovery (Szilagyi et al, 1970).

Anaesthesia

Paraplegia is a rare but recognised complication of intercostal blocks and of spinal and epidural anaesthesia but many of the episodes reported were due to the toxic nature of drugs no longer used.

The development of permanent paraplegia in an ambulant patient immediately after the injection of efocaine to produce an *intercostal block* was described by Moore (1954). The drug — which is corrosive and can cause cellulitis and sloughing — is thought to have reached the cord via the intercostal vessels (Angerer et al, 1953).

Ischaemic myelopathy appearing some time after a *spinal anaesthetic* was reported by Brain & Russell in 1937. This is a controversial subject for although Dripps et al (1954) gave over 10 000 such anaesthetics without mishap, there is a risk of paraplegia. Some substances are more dangerous than others and the concentration of the drug is probably more important than the quantity used (Payne & Bergentz, 1956). The contention that the onset of paraplegia in two patients on a single theatre list was due to phenol seeping into ampoules in which the anaesthetic was stored was attacked by Walshe after a well known High Court case (Macintosh, 1956; Walshe, 1956). Complications have also been attributed to detergents used to wash syringes (Wolman, 1966). Paraplegia after an *epidural anaesthetic* may develop insidiously or abruptly. The volume of anaesthetic used is much larger than that required for a spinal (500 as against 40 ml) and the gradual onset of paraplegia, which is associated with dense arachnoiditis, has been attributed to leakage into the subarachnoid space (Braham & Saia, 1958). Paraplegia which appears suddenly is associated with necrosis in the territory of the anterior spinal artery. It is not caused by adhesions or thrombosis and has been attributed to hypotension or to the effects of adrenalin (Davies et al, 1958).

Radiography

The neurological complications of aortography range in severity from spasm in the muscles of the legs through transient and permanent paraplegia to death. Such cases were first reported in 1949, 20 years after the introduction of the technique, by which time accidental damage to other organs was well known. It is hard to tell how often spinal cord symptoms, which usually appear during the investigation of non-neurological disorders, occur. By 1965 Hughes was aware of 43 cases and in one series of 17 494 examinations serious complications occurred in 0.5 per cent and the cord was damaged twice (Szilagyi et al, 1978). However, Mishkin (1973) heard of five cases of paraplegia with two deaths in that year and is almost certainly correct in believing that the overall incidence is much higher.

The paraplegia may be due to the manipulation and position of the catheter or to the toxic effects of the contrast medium. *Injection of contrast into the theca* is particularly dangerous. This seemingly improbable accident can occur in various ways. One radiologist aspirated clear fluid (c.s.f.) while doing an aortogram on an obese patient with a non-functioning left kidney. Thinking he had entered a hydronephrosis he then injected 30 ml of hypaque. The patient developed spasms and died within 45 minutes (Doroshow et al, 1962). Another, seeking the vertebral artery in a patient who had had a subarachnoid haemorrhage, was misled by blood stained c.s.f. aspirated from a root pocket (McCleery & Lewtas, 1963). Faced with such an emergency these authors recommend sitting the patient up, draining off the c.s.f. and irrigating the subarachnoid space from a cisternal puncture with normal saline. A tracheotomy should be done and relaxants should be given if spasms develop as they often do after 30 minutes. Patients who have had a subarachnoid haemorrhage should be given a hypotensive if the blood pressure rises but short-acting drugs should be selected because the rise is often transient.

Passing a catheter up an atheromatous aorta produces *cholesterol emboli* (Harrington & Amplatz, 1972). Patients often complain of pain in the legs and back and develop livedo reticularis at the level of the lesion. The tip of the catheter may also *penetrate the inner wall* of the aorta. To some extent this accident is unavoidable and in one series of 425 patients it happened in 42, three of whom died. Films taken after a small exploratory injection will usually show what has occurred and prevent the confusion which arises when massive dissection and obstruction of the aorta is caused by the investigation and not by the disease (Boblitt et al, 1959).

The *contrast medium* itself can cause a paraplegia because it is toxic, because the patient is allergic to it or because an excessive amount reaches the cord. The drugs are all dangerous in high concentration

but the most toxic ones have been withdrawn. The relevance of *allergy* is debatable. Kardjiev et al (1974) did not think it was important for their five patients had all had uneventful bronchial arteriograms. By contrast Szilagyi et al (1978) could only account for the paraplegia that sometimes appeared after the injection of a modest amount of contrast on the basis of a hypersensitivity reaction.

Inadequate dilution of an otherwise satisfactory substance is potentially dangerous but most incidents seem to occur when an *excessive amount* of an acceptable preparation enters an important radicular vessel. The drug may be accidentally injected directly into the artery during cerebral, bronchial or mediastinal angiography. Alternatively it may go preferentially into the spinal circulation because of occlusion of vessels, compression of the abdomen by a support, vasoconstrictors given to improve opacification of visceral arteries or suspension of respiration while X-rays are taken cause it to linger in the aorta. A supine position which leaves the mouths of the vessels on the 'floor' of the aorta and repeated injections which cause them to dilate may aggravate the situation (Margolis, 1970; Kardjiev et al, 1977; Ramirez Lassepas et al, 1977). In toxic paraplegia the lesion is usually in the thoracolumbar region but injury to the cervical cord has been reported (Ramirez Lassepas et al, 1977). Little is known about treatment but if spasms appear in the legs during angiography the procedure should be stopped and diazepam injected into the catheter (Szilagyi et al, 1978). The c.s.f., which may be xanthochromic, contains an excess of iodine and by sitting the patient up and replacing it with isotonic saline damage may be minimised (Mishkin et al, 1973). The prognosis is uncertain but paraplegia is likely to be permanent in those who have a flaccid paraplegia while those who only have spasms usually recover.

Intrathecal injections

Paraplegia due to arterial or venous thrombosis can occur after a variety of intrathecal injections. Apart from the anaesthetics and contrast media already mentioned, minute amounts of *methylene blue* used to trace leakage of c.s.f. can cause necrosis of the spinal cord in susceptible individuals. In the opinion of Sharr et al (1975) the technique should be abandoned. Thrombosis of the anterior and of the posterior spinal arteries may occur after the intrathecal injection of *phenol* to relieve intractable pain (Totoki et al, 1979; Hughes, 1970) and anterior spinal artery thrombosis has been reported after the use of phenol to produce a stellate ganglion block (Sovak et al, 1975). *Alcohol* and certain *antibiotics* are also potentially dangerous as Wolman (1966) explained in an extensive review of the subject.

Transient ischaemic attacks and intermittent claudication

Ischaemia of the spinal cord, like cerebral ischaemia, may cause *transient* symptoms. These can occur in isolation or as a prelude to infarction. The pathogenesis of such episodes is debatable but many are attributed to emboli which fragment. The opening of collaterals after occlusion of a vessel may also be significant but occlusion of the anterior spinal artery and its branches could not be circumvented in this way. The adverse effect of hypotension and nicotine (Buskirk & Davidson, 1960) and the relief of symptoms with large doses of hydergine and aminophylline (Zulch & Kurth-Schumacher, 1970) suggest that the temporary inability of diseased vessels to sustain an adequate flow is sometimes responsible.

Defective perfusion is certainly responsible for Dejerine's *intermittent claudication of the spinal cord.* At rest, these patients have no symptoms, but during exertion one or both legs become 'weak' and 'heavy', signs of spasticity appear and control of the sphincters may be lost. By degrees the patients' exercise tolerance decreases and ultimately, more or less abruptly, many become paraplegic. Dejerine's patients had syphilitic arteritis and responded to appropriate treatment but contemporary cases are usually attributed to degenerative changes in the blood vessels. (Zulch & Kurth-Schumacher, 1970).

Unlike 'ordinary' intermittent claudication, intermittent claudication of the spinal cord rarely causes discomfort. A form which affects the posterior aspect causing violent pain of the type seen in tabes has however been described (Bergmark, 1950). Characteristically it also differs in that the peripheral circulation is good — a fact which Bergmark confirmed with oscillography in his first case. However, it is to be expected that some patients with vascular disease severe enough to impair the function of the cord will have a poor blood supply to the lower limbs. Intermittent claudication of the cord must also be distinguished from *intermittent claudication of the cauda equina* (Blau & Logue, 1961). This condition is thought to be due to stenosis of the spinal canal which causes ischaemia in the lumbosacral roots during exertion by preventing dilation of vessels on their surfaces. Most patients have some evidence of a cauda equina lesion and develop a (potentially painful) numbness or burning that spreads over the surface of the limbs when they walk. Simultaneously reflexes, which in claudication of the cord become more active, disappear. Theoretically it is easy to distinguish between this condition and 'ordinary' intermittent claudication but defective peripheral circulation in the former, and wasting and a tendency for cramps to spread from calf to thigh in the latter can cause confusion. In such patients contrast studies may be required.

Chronic ischaemia

In 1881 Gowers suggested that the insidious development of paraplegia in elderly patients might sometimes be due to chronic ischaemia of the spinal cord. This idea has never been widely recognised but has been amply confirmed. After studying 26 patients of this sort Jellinger & Neumayer (1962) and Hughes & Brownell (1966) reached almost identical conclusions. Patients are over the age of 65, have severe aortic disease and present with a para or tetraplegia. Some subsequently develop wasting, fasciculation, areflexia and impairment of bladder function but sensation is usually intact. On average they survive for three years but some live ten and others die within months. The cord and anterior roots are wasted and there are degenerative changes in the anterior and lateral columns with patchy cavitation in the grey matter. The anterior spinal artery is intact. Similar signs, which resolved after treatment with chlorambucil, were reported in a 63 year old man with macroglobulinaemia (Peters & Clatanoff, 1968) but this cause of 'motor neurone disease' seems unfortunately to be exceptional.

Venous thrombosis

For the sake of simplicity diseases of the spinal veins can be considered under the headings of subacute necrotic myelitis, the effects of compression and 'true' thrombosis.

Subacute necrotic myelitis (Mair & Folkerts, 1953) is mentioned merely to exclude it for the slowly progressing paraplegia, loss of sphincter control and impairment of sensation seen in this condition are caused by an arteriovenous malformation. This lesion, which is often mistaken for a venous thrombosis, causes spinal necrosis by altering the haemodynamics of the blood supply of the cord.

The importance of *venous stasis* in the pathogenesis of paraplegia associated with intraspinal masses must not be overlooked. Writing about metastatic lesions Barron et al (1959) observed that 'simple direct pressure is not the whole answer nor do the usual lesions appear to be the result of arterial occlusion'. Pathological studies showed sparing of the grey matter and an 'oedematous type of malacia distinct from infarction — and more consistent with impairment of the venous return'. Gillilan (1970) makes the same observation about the myelopathy associated with cervical spondylosis.

Massive *thrombosis* of the veins of the spinal cord which presents with back pain quickly followed by paraplegia, loss of sphincter control and impairment of sensation is an uncommon but devastating event. It has been described in association with polycythaemia (Grunberg et al, 1950), various infections, spinal tumours and a clotting tendency due to the presence of a pancreatic tumour (Hughes, 1971). The poor prognosis is easily understood in the light of the vast haemorrhagic infarct extending over 15 consecutive segments which was found in the last of these patients.

HYPOTENSION

Experimental studies have shown that by reducing the blood pressure, animals in which certain radicular vessels have been ligated can be rendered paraplegic (Mosberg et al, 1954). Hypotension can also produce symptoms of cord ischaemia in man. A patient described by Wells (1966) became paraplegic when his hypertension was treated, recovering 'when his blood pressure was allowed to soar' and one described by Reichert et al (1934)

developed intermittent claudication of the spinal cord whenever his blood pressure fell. Severe haemorrhage (Levy & Strauss, 1942) coronary thrombosis, cardiac arrest and arrhythmias (Silver & Buckston, 1974) have also been incriminated, and in some patients a combination of factors seems to be responsible. Thus a patient described by Albert et al (1969) had a vagotomy (which might have damaged a spinal tributary) and later became paraplegic after a coronary thrombosis. The phenomenon is not confined to elderly arteriopaths for in intensive care units 'it is not uncommon to see evidence of cord disease in many young people who have been unconscious for some time after an overdose' (Lancet, 1974) and Gilles & Nag (1971) have reported six cases of myelopathy due to hypotension in infancy.

HAEMORRHAGE

Haemorrhages in the spine like those in the head may be extradural, subdural, subarachnoid or in the substance of the neuraxis. Both may be spontaneous or traumatic and spontaneous haemorrhages at both sites are often caused by vascular malformations. But the analogy ends there for within the skull the delicate unsupported veins which run from the brain to the sagittal sinus rupture readily to produce a subdural haematoma. The subdural veins in the cord are barely visible. Conversely extradural vessels in the skull are held firmly between the dura and the bone and protected from all but the most violent injuries. In the spine the mass of thin-walled poorly supported veins in the extradural space (Batson's plexus) is easily damaged and the most common haemorrhagic disorder is an extradural haematoma.

Extradural spinal haematomas usually occur in adults who present with severe back pain followed within hours by paraplegia and loss of sphincter control. The clinical picture is very variable and there are reports of children with haematomas, of painless lesions, of lesions causing hemisection of the cord or a radiculopathy and of the patients in whom symptoms took months to develop (Robertson et al, 1979; Senelick et al, 1976; Fosselle et al, 1978; Devadega et al, 1973). Predisposing factors such as hypertension or a haemorrhagic diathesis can often be identified and about 30 per cent of the patients reported were taking anticoagulants. In some the haemorrhage was evidently precipitated by twisting or trauma, including lumbar puncture and epidural anaesthesia, (de Angelis, 1972) or by straining as in labour and whooping cough. In others the illness appears to have started spontaneously during sleep. The definitive investigation is myelography which reveals the lesion in more than 90 per cent (Packer & Cummins, 1978) and decompression is a matter of urgency for the response depends on the speed with which this is done. Thus after six months McQuarrie (1978) found that 15 of the 29 patients operated on within three and a half days were walking whereas the six treated at a later stage made no recovery. Patients with haemophilia, who do not seem to respond to surgery, pose a formidable problem. Purely medical treatment may be more effective (Harvie et al, 1977).

Subdural haematomas which produce symptoms are rare for the subdural vessels are small and, unlike those in the brain, are not exposed to damage as they cross the subarachnoid space (Edelson et al, 1974). It has even been argued that subdural haematomas are merely a complication of subarachnoid haemorrhage (see below). Most patients have a defective clotting mechanism as a result of anticoagulant treatment, haemophilia or, more frequently, thrombocytopenia secondary to malignancy and many have had several lumbar punctures. Lumbar puncture should therefore be avoided in thrombocytopenia unless there is a strong indication. It should certainly be avoided if the platelet count is below 20 000 cu mm or is falling rapidly, unless platelets can be given just before the procedure. In any case the puncture must be done as neatly as possible using a small needle and the patient must subsequently be kept under careful observation (Dunn et al, 1979). The literature gives no clear indication about management but it is evident that surgery and even myelography and aspiration are potentially dangerous.

Subarachnoid haemorrhages in the spine, like those in the skull, are usually due to vascular malformations (which will be considered elsewhere) but may also be caused by tumours and by lumbar puncture. When Rice et al reviewed the literature in 1978 there were 31 reports of subarachnoid haemorrhages due to tumours, mostly ependymomas, many of which seem to have been precipitated by exertion. In their patient the haemorrhage occurred after myelography done to demonstrate a neurofibroma and the authors suggest that small feeding vessels may have been ruptured by movement of the tumour due to changes in the c.s.f. pressure.

A report of two patients with subarachnoid haematomas due to lumbar puncture is of considerable theoretical interest. The main subarachnoid vessels are thought to evade a (midline) lumbar puncture needle because they are small and because they enter alongside nerve roots in the upper lateral part of the canal. Traumatic taps are therefore attributed to damage to the epidural venous plexus. In these patients, however, there was no blood in the epidural space and it was clear that in one a subarachnoid vessel near the thrombus had been damaged. The authors point out that subarachnoid haematomas and combined subarachnoid and subdural haematomas have been found in autopsies done soon after lumbar puncture but that there are no reports of purely subdural haematomas at this stage. From this information they argue that a 'traumatic tap' is caused by injury to a radicular vessel in the subarachnoid space and that laceration of the membrane by the lumbar puncture needle may allow the blood to escape into the subdural space. If the autopsy is done some time after the lumbar puncture the subarachnoid haemorrhage will have resolved leaving a 'primary' subdural haematoma. But because purely subdural haematomas have not been observed in the acute stage it seems reasonable to suppose that the chronic ones reported arise in this way, i.e., they are part of a resolving subarachnoid haemorrhage and not the result of haemorrhage from the small subdural vessels (Masdeu et al, 1979).

REFERENCES

Adams R D, Merritt H H 1944 Meningeal and vascular syphilis of the spinal cord. Medicine (Baltimore) 23:181–214

Ahmann P A, Smith S A, Schwartz J F, Clark D B 1975 Spinal cord infarction due to minor trauma in children. Neurology (Minneapolis) 25:301–307

Albert M L, Greer W E R, Kantarowitz W 1969 Paraplegia secondary to hypotension and cardiac arrest in a patient who has had previous thoracic surgery. Neurology (Minneapolis) 19:915–918

Angerer A L, Su H H, Head J R 1953 Death following use of efocaine. Journal of the American Medical Association 153:550–551

Aszkanazy C L 1952 Sarcoidosis of the central nervous system. Journal of Neuropathology and Experimental Neurology 11:392–400

Backs A, Barraquer Bordas L, Barraquer Ferre L, Canadeu J M, Modolell A 1955 Delayed myelopathy following atlantoaxial dislocation by separated odontoid process. Brain 78:537–552

Barr R 1966 Human trichinosis. Canadian Medical Association Journal 95:912–917

Barré J A, D'Andrade C 1938 Paraplégie par ramollissement aigu unisegmentaire de la moelle survenue au cours de la grossesse. Revue Neurologique 69:133–135

Barron K D, Hirano A, Arahi S, Terry R D 1959 Experiences with metastatic neoplasms involving the spinal cord. Neurology (Minneapolis) 9:91–106

Bastian H C 1882 Quains Dictionary of Medicine. Longman Green and Co, London, 1459, 1479

Bergmark G 1950 Intermittent spinal claudication. Acta Medica Scandinavica Supp 246:30–36

Blau J N, Logue V 1961 Intermittent claudication of the cauda equina. Lancet 1:1081–1086

Boblitt D E, Figley M M, Wolfman E F 1959 Roentgen signs of contrast material dissection of aortic wall in direct aortography American Journal of Roentgenology 81:826–834

Braham J, Saia A 1958 Neurological complications of epidural anaesthesia. British Medical Journal 2:657–658

Brain R, Russell D 1937 Myelomalacia following spinal anaesthetic. Proceedings of the Royal Society of Medicine 30:1024–1030

Buskirk V, Davidson M 1960 Vascular insufficiency of the spinal cord. Southern Medical Journal 53:162–169

Carrot E, Pecker J, Le Menn G 1959 Paraplégie à rechutes due à la compression de l'artère du renflement lombaire par un minuscule méningioma. Revue Neurologique 101:584–586

Chakravorty B G 1969 Arterial supply of the cervical spinal cord and its relation to the cervical myelopathy in spondylosis. Annals of the Royal College of Surgeons 45:232–251

Cook A W 1959 Occlusion of the abdominal aorta and dysfunction of the spinal cord. Bulletin of the New York Academy of Medicine 35:47–489

Crawford E S, Fenstermacher J M, Richardson W, Sandiford F 1970 Reappraisal of adjuncts to avoid ischaemia in the treatment of thoracic aortic aneurysms. Surgery 67:182–196

Darwish H, Archer C, Modin J 1979 The anterior spinal artery collateral in coarctation of the aorta. Archives of Neurology 36:240–243

Davies A, Solomon B, Levene A 1958 Paraplegia following epidural anaesthesia. British Medical Journal 2:654–657

Day A L, Sypert G W 1977 Spinal cord sarcoidosis. Annals of Neurology 1:79–85

De Angelis J 1972 Hazards of subdural and epidural anaesthesia during anticoagulant therapy; a case report and review. Anaesthesia and Analgesia 51:676–679

de Sèze S, Guillaume J, Desproges-Gotteron R, Jurmand S H, Maitre M 1957 Semaine des hôpitaux de Paris 33:1767–1796

Devadiga K V, Gass H H 1973 Chronic lumbar extradural haematoma simulating disc syndrome. Journal of Neurology, Neurosurgery and Psychiatry 36:255–259

Di Chiro G, Fried L C 1971 Blood flow currents in spinal cord arteries. Neurology (Minneapolis) 21:1088–1096

Doroshow L W, Yoon H Y, Robbins M A 1962 Intrathecal injection: an unusual complication of translumbar aortography. Journal of Urology 88:438–439

Dripps R D, Vandam L D 1954 Long term follow up of patients who received 10098 spinal anaesthetics. Journal of the American Medical Association 156:1486–1491

Dunn D, Dhopesh V, Mobina J 1979 Spinal subdural hematoma: a possible hazard of lumbar puncture in an alcoholic. Journal of the American Medical Association 241:1712–1713

Edelson R N, Chernik N L, Posner J B 1974 Spinal subdural haematomas complicating lumbar puncture. Archives of Neurology 31:134–137

Ferguson L R J, Bergan J J, Conn J, Yao J S T 1975 Spinal ischaemia following abdominal aortic surgery. Annals of Surgery 181:267–272

Ford F R 1925 Breech delivery in the possible relations to injury of the spinal cord. Archives of Neurology and Psychiatry 14:742–750

Fosselle E, Vander Eecken H 1978 Idiopathic spinal epidural haematoma. Lancet 2:42

Gang D L, Dole K B, Adelman L S 1977 Spinal cord infarction following therapeutic renal artery embolization. Journal of the American Medical Association 237:2841–2842

Garland H, Greenberg J, Harriman D G F 1966 Infarction of the spinal cord. Brain 89:645–662

Gilles F H, Nag D 1971 Vulnerability of human spinal cord in transient cardiac arrest. Neurology (Minneapolis) 21:833–839

Gillilan L A 1970 Veins of the spinal cord. Neurology (Minneapolis) 20:860–868

Gowers W R (1881) The diagnosis of diseases of the spinal cord 2nd edition. P Blakiston's Son and Company, Philadelphia

Grant F C (1945) Epidural spinal abscess. Journal of the American Medical Association 124:509–512

Grinker R R, Guy L G 1927 Sprain of cervical spine causing thrombosis of anterior spinal artery. Journal of the American Medical Association 88:1140–1142

Grunberg A, Blair J L, Rawcliffe R M 1950 Unusual neurological symptoms in polycythaemia rubra vera. Edinburgh Medical Journal 57:305–308

Hallenbeck J M, Bove A A, Elliott D H 1975 Mechanisms underlying spinal cord damage in decompression sickness. Neurology (Minneapolis) 25:308–316

Harrington A 1925 Embolism of the spinal cord. Glasgow Medical Journal 103:28–32

Harrington D, Amplatz K 1972 Cholesterol embolization and spinal infarction following aortic catheterization. American Journal of Roentgenology 115:171–174

Harvie A, Lowe G D O, Forbes C D, Prentice C R M, Turner J 1977 Intraspinal bleeding in haemophilia: successful treatment with factor VIII concentrate. Journal of Neurology, Neurosurgery and Psychiatry 40:1220–1223

Hassler O 1966 Blood supply to human spinal cord. Archives of Neurology 15:302–307

Henson R A, Parsons M 1967 Ischaemic lesions of the spinal cord. Quarterly Journal of Medicine 36:205–222

Hilal S K, Keim H A 1972 Selective spinal angiography in adolescent scoliosis. Radiology 102:349–359

Hirose G, Kosoegawa H, Takado M, Shimazani K, Murakami E 1979 Spinal cord ischaemia and left atrial myxoma. Archives of Neurology 36:439

Hubert J P, Ectors M, Ketelbant-Balasse P, Flament-Durand J 1974 Fibrocartilaginous venous and arterial emboli from the nucleus pulposus in the anterior spinal system. European Neurology 11:164–171

Hughes J T 1964 Spinal cord infarction due to aortic trauma. British Medical Journal 2:356

Hughes J T 1965 The pathology of vascular diseases of the spinal cord. Paraplegia 2:207–213

Hughes J T 1970 Thrombosis of the posterior spinal arteries. Neurology (Minneapolis) 20:659–664

Hughes J T 1971 Venous infarction of the spinal cord. Neurology (Minneapolis) 21:794–800

Hughes J T, Brownell B 1964 Cervical spondylosis complicated by anterior spinal artery thrombosis. Neurology (Minneapolis) 14:1073–1077

Hughes J T, Brownell B 1966 Spinal cord ischaemia due to arteriosclerosis. Archives of Neurology 15:189–202

Hughes J T, Macintyre A G 1963 Spinal cord infarction occurring during thoracolumbar sympathectomy. Journal of Neurology, Neurosurgery and Psychiatry 26:418–421

Jellinger K 1967 Spinal cord arteriosclerosis and progressive vascular myelopathy. Journal of Neurology, Neurosurgery and Psychiatry 30:195–206

Jellinger K, Neumayer E 1962 Myélopathies progressives d'origine vasculaire. Revue Neurologique 106:666–669

Judice D J, Le Blanc H J, McGarry P A 1978 Spinal cord vasculitis presenting as a spinal cord tumour in a heroin addict. Journal of Neurosurgery 48:131–134

Kardjiev V, Symeonov A, Chankov I 1974 Etiology pathogenesis and prevention of spinal cord lesions in selective angiography of the bronchial and intercostal arteries. Radiology 112:81–83

Kewalramani L S, Saleem S, Bertrand D 1978 Myelopathy associated with systemic lupus erythematosus. Paraplegia 16:282–294

Laguna J, Cravioto H 1973 Spinal cord infarction secondary to occlusion of the anterior spinal artery. Archives of Neurology 28:134–136

Lancet leading article 1974 Spinal stroke 2:1299–1300

Leonard J C 1979 Thomas Bevill Peacock and the early history of dissecting aneurysms. British Medical Journal 2:260–262

Leonard J C, Hasleton P S 1979 Dissecting aortic aneurysms: a clinicopathological study. Quarterly Journal of Medicine 48:55–63

Levy N A, Strauss H A 1942 Myelopathy following compression of abdominal aorta for postpartum haemorrhage. Archives of Neurology and Psychiatry 48:85–91

Lindemulder F G 1931 Myelitis occurring in the primary and in the secondary stage of syphilis. Archives of Neurology and Psychiatry 26:167–169

Logue V 1952 Thoracic intervertebral disc prolapse and spinal cord compression. Journal of Neurology, Neurosurgery and Psychiatry 15:227–241

McCleery W N C, Lewtas N A 1966 Subarachnoid injection of contrast medium. British Journal of Radiology 39:112–114

Macintosh R 1956 Paraplegia following spinal anaesthesia. Lancet 1:807, 961, 1073

McQuarrie I G 1978 Recovery from paraplegia caused by spontaneous spinal epidural hematoma. Neurology (Minneapolis) 28:224–228

Mair W G P, Folkerts J F 1953 Necrosis of the spinal cord due to thrombophlebitis. Brain 76:563–575

Margolis G 1970 Pathogenesis of contrast media injury: insights provided by neurotoxicity studies. Investigative Radiology 5:392–406

Masdeu J C, Breuer A C, Schoene W C 1979 Spinal subarachnoid haematomas: clue to a source of bleeding in traumatic lumbar puncture. Neurology (Minneapolis) 29:872–876

Mishkin M M, Baum S, Di Chiro G 1973 Emergency treatment of angiography induced paraplegia and tetraplegia. New England Journal of Medicine 288:1184–1185

Moore D C 1954 Complications following the use of efocaine. Surgery 35:109–114

Mosberg W H, Voris H C, Duffy J 1954 Paraplegia as a complication of sympathectomy for hypertension. Annals of Surgery 139:330–334

Moxon W 1881 Influence of the circulation of the nervous system. Lancet 1:527–531

Mozingo J R, Denton I C 1975 The neurological deficit associated with sudden occlusion of abdominal aorta due to blunt trauma. Surgery 77:118–125

Packer N P, Cummins B H 1978 Spontaneous epidural haemorrhage; a surgical emergency. Lancet 1:356–358

Palmer J L 1972 Radiation myelopathy. Brain 95:109–122

Payne J P, Bergentz S E 1956 Paraplegia following spinal anaesthesia. Lancet 1:666–668

Pennybacker J 1958 Discussion on vascular disease of the spinal cord. Proceedings of the Royal Society of Medicine 51:547–550

Peters B H, Levin H S, Kelly P J 1977 Neurologic and psychologic manifestations of decompression illness in divers. Neurology (Minneapolis) 27:125–127

Peters H A, Clatanoff D V 1968 Spinal muscular atrophy secondary to macroglobulinaemia: reversal of symptoms after chemotherapy. Neurology (Minneapolis) 18:101–108

Ramirez-Lassepas M, McLelland R R, Snyder D B, Marsh D G 1977 Cervical myelopathy complicating cerebral angiography. Neurology (Minneapolis) 27:834–837

Reichert F L, Rytand D A, Bruch E L 1934 Arteriosclerosis of the lumbar segmental arteries producing ischaemia of the spinal cord and consequent claudication of the thighs. American Journal of Medical Science 187:794–806

Rice J F, Shields C B, Morris C F, Neely B D 1978 Spinal subarachnoid haemorrhage during myelography. Journal of Neurosurgery 48:645–648

Robertson W C, Lee Y E, Edmondson M B 1979 Spontaneous spinal epidural heamatoma in the young. Neurology (Minneapolis) 29:120–122

Rouquès L, Passelecq A 1957 Syndrome de Brown Séquard après thoracoplastie. Revue Neurologique 97:146–147

Rozsahegyi I 1959 Late consequences of the neurological forms of decompression sickness. British Journal of Industrial Medicine 16:311–317

Ruhberg G N, Noble J F 1941 Diabetes with infarction of the cord. Minnesota Medicine 24:495–496

Schneider R C, Crosby E C 1959 Vascular insufficiency of brain stem and spinal cord in spinal trauma. Neurology (Minneapolis) 9:643–656

Schott B, Cotte L, Tommasi M 1959 Ramollissement spinal postérieur en D7 D8 par myéloma osseux plasmocytaire D11–L1. Revue Neurologique 101 : 16–27

Senelick R C, Norwood C W, Cohen G H 1976 'Painless' spinal epidural haematoma during anticoagulant therapy. Neurology (Minneapolis) 26 : 213–215

Sharr M M, Weller R O, Brice J C 1978 Spinal cord necrosis after intrathecal injection of methylene blue. Journal of Neurology, Neurosurgery and Psychiatry 41 : 384–386

Siddorn J A 1978 Schistosomiasis and anterior spinal artery occlusion. American Journal of Tropical Medicine and Hygiene 27 : 532–534

Silver J R, Buxton P H 1974 Spinal stroke. Brain 97 : 539–550

Sovak B S, Rasminsky M, Finlayson M H 1975 Complications of phenol neurolysis. Archives of Neurology 32 : 226–228

Strauss R H, Prockop L D 1973 Decompression sickness among scuba divers. Journal of the American Medical Association 223 : 637–640

Symonds C P, Meadows S P 1937 Compression of the spinal cord in the neighbourhood of the foramen magnum. Brain 60 : 52–84

Szilagyi D E, Hageman J H, Smith R F, Elliott J P 1978 Spinal cord damage in surgery of the abdominal aorta. Surgery 83 : 38–56

Thenabadu P N, Wickremasinghe H R, Rajasuriya K 1970 Acute ascending ischaemic myelopathy in polyarteritis nodosa. British Medical Journal 1 : 734

Thomas P, Dwyer C S 1950 Postoperative flaccid paraplegia. Anesthesiology 11 : 635–636

Tokoti T, Kato T, Nomoto Y, Kurakazu M, Kanaseki T 1979 Anterior spinal artery syndrome — a complication of cervical intrathecal phenol injection. Pain 6 : 99–104

Turnbull I M, Brieg A, Hassler O 1966 Blood supply of cervical spinal cord in man. Journal of Neurosurgery 24 : 951–965

Walshe F M R 1956 Paraplegia following spinal anaesthesia. Lancet 1 : 859, 1015

Wells C E C 1966 Clinical aspects of spinovascular disease. Proceedings of the Royal Society of Medicine 59 : 790–796

Wikler A, Marmor J, Hurst A 1937 Air embolism of the spinal cord following attempted pneumothorax. Journal of the American Medical Association 109 : 430–431

Wolman L 1966 The neuropathological effects resulting from the intrathecal injection of chemical substances. Paraplegia 4 : 97–115

Wolman L, Hardy A G 1970 Spinal cord infarction associated with the sickle cell trait. Paraplegia 7 : 282–291

Zulch K J, Kurth-Schumacher R 1970 The pathogenesis of 'intermittent spinovascular insufficiency' ('spinal claudication of Dejerine') and other vascular syndromes of the spinal cord. Vascular Surgery 4 : 116–136

23

Stroke rehabilitation

R. Langton-Hewer

A stroke is a catastrophic event both for the patient and his relatives. A previously normal, intelligent person may be suddenly rendered aphasic, paralysed and incontinent. The shock is total. All too often nothing can be done, medically or surgically, to improve the situation in the acute phase. The quality of the remainder of the patient's life will thereafter largely depend upon the degree of functional recovery which occurs. It is the aim of rehabilitation to help the patient make the best of his residual capabilities.

The yearly incidence of stroke is approximately 2 per 1000 in the general population, and it is probable that approximately one-third will be left with some degree of neurological disability — usually a hemiparesis or a hemiplegia. Some of these patients will be left with severe handicap, and Harris et al (1971) found that stroke is the commonest cause of severe physical handicap in the community. They estimated that there are 130 000 impaired stroke survivors living in private households in Great Britain. It needs to be remembered, however, that stroke is only one cause of neurological disability. Others include head injury, multiple sclerosis, spinal injury, muscular dystrophy, spina bifida, cerebral palsy and various 'system degenerations' such as Parkinsonism and motor neurone disease. Important non-neurological causes of physical disability include rheumatoid arthritis, other diseases of the osteoarticular system and emphysema. At least 56 per cent of patients aged between 15 and 59 who are receiving long term care in Younger Chronic Sick Units are disabled as a result of neurological disease (Circular London, Ministry of Health, 1968).

The term rehabilitation implies the restoration of patients to their fullest physical, mental, and social capability and embraces the many physical, social and organisational aspects of the after-care for patients who require more than acute short-term definitive care. The problem has been the subject of two reports (Department of Health and Social Security Welsh Office, 1972; Scottish Home and Health Department, 1972) and it is perhaps sad that there were no neurologists on either of the relevant subcommittees. Nichols (1974) has briefly reviewed the practice of rehabilitation and includes the following principles:

1. A clear definition of the clinical problem and *likely outcome* must be made and discussed with all concerned as early as possible (the patient included).

2. A realistic programme for *hospital admission* and returning home and to work should be agreed as soon as possible.

3. Appropriate *industrial or domestic resettlement* must be phased in with physical treatment as soon as possible.

4. There must be *no gaps in treatment* — even for a few days.

5. Skilled *assessment* of the environmental needs, aids and appliances, and the social support needed for people with long-term disabilities.

If such a programme is to be implemented, there must be close co-operation between a large number of people from various disciplines — including doctors, social workers and physical therapists. They must work together assessing, planning, and implementing a management programme.

A number of workers in the United Kingdom have reported on supervised programmes of rehabilitation for stroke patients (Adams, 1974; Isaacs & Marks, 1973; Millard, 1973; Somerville et al,

1974; Wilkinson, 1973). The reports originate either in departments of geriatrics or in special rehabilitation units.

It is a common view that stroke patients in hospital do not always receive the optimal level of rehabilitation (Blower & Ali, 1979). Recently a number of specialised Rehabilitation Units have been established in the United States (Feigenson et al, 1979) and in the United Kingdom (Blower & Ali, 1979; Garraway et al, 1980). Enthusiasm for these is high, but published assessments of their value are rare. A recent randomised controlled trial in Scotland showed an initial benefit when stroke unit care was compared with management in a medical ward. However, this benefit was lost at a one year follow-up (Garraway et al, 1980).

Stroke is commonly thought of as being a hospital-based problem, but in pratice the admission rate appears to vary widely throughout the country. The National Survey of General Practitioners (1974) found that only 42 per cent of all new episodes of cerebrovascular disease were referred for admission. Cochrane (1970) in South Wales estimated that 60 per cent of stroke patients were kept at home. Weddell (1979) in Surrey found that at four days only 25 per cent of patients were still at home. The most comprehensive study of present management was given by Brocklehurst et al (1978). This group noted that the main reason for hospital admission was the need for nursing care. They found that even if a patient was admitted to hospital very few investigations were undertaken.

There have been no controlled trials to assess the value of domiciliary care for acute strokes. Various authors have commented on the need for this (Mulley & Arie, 1978; Weddell & Beresford, 1979). This is surprising since hospitals are such expensive items. Weddell (1973) summarises the problem neatly:

The rehabilitation of people after a stroke must be considered first as a problem involving people, and people at home, rather than in hospital. Rehabilitation to achieve the fullest possible life at home must always be the target. Whether hospital services have a significant part to play needs to be questioned. It may be that the most effective measures are those that increase people's capabilities in their own homes, for example, the installation of aids and adaptations as soon as possible after the stroke, together with much improved co-ordination between medical services and the local authorities and voluntary agencies.

A controlled trial using a Domiciliary Care Team is now being undertaken in Bristol.

In addition to its obvious practical, economic, and humanitarian importance the subject of recovery following a stroke is of interest to all those who wish to find out how the nervous system compensates for damage. This subject has recently been reviewed in a remarkable book edited by Paul Bach-y-rita (1980). Wall, in this book, makes a strong case for 'unmasking' as the mechanism for late recovery. Rosenzweig (1980) reviewed the considerable literature relating to recovery in animals, and showed that there is indeed evidence that 'complex stimulation and opportunities for experience' are important for maximal recovery. In humans, there is little published evidence that therapy alters the ultimate level of physical recovery. This view requires to be challenged by a larger number of properly controlled trials. Natural recovery makes it difficult to prove the efficacy of therapy. During the last few years there has been much interest in the possibility of constructing recovery curves and of predicting outcome (Hiorns & Newcombe, 1979).

The subject of stroke rehabilitation is a large one. This chapter seeks to outline the size and scope of the problem, and to discuss the assessment and management of the patient.

THE SIZE OF THE STROKE-INDUCED DISABILITY PROBLEM

When planning rehabilitation services, it is desirable to know the number of disabled persons who are likely to exist in the area of study.

The yearly incidence of stroke varies between 1.65 and 2.45 per 1000 in six studies surveyed by Marquardsen (1978). It is generally accepted that the figure is approximately 2 per 1000 persons. The incidence rises markedly with age and about 70 per cent occur in persons aged 65 and over. (Marquardsen, 1969).

Data relating to the occurrence of *disabled* stroke survivors is sparse. Weddell (1979) found that just under half (46 per cent) of the three week survivors were partially of completely dependent in transferring. Our own unpublished figures also indicate that approximately 50 per cent of survivors will be left with a substantial neurological deficit which usually includes a hemiplegia. If it is assumed that one-third to one-half of stroke victims survive three weeks with a disability, then the average general practitioner (with a list of 2500) would have two or three new disabled patients per year added to his list. The quarter of a million population served by an 'average' District General Hopsital would produce 170–250 cases yearly. The survivors are, in the main, elderly. Weddell (1979) found that 67 per cent of the men and 80 per cent of the women who survived three months were over the age of 65.

The overall prevalence of stroke survivors is between 4.4 and 6.7 per thousand (Petlund, 1970; Whisnant et al, 1971); 50–60 per cent will be disabled as a result of the stroke. This represents approximately 6–8 persons on the list of the 'average' general practitioner, and 550–820 persons per quarter of a million population. The yearly incidence of stroke-induced dysphasia is probably about 50 cases per quarter of a million. The prevalence rate in the same population is about 130 (Matsumoto et al, 1973; Hopkins, 1975).

Definition of quantification in stroke rehabilitation

One of the main difficulties in evaluating rehabilitation methods used in stroke rehabilitation is the lack of agreed criteria of assessment. If comparisons are to be made between treatment in hospital and at home, between one unit and another, or between the effects of different treatment regimes, it is necessary to know whether the patients were comparable and whether the criteria were the same. At present, there is no general agreement even about the definition of stroke, there is no standard method of reporting the nature, severity, cause or duration of neurological deficit. Furthermore, there are no agreed methods for evaluating outcome, other than death or survival.

The problem of definition has been discussed by Capildeo et al (1978). Marquardsen (1978) gives the recommmended WHO definition — 'rapidly developed signs of focal (or global) disturbance of cerebral function, leading to death, or lasting more than 24 hours, with no apparent cause other than vascular.' A similar definition was given by the WHO in 1971 and by the Royal College of Physicians (RCP) Working Group on Strokes (1974). However, two important recent studies (Weddell, 1974; Brocklehurst et al, 1978) have both used definitions which omit any reference to a vascular aetiology. No two stroke patients are precisely the same, and a number of different types of stroke can occur. Most, however, have a hemiplegia. The RCP Working Group (1974) considered that in describing the deficit note should be taken of:

1. The side of the stroke.
2. Whether the neurological deficit resulted in motor loss only (or predominantly) or whether this was accompanied by major perceptual, cognitive or language deficit.
3. Whether the patient was in good, or fairly good health apart from the stroke, or whether he suffered from one or more complicating conditions known to affect prognosis adversely, for example, previous stroke or heart disease.

Isaacs & Marks (1973) suggested a simple classification using the first two items mentioned above. This classification was:

1. Right hemiplegia with communication disorder.
2. Right hemiplegia, no communication disorder.
3. Left hemiplegia, perceptual loss.
4. Left hemiplegia, no perceptual loss.

They divided the cases into two main groups — complex and simple. The complex cases had a major communication or perceptual disturbance, simple cases had not.

Various attempts have been made to quantify the various perceptual and intellectual abnormalities in elderly patients (Adams, 1974; Denham & Jeffreys, 1972; Hodkinson, 1972; Isaacs & Marks, 1973; Wilson & Brass, 1973). The functional results can be described in various ways. The most usual appears to be that of Rankin (1957). His scaling system is used by Marquardsen (1969):

Grade I   No significant disability. Able to carry out all usual activities.

Grade II   Slight disability. Unable to carry out some previous activities, but able to look after own affairs without assistance.

Grade III   Moderate disability. Able to walk without assistance but requiring some help with dressing.

Grade IV   Moderately severe disability. Incapable of walking alone and unable to attend to own bodily needs without assistance.

Grade V   Severe disability. Bed-fast or chair-fast. Usually incontinent, requiring constant nursing care and attention.

Adams (1974) used a slightly different system:

Recovered Grade I   Fully independent. Intellect clear. Some use of hand. Confident gait.

Grade II   Handicapped. Mental clouding. Arm disabled. Walks unaided.

Long Stay   Confined to chair or bed. May be confused. May be incontinent.

The above mentioned systems may be made compatible (Report of the RCP Working Group on Strokes 1974): Adam's grades I and II would include all patients in Rankin's grades I, II and III. The long-stay patients of Adams were made equivalent to Rankin's categories IV and V. No system is perfect and a balance has to be struck in dealing with a complex problem.

Degrees of independence can also be described in terms of ADL (activities of daily living). Katz et al (1963) reported on an index of ADL which was developed to study the results of treatment and prognosis in the elderly and chronically sick. Grades of the index summarise performance in bathing, dressing, going to the toilet, transferring, continence and feeding. There are thus six grades (A-F), A being independent in the six activities listed above and F being dependent in all six functions. This scale has been extensively used by many workers to measure the abilities of patients disabled by a variety of causes.

Another much used functional evaluation system was described by Mahoney & Barthel (1965) and is known as the Barthel Index. This has a 10 point scale which includes feeding, transferring, personal toilet, getting on and off the toilet, bathing oneself, walking on a level surface, ascending and descending stairs, dressing, controlling bowels and controlling bladder. Schoening & Iversen (1968) gave details of the Kenny self-care evaluation. This is a numerical rating system utilising a five point scale of the patient's abilities in six categories of self care activities. Included in the six categories are 17

specific activities — thus 'locomotion' includes three subgroups, walking, stairs, and wheelchairs. This is a particularly detailed system and has been used for the construction of 'learning curves' for several groups of patients, including hemiplegics (Schoening & Iversen, 1968).

There are thus three main ADL scales in current use. The subject is discussed by Diller (1970), Nichols (1976) and by Sheikh et al (1979). The last authors highlight the problem that many patients do not always undertake certain activities although they can do so. ADL scales do not give much information about the quality of life or about how the patient participates in everyday activities inside and outside the home.

Sarno et al (1973) presented a detailed functional life scale. This scale was later simplified, validated and published as Level of Rehabilitation Scale — LORS (Carey & Posavac, 1978). The scale includes 47 items which are divided into five groups — ADL, cognition (e.g., reading and writing), home activities (e.g., preparing food, use of telephone, etc.), outside activities (e.g., shopping and use of public transport), social interaction (going to work or school, and visiting friends). The authors claim that the scale, which depends upon an interview with a person who knows the patient well, can usually be completed in 15 minutes. The results are expressed as a percentage of normal function.

An important recent study (Labi et al, 1980) indicates that a significant proportion of stroke survivors manifest social disability despite complete physical restoration.

Medical assessment

Whereas most stroke survivors have a hemiplegia, this is not necessarily the most important result of a stroke. Adams & Hurwitz (1963) have reviewed a group of 45 bed-fast, hemiplegic patients in order to determine why they were unable to recover the ability to walk and look after themselves. Physical disabilities, such as dense paralysis complicated by severe sensory loss or limited exercise tolerance, were responsible in only half the patients. The others had cerebral deficits which the authors classified into four groups — impaired learning ability, disturbed awareness of self or space, disordered integrative action and emotional disorders. Within these groups they identified a number of 'mental barriers to recovery from strokes':

1. Inability to learn (clouded consciousness, aphasia, memory defects, dementia).

2. Disturbed perception and attitude towards illness (e.g., neglect or denial of the hemiplegic limbs or disordered spatial orientation).

3. Disordered integrative action (imparied postural function, agnosia, apraxia, perseveration and synkinesia).

4. Disturbance of emotional behaviour (emotional instability, apathy, loss of confidence, fear, unwillingness to try, catastrophic reactions, depression).

It was pointed out that the patient seldom has the insight to appreciate these barriers. Unless the physician is aware of these problems and plans his examination appropriately and systematically, it is possible that these all-important deficits will be overlooked. Adams (1974) gives six general points which should be considered when assessing stroke survivors. What follows is based mainly on his account.

It is first necessary to known something about the patient's personality and premorbid state of health. Such information usually needs to be acquired from a relative or friend.

Exercise tolerance

It is particularly important to know about the presence of associated vascular symptoms such as angina, claudication, and possible postural hypotension, chronic bronchitis, emphysema, and osteoarthritis, which may alter the patient's mobility.

Motivation

In assessing motivation it is important to know what the patient was like before the stroke. Information will be required about his interests, his energy and drive, and his psychological stability — particularly his reaction to previous stressful situations. It is important to recognise that the patient's apparent unwillingness to help himself may in fact be due to associated disorders such as severe depression or defective memory. Such

patients may be wrongly blamed for 'not trying'. Adams (1974) stresses the importance of reassurance; the patient should be told that he stands a good chance of eventually becoming independent and that the various humiliating features of the early weeks following the stroke may not persist.

Sensory deficits

Gross disturbances of memory, abnormalities of visuo-spatial orientation, and other high level visual defects with preserved visual acuity, are examples of the type of sensory abnormality which may not be obvious at first glance, but which profoundly affect the patient's ability to undertake everyday tasks. All too frequently such deficits go unnoticed, thus making the efforts of the rehabilitation team both illogical and frequently unsuccessful. In general, lesions of the left hemisphere produce verbal disorder, notably dysphasia, whereas lesions of the right hemisphere tend to produce defects of visual perception and spatial integration. Some of the main deficits are outlined in Table 23.1.

The method of assessment proposed by Adams is unconventional in that sensory function is tested before motor function. Adams makes out a good case for grouping together all sensory modalities, vision and hearing being included with disorders of proprioception and spatial integration.

Mental capacity

Any method of assessment for brain damaged patients must include a test battery which will identify the important deficits mentioned in Table 23.2. The method should be comprehensive. It must also be simple to use, capable of being administered by a wide range of persons (not only psychologists), capable of being performed without complex apparatus and unlikely to cause stress or embarrassment to the patient. It should also give a quantifiable estimate of impairment and must be capable of validation.

It may be argued that it would be impossible to meet all these requirements. Therefore a number of test batteries have been devised in an attempt to meet them all. These include those of Adams (1974), Hodkinson (1972), Isaacs (1971), and

Table 23.1 Table of principal 'sensory deficits'

	Deficit	Comment
Vision	Refractive errors	Ask the relatives to get the patient's glasses.
	Hemianopia	The patient may ignore people and objects placed in the blind field. The relatives and staff should stand, in the early stages at least, in the 'seeing field'. Bed lockers and food should be similarly placed. Some patients with a right hemisphere stroke may deny the existence of a left homonymous hemianopia. Such patients, if asked to draw, may leave out the left side of what they are drawing. They may also ignore food placed on the left side of the plate.
	Cortical blindness	This usually results from vascular or anoxic changes occurring bilaterally in the occipital cortex. Denial of blindness sometimes occurs.
	Visual agnosia (mind blindness)	The patient is not blind but is unable to recognise what he sees. He is unable to assess the size, shape, and position of objects, although he may be able to do so if he is able to use a non-visual modality such as touch or hearing.
Hearing	Deafness	Removal of wax or the provision of a hearing aid are simple remedies which should not be forgotten. Social isolation and depression are fostered by deafness.
Disorders of body image and spatial orientation	Auditory agnosia Agnosia for the paralysed side	In this condition the patient can hear satisfactorily but cannot interpret what is said. In some patients there is loss of the normal awareness of the integrated representation of body segments. Some such patients may cease to be aware of the paralysed side of the body and may deny the existence of paralysis (anosagnosia). Such patients are frequently unable to draw symmetrical objects such as a house, a person or a clock-usually omitting, or poorly representing, objects on the affected side. A few patients experience complex delusions about the paralysed limbs, sometimes describing them as being longer or shorter than normal, covered with hair, or having a highly abnormal shape. Such delusions are frightening to the patient, who may be unwilling to acknowledge them.
	Impairment of space perception	Disturbances of the perception of the horizontal and vertical have been described in a series of papers, and it is likely that such disturbances are important barriers to recovery (Bruell et al, 1957; Birch et al, 1961; Birch et al, 1960).
Tactile and postural sensation in the limbs		Pin-prick sensation, touch localisation, and the ability to recognise objects placed in the hand are tested in the conventional way. Loss of proprioceptive sensation is usually easily detected by getting the blindfolded patient to put the index finger of the good hand on to that of the paralysed hand, which is held in different positions by the physician. The results of this test need to be interpreted with caution in patients who have disorders of body image.

Denham & Jeffreys (1972). Some of the tests involve the use of simple toys such as a post box or paper board. All involve a simple scoring system. It will be readily appreciated that any test will depend on a number of different factors. Thus, the ability to read and to paraphrase a sentence depends upon the intactness of vision, the ability to recognise the relevant letters and words, the ability to understand the concepts and subtleties of what is written, and the ability to remember what has been read. Even the simplest test will frequently depend upon several different modalities. The 'ultimate' test has yet to be devised but it is to be hoped that before long some degree of standardisation will become apparent so that the results of therapy in different centres can be compared.

Motor deficit

Some of the observations required when assessing recovery from motor deficit in hemiplegia are itemised in Table 23.3. The subject is discussed more fully in a later section.

Postural control

The control of posture is frequently defective following a stroke. The patient may not be able to sit straight and in this event will not be able to stand or to walk. This problem is particularly common during the first days and weeks after onset. Sometimes the patient appears to be quite oblivious of the problem; some probably have disturbances of spatial orientation. When the problem persists it is sometimes due to spasticity of trunk muscles on the affected side.

The deficits which occur after a stroke are frequently complex. It is of great importance that the assessment should be carefully undertaken so that no important deficits are overlooked. Failure to do this will probably result in misdirection of

Table 23.2 Mental capacity

	Deficit	Comment
General assessment of appearance and mood	Dysphasia	The patient's ability to understand and to express himself must be tested initially, as much of what follows will depend on this. If dysphasia is present, detailed testing will need to be undertaken at a later state.
	Perseveration	The patient persists in making the same response to different stimuli — for example, when asked to add two and two he will correctly say four, but if asked to add two and three he will still say four.
	Level of alertness	
	Comprehension and insight. Ability to concentrate	Distractability and inattentiveness make rehabilitation difficult.
	Reasoning ability	This is easily tested by setting the patient a simple problem or getting him to paraphrase proverbs.
	Arithmetic	Simple addition and subtraction.
Speech		Detailed testing will be undertaken at this stage, if relevant.
Memory		Both registration and recall should be tested. Tests include digit retention, forwards and backwards and the ability to repeat the salient features of a simple story or to remember an address correctly.
Behaviour and mood	Initiative Spontaneity Sense of humour Continence	Does the patient spontaneously attempt to do things himself or does he wait to have everything done for him?
	Emotional state	Depression is common and is a very important cause of lack of progress. Some patients show marked emotional lability.
Performance		The patient's capacity to undertake self-care and other activities would usually be assessed by the nursing staff and others.

the efforts of the rehabilitation team. A systematic approach to the problem such as that outlined by Adams (1974) is clearly desirable.

Practical management

The first medical person to be involved when a patient has a stroke is usually the general practitioner. He will have to decide whether or not to admit the patient to hospital. Factors influencing his decision include doubt about the diagnosis, the possibility of providing treatment in the acute phase, and nursing and social factors. Frequently, the patient's immobility is the reason for admission e.g., the elderly spouse is unable to lift the patient in and out of bed.

If the patient is not admitted to hospital, the family will require practical help and advice immediately. Advice needs to be given, amongst other things, about:

1. *Lifting and transferring*. They must be shown how to help the patient to get from one side of the bed to another and from the bed to the chair or commode, and vice versa.

2. *Management of incontinence*. This may involve fluid restriction in the evening, deliberate waking in the night in order to pass urine, and/or the supply of appropriate incontinence garments.

3. *Management of dysphasia*. Some assessment of the patient's dysphasic difficulty must be made and the relatives shown how to communicate with the patient.

It may be necessary to get the local authority to supply a commode and other relevant aids. If physiotherapy treatment is to be given the patient will usually have to attend hospital on a daily basis, but this may involve long ambulance journeys which are frequently poorly tolerated by the patient. It must be conceded that in practice it is currently difficult to achieve efficient management of the severely disabled stroke patient in a purely home environment.

If the patient is admitted to hospital even for a short while, it should be possible to plan the rehabilitation programme. This programme involves a number of distinct but interrelated stages. These are assessment, definition of objectives, planning and implementation of a treatment programme, and long-term follow-up. When carrying out this programme it is important that the various members of the team should work closely together.

Assessment

Assessment involves finding out as much about the patient as possible, so that realistic objectives can be defined. This includes information about his previous employment, his interests, his personality, how he has reacted to previous stress and about his family. Because recovery is often a lengthy process it may be necessary to carry out several assessments over a period of months.

Objectives

The first objective is usually independence — the ability to wash, dress, feed, and manage his own toilet together with some degree of independent mobility. Sometimes the objectives are less ambitious. They may be limited to being able to feed, transfer from bed to a chair and regain some degree of continence. Other patients who may be more ambitious may eventually return to work. Objectives need to be reviewed from time to time as recovery occurs.

Planning and implementation of treatment programme

All too often the stroke patient is given only a few minutes of physiotherapy, occupational therapy and speech therapy per day, usually at irregular intervals. He spends much of his time in the ward or at home doing nothing. Such a haphazard approach is demoralising for all concerned. A planned and integrated management programme needs to be worked out for each patient. The patient should be consulted and told what is planned for him. He should be given a weekly written timetable, so that he and his family know what to expect.

The various members of the rehabilitation team need to work closely together and ideally there should be shared responsibilities between the hospital and the community. It is particularly important to involve the community services at an early stage, so that the transfer of the patient from hospital to home is smooth. Home adaptations must be organised and 'aids' ordered at an early stage.

Long-term follow-up

Reliable data relating to the rate of recovery depend upon the availability of well-validated and sensitive measures of outcome. Twitchell (1951) described the course of motor recovery following stroke. This classical paper gives details of the physiological sequence of recovery in the limbs. An important recent contribution is that of Brocklehurst et al (1978), who studied 139 patients who had suffered a recent stroke and survived two weeks. These workers studied several parameters of recovery, including mobility, ADL, and mental confusion. Most recovery occurred within eight weeks. However, 12 per cent showed improvement in their walking score beyond eight weeks, and 28 per cent showed improvement in their ADL score beyond this time. The study indicates that apart from some patients with minimal disability, little further recovery can be expected beyond six months from the date of the stroke. The findings suggest that a major investment in physical therapy beyond six months is probably wasteful.

For those who are left with a substantial disability it will probably be necessary to provide long-term support. Following discharge from active treatment remedial staff can participate in the patient's and family's adjustment by providing continued support through the telephone and direct contact. Some Units have established Stroke Clubs (Isaacs, 1977). The Chest, Heart and Stroke Association has supported the formation of Stroke Clubs throughout the United Kingdom and there are now 260 such Clubs in existence. There is also a network of Speech Groups (Griffith, 1975). A variety of hobbies and other activities are open to younger stroke patients. Examples include gardening, golf and even archery (Guttman, 1976; Hale, 1979). These activities can all be used to implement the general principle that disabled patients should not, if possible, be allowed to remain socially isolated.

COMPOSITION OF THE REHABILITATION TEAM

A large number of people are involved in attempting to get the stroke patient to make the best of his residual capabilities. The patient's own family, notably the husband or wife and the children, are amongst the most important. They are easily forgotten, in spite of the fact that it is they who will probably eventually have to shoulder a large part of the burden. Similarly, the family doctor is in a unique position because of his knowledge of the patient and his background.

Members of the rehabilitation team will each have their own defined areas of responsibility, but inevitably there will be a considerable amount of overlap. Thus, the nursing staff, the physiotherapist and the occupational therapist will all be involved in helping the patient to stand and walk. The hospital rehabilitation team will usually include:

1. The *consultant* and his junior supporting staff. They will be responsible for making a medical assessment and for co-ordination of the activities of the team.

2. *Nursing staff* (see below).

3. *Social worker.* The social worker's main functions include home assessment, co-ordination of the various 'helping agencies' in the community (both statutory and voluntary), and follow-up visits, as necessary. The social worker is well placed to assess the various stresses and problems faced by the patient and his family. In addition, he or she will need to be aware of legislation relevant to the care of the handicapped.

4. *Physiotherapist.* The physiotherapist will be responsible for helping the patient to regain control over the paralysed limbs and to achieve some degree of independent mobility. The question of which techniques of physical therapy should be used are discussed in the next section. It is essential that the various members of the team should use the same methods of treatment. Different and possibly contradictory treatment methods will only confuse.

5. *Occupational therapist* (see below).

6. *Speech therapist* (see below).

7. *Neuropsychologist.* Unfortunately, there are very few neuropsychologists. There is little doubt that such a person is a very valuable member of the team, both in identifying cognitive and other disorders and also in developing treatment methods for those conditions, which are not always obvious but very important. In practice the doctor, with the help of other members of the team, will usually undertake the psychological assessments.

8. *Psychiatrist.* Depression is a particularly important complication of stroke. The psychiatrist may be able to give valuable advice on the management of this and other psychiatric complications.

9. *Orthotist.* The provision of orthotic devices, e.g., foot drop support, is a specialised task, and the orthotist, if one is available, should be consulted.

10. *Orthopaedic surgeon.* The place of surgery in the management of hemiplegic patients is briefly discussed below. Surgery may be indicated for the correction of contractures and the alleviation of spasticity.

Nursing

The patient in hospital, and his family, are more likely to confide in the nurse than anyone else; certainly, they see a great deal of her. The nurse will be partly responsible for helping the patient to regain independence and for teaching him, for instance, to feed and wash. Similarly, the district nurse will be closely involved with the patient's home management. Some general points relevant to the nursing of stroke patients may be mentioned.

Correct positioning in bed

The patient should not remain in bed during the day without a very good reason. It is usually possible to get the patient sitting up within a few days of the acute event.

The bed itself should be neither too high nor too low; ideally it should be of variable height. The height of the bed is particularly important when the patient is being nursed at home. A bed that is at the wrong height may make if impossible for the patient to be got in and out of bed (see Fig. 23.1). The mattress should be firm and should not sag in the middle. There should be a backrest.

The patient should be nursed in such a way as to minimise the likelihood of deformities. Failure to

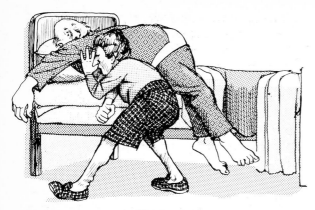

Fig. 23.1

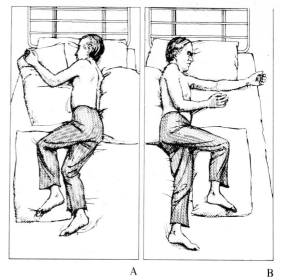

A   B

Fig. 23.3

do so may result in deformities of the type shown in Figure 23.2. In particular, the arms should be maintained on a pillow in a partially abducted position, with the elbow slightly flexed. The leg should be kept in an extended position with a cradle over the foot, to eliminate pressure by the bedclothes (Fig. 23.3A and B).

and involve the dangers of flexion contractures of hips and knees. The back of the chair should have a variable rake so that the patient can, if necessary, fall asleep without being awakened by his head falling forwards or sideways due to lack of support. The arm should be supported on a pillow or specially designed armrest, with the shoulder partially abducted and the elbow partially flexed (Fig. 23.4).

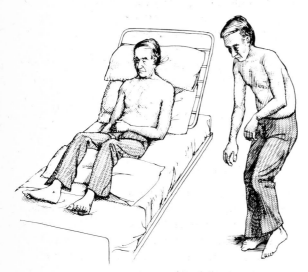

Fig. 23.2

If a hemianopia is present, relatives should be instructed to sit on the normal side. Similarly, bed lockers and food should be placed within the 'seeing' field.

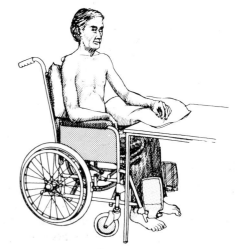

Fig. 23.4

Lifting and transferring

The nursing staff and physiotherapist must adopt a standardised approach to lifting and transferring (see Figs. 23.5 and 23.6).

Correct positioning in chair

The height of the chair and the depth of the seat should be correct. Many chairs are much too low

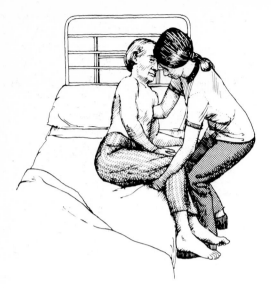

Fig. 23.5

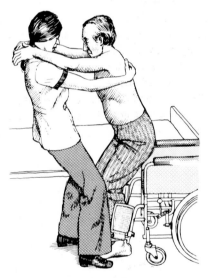

Fig. 23.6

Feeding

Initially, the patient will need to use his good arm for feeding. The nursing staff must be particularly alerted if there is a hemianopia and if there is anisognosia. Such patients may ignore food placed on the affected side.

Sphincters

Bladder training is a vital nursing function. Walking is very difficult when there is a catheter, or Paul's tube and the urinary bag, in situ. Training is likely to involve regular attempts at micturition, hourly in some cases. Bowel training is not usually a major problem. Faecal incontinence may be due to faecal impaction.

Avoidance of pressure sores

Pressure sores delay rehabilitation and can usually be avoided. Frequent turning of the patient by day and night is essential. Sores are particularly liable to occur on the heels and over the malleoli as well as in the lumbosacral area and over the greater trochanters. Heel sores may be prevented by using a specially shaped calf pad and by enclosing the heel in tube gauze.

Dressing

Pyjamas or a nightdress are probably the least suitable clothing for patients undergoing active rehabilitation. Frequently the donning of ordinary day clothes affects a remarkable psychological change in previously depressed patients. For a man, trousers and shirt are usually satisfactory. Alternatively, a track suit could be worn as this fosters the idea that something active is expected. Proper lace-up shoes should be provided when the patient first starts to walk. Bedroom slippers are quite unsuitable.

Occupational therapy

The occupational therapist must cooperate closely with the physiotherapist, nursing staff and speech therapist. Much of her work will be undertaken in the patient's home. Her duties will include:

ADL activities. The occupational therapist will be involved with the retraining of basic self-care activities such as feeding, dressing and washing. She will do this in collaboration with the spouse and with the nursing staff.

Assessment in the patient's home. The occupational therapist will need to look at such practical points as the presence or absence of a handrail on the stairs, the height of the cooker, whether the doors are wide enough to take a wheelchair and whether there are steps in the house which make mobility difficult. Having made her assessment, she would need to liaise with the local authority in arranging to get the necessary alterations undertaken as quickly as possible, so that the patient's discharge from hospital is not delayed.

Aids and appliances. Examples of practical aids which may help the disabled stroke patient include 'Velcro' instead of buttons, elastic shoelaces instead of the conventional type which need to be tied, one-hand potato peelers, and non-slip mats to be used under plates. The occupational therapist must be in a position to select such aids and to teach the patient and his relatives in their use. It should, however, be noted that many patients dislike 'gadgets', feeling that they emphasise the fact of disability. The number of aids should be kept to a minimum.

Providing the patient with something interesting to do. Inevitably, the range of activities available to the severely disabled patient is limited. It requires considerable imagination to find things that he can do and enjoy. It is all too easy to sit the patient down in front of the television screen. An activity enjoyed by many disabled people is gardening (see above).

Hand exercises. The occupational therapist is usually responsible for teaching hand exercises to hemiplegic patients. Regretfully, however, many patients never reach the stage of being able to use the affected hand usefully.

TREATMENT OF HEMIPLEGIA BY PHYSICAL METHODS

Despite the evident importance of physical therapy in the management of hemiplegia, there is considerable disagreement about which methods are best. A number of techniques are advocated (see Bobath, 1978; Knott, 1967; Rood, 1969; Brunnstrom, 1970). To date, however, little attempt has been made at validation. Amongst the factors which have influenced the development of techniques of physical therapy are the following:

1. The importance of sensory input to movement.
2. The presence of abnormal patterns of movement.
3. Spasticity.

4. The phenomena of inhibition and facilitation of movement.

Sensory input and movement

Mott & Sherrington (1895) studied monkeys with complete sensory denervation of a limb produced by section of the posterior nerve roots. The limb was rendered useless. This devastating effect, however, only occurred when denervation was complete; if one root was spared, the motor deficit was much less. Twitchell (1951) repeated and extended these experiments and noted, in particular, the loss of the ability to use the hand when denervation was complete. However, when one sensory root supplying a portion of the hand was spared, the animal was able to use the limb in a nearly normal manner, for walking, climbing, feeding and grooming. Twitchell emphasised the importance of both exteroceptive and proprioceptive impulses in motor function.

Brodal (1973), in describing his own stroke, noted the value of passive movement in training. Initially, he was unable to make a voluntary movement at a joint. However, when the movement had been made passively several times by the therapist, he was able to perform the movement, albeit with minimal force.

Practically all physiotherapists use passive movement and emphasise its importance. The fact remains that for at least 23 hours out of 24, the totally paralysed hemiplegic limb is lying perfectly still. It is possible that recovery might be hastened if passive movement, providing some degree of sensory feedback, could be given for several hours daily.

The presence of abnormal patterns of movement: the existence of 'limb synergies'

The flaccidity that follows the stroke is, within a matter of weeks, usually replaced by spasticity. During this phase the hemiplegic 'synergies' make their appearance. These synergies are stereotyped movements consisting either of a gross flexion or extension movement. The muscles activated in each synergy cannot, in the early stages, be recruited for different movement patterns. There is a 'loss of selective movement patterns' (Bobath, 1978). The sequence of recovery in the hemiplegic limb was described in Twitchell's classic paper (1951), which has greatly influenced the development of various physiotherapy techniques.

It has been argued (Bobath, 1978) that pathological reflex responses of the type mentioned above should not be employed in training for fear that they will prevent the return of normal movement. According to this view, the patient should not be allowed to use the basic limb synergies of flexion and extension, but rather attempts should be made, from the beginning, to develop normal motor responses. Any movement in the direction of the abnormal response should be prevented, and the patient's limbs, at rest, should be placed in a 'reflex-inhibiting posture' — usually the opposite position of the dominant synergy.

Brunnstrom (1970), after a review of the evidence, comes to the opposite conclusion and considers that the patient should be encouraged to gain control of basic limb synergies. She considers that once the synergies can be performed it should be possible to train the patient to modify the pattern of movement. She notes that the synergies appear to constitute a necessary intermediate stage of further recovery and cites the work of Twitchell (1951) in support of the view that the gross movement synergies of flexion and extension always precede the restoration of advanced motor function following hemiplegia in man. Brunnstrom makes use of 'associated reactions' in training. Thus, for example, a strong voluntary effort involving the normal arm may produce an involuntary movement on the paralysed side. Unfortunately, the studies of Twitchell have never been repeated and extended; it is clear that much basic work needs to be done in order to establish the stages through which the weak limbs pass during recovery.

Spasticity

Spasticity, when severe, can obscure residual movement; all major physiotherapy techniques involve some method of trying to reduce spasticity. Bobath (1978) considers that the physiotherapist should not allow an active movement until she has made sure that it will not be resisted by spastic muscle groups. She describes various manoeuvres for inhibiting spasticity.

Inhibition and facilitation of movement

Voluntary movement can be inhibited by many factors, some of them 'psychological'. For example, a long and tedious ambulance journey, or contact with a bad-tempered member of staff, may make the patient tense, unable to relax and thus not able to benefit from treatment. It is known that certain stimuli can be used to produce excitation and inhibition of different muscle groups. Thus, for example, Hagbarth (1960) studied electromyographically, the effects of stimulation of the skin of the lower limb in terms of excitation and inhibition of flexor and extensor motoneurones. Skin stimulation in certain specific areas causes excitation of extensor motoneurones and inhibition of flexor motoneurones. Skin stimulation may be used therapeutically, for instance, by brushing the skin of the relevant segment (Rood, 1969).

Another example of facilitation is given by Twitchell (1951). He showed that the relaxation phase of a finger jerk could be much prolonged by the willed effort of the patient, despite the absence of voluntary movement. In some patients the attempts to pull against the fingers of the examiner whilst intermittent finger jerks were being delivered produced flexion of the wrist, elbow and shoulder. These and other responses he called proprioceptive facilitation. A series of clinical therapeutic techniques involving PNF (proprioceptive neuromuscular facilitation) have been described (Knott, 1967).

Thus there are several approaches to the treatment of spastic hemiplegia. These are summarised by Manning (1974) and Johnstone (1980). The patient can be trained to use the unaffected side for all tasks previously undertaken by both together, the affected side being neglected and the leg being used purely as a prop. Alternatively, an attempt can be made to retrain the affected side — as much as the patterns of spasticity will allow.

The Bobath techniques are widely used, partly because they deal specifically and effectively with the problems of spasticity. They aim to suppress abnormal movement patterns produced as a result of spasticity before allowing normal movement to occur. The techniques of PNF are also employed in combination with those of Bobath. The techniques of Brunnstrom, however, are not so much used in the U.K.

EVALUATION OF THERAPEUTIC TECHNIQUES

A number of attempts have been made to ascertain the usefulness, or otherwise, of different methods of physical rehabilitation.

In 1961 Feldman et al reported on a controlled study of the rehabilitation of an unselected group of 82 stroke patients admitted to Bellvue Hospital with a hemiplegia or hemiparesis. The control group of 40 patients was given functionally-orientated medical care including training in sitting, standing, balancing, walking and self-care activities. The other 42 comprising the rehabilitation group were given a programme which was 'prescribed individually' and was varied according to the patient's needs and progress. Forty-two and a half per cent of the controls and 45 per cent of the rehabilitation group achieved a level of function at which they were able to perform the activities of daily living independently in a satisfactory manner. Fifty-five per cent of the control group were discharged home compared with 66 per cent of the rehabilitation group. The authors conclude that 'the results suggest that the great majority of hemiparetic stroke victims can be rehabilitated adequately on medical and neurological wards, without formal rehabilitation services, if proper attention is given to ambulation and self-care activities'.

Marquardsen (1969) after reviewing the literature and his own large series, concludes that 'it would seem, therefore, that few stroke patients would benefit from long continued and extensive treatment in rehabilitation institutions'.

Stern et al (1970) reported on the effects of facilitation exercise techniques in stroke rehabilitation. Sixty-two patients with hemiplegia were divided randomly into two groups. The control group received no specialised therapy. The 'exercise group' was given a special exercise programme which included proprioceptive neuromuscular facilitation. The motility index test of knee-flexion and extension strength and the Kenny Rehabilitation Institute Self Care Evaluation were the measurements used to determine improvements. The authors concluded that no significant difference existed in improvement between the control and the 'exercise group'. The results have been questioned (Inaba et al, 1973) on various grounds including the nature of the evaluation methods used which, with the exception of the assessment of activities of daily living, are poor measures of improvement in patients with hemiplegia.

Peacock et al (1972) reported on an epidemiological study undertaken in Birmingham, Alabama. Fifty-two patients were included in this study on rehabilitation. They were first assessed by a multidisciplinary team on their personal care and occupational status and potential. Then they were randomised into a control group of 23, who were given standardised hospital care, and an experimental group of 29, who were given intensive rehabilitation. Re-evaluation at the time of maximum improvement showed little or no advantage for the group receiving intensive rehabilitation.

Inaba et al (1973) studied 77 hemiplegic patients. The patients were divided into three treatment groups. Group I patients served as a control group and received functional training only and 'selective stretching'. Group II patients received active exercises in addition to functional training and 'selective stretching'. Group III patients received progressive resistive exercises, as well as functionally-orientated training and 'selective stretching'. The results indicated that a one month programme of progressive resistive exercises and training in ADL is more effective than a programme of ADL alone, or when this is combined with simple active exercises. However, following two months of treatment, no difference was evident between the groups in levels of achievement in activities of daily living. The results were claimed to demonstrate that the same level of function can be achieved in half the time, providing the most effective treatment procedures are utilised.

A useful review on the subject was published by Lehmann et al in 1975 under the title 'Stroke: does rehabilitation affect outcome?' This paper reviews the literature up to that time. The authors reported on a sample of 114 consecutive stroke admissions to a rehabilitation centre. The mean time from onset to admission was 9.9 months. It was found that with intensive therapy significant gains were achieved which could not be attributed merely to spontaneous recovery.

A recent important study has been published by Smith et al (1981). Of 1094 patients with a confirmed stroke admitted to Northwick Park Hospital, London, 121 (11 per cent) were suitable for intensive treatment. They, and 12 patients referred directly to outpatients, were allocated at random to one of three different courses of rehabilitation. Intensive was compared with conventional rehabilitation and with a third regimen which included no routine rehabilitation, but under which patients were encouraged to continue with exercises taught while in hospital and were regularly seen at home by a health visitor. Progress at 3 months and 12 months was measured by an Index of Activities of Daily Living. Improvement was greatest in those receiving intensive treatment, intermediate in those receiving conventional treatment and least in those receiving no treatment. Decreasing intensity of treatment was associated with a significant increase in the proportion of patients who deteriorated and in the extent to which they deteriorated. It was concluded that probably only a few patients, mostly men, are suitable for intensive outpatient rehabilitation, but for those patients the treatment is effective and realistic.

The above studies still do not give clear answers about the usefulness or otherwise of rehabilitation procedures. Further controlled studies are required and these must include sensitive and relevant assessment techniques and a clear idea of what procedures are being evaluated. It has not yet been established that any one physical technique is better than another, or indeed that any particular treatment method is better than simple functionally-orientated therapy. It is perhaps surprising that there have been no attempts to validate the very widely used Bobath techniques. In assessing the usefulness or otherwise of therapeutic techniques, it must be remembered that rehabilitation inevitably involves a 'package deal'. A large number of different factors are involved.

For many years there has been interest in the problem of exciting peripheral nerves electrically for the purpose of producing a functional muscle contraction. In particular, several devices have been developed to stimulate the common peroneal nerve by superficial surface stimulation in order to correct the 'foot drop' occurring in hemiplegic patients. This and other aspects of the problem were reviewed in 1972 (Functional Neuromuscular Stimulation, 1972). The use of proportionally controlled functional electrical stimulation at the hand has been reported (Rebersek & Vodovnik, 1973). Programmed electrical stimulation of areas of the brain in order to produce skilled movements have been investigated in monkeys (Pinneo et al, 1972). The applicability of this technique to man is still uncertain and little progress appears to have been made during the last number of years.

The possibility of using biofeedback techniques in training has been investigated by a number of workers. Recent important contributions include those of Brudny et al (1976 & 1979) and Wolf et al (1980). The subject of biofeedback and visceral learning generally has been the subject of an important review (Miller, 1978). Most workers have used e.m.g. signals obtained from limb muscles, which are then appropriately amplified, rectified, integrated and displayed in a visual or auditory manner. Some workers claim to have produced an improvement in functional recovery in the upper limb, but the technique has not yet been widely explored in the U.K.

COMMUNICATION DISORDERS AND APHASIA

Inability to communicate is one of the most serious results of a stroke for many patients and their families. This section briefly discusses the natural history of aphasia, the effectiveness of speech therapy, the measurement of change and the various types of therapy that are available.

Natural history of aphasia

It is recognised that most patients show some degree of spontaneous recovery. Important contributions to this subject include those of Culton (1969), Kenin & Swisher (1972) and Kertesz &

McCabe (1977). Most improvement occurs during the first three months, but demonstrable recovery can occur up to six months post-stroke, and possibly longer (Sands et al, 1969). Recovery rates are higher for post-traumatic cases than for stroke patients; global aphasia has a poor prognosis and younger patients usually recover better than older ones. There is disagreement as to the relative outlooks of comprehension and expressive language (Kertesz & McCabe, 1977).

Effectiveness of speech therapy

The rationale of speech therapy remains unclear, but must be investigated if resources are to be rationally used (British Medical Journal, 1977). The problem of undertaking studies in this field has been reviewed by Darley (1972); Hopkins (1975) and Sarno (1976). Factors requiring consideration include:

1. The small number of cases likely to be available for study.
2. The effect of spontaneous recovery.
3. The difficulty of specifying the amount and details of treatment given.
4. The impossibly large number of variables including sex, age, site of lesion, and type and severity of aphasia.

Firm evidence for the efficacy of speech therapy can only be obtained by controlled trials involving random assignment of patients to treatment and non-treatment groups. Ethical considerations currently preclude the total withholding of therapy and for this reason the control group is usually given either non-specific general encouragement or is managed by untrained volunteers (see below).

Sarno (1976) reviewed the literature and could only find six studies in English which had addressed themselves specifically to recovery with rehabilitation in post-stroke aphasic patients. The only attempt at a control trial was that of Sarno et al (1970). This study can be criticised on the grounds that it was non-random; only 31 patients were involved. Only patients with severe aphasia were studied and there was no attempt to match the patients for certain important variables such as site and size of the lesion.

The problems faced by aphasic patients and their families are considerable and the resources of speech therapy departments are limited. Furthermore, little is known about the most effective way of deploying the skills of professional speech therapists. As a result of this disparity, which was pointed out by Hopkins in 1975, Griffith (1975) has pioneered the use of volunteer helpers. Many volunteer schemes based on her methods now exist in the U.K., using non-professional helpers for aphasic subjects. The efficacy of such schemes has not yet been determined, although there is some evidence that social confidence does increase (Lesser & Watt, 1978).

Two recent U.K. studies (Meikle et al, 1979; David et al, 1979) compared the results of treatment by trained speech therapists with those obtained by volunteers. The first study showed no important differences between the two groups. However, the total number of patients in this study was only 31. The Bristol group have recently published details of their feasibility study (David et al, 1979). Patients were allocated randomly to either individual speech therapy or to an equal amount of intervention from untrained volunteers. Their progress was closely followed for 12 weeks of treatment, then subsequently until the end of one year. After some minor changes to the protocol this study is now continuing as a large project involving about 20 centres.

Measurement of change

Reliable and well-validated test procedures are required for describing both the natural history of aphasia and the possible efficacy of therapy. Several such procedures are in everyday use and the most frequently used is probably the Minnesota Test for differential diagnosis of aphasia (Schuell, 1965). The Porch Index of Communicative Ability (Porch, 1967) is another detailed test which is becoming increasingly popular, as it enables the assessor to record such important items as the latency of response and the ability to use substitute words, self-corrections and the use of gesture with minimal cues.

The Functional Communication Profile (Sarno & Sands, 1970), is being increasingly used as a short test which can be completed in 15–20 minutes. This is based on a structured conversation between examiner and patient and provides quantification in percentage terms of the patient's ability to function in a variety of language activities of daily life including speech, understanding and writing.

Types of therapy

It has been said that there are probably as many methods of aphasia therapy as there are aphasic patients. This overstatement reflects the many theories about language recovery in aphasia. The subject has been reviewed by Darley (1972) and Sarno (1976). Space does not allow a detailed discussion here. Some of the techniques currently being used are listed below. There is considerable overlap between them:

1. *General stimulation.* The patient is encouraged to speak, whatever the content. Great importance is attached to taking note of the patient's interests and premorbid personality. Some workers make use of filmstrip to stimulate the patient's interest.

2. *Programmed instruction* (Sarno et al, 1970). This views language rehabilitation as an educative process and applies operant conditioning methods drawn from learning theory and principles drawn from psycholinguistic analysis. Some workers use the language laboratory in much the same way as when used for teaching normal people foreign languages.

3. *Melodic intonation* (Albert et al, 1973). This makes use of an assumed residual melody through a series of carefully graduated steps in which the patient, in unison with the therapist, intones a melody with meaningful words or phrases.

4. *Visual communication therapy* (Velletri-Glass et al, 1973). This system derives from the observation that severe aphasics usually use the visual system without difficulty. Patients are taught to recognise symbols drawn on cards to represent words and then to manipulate these in order to make appropriate responses.

Other experimental techniques include exposure to hyperbaric oxygen, drugs, psychotherapy and hypnosis.

Table 23.3 gives practical advice on helping the aphasic patient to communicate and on helping patients with problems of comprehension.

Table 23.3 Practical advice on helping the aphasic patient to communicate

Never hurry the patient. Remember that he may take much longer than normal to understand what is said, and to formulate his reply.

Any attempt at communication by the patient should be encouraged — if only with a 'thumbs-up' sign.

Do not 'talk over' the patient when he is able to answer questions himself. Avoid 'Does he take sugar in his tea?' Speak TO the patient. Do not leave him out; for example, he should not be left out on a ward round.

Any attempt on the part of the patient should be accepted and encouraged. Remember that many patients feel embarrassed, humiliated, and frustrated.

Find out what interests the patient and centre discussion around these. The patient will probably perform best when talking about things that are familiar to him.

If the patient uses a one word sentence, e.g., 'toilet', encourage him to expand the sentence by saying 'I want to go to the toilet'.

Remember that fatigue and emotional disturbance adversely affect both comprehension and expression. Make sure that the patient is relaxed. He may perform best if there is nobody else in the room.

Aphasic patients are highly distractable. Avoid background noise.

Practical advice on helping patients who have a problem with comprehension

Remember that most patients have, at the least, a mild receptive disability.

Never under-estimate the patient's comprehension.

Avoid long, rambling conversations — the patient will not understand.

Speak a little slower than normal. Do NOT shout!

Stand in front of the patient so that he can see your facial movements and expression.

COMPLICATIONS

Complications are those events which occur at some point after the onset of the stroke. Those that affect rehabilitation can conveniently be divided into those that are primarily cerebral and those that involve the limbs. These subjects have been thoroughly reviewed by Moskowitz (1969). Some of the more important complications are listed below.

Depression

Depression is very easily overlooked or misdiagnosed as 'poor motivation', particularly in patients with a significant communication disorder. Indeed, it seems likely that most patients with a severe stroke do become depressed at some point.

An attempt must be made to understand the patient's problems, which may be highly complex. Problems include worries about finance, employment, the possibility of permanent disablement and marital relations. One member of the stroke team must be responsible for establishing rapport with the patient and must be prepared to spend time helping sort out the patient's problems. Antidepressive drugs may be used in some cases but cannot be regarded as a panacea.

Epilepsy

The prevalence of epilepsy was noted to be 6 per cent in Marquardsen's series (1969) and 7.7 per cent in that of Louis & McDowell (1967). Moskowitz (1969) quotes a prevalence of over 15 per cent in a long-term follow-up of older patients.

Venous thrombosis in the hemiplegic leg

Cope et al (1973) undertook a phlebographic study of patients who had survived the acute stroke and found a 33 per cent prevalence of acute venous thrombosis in the hemiplegic leg. In about one-third, the thrombosis was undiagnosable by clinical examination. The practical importance of this complication has not yet been fully explored.

Painful stiff shoulder

Pain and stiffness in the shoulder of a hemiplegic arm is very common. It is frequently the result of faulty lifting technique and poor positioning of the limb in the early flaccid stage. Any attempt to assist the patient into a sitting or standing position must avoid load-bearing on the affected joint. In addition, the weight of the arm itself tends to distract the shoulder capsule, and for this reason it may be helpful to put the arm into a sling when the patient is walking. Pain and stiffness can sometimes be alleviated by local injections of hydrocortisone. Other causes of a painful shoulder are:

1. Fracture of the neck of the humerus.
2. Dislocation of the shoulder joint (particularly liable to occur in the flaccid stage).
3. Contracture due to the later development of spasticity. In some cases this may necessitate surgical division of the major muscles which cause internal rotation and adduction of the shoulder (Braun et al, 1971).
4. Shoulder/hand syndrome. This complication has been also named 'post-hemiplegic reflex sympathetic dystrophy' (Moskowitz et al, 1958). This problem occurs in about five per cent of stroke patients. In severe cases there is demineralisation of the head and neck of the humerus. Oral steroids and vigorous passive exercises are usually effective.
5. Inflammation in soft tissues around the shoulder joint. Inflammation may occur in a number of different sites including the acromio-clavicular and glenohumeral joints, the biceps tendon and in the subdeltoid bursa (Braun et al, 1971).
6. Ectopic calcification in the periarticular structures. This is a rare complication and the diagnosis can only be made by X-ray.

Gross spasticity

Mild degrees of spasticity are the rule in the later stages of hemiplegia and there are various physiotherapeutic techniques available for its reduction (Bobath, 1978). Sometimes, however, the spasticity cannot be controlled by simple positioning and relaxing techniques and other measures may need to be adopted. These include:

Cooling. A temporary reduction in the severity of spasticity can often be achieved by applying ice-bags or by immersing the spastic limb in cold water (Hedenberg, 1970; Lee & Warren, 1974).

Drugs. A large number of drugs have been used to reduce spasticity. The use of diazepam was evaluated in various neurological conditions by Nathan (1970). The practical experience of most workers is that drugs are of very limited value in the management of spasticity occurring in the hemiplegic patient.

Intraneural, intramuscular and intrathecal phenol injections. A temporary reduction in spasticity lasting for about six months can sometimes be achieved by selective injections of phenol into the nerve sheaths of peripheral nerves (Braun et al, 1973). Phenol injections can be a valuable supplementary form of treatment when combined with tendon transplant or vigorous physical therapy.

Similar results have been reported with intramuscular motor point injections (Halpern & Meelhuysen, 1966; Awad, 1972). When spasticity in the leg is very severe, rendering nursing impossible, it may occasionally be necessary to resort to intrathecal phenol injections (Roper, 1975). Such procedures are usually reserved for incontinent patients.

Destructive surgery. Occasionally, spasticity can only be overcome by destructive surgery involving division of muscles, tendons or nerves. For example, where there is severe finger flexion there can be odoriferous maceration in the palm of the hand. Division of the flexor tendons at the wrist will relieve this. (Roper, 1975).

Contractures and deformities

Contractures are liable to follow prolonged unrelieved severe spasticity — the result of irreversible changes in the soft tissues around the joints. Contractures may occur at all the main limb joints. Sometimes there is a combination of spasticity and contracture. Two examples may be given:

Equinovarus deformity. In moderate cases this can be controlled with a short leg brace which must not incorporate a spring as this will accentuate the stretch reflex. In other cases the deformity can be corrected by elongation of the Achilles tendon and transfer of half of the tibialis anterior to the outer border of the foot (Roper, 1975).

Pronation-flexion deformity of the forearm and hand. This can sometimes be partially corrected, in carefully selected cases, by surgical release of the flexor origins of the relevant muscles (Braun et al, 1970). The potential for surgery of hemiplegic deformities has been pioneered at Rancho Los Amigos Hospital, Downey, California (Nickel, 1969; Roper, 1975).

Splinting and calipers

Lightweight splints are sometimes used in order to maintain the flaccid paralysed limb in a satisfactory position. Splints alone are useless when there is marked spasticity. One of the most used devices is a below-knee brace sometimes combined with a T strap. The usefulness of this brace is debated and many physiotherapists claim that there is rarely a need for any type of foot-drop support. The author's experience, however, is that a brace can sometimes be very useful, particularly in the early stages before marked spasticity has developed.

Fracture of long bones

Fractures of the neck of the femur are particularly likely to occur in patients with an equinovarus deformity of the ankle because of the obvious tendency for the foot to catch on the ground (Treanor, 1969).

Peripheral nerve palsies

A variety of root and nerve compression lesions can occur, particularly if the paralysed limbs are allowed to rest in an incorrect position (Moskowitz, 1969). Nerve palsies readily go undiagnosed when they occur in an already partially paralysed limb. Lesions of the C5-6 root, the long thoracic nerve and the radial nerve all occur if the unsupported arm is allowed to hang out of bed. In the case of the radial nerve the back of the upper arm may rest against the hard edge of the bed. Ulnar nerve lesions can occur if the inner side of the elbow is allowed to rest on the unpadded rail of a wheelchair. Common peroneal and sciatic nerve lesions can both occur with faulty positioning.

OUTCOME

Mortality

Marquardsen (1969) has pointed out that, whereas no sharp distinction can be made between immediate and later mortality after cerebrovascular accident (CVA) — the shape of the survival curve indicates that the majority of early deaths have occurred within three weeks of the stroke. Most publications give early mortality at either three or fours weeks from the ictus. Marquardsen (1969) found that 50.5 per cent of men and 44.8 per cent of women in his retrospective hospital series had died by three weeks. Early mortality figures derived from community studies vary widely — 33 per cent (Marquardsen, 1978); 44.7 per cent (Whisnant, 1971); 47.4 per cent (Weddell, 1974); 56.6 per cent (Eisenberg, 1964); and 57 per cent

(Acheson & Fairbairn, 1971). The prognosis is determined mainly by the age of the patient and the type, size, and anatomical site of the lesion. About 75 per cent of cerebral haemorrhages, but only 25–30 per cent of ischaemic strokes, are fatal. (Marquardsen, 1978).

The survival prospects of those patients still alive at the end of the first month are of particular interest to those involved in the planning of services for the disabled. The number of four-weeks survivors who will die within the first year ranges between 27–35 per cent (Eisenberg et al, 1964; Acheson et al, 1971; Marquardsen, 1976; Brocklehurst et al, 1978). By three years 56–63 per cent will be dead (Eisenberg et al, 1964; Brocklehurst, 1978), and 66 per cent by five years (Eisenberg et al, 1964).

Marquardsen (1969) followed 407 three-week survivors for between 10 and 23 years. Throughout the observation period, the mortality was much higher than that of the general population of similar age. The observed three-year mortality rate was 46 per cent, in contrast to an expected mortality rate of only 12 per cent. A median survival time was 3.5 years, as opposed to 10 years in the corresponding general population. The annual rate at which survivors decreased remained approximately constant for at least 10 years after the stroke — being 16 per cent for males and 18 per cent for females. Younger patients survived longer than older patients. The main causes of death in this series were recurrent strokes — 23 per cent; myocardial infarction — 10 per cent, and heart failure or broncho-pneumonia — 30 per cent.

It is apparent that the age at which the stroke occurs is an important prognostic feature. Marquardsen found that in males below the age of 60 the number of survivors decreased at an annual rate of about 10 per cent, wheras in the group aged 70–79 the rate was 25 per cent. The corresponding median survival time was 6.5 years and 2.2 years respectively. Marquardsen found that one of the most important prognostic factors was the ultimate functional capacity achieved by patients during their stay in hospital. Thus, for instance, a strikingly bad prognosis was found in the most severely disabled patients. Four-fifths had died within two years of the stroke. The mean expectation of life in this category was 1.5 years.

Risk of a further stroke

The problem was considered in detail by Marquardsen (1969), who made the following observations:

1. The annual risk of having a further stroke appears to be independent of the length of time which has elapsed since the primary stroke. The average annual recurrence rate was 8 per cent for males and 9 per cent for females.
2. The time interval between the primary stroke and the first recurrence ranged from a few weeks to 17 years (average 3.7 years).
3. The risk of having a further stroke is not significantly greater during the first 12 months after the initial stroke — 8.6 per cent for males, and 12.2 per cent for females.
4. Marquardsen calculated that 50 per cent of the survivors would have a second attack within 8 years and 75 per cent within 16.5 years. It is clear, however, that many patients will die from a different disease before having a further stroke.

Functional outcome

It is only in recent years that the functional outcome following stroke has been documented. Even now, there are very few properly conducted population studies. A major difficulty concerns the lack of standardised assessment techniques. The problem was discussed by the Royal College of Physicians' Working Group on Strokes (1974).

Five community-based series give information relating to the outcome of patients who have survived the first three-four weeks (Wallace, 1967; Marquardsen, 1969; Petlund, 1970; Matsumoto et al, 1973; and Gresham et al, 1975). The papers show a considerable degree of agreement, although the results given by Petlund show some divergence from the others, possibly because this was a prevalence rather than an incidence study. Of those working before the stroke 29–36 per cent were working, or were able to work, afterwards; 20–27 per cent could not walk unaided; 31–52 per cent were dependent in some aspect on self care activity; 12–21 per cent of stroke survivors will require long term institutional care in a hospital or nursing home. Overall the results of these community studies indicate that about 50 per cent of stroke survivors will achieve a full, or almost full, functional recovery. Marquardsen (1969) reviewed the literature relating to hospitalised stroke survivors, and found that 50–70 per cent were able to walk unaided and 20–30 per cent had to be transferred to institutions. The proportion who could go back to work was highly dependent upon the age structure of the series, varying between 1–25 per cent. The average duration of hospital stay of stroke survivors was 52 days for males and 73 days for females.

Prediction of outcome

Marquardsen (1969) found that there were a number of clinical manifestations which were associated with an unfavourable functional prognosis. Of the adverse factors already present at the time of admission, the most important were: — age over 70, severe motor impairment, impairment of consciousness of more than a few hours duration, conjugate ocular deviation and conceptual disorders. During the subsequent course the following factors were indicative of a poor recovery: — lack of improvement of motor function, persistent confusion or apathy, urinary or bowel incontinence and extracerebral complications.

The importance of mental confusion, memory loss, depression, and cognitive and visuo-spatial disorders has been emphasised by many authors (Adams, 1974). However, Isaacs (1973) found that language and perceptual disorders did not necessarily present an insuperable barrier to recovery, since with an appropriate treatment programme many patients with these disabilities regained functional independence and were able to return home.

Marquardsen found that right-sided cerebral lesions carried a less favourable prognosis than left-sided lesions. Patients with lesions confined to the brainstem did better than those with hemisphere abnormalities.

Rate of recovery

Reliable data relating to the rate of recovery depend upon the availability of well validated and sensitive measures of outcome. Twitchell (1951) described the course of motor recovery following stroke. This classical paper gives details of the physiological sequence of recovery in the limbs. All those who regained complete recovery of upper limb function had some voluntary hand movement by 15 days.

An important recent contribution is that of Brocklehurst et al (1978), who studied 139 patients who had suffered a recent stroke and survived two weeks. These workers studied seven parameters of recovery, including mobility, ADL, and mental confusion. Most recovery occurred within eight weeks. However, 12 per cent showed improvement in their walking score beyond eight weeks and 28 per cent showed improvement in their ADL score beyond this time. The study indicates that, apart from some patients with minimal disability, little further recovery could be expected beyond six months from the date of the stroke. The findings suggest that a major investment in physical therapy beyond six months is likely to be wasteful.

The future

It is clear that much still requires to be done in the field of stroke rehabilitation. The problems range from the organisation of care services, both in hospital and in the community, to the physiology of motor control. It is certainly a field in which collaboration can usefully be developed between people with widely differing skills.

REFERENCES

Acheson R M, Fairbairn A S 1971 Record linkage in studies of cerebrovascular disease in Oxford, England. Stroke 2:48–57

Adams G F 1974 Cerebrovascular disability and the ageing brain. Churchill Livingstone, Edinburgh and London

Adams G F, Hurwitz L J 1963 Mental barriers to recovery from strokes. Lancet ii:533–537

Albert M, Sparks R, Helm N 1973 Melodic intonation therapy for aphasia. Archives of Neurology 29:130–131

Andrews K, Stewart J 1979 Stroke recovery: he can but does he? Rheumatology & Rehabilitation 18:43–48

Awad E A 1972 Intramuscular neurolysis for stroke. Minnesota Medicine 55:711–713

Birch H G, Proctor F, Bortner M, Lowenthal M 1960 Perception in hemiplegia: 1. Judgement of vertical and horizontal by hemiplegic patients. Archives of Physical Medicine & Rehabilitation 41:19–27

Birch H G, Belmont I, Reilly T, Belmont L 1961 Visual verticality in hemiplegia. Archives of Neurology 5:444–453

Blower P, Ali S 1979 A stroke unit in a District General Hospital: the Greenwich experience. British Medical Journal 2:644–646

Bobath B 1978 Adult hemiplegia: evaluation and treatment. 2nd ed. William Heinemann Medical Books Ltd, London

Braun R M, Mooney V, Nickel V L 1970 Flexor-origin release for pronation-flexion deformity of the forearm and hand in the stroke patient. An evaluation of the early results in 18 patients. Journal of Bone and Joint Surgery 52A:907–920

Braun R M, West F, Mooney V, Nickel V L, Roper B, Caldwell C 1971 Surgical treatment of the painful shoulder contracture in the stroke patient. Journal of Bone and Joint Surgery 53A:7, 1307–1312

Braun R M, Hoffer M M, Mooney V, McKeever J, Roper B 1973 Phenol nerve block in the treatment of acquired spastic hemiplegia in the upper limb. Journal of Bone and Joint Surgery 55A:3, 580–585

British Medical Journal—leading article 1977 Recovery patterns and prognosis in aphasia. British Medical Journal 2:848–849

Brocklehurst J C, Andrews K, Morris P E, Richards B, Laycock P J 1978 Medical, social and psychological aspects of stroke — final report. University of Manchester

Brodal A 1973 Self observations and neuro-anatomical considerations after a stroke. Brain 96:675–694

Brudny J, Korein J, Grynbaum B B, Friedmann L W, Weinstein S, Sachs-Frankel G, Belandres P V 1976 EMG feedback therapy: review of treatment of 114 patients. Archives of Physical Medicine & Rehabilitation 57:55–61

Brudny J, Korein J, Grynbaum B B, Belandres P V, Gianutsos J G 1979 Helping hemiparetics to help themselves: sensory feedback therapy. Journal of the American Medical Association 241:8, 814–818

Bruell J H, Peszcynski M, Volk D 1957 Disturbance of perception of verticality in patients with hemiplegia: 2nd Report. Archives of Physical Medicine and Rehabilitation 38:776–780

Brunnstrom S 1970 Movement therapy in hemiplegia: a neurophysiological approach. Harper and Row, New York

Capildeo R, Haberman S, Rose F C 1978 The definition and classification of stroke. Quarterly Journal of Medicine, New Series XI vii 186:177–196

Carey R G, Posavac E J 1978 Program evaluation of a physical medicine and rehabilitation unit: a new approach. Archives of Physical Medicine and Rehabilitation 59:330–337

Circular London, Ministry of Health 1968 Care of Younger Chronic Sick Patients in Hospitals. London: HMSO (68) 41

Cochrane A L 1970 Burden of cerebrovascular disease. British Medical Journal 3:165

Cope C, Reyes T M, Skversky N J 1973 Phlebographic analysis of the incidence of thrombosis in hemiplegia. Radiology 109:No. 3, 581–584

Culton G 1969 Spontaneous recovery from aphasia. Journal of Speech and Hearing Research 12:825–832

David R M, Enderby P, Bainton D 1979 Progress report on an evaluation of speech therapy for aphasia. British Journal of Disorders of Communication 14:85–88

Darley F C 1972 The efficacy of language rehabilitation in aphasia. Journal of Speech and Hearing Disorders 37:3–21

Denham M J, Jeffreys P M 1972 Routine mental testing in the elderly. Modern Geriatrics 2:275–279

Department of Health and Social Security Welsh Office 1972 Rehabilitation. Report of a sub-committee of the standing medical advisory committee (Tunbridge Report).

Diller L 1970 Behavioural change in cerebrovascular disease. Benton A L (ed) Harper & Row, New York and London

Eisenberg H, Morrison J T, Sullivan P, Foote F M 1964 Cerebrovascular accidents — incidence and survival rates in a defined population. Middlesex County, Connecticut. Journal of the American Medical Association 189:883–888

Feigensen J S, Gitlow H S, Greenberg S D 1979 The disability orientated rehabilitation unit — a major factor influencing stroke outcome. Stroke 10:5–8

Feldman D J, Lee P R, Unterecker J, Lloyd K, Rusk H A, Toole A 1971 A comparison of functionally orientated medical care and formal rehabilitation in the management of patients with hemiplegia due to cerebrovascular disease. Journal of Chronic Diseases 15:297–310

Garraway W M, Akhtar A J, Prescott R J, Hockey C 1980 (a) Management of acute stroke in the elderly: preliminary results of a controlled trial. British Medical Journal 1:1040–1043

Garraway W J, Akhtar A J, Hockey C, Prescott R J 1980 (b) Management of acute stroke in the elderly: follow-up of a controlled trial. British Medical Journal ii:827–829

Gresham G E, Fitzpatrick T E, Wolf P A, McNamara P M, Kannel W B, Dawber T R 1975 Residual disability in survivors of stroke — the Framingham Study. New England Journal of Medicine 293:954–956

Griffith V E 1975 Volunteer scheme for dysphasia and allied problems in stroke patients. British Medical Journal 3:633–635

Guttman Sir L 1976 Textbook of sport for the disabled. H M & M Publishers, Aylesbury, England

Hagbarth K E 1960 Spinal withdrawal reflexes in human lower limb. Journal of Neurology, Neurosurgery and Psychiatry 23:222–227

Hale G 1979 The source book for the disabled. Paddington Press Ltd, New York, London

Halpern D, Meelhuysen F E 1966 Phenol motor point block in the management of muscular hypertonia. Archives of Physical Medicine and Rehabilitation 47:659–664

Harris A I, Cox E, Smith C H W 1971 Handicapped and impaired in Great Britain: Part 1. Office of Population Censuses and Surveys, London, HMSO

Hedenberg L 1970 Functional improvement of the spastic hemiplegic arm after cooling. Scandinavian Journal of Rehabilitation Medicine 2:154–158

Hiorns R W, Newcombe F 1979 Recovery curves: uses and limitations. International Rehabilitation Medicine 1:173–176

Hodkinson H M 1972 Evaluation of a mental test score for assessment of mental impairment in the elderly. Age and Ageing 1:233–238

Hopkins A 1975 The need for speech therapy for dysphasia following stroke. Health Trends 7:58–60

Inaba M, Edberg E, Montgomery J, Gillis M K 1973 Effectiveness of functional training, active exercises, and resistive exercise for patients with hemiplegia. Physical Therapy 53:28–35

Isaacs B 1971 Identification of disability in the stroke patient. Modern Geriatrics 1:390–402

Isaacs B, Marks R 1973 Determinants of outcome of stroke rehabilitation. Age and Ageing 2:139–149

Isaacs B 1977 Five year experience of a stroke unit. Health Bulletin 35:94–98

Johnstone M 1980 Home care for the stroke patient. Churchill Livingstone, Edinburgh, London, New York

Katz S, Ford A B, Moskowitz R W, Jackson B A, Jaffe M W 1963 Studies of illness in the aged: the index of ADL; a standardised measure of biological and psychosocial function. Journal of the American Medical Association 185:914–919

Kenin M, Swisher P L 1972 A study of pattern of recovery in aphasia. Cortex 8:56–68

Kertesz A, McCabe P 1977 Recovery patterns and prognosis in aphasia. Brain 100:1–18

Knott M 1967 Introduction to and philosophy of neuromuscular facilitation. Physiotherapy 53:2–5

Labi M L L, Phillips T F, Gresham G E 1980 Psychosocial disability in physically restored long-term stroke survivors. Archives of Physical Medicine & Rehabilitation 61:561–565

Lee J M, Warren M P 1974 Ice, relaxation and exercise in reduction of muscle spasticity. Physiotherapy 60:296–302

Lehmann J F, Delateur B J, Fowler R S, Warren C G, Arnhold R, Schertzer G, Hurka R, Whitmore J J, Masock A J, Chambers K H 1975 Stroke: does rehabilitation affect outcome? Archives of Physical Medicine & Rehabilitation 56:375–382

Lesser R, Watt M 1978 Untrained community help in the rehabilitation of stroke sufferers with language disorder. British Medical Journal 2:1045–1048

Louis S, McDowell F 1967 Epileptic seizures in nonembolic cerebral infarction. Archives of Neurology 17:414–418

Mahoney F I, Barthel D W 1965 Functional evaluation: the Barthel Index. Maryland State Medical Journal 14:61–65

Manning J 1974 Hemiplegia. In: Cash J (ed) Neurology for physiotherapists. Faber and Faber, London

Marquardsen J 1969 The natural history of acute cerebrovascular disease. Munksgaard, Copenhagen

Marquardsen J 1976 An epidemiological study of stroke in a Danish urban community. In: Gillingham F J, Mawdsley C, Williams A E (eds) Stroke. Churchill Livingstone, Edinburgh, London, New York

Marquardsen J 1978 The epidemiology of cerebrovascular disease. Acta Neurologica Scandinavica Supplement 67:57–75

Matsumoto N, Whisnant J P, Kurland C T, Okazaki H 1973 Natural history of stroke in Rochester, Minnesota. Stroke 4:20–29

Meikle M, Wechsler E, Tupper A, Benenson M, Butler J, Mulhall D, Stern G 1979 Comparative trial of volunteer and professional treatments of dysphasia after stroke. British Medical Journal 2:87–89

Millard J B 1973 Medical rehabilitation and hemiplegia. Proceedings of the Royal Society of Medicine 66:1003–1008

Miller N E 1978 Biofeedback and visceral learning. Annual Review of Psychology 29:373–404

Moskowitz E, Bishop H F, Shibutani K 1958 Posthemiplegic reflex sympathetic dystrophy. Journal of the American Medical Association 167:836–838

Moskowitz E 1969 Complications in the rehabilitation of hemiplegic patients. Medical Clinics of North America 53:541–59

Mott F W, Sherrington C S 1895 Experiments upon the influence of sensory nerves upon movement and nutrition of the limbs. Proceedings of the Royal Society of Medicine 57:481

Mulley G, Arie T 1978 Treating stroke: home or hospital? British Medical Journal 2:1321–1322

Nathan P W 1970 The action of diazapam in neurological disorders with excessive motor activity. Journal of the Neurological Sciences 10:33–50

Morbidity Statistics from General Practice 1974 Second national study 1970–71. Studies on medical and population subjects No. 26. Office of Population Censuses & Surveys, London HMSO

Nichols P J R 1974 Rehabilitation in the reorganised National Health Service. A King's Fund centre talk. Occupational Therapy, July 1974, 113–116

Nichols P J R 1976 Are ADL indices of any value? Occupational Therapy 39:160–163

Nickel V L (ed) 1969 Symposium on the orthopaedic management of stroke. Reprinted from Clinical Orthopaedics No. 63. Philadelphia: J B Lippincott

Peacock P B, Riley C P, Lampton T D, Raffel S S, Walker J S 1972 The Birmingham stroke, epidemiology and rehabilitation study. In: Stewart G T (ed) Trends in epidemiology. Charles C Thomas, Springfield, Illinois

Petlund C F 1970 Prevalence and invalidity from stroke in Aust Agder County of Norway. Norwegian Monographs on Medical Science, Oslo

Pinneo L R, Kaplan J N, Elpel E A, Reynolds P L, Glick J H 1972 Experimental brain prosthesis for stroke. Stroke 3:16–26

Porch B 1967 The Porch index of communicative ability. Palo Alto, Consultant Psychologists

Rebersek S, Vodovnik L 1973 Proportionally controlled functional electrical stimulation of the hand. Archives of Physical Medicine & Rehabilitation 54:378–82

Report of Working Group on Strokes 1974 Royal College of Physicians, London

Report of WHO Meeting 1971 Cerebrovascular diseases: prevention, treatment and rehabilitation. Geneva

Rood M 1969 Unpublished observations

Roper B A 1975 Surgical aspects of stroke rehabilitation. Modern Geriatrics 5:4–9

Rosenzweig M R 1980 Animal models for effects of brain lesions and for rehabilitation. In: Bach-y-Rita P (ed) Recovery of function: theoretical considerations for brain injury rehabilitation. Hans Huber Publishers, Bern, Stuttgart, Vienna

Sands E, Sarno M T, Shankweiler D 1969 Long-term assessment of language function in aphasia due to stroke. Archives of Physical Medicine and Rehabilitation 50:202–206

Sarno J E, Sarno M T, Levita E 1973 The functional life scale. Archives of Physical Medicine & Rehabilitation 54:214–220

Sarno M T, Silverman M, Sands E 1970 Speech therapy and language recovery in severe aphasia. Journal of Speech & Hearing Research 13:607–623

Sarno M T 1976 The status of research in recovery from aphasia. In: Lebrun Y, Hoops R (eds) Recovery in aphasics. p 13–30

Sarno M T, Sands E 1970 An objective method for the evaluation of speech therapy in aphasia. Archives of Physical Medicine & Rehabilitation 51:49–54

Schuell H 1965 Differential diagnosis of aphasia with the Minnesota Test. Minneapolis, University of Minnesota Press

Schoening H A, Iversen I A 1968 Numerical scoring of self-care status: a study of the Kenny Self-Care Evaluation.

Archives of Physical Medicine and Rehabilitation 49:221–229

Scottish Home and Health Department 1972 Medical rehabilitation: the pattern for the future (Mair Report). HMSO Edinburgh

Sheikh K, Smith D S, Meade T W, Goldenberg E, Brennan P J, Kinsella G 1979 Repeatability and validity of a modified activities of daily living (ADL) Index in studies of chronic disability. International Rehabilitation Medicine 1:51–58

Smith D S, Goldenberg E, Ashburn A, Kinsella G, Sheikh K, Brennan P J, Meade T W, Zutshi D W, Perry J D, Reeback J S Remedial therapy after stroke: a randomised controlled trial. British Medical Journal 282:517–520

Somerville J G, Wilkinson M, Canning M, D'Alton A, Langridge J C, Keane W, Wycherley J, Draper J 1974 A symposium on the rehabilitation of the stroke patient. Nursing Mirror, August 9, 57–78

Spern P H, McDowell F, Miller J M, Robinson M 1970 Effects of facilitation exercise techniques in stroke rehabilitation. Archives of Physical Medicine & Rehabilitation 51:526–531

Rankin J 1957 Cerebral vascular accidents in patients over the age of 60. II Prognosis. Scottish Medical Journal (ii):200–215

Treanor W J 1969 The role of physical medicine treatment in stroke rehabilitation. Clinical Orthopaedics 63:14–22

Twitchell T E 1951 The restoration of motor function following hemiplegia in man. Brain 47:443–480

Velletri-Glass A, Gassaniga M, Premack D 1973 Artificial language training in global aphasics. Neuropsychologia 11:95–103

Wall P D 1980 In: Bachy-y-rita P (ed) Recovery of function: theoretical considerations for brain injury rehabilitation. Hans Huber, Bern, Stuttgart, Vienna

Wallace D C 1967 A study of the natural history of cerebral vascular disease. Medical Journal of Australia 1:90–95

Weddell J M 1974 Rehabilitation after stroke — a medicosocial problem. Skandia international symposium on rehabilitation after central nervous system trauma. Bostrom H, Larsson T, Ljungstedt N (eds). Nordiska Bokhandelns Forlag, Stockholm

Weddell J M, Beresford S A A 1979 Planning for stroke patients. A 4-year descriptive study of home and hospital care. HMSO, London

Whisnant J P, Fitzgibbons J P, Kurland L T, Sayre G P 1971 Natural history of stroke in Rochester, Minnesota, 1945 through 1954. Stroke 2:11–21

Wilkinson M 1973 Rehabilitation after stroke. British Journal of Hospital Medicine 10:278–283

Wilson L A, Brass W 1973 Brief assessment of the mental state in geriatric domiciliary practice. Age and Ageing 2:92–101

Wolf S L, Baker M P, Kelly J L 1980 EMG Biofeedback in stroke: a one-year follow-up on the effect of patient characteristics. Archives of Physical Medicine & Rehabilitation 61:351–355

24

Management of cerebrovascular disease: a community perspective

Michael Garraway

It has been suggested that no single medical measure could make such a contribution to the quality of life in old age as the prevention of stroke (WHO, 1971). Unfortunately the difficulty of achieving this at a community level, for example the detection and effective treatment of hypertension, means that stroke will continue to be a major burden on the family and on the resources of health and social services.

The burden on the family

It has been estimated that up to 130 000 persons live at home in Great Britain handicapped to some degree by stroke (Harris, 1971). Thirty per cent of such persons are in need of special care, being dependent on someone else for daily living activities. This reservoir of disability has important implications for relatives and friends and for the provision and use of community, health and social services. A stroke is a massive blow not only to the patient, but to his family. It forces a dramatic change in life style and in the patient's role within the family. Borden (1962) has highlighted the psychological stigma and loss of self esteem following stroke which can be such a burden.

Particular strain arises when patients have deteriorated mentally following stroke (Collins et al, 1960). The family may have feelings of guilt over the stroke, which in turn can lead to overprotection of the patient and increase his dependency. Yet the family have an important role in providing support to the patient (Litman, 1964) and this can augment his response to treatment. One might expect that the policy of understanding what is involved for the family in coping with long-term illness such as stroke would be widely adopted, particularly since the adjustment which the patient and family can make to their new situation may determine the patient's ability to live in the community (Hyman, 1975). However, one study concluded that often little effort is made to involve the family following admission to hospital, social and emotional issues being pushed into the background by frenetic physical activity. Neither the patient nor his family may understand the nature of his illness or treatment because of inadequate communication (Mykyta et al, 1976).

The burden on the health service

A report issued by the World Health Organisation (1971) stated that acute stroke should be a medical emergency and require hospital admission; but there is dispute as to what proportion of strokes are admitted. Langton-Hewer (1976) estimated that only 40 per cent of patients are admitted to hospital in Bristol within the first week. This estimate is similar to that given by Cochrane (1970) who stated that 60 per cent of all 'clinical' strokes in South Wales do not go to hospital although they are similar in severity and fatality to those who are hospitalised. The most reliable way of estimating the proportion of strokes receiving hospital care is to establish a stroke register based on a defined population (Harmsen & Tibblin, 1972). Such a study has been done in South East England (Weddell, 1979). All persons in the area of Frimley and Farnham who had a stroke due to any underlying condition and of sufficient severity to necessitate medical or nursing care at home or in hospital were included. Of those registered within three weeks of occurrence, 73 per cent were receiving hospital care. The difference between

Bristol and South Wales on the one hand, and Frimley and Farnham on the other, may be due to incomplete case ascertainment. It may also depend on the policy which is adopted towards the hospital admission of stroke in a particular locality. This in turn may be influenced by the levels of provision of hospital and community-based health and social services.

Evidence that stroke is creating a burden on the hospital service comes from both ends of the hospital spectrum; at admission and on discharge. Warren et al (1967) studied referrals for urgent admissions to hospital by general practitioners made through the Emergency Bed Service (EBS) in London. Only 20 per cent of patients were placed without difficulty, 35 per cent had to be mandated into hospital by the Regional Medical Admissions Officers, and the remaining 45 per cent were refused emergency admission and were referred back to their general practitioner. On the other hand, a study of the use of medical wards in Aberdeen (Sutherland, 1972) found that long-stay patients occupied one-third of all acute medical bed days. A diagnosis of cerebrovascular disease was closely associated with this group of patients who constituted 'bed blockers', although this term was not specifically defined.

Hospital resources used by stroke patients

The contribution which stroke makes to the use of hospital resources is considerable. The proportion of hospital bed occupancy attributable to stroke in Scotland is summarised in Table 24.1. In 1976, cerebrovascular disease had the highest occupancy of hospital bed days of any diagnostic group, using no less than 1 070 998 bed days. This represents 11.1 per cent of all bed days in all specialities for that year (excluding mental illness, mental deficiency and maternity). The prospects for the future are alarming. The trend over the past few years in Scotland shows a relative increase in the proportion of hospital bed days devoted to the care of stroke patients in relation to total available resources, particularly in the elderly age groups (Garraway, 1976). This is illustrated in Table 24.2.

Table 24.2 Trend in hospital bed utilisation, Scotland, 1968–1976: projected to 1981, 1991 and 2001

| | Bed days used (or projected) (%)* | |
	Males	Females
1968	319 772 (7.4)	545 235 (10.2)
1976	328 477 (8.6)	742 521 (12.8)
1981	355 213 (9.3)	829 535 (14.3)
1991	404 867 (10.6)	997 762 (17.2)
2001	454 521 (11.9)	1 165 990 (20.1)

*Percentage relate to actual or projected bed day use
Source: Derived from Scottish Hospital Inpatient Statistics adhoc tabulations MORA 8/218B. Information Services Division of the Common Services Agency, Scottish Health Service, Edinburgh, 1979

If the average annual percentage increase in the use of bed days during the period 1968–1976 applies in the future, patients with stroke will occupy 12 and 20 per cent of all male and female hospital bed days respectively (excluding mental illness and maternity) by the year 2001. This assumes that hospital admission and discharge criteria remain the same and the number of available beds is constant. The incidence of stroke rises rapidly with age, and the trend will be further accentuated by the expected relative increase in the elderly, particularly the very elderly, for the rest of this century (Office of Population Censuses and Surveys, 1978).

Table 24.1 Leading causes of hospital bed utilisation*, Scotland; 1976

| Disease | Bed days used (%) | | |
	Male	Female	Total
Cerebrovascular disease	3.4 (328 477)	7.7 (742 521)	11.1 (1 070 998)
Pneumonia	2.4 (232 692)	5.2 (497 032)	7.6 (729 724)
Acute myocardial infarction	1.5 (149 081)	1.6 (149 516)	3.1 (298 597)
Fractured neck of femur	0.3 (31 958)	1.5 (137 139)	1.8 (169 097)
Bronchitis and emphysema	1.1 (102 668)	0.6 (58 722)	1.7 (161 390)

Figures in parenthesis are numbers of bed days
*Excluding maternity and mental illness
Source: Scottish Hospital Inpatient Statistics, 1976. Information Services Division of the Common Services Agency, Scottish Health Service, Edinburgh, 1978.

Intensive care facilities for acute stroke patients

What can be done to alleviate the important and increasing burden which stroke is placing on health services and, in particular, on the hospital sector? There is broad agreement on the kind of supportive care which is required for the stroke patient during the acute phase (United States Department of Health, Education and Welfare, 1976). Guidelines have also been suggested for the use of special procedures, equipment and consultative medical services (Report of the Joint Committee for Stroke Facilities VI, 1973). What is not clear is whether care of patients with acute stroke should be in the hands of a general medical service, or should be the responsibility of a specialised hospital unit.

Several attempts have been made to clarify this issue. An appropriate way of demonstrating an effect of specialist care in the acute stage of stroke is to compare results prospectively with a similar group of patients treated in a general hospital setting. Not all studies claiming advantages for stroke intensive care units have done this. For example, although secondary complications such as pneumonia, pulmonary embolism, pressure sores and urinary tract infection appeared to show a sharp decline during the first year of operation of an intensive care stroke unit in Toronto, there was minimal impact on death from the primary cerebral lesion in the early phase (Norris & Hachinski, 1976). Unfortunately no comparative group was assessed. A similar study took the form of a 'before' and 'after' comparison (Drake et al, 1973). Three hospitals in the San Francisco Bay Area developed acute neurovascular care units (NCUs). The emphasis was on personnel and services rather than special equipment. Comparisons of 'before' and 'after' outcomes revealed no difference in immediate mortality, but a 50 per cent reduction in secondary complications such as pneumonia, pulmonary embolism and congestive cardiac failure. It was concluded that the NCU was a useful and practical method for improving care of acutely ill stroke patients. Another report from an intensive stroke unit in Memphis, Tennessee (Pitner & Mance, 1973) used controls matched by diagnosis from an adjacent neurological ward in the same hospital. It was confirmed that there was no difference in overall mortality between stroke patients admitted to the intensive care unit and those in the ward. A further study was undertaken in Pittsburgh (Kennedy et al, 1970). The outcome of admissions to a stroke intensive care unit (SICU) was compared with control stroke patients admitted to local community hospitals. No overall reduction in stroke mortality was demonstrated for patients receiving intensive medical and nursing care. The study concluded that acute stroke care could not be equated with acute coronary care and that expectations similar to those being claimed for coronary care units would not be realised.

Intensive care makes little or no improvement to the natural history of stroke. The focus on changes in the organisation of health services should be shifted to those patients who survive the immediate period, and the most effective means of organising the rehabilitation of stroke needs to be determined.

Management of stroke during the acute phase of rehabilitation

The rationale of admitting patients with stroke to medical units has been described (Sutherland, 1972). It is to enable patients to have their diagnoses confirmed by all the necessary investigative techniques, skills and equipment. However, is the general physician the best person to provide optimal long term care for the stroke patient? It can be postulated that medical units with their emphasis on diagnosis and 'cure' of disease are not equipped in terms of staff or facilities to handle the 'care' problems inherent in stroke rehabilitation. Adams & McComb (1953) concluded that the prognosis of the hemiplegic patient was better in a geriatric unit than in the average medical unit. They evolved a ward routine, adapted to the capacity of the patients which, together with the encouragement and competitive stimulus of group treatment with similarly afflicted patients, was an important factor in prognosis. The report of a Royal College of Physicians' Working Party on Geriatric Medicine (1972) concluded that it would be appropriate for some departments of geriatrics to develop special stroke rehabilitation units. Sutherland (1972) in her study of problems created by the admission of elderly patients to medical units in Aberdeen, suggested that one answer to the 'blocked bed' situation might be to create a stroke rehabilitation unit.

The components of a stroke rehabilitation unit

What are the components of a stroke rehabilitation unit? These have been defined as either: a team of specialists who are knowledgeable about the care of the stroke patient and who consult throughout a hospital, or a special area of a hospital designated for stroke patients who are in need of rehabilitation services and skilled professional care. (McCann & Culbertson, 1976). A major advantage of a special unit is the opportunity of developing a collaborative policy for stroke rehabilitation (Isaacs, 1977). Such a policy should include a comprehensive assessment of all aspects of patients' illness, collaboration between the different disciplines, identification of the objectives of rehabilitation and an educational role (Isaacs, 1977). The components of a stroke rehabilitation team have been described in Chapter 23. Simply assembling a team will not in itself provide optimal conditions for rehabilitation. Co-ordinated action is required to formulate an integrated rehabilitation plan suited to each patient. This will involve staff conferences and ward rounds with each member of the team participating in all the activities of the stroke unit (Feigenson & McCarthy, 1977). To be effective, a stroke rehabilitation programme requires adequate physical facilities although these are of secondary importance to a properly organised team. (Department of Health, Education and Welfare, 1976).

The stroke unit as a therapeutic community

An important factor is the psychological and therapeutic effect which the rehabilitation unit could have on patients (Lee, 1958). The concept of the therapeutic community has been put forward as a reason why stroke units may get better results than medical units (Abramson et al, 1963). The rehabilitation unit is visualised as a community where the close relationship between staff and patients has a profound effect in maintaining the gains produced by hospital care. These authors

were also concerned that conventional institutional treatment could result in the patient becoming an isolated unit within the medical ward, depending on hospital staff, and gradually losing his ability to respond to his disability as motivation declines. Patient and family may become increasingly alienated from each other and come to view the hospital as the only place where the patient can be properly cared for. Moreover, in the conventional institutional setting, treatment plans may not be based on a firm knowledge of the environment to which the patient will return, resulting in overtreatment or undertreatment. Another advantage which has been claimed for the stroke unit is the creation of an atmosphere of stroke awareness in the hospital or community (Borhani, 1974).

Involving the family

It has been suggested that the family is the most important resource available to the stroke patient and to the rehabilitation team. (Joint Committee for Stroke Resources II, 1972). Family members can provide motivation to help him reach rehabilitation goals. To utilise fully this crucial asset requires active involvement of family members by professional personnel who care for the patient. Discussion may include reassurance, prognosis and a description of the plan of treatment with emphasis on the need to exploit spontaneous recovery and to use ingenuity in obtaining cooperation from the patient. Programmes of family education have been devised (Wells, 1974; Overs & Belknap, 1967), in which the value of personal contact between each member of the rehabilitation team and members of the family has been stressed, as well as informal question and answer sessions in which families can participate. Audio-visual aids may stimulate questions and can be used to complement personal contact. The formation of stroke clubs may be a useful way of continuing support to the relatives of stroke patients after discharge from hospital (Isaacs, 1977). A real measure of success in involving the family as a rehabilitation resource has been the emergence of self-help groups (Hurwitz & Adams, 1972). These may promote social integration of patients and relatives, co-ordinate transport arrangements, and initiate voluntary work.

The controversy over stroke units

Several studies have attempted to assess the effectiveness of stroke rehabilitation units, but deficiencies in methods employed make it difficult to interpret the conclusions. Opinion is divided: on the one hand, Waylonis et al (1973) found that a stroke rehabilitation team introduced into a small community hospital did not have any effect on the functional outcome of patients. A randomised controlled trial compared standard University Hospital care with intensive rehabilitation (Peacock et al, 1972). Numbers admitted to the study were too small to give a reasonable chance of reaching statistical significance and there were many dropouts in the control group. The conclusion reached was that although the results of short-term intensive rehabilitation were encouraging, lengthy rehabilitation gives little additional benefit.

Conversely, several other studies have concluded that a special unit does have some value in stroke rehabilitation. Isaacs & Marks (1973) in Glasgow concluded that severely disabled stroke patients can respond to prolonged rehabilitation. This was a descriptive study with no patients available for comparison. A stroke rehabilitation unit was established in Portland, Oregon in 1969 (Dow et al, 1974). The proportion of patients, equally severely affected, who were able to go home rose from 13 per cent to 56 per cent as a result of being in the unit, with no corresponding increase in the proportion of controls going home from other hospitals. Another report compared two groups of patients treated 'before' and 'after' a stroke rehabilitation unit had been commissioned (Adams, 1974). During the period 1948–56 when elderly stroke patients were rehabilitated in the geriatric wards, approximately 40 per cent of patients regained sufficient independence to enable them to be discharged home. During the period 1956–58, a stroke rehabilitation unit was established and stroke patients transferred there from medical units one or two weeks following onset. Adams demonstrated that the proportion of patients discharged home rose to 60 per cent, with a lowering of both the proportion of patients requiring long-stay care and those dying within two months of onset. McCann & Cuthbertson (1976) compared a stroke rehabilitation unit with the medical service of a general hospital in Rhode Island. The difference in treatment in the stroke unit was an aggressive philosophy of rehabilitation, with 'specialisation' of nursing and therapy personnel who were concerned only with stroke patients. There was also an emphasis on family involvement. Comparison was made between 224 patients treated in the unit and 110 similar patients treated in medical wards. A patient was considered to have improved if his condition decreased in severity between the time of admission and the time of discharge. Functional status of patients on admission was expressed as mild, moderate and severe disability. No significant difference was found between the two treatment systems for mild or severe gradings, but the stroke unit attained significantly better results for strokes presenting with moderate disability.

An attempt to resolve the controversy surrounding stroke rehabilitation units has recently been made through a randomised controlled trial carried out in Edinburgh which compared the management of elderly patients with acute stroke in a stroke unit and medical units (Garraway et al, 1980). The stroke unit was created by changing the function of a ward of 15 beds within a geriatric unit (Isaacs, 1977). Almost all general practitioners serving a catchment population of 470 000 notified patients aged 60 years and over, using as the definition of stroke, a focal neurological deficit of presumed vascular origin that had been present for at least six hours but no longer than three days. Medical staff were on call 24 hours a day to undertake home visits to confirm the practitioners' diagnosis. The outcome of the acute phase of rehabilitation was assessed when discharge was imminent or at a cut-off point of 16 weeks after admission, using an activities of daily living unit designed to reproduce the home. (Smith et al, 1977). A higher proportion of patients discharged from the stroke unit were assessed as independent (62 per cent of survivors) compared with patients discharged from medical units (45 per cent of survivors). The study concluded that the stroke unit improved the natural history of stroke during the acute phase of rehabilitation by increasing the proportion of patients who were returned to functional independence.

The over-straining of therapeutic resources that

might have followed the creation of the stroke unit did not occur. What was achieved was wider use of physiotherapy and occupational therapy and much shorter delays before commencing treatment. Although these differences might have contributed to the improved outcome of patients admitted to the stroke unit, this study cannot say whether the optimal mix of treatment was used. This information can only come from a series of controlled trials examining each component of stroke rehabilitation in turn.

The triage of stroke rehabilitation

The humanitarian spirit in medicine is to support the course of maximum effort for all patients, even when a proportion of patients will respond poorly to such efforts. This is an appropriate approach when services and facilities are abundant, but when time or resources are scarce it may be more rational to concentrate on those patients who are likely to respond most readily, while providing less intensive care to those persons who are likely to be poor responders whose condition does not warrant intensive treatment (Wylie, 1968). This concept of triage has been widely used by military surgeons. The recently completed Edinburgh trial of stroke unit versus medical units in the management of acute stroke adopted this concept in the selection of patients for the study (Garraway et al, 1980). Stroke presentations seen on home visits were divided into a triage of three bands: 'upper', 'middle' and 'lower', using selection criteria derived from previous studies of the natural history of stroke. Patients placed in the 'middle' band of strokes using the criteria illustrated in Table 24.3, were eligible for the study. The 'upper' band contained patients who were likely to do poorly whether they were rehabilitated or not. The 'lower'

band contained patients who were likely to recover spontaneously and who would not require a sustained period of rehabilitation. Concentrating on the 'middle' band of strokes allowed a more realistic comparison to be obtained of the relative effectiveness of a stroke unit and medical units in rehabilitating those patients whose prognosis in terms of years of life was good, but who were likely to have residual disability which would require ongoing support.

The size of a stroke rehabilitation unit

Including epidemiology in the study of health services enabled results to be applied to whole populations once it has been demonstrated that changes in the organisation or use of health services can alter the natural history of disease for the better. Thus, basing the Edinburgh trial of stroke management on hospital admissions from a defined population and completing the triage of stroke rehabilitation for all such admissions enabled the number of beds which would be required for a stroke unit per unit of population to be estimated. A stroke unit for a standard population would require four beds per 10 000 persons aged 60 years and over, or 14 beds for a stroke unit located in a District General Hospital serving a population of 250 000 of whom 18 per cent were aged 60 years and over. The steps taken and the assumptions made in making this estimate have been described elsewhere (Garraway et al, 1980).

Management of stroke during the continuing phase of rehabilitation

It is necessary to ensure that the gains made during the initial hospital phase of rehabilitation are

Table 24.3 Management of acute stroke: a community perspective

	Stroke presentation	Prognosis	Eligibility
'Upper band'	Unconscious at onset	Bad for survival	
	Prestroke dependency	Likely to remain dependent	Excluded
'Middle band'	Conscious at onset	Good for survival	
	Established or developing hemiplegia	Spontaneous recovery of independence unlikely	Included
'Lower band'	Conscious at onset	Good for survival	
	No demonstrable hemiplegia	Spontaneous recovery of independence likely	Excluded

maintained once the patient has been discharged. A recent follow-up study of stroke patients who had been in the Rehabilitation Centre at the University of Minnesota Hospital revealed that the results achieved by rehabilitation were maintained or improved over the following seven or eight years (Anderson et al, 1977). It was concluded that this was due as much to the education of the patient and his family as through the use of community resources. Functional loss, when it did occur, was usually secondary to a superimposed health problem. It is generally accepted that functional recovery following stroke takes a long time. Hurwitz & Adams (1972) have suggested that up to two years may elapse before the full capacity of the patient to participate in social activities can be realised. This observation is supported by other studies such as those undertaken by Rosenthal (1962) and by Miglietta et al (1976).

It has also been suggested that the patient who has been rehabilitated may regress to a state of disability after returning home if he and his family have not been given adequate orientation and instruction as to the need for continued effort, and do not receive encouragement and supervision (Report of the Joint Committee on Stroke Facilities, X, 1974). This was confirmed by the results of the follow-up conducted over a period of one year amongst survivors who participated in the Edinburgh trial management of acute stroke in the elderly. The improvement in functional outcome at the time of discharge from hospital that had been achieved through establishing a stroke unit had disappeared by one year (Garraway et al, 1980). One factor that might have contributed to this was overprotection by the families of patients who had been treated in the stroke unit and who were not permitted to carry out activities of daily living in which they were independent. Relatives and friends must have had a heightened awareness of patients' disabilities as a result of the better communication that existed with members of the staff of the stroke unit (Murray et al, 1980). The opportunity was available to give adequate orientation and instruction to the families of patients in the stroke unit about the need to maintain gains made during the acute phase of rehabilitation, but the extent to which this opportunity was taken and the reasons why families might have adopted a more protective role to the detriment of the long-term functional outcome of these patients are not known.

Community services for strokes

It has been suggested that a realistic goal in stroke rehabilitation is independent self-care and a return home (Marquardsen, 1969). In the elderly, this calls for a continuing multidisciplinary approach and the employment of a full range of community services once hospital discharge has been affected (Adams, 1974). There is general agreement on the importance of the community health team in giving impetus to ongoing rehabilitation and providing support to the family as they cope with the sudden and devastating change in their lifestyle which the return of the stroke patient brings with him on discharge from hospital (Report of the Joint Committee on Stroke Facilities, X, 1974).

The use of community services

Adams (1974) has given a broad outline of the place of community services in the continuing rehabilitation of elderly strokes. The problem in providing community services for stroke patients is the lack of real guidelines for the long-term management of the hemiplegic stroke (Moskowitz et al, 1972). It is not known whether the present use of community health and social services by stroke patients is appropriate because criteria used to provide services are not clearly established. In particular, it is not clear to what extent demands made by stroke patients on community services are related to the actual need for these services. Information on the use of community services is fragmented, but it is possible to gain some insight by examining the extent to which different studies have found community services to be provided or used.

A job definition for the general practitioner suggests that he should be regarded as the leader of the community health team and the person who is responsible for providing continuity of care for patients in family units in the community (Royal College of General Practitioners, 1972). It has been claimed that the physical, mental and social problems of handicapped people living at home are mainly solved by the individual general practitioner who makes the major and usually only contribution towards encouraging his patient to cope with residual disability (Yates, 1968). Evidence suggests that these obligations are not being entirely fulfilled with regard to stroke patients. Harris (1971), found that only 25 per cent of handicapped stroke patients living in private households and in need of special care had seen their general practitioner in the previous three months. Only three out of the 29 patients followed up in a Glasgow series (Isaacs et al, 1976) were visited by the general practitioner as a result of notification by the hospital that the patient had been discharged. One of the consequences of this lack of contact has been highlighted by Anderson (1978). She found that the most common reason for outcomes which did not reach expectations was inadequate follow-up. There were missing links between the family doctor and the use of follow-up care resources. Wylie (1964) in a study of referral patterns of stroke patients from general practitioners to a physical medicine and rehabilitation unit in Baltimore concluded that improved medical school teaching of rehabilitation would be the long-term remedy for more appropriate participation by general practitioners in stroke rehabilitation.

The extent of community nurse involvement in the continuing care of stroke patients does not appear to be very extensive either. Data on home nursing in Scotland (Carstairs, 1966) showed that only nine per cent of nursing workload was associated with stroke patients. The only source of data on other community service involvement with stroke patients comes from a descriptive study set up to identify the pathways of rehabilitation followed by patients who had suffered an acute stroke in Manchester (Brocklehurst et al, 1978). Stroke patients comprised only one per cent of health visitors' workload. More than half the patients in this study had contact with social services, divided almost equally between hospital and community based social workers. Contacts with social workers were mainly requests for provision of aids and adaptations or assessments in relation to possible services. Less than one in ten patients received meals on wheels and only one in every seven patients had a home help. Eight per cent of patients who survived to one year after onset were in receipt of chiropody services.

The follow-up of the Edinburgh controlled trial of stroke unit versus medical units in the management of acute stroke found that there were no major differences between stroke unit and medical unit patients in the levels of contact which occurred with individual community services (Garraway et al, 1980). The overall level of contact with virtually all services was low and confirmed the findings of a previous study which recorded the support and care given to stroke survivors in home or hospital care (Weddell & Beresford, 1979) that the involvement of health and social services in the long-term management of stroke patients is not very extensive. The Edinburgh study also found that criteria used to allocate community services did not take into account the functional performance of patients in carrying out activities of daily living. It was concluded that although there was an important role for community services in providing support for the stroke patient and his family in their own home, the contribution which these services can make in maintaining gains in the functional performance of stroke patients made during the acute phase of rehabilitation is restricted because criteria used to provide services are not yet clearly established.

Balancing the cost equation of stroke rehabilitation

Although estimates of the direct cost of stroke illness to the community have been made (Carstairs, 1976), there is a lack of data on the cost-benefit of rehabilitating strokes and on the cost-effectiveness of different methods of organising stroke rehabilitation. It has been suggested that the costs of stroke rehabilitation with its labour intensive team approach may be high, but the costs of maintaining strokes in a dependent state because they do not receive rehabilitation are even higher (Kottke, 1974). Lehmann and his colleagues (1975) described a cost-benefit ratio to assess the economics of rehabilitating a stroke victim and concluded that a substantial net saving resulted from rehabilitation. Neither of these studies which tried to make the economic case for devoting rehabilitation resources to stroke patients adequately tackled the financial equation which urgently requires to be solved, viz.: if resources are devoted to stroke rehabilitation at an early stage after onset, resulting, as evidence suggests, in a higher proportion of patients becoming functionally independent, does this mean a lower input of resources from community services will be required in the long term? No satisfactory answer to this crucial question has been found.

REFERENCES

Abramson A S, Kutner B, Rosenberg P, Berger R, Weiner H J 1963 A therapeutic community in a general hospital: adaptation of a rehabilitation service. Journal of Chronic Disease, 16:179–186

Adams G F, McComb S G 1953 Assessment and prognosis in hemiplegia. Lancet, ii, 266–269

Adams G F 1974 Prognosis and prospects of strokes In: Cerebrovascular disability and the ageing brain. Churchill Livingstone, Edinburgh, London

Anderson E, Anderson T P, Kottke F J 1977 Stroke rehabilitation: maintenance of achieved gains. Archives of Physical Medicine and Rehabilitation, 58:345–352

Anderson T W, McLure W J, Athelstan G et al 1978 Stroke rehabilitation: evaluation of its quality by assessing patient outcomes. Archives of Physical Medicine and Rehabilitation 59:170–175

Borden W A 1962 Psychological aspects of stroke: patients and family. Annals of Internal Medicine 57:689–692

Borhani N O 1974 Stroke surveillance: the concept of a stroke team in diagnosis, treatment and prevention Stroke 5:78–80

Brocklehurst J C, Andrews K, Richards B, Laycock P J 1978 How much physical therapy for patients with stroke? British Medical Journal 1:1307–1310

Carstairs V 1966 Home nursing in Scotland. Scottish Health Service Studies, No. 2. Edinburgh Scottish Home and Health Department.

Carstairs V 1976 Stroke: resource consumption and the cost to the community. In: Gillingham F J, Mawdsley C, Williams A E (eds) Stroke, Proceedings of the Ninth Pfizer International Symposium. Churchill Livingstone, Edinburgh, London

Cochrane A L 1970 Burden of cerebrovascular disease. British Medical Journal 3:165

Collins Patricia, Marshall J, Shaw D A 1960 Social rehabilitation following cerebrovascular accidents. Gerontologica Clinica 2:246–256

Dow R S, Dick H L, Cromwell F A 1974 Failures and successes in a stroke program. Stroke 5:40–47

Drake W E, Hamilton M J, Carlsson M, Blumenkrantz J 1973 Acute stroke management and patient outcome: The value of neurovascular care units (NCU) Stroke 4:933–945

Feigenson J S, McCarthy M L 1977 II; Guidelines for establishing a stroke rehabilitation unit. New York State Journal of Medicine 34:1430–1434

Garraway W M 1976 The size of the problem of stroke in Scotland. In: Gillingham F J, Mawdsley C, Williams A E (eds) Stroke: Proceedings of the Ninth Pfizer International Symposium

Garraway W M, Akhtar A J, Prescott R J, Hockey L 1980 Management of acute stroke in the elderly: preliminary results of a controlled trial. British Medical Journal 280:1040–1043

Garraway W M, Akhtar A J, Hockey L, Prescott R J 1980 Management of acute stroke in the elderly: follow-up of a controlled trial. British Medical Journal 281:827–829

Garraway W M, Akhtar A J, Smith D L, Smith M E 1981 The triage of stroke rehabilitation. Journal of Epidemiology and Community Health 35:39–44

Garraway W M, Walton M S, Akhtar A J, Prescott R J 1981 The use of health and social services in the management of stroke in the community: results from a controlled trial. Age and Ageing 10:95–104

Harmsen P, Tibblin G 1972 A stroke register in Göteborg, Sweden. Acta Medica Scandinavica 191:463–470

Harris A I 1971 Handicapped and impaired in Great Britain. Part I. Social Survey Division of the Office of Population Censuses and Surveys. Her Majesty's Stationery Office, London

Hurwitz L J, Adams G F 1972 Rehabilitation of hemiplegia: indices of assessment and prognosis. British Medical Journal 1:94–98

Hyman M D 1975 Social psychological factors affecting disability among ambulatory patients. Journal of Chronic Diseases 28:199–216

Isaacs B, Marks R 1973 Determinants of outcome of stroke rehabilitation. Age and Ageing 2:139–149

Isaacs B, Neville Y, Rushford I 1976 The stricken: the social consequences of stroke. Age and Ageing 5:188–192

Isaacs B 1977 Five years' experience of a stroke unit. Health Bulletin, Edinburgh 35:93–98

Kennedy F P, Pozen T J, Gabelman E H, Tuthill J E, Zaeutz S D 1970 American Heart Journal 80, 188–196

Kottke F J 1974 Historia Obscura Hemiplegiae. Archives of Physical Medicine and Rehabilitation 55:4–13

Langton-Hewer R 1976 Stroke rehabilitation — a neurologist's view. In: Gillingham F J, Mawdsley C, Williams A E (eds) Stroke, Churchill Livingstone, Edinburgh, London

Lee P 1958 Rehabilitation programs. In; Wright I S, Millikan C H (eds) Cerebral vascular disease. Transactions of the Second Conference of the American Heart Association. Grune and Stratton, New York and London

Lehmann J F, DeLateur B J, Fowler R S et al 1975 Stroke: Does rehabilitation affect outcome? Archives of Physical Medicine and Rehabilitation 56:375–382

Litmann T J 1964 An analysis of the sociological factors affecting the rehabilitation of physically handicapped patients. Archives of Physical Medicine and Rehabilitation 45:9–16

McCann C, Culbertson R A 1976 Comparison of two systems for stroke rehabilitation in a general hospital. Journal of the American Geriatrics Society 24:211–216

Marquardsen J 1969 A natural history of acute cerebrovascular disease. A retrospective study of 769 patients. Munksgaard, Copenhagen

Miglietta O, Chung T-S, Rajeswaramma V 1976 Fate of stroke patients transferred to a long-term rehabilitation hospital. Stroke 7:76–77

Moskowitz W, Lightbody F E H, Freitag N S 1972 Long-term follow-up of the poststroke patient. Archives of Physical Medicine and Rehabilitation 53 167–172

Murray S K, Garraway W M, Akhtar A J, Prescott R J. Communication between hospital and home in the management of acute stroke in the elderly: results from a controlled trial. (Unpublished)

Mykyta L J, Bowling J H, Nelson D A, Lloyd E J 1976 Caring for relatives of stroke patients. Age and Ageing 5:87–90

Norris J W, Hachinski V C 1976 Intensive care management of stroke patients. Stroke 7:573–577

Office of Population Censuses and Surveys 1978 Demographic Review. A report on population in Great Britain. Series DR No. 1. Her Majesty's Stationery Office, London

Overs R P, Belknap E L 1967 Educating stroke patients' families. Journal of Chronic Diseases 20:45–51

Peacock P B, Riley C P, Lampton T D, Raffel S S, Walker J S 1972 The Birmingham stroke epidemiology and rehabilitation study. In: Stewart G T (ed) Trends in epidemiology. Application to health service research and training. Charles C. Thomas, Springfield, Illinois

Pitner S E, Mance C J 1973 An evaluation of stroke intensive care: results in a municipal hospital. Stroke 4:737–741

Report of the College Committee on Geriatric Medicine 1972 Royal College of Physicians, London

Report of Joint Committee for Stroke Facilities II 1972 Rehabilitation Study Group. Stroke 3:375–407

Report of the Joint Committee for Stroke Facilities, VI 1973 Special procedures and equipment in the diagnosis and management of stroke. Stroke 4:113–137

Report of the Joint Committee for Stroke Facilities, X 1974 Community Health Services for Stroke. Stroke 5:115–144

Rosenthal A M 1962 Five year follow-up study of the patients admitted to the rehabilitation centre of the hospital of the University of Pennsylvania. American Journal of Physical Medicine 41:198–211

Smith M E, Garraway W M, Akhtar A J, Andrews C J A 1977 Assessment unit for measuring the outcome of stroke rehabilitation. British Journal of Occupational Therapy 40:51–53

Sutherland A 1972 Scottish Health Service Studies, No. 22. A study of long-stay admission to the acute medical wards of the Aberdeen hospitals. Scottish Home and Health Department, Edinburgh

U. S. Department of Health, Education and Welfare 1976 Guidelines for stroke care. Johns A L, Hartman E C, Aronson S M (eds) U.S. Government Printing Office, Washington, D.C

Warren M D, Cooper Jane, Warren Joan L 1967 Problems of emergency admissions to London hospitals. British Journal of Preventive and Social Medicine 21:141–149

Waylonis G W, Keith M W, Aseff J N 1973 Stroke rehabilitation in the midwestern county. Archives of Physical Medicine and Rehabilitation 54:151–155

Weddell J M, Beresford S A A 1979 Planning for stroke patients. A four-year descriptive study of home and hospital care. Her Majesty's Stationery Office, London

Wells R 1974 Family stroke education. Stroke 5:393–396

Working party of the Royal College of General Practitioners on learning and teaching 1972 The educational process and vocational training. In: The future general practitioner. British Medical Association for the Royal College of General Practitioners, London

World Health Organisation 1971 Cerebrovascular diseases: prevention, treatment and rehabilitation. World Health Organisation Technical Report Series, No. 469. World Health Organisation, Geneva

Wylie C M 1964 Age and long-term hospital care following cerebrovascular accidents. Journal of American Geriatrics Society 12:763–770

Wylie C M 1968 Age and the rehabilitative care of stroke. Journal of the American Geriatrics Society 16:428–435

Yates G 1969 Rehabilitation and the General Practitioner. Journal of the Royal College of General Practitioners 17:292–298

Index

487